Sixth Edition

Parasitic Diseases

Despommier
Griffin
Gwadz
Hotez
Knirsch

Parasites Without Borders, Inc. NY

Dickson D. Despommier, Daniel O. Griffin, Robert W. Gwadz, Peter J. Hotez, Charles A. Knirsch

Life Cycles by
John Karapelou

Photographs by
Dickson D. Despommier

Parasitic Diseases
Sixth Edition

With over 400 illustrations in full color

~3,000 references

Parasites Without Borders, Inc. NY

Dickson D. Despommier, Ph.D. Professor Emeritus of Public Health (Parasitology) and Microbiology, The Joseph L. Mailman School of Public Health, Columbia University in the City of New York 10032

Daniel O. Griffin, M.D., Ph.D. Clinical Instructor of Medicine, Department of Medicine-Division of Infectious Diseases, Associate Research Scientist, Department of Biochemistry and Molecular Biophysics, Columbia University Medical Center New York, New York, NY 10032

Robert W. Gwadz, Ph.D. Captain USPHS (ret), Visiting Professor, Collegium Medicum, The Jagiellonian University, Krakow, Poland, Fellow of the Hebrew University of Jerusalem, Fellow of the Ain Shams University, Cairo, Egypt, Chevalier of the Nation, Republic of Mali

Peter J. Hotez, M.D., Ph.D., FASTMH, FAAP Dean, National School of Tropical Medicine, Professor, Pediatrics and Molecular Virology & Microbiology, Head, Section of Pediatric Tropical Medicine, Baylor College of Medicine, Texas Children's Hospital Endowed Chair of Tropical Pediatrics, Director, Sabin Vaccine Institute Texas Children's Hospital Center for Vaccine Development, President, Sabin Vaccine Institute, Baker Institute Fellow in Disease and Poverty, Rice University, University Professor, Baylor University, Co-Editor-in-Chief, PLoS Neglected Tropical Diseases, Chair, Technical Advisory Board, END Fund, United States Science Envoy

Charles A. Knirsch, M.D., M.P.H. Assistant Clinical Professor, Division of Infectious Diseases, Department of Medicine, College of Physicians and Surgeons, Columbia University in the City of New York, New York, NY 10032; Vice President, Pfizer Vaccines Clinical Research and Development, Pearl River, NY, 10965

A number of the drawings utilized herein are printed with the permission of Karapalou Medical Art, with all rights reserved. 3739 Pendlestone Drive, Columbus, Ohio. 43230.

Cover Design: Dickson Despommier and Daniel O. Griffin (*Toxoplasma gondii* infected cell)

Page layout and design: Dickson Despommier and Daniel O. Griffin

Library of Congress Cataloguing-in-Publication Data

Parasitic Diseases / Dickson D. Despommier, Robert W. Gwadz, Daniel O. Griffin, Peter J. Hotez, Charles A. Knirsch:
     - 6th edition

     p. cm.
     Includes bibliographical references and index.
     ISBN :978-0-9978400-0-1 (Hardcover)
     ISBN: 978-0-9978400-1-8 (PDF version)
     ISBN :978-0-9978400-2-5 (Kindle version)
     ISBN: 978-0-9978400-3-2 (iBook version)
     1. Parasitic diseases Dickson D. Despommier, Robert W. Gwadz, Daniel O. Griffin, Peter J. Hotez, Charles A. Knirsch.
     IV. Title. Parasitic Diseases
     . ©
Printed on paper made of pulp from trees harvested in managed forests.

Printing by Sentinel Printing, 250 North Highway 10, St. Cloud, MN 65302

We dedicate our 6th edition to President Jimmy Carter and William Campbell. We want to recognize President Carter's leadership and support for the eradication and elimination of neglected tropical diseases as central to alleviating suffering and improving life for the world's most disadvantaged populations. We want to recognize William Cambell as one of the people responsible for the miracle drug, ivermectin. For his excellent work, he was awarded the Nobel Prize in Physiology or Medicine in 2015.

Acknowledgements:

We acknowledge the contribution of John Karapelou for his elegant life cycle drawings. Thanks to David Scharf for granting us use of his stunning scanning electron micrographs of the very things that attract legions of new medical students to the field of tropical medicine. Thanks to all the course directors of parasitic diseases and parasitology who choose our book as the one to help guide their students through the complexities of life cycles, clinical presentations, and biology. We hope that the 6th edition proves even more useful for you and your students in the coming years.

Thanks to all the infectious disease experts (Justin Aaron, Sapha Barkati, Craig Boutlis, Mary Burgess, Matthew Cheng, Lucy Cheng, Elise O'Connell, Priya Kodiyanplakka, Atul Kothari, Michael Libman, Tim McDonald, Juan Carlos Rico, Jordan Rupp, Keyur Vyas, Johnnie Yates) who have volunteered their time and expertise to review this textbook prior to its publication. Thank you to all the donors who are making it possible for us to get this book into the hands of those who need it the most.

Preface

Remarkable achievements in parasitic disease research, both basic and translational, have occurred over the last ten years, and we have incorporated the majority of these into the 6th edition of Parasitic Diseases. We have added over 1,000 new references to document these advances. Innovative work in the laboratory has provided the clinician/research scientist with a much clearer understanding of the mechanisms of pathogenesis. The number of recently discovered interleukins and their cellular networks has completely re-ordered our comprehension of how parasites and our defense system works to produce protection against infection/reinfection, or in some cases, how it becomes subverted by the offending pathogen to enable it to endure inside us for long periods of time. A plethora of molecular-based diagnostic tests have found their way into the routine of the parasitology diagnostic laboratory, improving the ease at which the offending pathogen can be rapidly identified. Newer drugs, many with less harmful side-effects than the ones they replaced, have come on the market that make controlling parasite populations at the community level possible without the risk of harming the very ones we wish to help.

The Human Genome Project was completed in 2003. Now the genomes of a significant number of pathogens have also been determined, and many of the eukaryotic variety are featured in Parasitic Diseases, 6th edition. Furthermore, the genomes of some important arthropod vectors have also been published. Results from these efforts hold great promise for the development of effective new vaccines, drugs, and control programs based on identifying unique molecular pathways essential to each pathogen in question. These on-going projects serve as a living testament to the perseverance of a small, dedicated band of talented parasitologist/parasitic disease researchers, whose sole wish is to help stem the tide regarding the spread of these life-threatening entities.

Political will and strong social support have combined to severely limit the spread of some parasites without the use of vaccines or drugs. For example, dracunculosis has been brought under control in all but a few regions of Africa, and the southern cone initiative of South America has resulted in fewer and fewer cases of Chagas Disease. The use of ivermectin has greatly reduced the burden of River Blindness in many countries in West Africa. While there are no new classes of drugs for treating resistant malaria, artemesinin derivatives continue to be effective in reducing the mortality of the world's most devastating infectious disease wherever that chemotherapeutic agent is available.

As encouraging and inspiring as these research efforts are, they are the only bright spots on an ever increasingly depressing picture of world health, revealing the lack of control of many species of eukaryotic parasites that significantly detract from our ability to carry out a decent day's work. For example, worm infections continue to exact their toll on the normal development of the world's children, who are forced, simply by where they live, to co-exist with these intestinal helminths. In addition, diarrheal diseases caused by a variety of infectious agents, including *Entamoeba histolytica, Giardia lamblia, Cryptosporidium parvum* and *Cyclospora cayatenensis*, round out the list of miseries to be dealt with by all those living in poverty in the less developed world. The seemingly simple employment of basic sanitation, safely sequestering feces and urine away from our drinking water and food supply, remains high on the list of things to do for those countries in which these two human by-products serve as the only source of fertilizer.

Political instability of vast regions of Africa and the Middle East has led to the re-emergence of many infectious diseases, including leishmaniasis and African trypanosomiasis. This has been largely due to environmental destruction, abandonment of control programs, and forced migration of tens of thousands of individuals from regions that were relatively safe in which to live, to places that no one should have to occupy, no matter how short the duration. These seemingly intractable situations require more than vaccines and drugs to affect a cure. Social equity, economic development, and long-term planning are the drugs of choice. The impact of HIV/AIDS in resource-constrained geographic areas has significantly reduced overall life expectancy. The interplay of immunosuppression caused by this disease and the impact on other parasitic diseases is still poorly understood, and requires careful monitoring. As access to antiretroviral therapy improves due to the Global Fund and other non-governmental entities, new clinical syndromes are likely to emerge due to parasites behaving differently in hosts with an ever-changing immune status.

It is our intent that readers of this text will be adequately armed with basic knowledge of parasites and the clinical disease states they cause, to allow them to join in a global effort already underway that has everything to do with improving the fitness and survival of the vast majority of the human species.

Contents

III. Eukaryotic Parasites

Eukaryotic parasites encompass subsets of organisms within the protozoan and helminth (parasitic worm) groups. In addition, medically important arthropods have been included in discussions of eukaryotic parasites, since so many of these pathogens are transmitted to humans by arthropod vectors. Besides, some medically relevant arthropods cause disease on their own.

From a biological perspective, a phylogenetic presentation of eukaryotic parasitic organisms would undoubtedly satisfy those specialists who strictly adhere to the zoological literature, while most medical students and practicing clinicians would have little or no use for this information. The physician is more inclined to group them according to their syndromes, if they were to classify them at all. We have settled upon a compromise, in which these organisms are encountered by the reader in a somewhat biologically correct order, together with an outline of their classification and clinical presentations. Nonetheless, it is in some sense intellectually satisfying to review parasitic organisms with a semblance of evolutionary precision, allowing each student to learn about them in a sequence that most experts in the field of parasitology have agreed upon, going from the single-cell parasites to the worms and beyond. We present protozoans first, followed by the helminths, and finally round out the synopsis with medically relevant arthropods.

The last half of the twentieth century has been a remarkable one for the community-based control of pathogenic organisms. New vaccines and antibiotics have also helped reduce the incidence of numerous pathogenic organisms. At the same time, it has also heralded the emergence and re-emergence of a wide spectrum of infectious agents: viruses (e.g., SARS, HIV, monkey pox, avian influenza, dengue, chikungunya, Zika), bacteria (e.g., *Legionella pneumophila*, *Borrelia burgdorferi*, *Escherichia coli* strain OH157), protozoa (e.g., *Cryptosporidium parvum*, *Cyclospora cayetanensis*), and helminths (e.g., *Echinococcus multilocularis*, *Angiostrongylus cantonesis*, *Trichinella spiralis*). Viewed from an evolutionary perspective, humans represent a highly successful system of essential niches, of which an astonishingly wide variety of eukaryotes have been able to take advantage.

The number of individuals infected with any given parasite rarely makes but little impression on even the most attentive medical student, especially when it is a very large number, as is the case for *Ascaris lumbricoides,* which infects hundreds of millions of people around the world. So when one hears for the first time that 100s of millions of people are infected with malaria each year, and over ½ a million children per year die in Africa alone from this infection, these facts seem somehow remote, even abstract. Yet, when a single child suffering from the cerebral form of this disease-causing entity is admitted into a modern hospital in critical condition, and, regardless of treatment, that young person dies, the health care community of that institution is put into collective shock. If the death occurred at a teaching hospital, a grand rounds is the usual outcome, perhaps motivated by some vague sense of guilt, in an attempt to see if anything could have been done to spare that life. Unfortunately the most lethal species of malaria, *Plasmodium falciparum*, is evolving more and more resistance to the medications in our arsenal.

Parasitic Protozoa

What is a protozoan? Which ones cause disease? How do those that are parasitic differ from their free-living counterparts? What are the pathogenic mechanism(s) by which they cause disease? There are over 200,000 named species of single-celled organisms that fall under the category protozoa, while many more, no doubt, await discovery. Only some small fraction of these are parasitic for the human host, yet some can cause great harm (e.g., malaria), especially when they are encountered for the first time.

Protozoans are single-cell organisms inside of which usually resides one membrane-bound nucleus, with a few exceptions, such as *Giardia lamblia* and *Dientamoeba fragilis*. Most protozoa have one type of organelle that aids in their movement (e.g., flagella, undulating membrane, cilia). Metabolic pathways also vary from group to group, with both anaerobic and aerobic energy metabolisms being represented among the parasites to be discussed. In the case of parasitic organisms, the host provides the energy source. There are a variety of drugs that take advantage of the dependence of parasites on host energy metabolism.

The following sections are organized in such a way as to enable the student or clinician easy access to a highly distilled body of information relating to the general schemes employed when these organisms interact with the human host to produce disease. Thus, rather than being an exhaustive text, only biological information essential to the understanding of clinical aspects of a given disease-causing organism will be emphasized.

The following topics are deemed medically relevant; 1. mechanisms of entry, 2. niche selection, 3. reproduction, 4. mechanisms of survival (i.e., virulence factors), and 5. mechanisms of pathogenesis. All single-cell organisms have complex biochemistries, often employing unique pathways that give some of them remarkable evolutionary advantages. These include the ability of a given population to vary their protein surfaces, edit their mRNA transcripts, secrete peptides that prevent the fusion of lysosomal membranes to the parasitophorous vacuole, and give off substances that inhibit host protective immune responses. A plethora of unique molecular pathways have been described for this diverse group of parasites, but a comprehensive description of them is beyond the scope of this book. Some attention to both the biochemical and molecular biological findings for a given organism will be presented whenever they have relevance to the understanding of the mechanisms of pathogenesis or parasite survival strategies.

Mechanisms of Entry

Protozoans gain entry into their host in one of several ways; oral, sexual, inhalation, direct contact, and through the bites of blood-sucking vectors. Avoidance or prevention of infection requires an intimate knowledge of its transmission cycle, and knowing the route of entry into the host is one of the most important aspects in that regard. Many species of parasitic protozoa have evolved stages that facilitate their dispersal into the environment, increasing their chances of encountering a host. Some intestinal protozoa produce a resistant cyst enabling them to lie dormant in the environment for long periods of time, months to years, in some cases. Others depend upon human activities for their dispersal, as in the case of *Trichomonas vaginalis*, which is sexually transmitted. Certain ameoba may infect humans through inhalation or direct contact. Vector-borne organisms rely on the biology of blood sucking insects, for the most part. Mosquitoes transmit all species of malaria (*Plasmodium* spp.), tsetse flies transmit African Sleeping Sickness (*Trypanosoma brucei* spp.) and sandflies transmit all species of *Leishmania*. In these instances, the organism is injected directly into the host's blood stream or interstitial tissue fluids where they proceed to undergo complex developmental life cycles culminating in numerous cycles of asexual division once they achieve their essential niche.

A more complex strategy is employed by *Trypanosoma cruzi*, an organism transmitted by a large hemipteran with ferocious looking biting mouth parts. In this instance, the organisms are excreted along with the fecal exudate at the time of the second blood feeding. We become infected unknowingly by rubbing the organisms into the bite wound or into a mucous membrane after the insect withdraws its mouth parts.

Niche Selection

Each protozoan has been selected for life in a specific essential niche, which can only be defined by a comprehensive knowledge of the anatomical, physiological, and biochemical features of that site. To gain some measure of the difficulties associated with attempting to describe the essential niche, be it that of a parasite or any other organism, let us consider the intracellular milieu of the normal red blood cell. This site represents one of the best studied of all intracellular environments. Yet for the most part, we still do not understand precisely how that anucleate cell's membranes interact with vascular endothelial cells when the cell traverses the capillary and exchanges gases with the surrounding tissues. To make matters worse, a red blood cell that is infected with *Plasmodium falciparum* behaves quite differently from that of a normal one, failing to deform as it enters the capillary bed. This single aspect of the infection has serious pathological consequences for the host, as will be detailed in the section dealing with the clinical aspects of malaria. The internal molecular environment of the infected red cell must be considered as a "hybrid," consisting of both host and parasite elements. Proteins, produced by the developing merozoite, locate to the cytoplasm of the host cell, and some even integrate at the red cell membrane surface, forming complexes with host structural proteins such as spectrin and glycophoran. Others remain in the general region of the red cell cytoplasm. Over the entire period of the developmental cycle of the parasite, new proteins are produced that locate to specific regions of an ever-changing host cell environment. The infected red cell represents a very dynamic situation; even with the most sophisticated instrumentation, it has been impossible to fully appreciate the setting in which this important pathogen lives out its life. Finally, no two species of *Plasmodium* behave the same in their erythrocytic niche, due largely to dramatic genetic differences between the major species infecting humans. Hence, it is likely that we will never gain a "full face-on" view of this or any other pathogen in order to sufficiently design new therapeutics that would prevent the organism from taking full advantage of its ecological setting. The complexities presented to the research parasitologist by just this single organism continue to challenge them to design innovative experiments that may allow us one day more than a glimpse into its secret life.

At the other end of the scale is *Toxoplasma gondii*, a protozoan capable of infecting virtually any mammalian cell and reproducing within it. *Toxoplasma gondii's* lack of host restriction makes it the most widely distributed parasite on earth.

Migration to favorable sites within the host often requires an active role for the pathogen, but frequently they "hitch a ride" in our bloodstream or through our intestinal tract. Some are capable of infecting cells that under most circumstances would serve to protect us from these kinds of organisms. The macrophage is a permissive host cell for *Toxoplasma gondii* and for all species of *Leishmania*. In these infections, the very cell type we depend upon for innate protection against invaders turns out to be the culprit, aiding in their dispersal throughout the body.

Division and Reproduction

Multiplication within the human host is the rule for protozoans, in contrast to most helminth species, in which infection usually results in a single adult parasite. The definitive host is the one harboring the sexual stages or the adult stages of a given parasite. Hence, the human is not the definitive host for a wide range of protozan infections, including the Plasmodia and *Toxoplasma gondii*. Female anopheline mosquitoes are the definitive hosts for all malaria species infecting humans, while the domestic cat is the permissive host for the sexual stages of *T. gondii*. Humans are the definitive host for *Cryptosporidium parvum*. It should be emphasized, however, that not all parasitic protozoa have sexual cycles.

As pointed out, all protozoans reproduce asexually after gaining entrance into the human host. Pathological consequences result directly from their increasing numbers. During the height of the infection, they place ever-increasing demands upon their essential niches. The mechanisms by which protozoa divide asexually are numerous, with binary fission being the most common. Malarial parasites reproduce within the red cell by a process called schizogony, in which the organism undergoes nuclear division within a common cytoplasm (karyokinesis). Just before rupturing out of the hemoglobin-depleted red cell, the parasite's cytoplasm divides to accommodate each nucleus, leaving its toxic waste product, crystals of haemazoin, in the now empty red cell stroma.

Mechanisms of Survival

Each species of parasite has been selected for life within the human host by evolving strategies that; (A) inhibit or divert our immune system, (B) avoid or inhibit intracellular killing mechanisms, and (C) infect regions of the body that are incapable of protective immune responses. For example, the African trypanosomes produce "smoke screens" of surface antigens whose sole purpose seems to be to keep the immune system busy, while a small select population changes its protein coat to a different antigenic variant, thus temporarily escaping the host's immune surveillance system. Certain stages of the malaria parasite and *Giardia lamblia* can also vary their surface proteins, presenting our immune system with a bewildering array of antigenic determinants to deal with as an infection progresses. *Toxoplasma gondii* inhibits the fusion of lysosomal vesicles with the parasitophorous vacuole, thus escaping the killing effects of acid hydrolases. *Cryptosporidium parvum* and all species of malaria occupy immunologically "silent" niches. *Trypanosoma cruzi* actually penetrates out of the parasitophorous vacuole into naked cytoplasm, escaping the ravages of lysosomal enzyme activity. There are numerous other examples and they will be discussed whenever relevant. Independent of the biochemical strategy employed by the protozoan parasite, the result is tissue damage, often severe.

Mechanisms of Pathogenesis

Regardless of the mechanism employed by the parasite to escape being killed, the usual consequence of infection from the perspective of the human host is tissue damage. The extent of cellular damage inflicted by a given parasite is related to the location of their essential niche, the metabolic requirements of the parasite, and their population density throughout the infection. Energy is derived from the host, placing a burden on infected hosts for providing this essential ingredient. The penchant of the parasite for killing the cell it invades, or eroding away the tissue it occupies while feeding on our cells, results in measurable pathological consequences that translate directly into clinical signs and symptoms. For example, when the malaria parasite exits from the red cell at the end of its division cycle, the rupture of the stroma results in the release of toxic waste products (haemazoin) that elicit fever. *E. histolytica*, as its name implies, attaches to, then ingests living cells. It then digests them, using acid hydrolases to do so, and in the process induces bloody diarrhea (dysentery).

Infection with *T. gondii* results in lymphedema and fever due to the death of large numbers of host cells throughout the body. The molecular basis for these pathological effects will be discussed in detail at the appropriate time. Suffice it to state here that we do not know any parasite's *modus operandi* completely, and the scientific literature will undoubtedly continue to bring with it new surprises and revelations in the near future.

Parasitic Helminths (worms)

Helminths belong to four phyla: Nematoda (roundworms), Platyhelminthes (flatworms), Acanthocephala (spiny-headed worms), and Nematophora (hairworms). Only worms belonging to the first two are endoparasitic to humans. Both the Nematoda and Platyhelminthes have many free-living species as well. A general description of each major group precedes each section. What follows is a general description of their biology.

Mechanisms of Entry

Helminths have evolved multiple strategies for entering the host and establishing infection. Among the nematodes, infection is usually established by exposure to an environmentally resistant stage.

For many of the common intestinal nematodes such as *Ascaris lumbricoides* or *Trichuris trichiura*, this occurs via the ingestion of embryonated eggs in the soil, or on fecal-contaminated fruits and vegetables. In many tropical countries helminth eggs have been isolated from nearly all environments. They have even been recovered from paper currency. For other nematodes, infection is established when larval stages, living in the soil, enter the host. Sometimes infection is strictly food-borne and occurs only when larvae are ingested in uncooked meat. Many species of nematode are transmitted by arthropods, such as lymphatic filariasis (mosquito), loaiasis (deer fly), onchocherciasis (black fly) and guinea worm infection (copepods).

Trematodes spend a portion of their life cycle in a wide variety of snail intermediate hosts. After exiting the snail, the larval stage, known as a cercaria, typically attaches to a second intermediate host, such as a fish, a crab, or aquatic vegetation. For this reason, most trematode infections are food-borne. The exception are the schistosomes, which cause a spectrum of illnesses. The schistosome cercariae are able to penetrate skin via a hair shaft.

Cestodes are acquired via the oral route, regardless of the stage that ends up causing the infection. Most adult tapeworm infections of humans result from the ingestion of inadequately cooked contaminated fish, beef, or pork. Two clinically significant juvenile tapeworm infections, cysticercosis and echinococcosis, result from accidental ingestion of the eggs.

Niche Selection

Unlike protozoans, most species of parasitic helminths occupy more than a single niche in their human host during their life cycle. For example, although hookworms live as adults in the small intestine, in order to arrive there, the infective larvae frequently must first pass through the skin and lymphatics before spending time in the bloodstream and lungs. Similarly, *Ascaris* eggs hatch in the intestine before the emerging larval stage enters the portal circulation; the larvae enter liver and lungs prior to re-entry into the gut. As adults, helminths have been recovered from almost every organ including liver, lungs, lymphatics, bloodstream, muscle, skin, subcutaneous tissues, and brain.

Many species of parasitic helminths (nematodes, cestodes, and trematodes) live as sexually mature adults in the gastrointestinal tract. In many underdeveloped countries, it is usual to find school-aged children who harbor three or four different species of helminths in their intestine, with each species occupying a different portion of the gut track. Symptoms arising from heavy infection with a given helminth are associated with a particular region of the GI tract.

Reproduction

Nematode parasites that live in the GI tract produce eggs or larvae that exit the host with the fecal mass. Nematodes living in blood or lymphatic vessels produce larvae that circulate in the bloodstream and must be ingested by the appropriate arthropod vector in order to exit the host.

In the cestodes, the situation is somewhat different as each proglottid segment of the adult cestode tapeworm is hermaphroditic. Because there is usually only one adult worm present, the worm self-fertilizes adjacent segments. Adult tapeworms shed segments into the lumen of the small intestine and they can exit the host under their own power. Other adult tapeworms produce segments that then disintegrate releasing their eggs into the fecal mass for export. Juvenile tapeworm infections remain as such and produce no diagnostic stage. These infections present real problems for the clinician seeking a definitive diagnosis for their patient.

Except for the schistosomes, the trematodes (flukes) are all hermaphroditic. Despite this all-in-one reproductive arrangement, cross-fertilization between two trematodes of the same species is common. Intestinal trematodes produce eggs that exit with the feces, as for example, with the eggs of *Heterophyes heterophyes*. Eggs of the lung fluke, *Paragonimus westermani*, exit the host either when they are coughed up in sputum or after they are swallowed, in which case they exit in the feces. Some helminths have evolved elaborate adaptations in order to ensure that their eggs leave the human host. For instance, schistosome eggs are deposited against the inside wall of a blood vessel. These eggs are equiped with sharp spines and a battery of lytic enzymes that allow them to traverse the vessel endothelium and gut wall. The eggs break through the serosal surface of either the intestine or bladder (depending upon the species), before entering the muscularis and then the lumen. Adult schistosomes and *Paragonimus,* that locate to ectopic sites (e.g., nervous system), produce eggs that remain at the site of infection, often resulting in serious pathological consequences for the host.

Mechanisms of Survival

Like the protozoa, the helminths occupy habitats which most of us would consider highly inhospitable. The selective pressures that led to their elaborating mechanisms for survival in these environments are still poorly understood. Adult schistosomes live in the bloodstream, a place where one might expect to encounter the constant bombardment of the immune system's slings and arrows of antibody molecules and leukocytes of various types. Yet, there the worms can remain for up to twenty years in that niche. The molecular basis by which this happens is not known, although a number of immune evasion and immunological masking mechanisms have been described. Important for helminth survival is their unique array of natural products elaborated and released into the host. Hookworms can freely ingest blood in the intestinal mucosa and submucosa because they produce peptides and eicosanoids that block host clotting, host platelet aggregation, and host inflammation. Many of these peptides themselves have proven to be useful as new potential therapeutic agents for human coronary artery disease, stroke and autoimmune disorders. *Trichuris trichiura* releases a pore- forming protein that promotes cell fusion around the anterior end of the organism, allowing it to become embedded in epithelial tunnels. Indeed, the argument has been made that parasitic helminths are themselves equivalent to small biotechnology companies, which, through research and development in the form of millions of years of evolutionary selection, now produce a wide array of pharmacologically active compounds which we may find useful, as well.

Mechanisms of Pathogenesis

Helminths injure their human host both through mechanical and chemical mechanisms. Large helminths, such as *Ascaris lumbricoides*, can cause physical obstruction of the intestine, or exert damage when they migrate into the biliary tree. As already noted, helminths release peptides and eicosanoids that down regulate host inflammatory processes. In some cases, helminths bias host immunity to produce Th-2-like responses that may make the host less likely to eliminate the parasite. Immune regulation on the part of the parasite may also have consequences for the host regarding a wide variety of viral infections. There is some evidence to support the role of helminths as co-pathogens that promote susceptibility to HIV infection and AIDS. In many cases, some of the most important mechanisms of pathogenesis are still not known. Heavy infection with some intestinal nematodes (e.g., hookworm) are considered to be the major cause of stunted growth during childhood as well as inducing impaired cognitive behavior and intellectual development. While intuitively we might suspect that parasite-induced malnutrition plays an important role in this process, the true basis by which these processes occur is not known.

Host-mediated immunopathology accounts for a large measure of the damage that occurs during some helminth infections. This is particularly true for infection with the schistosomes. However, current evidence suggests that in the case of infection with a number of filarial worm species, an endosymbiont, *Wolbachia* sp. of bacteria, may be responsible for most of the pathological consequences of the infection. Brain parenchymal inflammation and seizures in cysticercosis are well documented.

The genomes of many of these important pathogens of humans are now available, so new approaches to the clinical management of patients suffering from them are surely to emerge from the laboratory and find their way to the bedside. At least that is the hoped for outcome of such research.

IV. The Protozoa

Over 200,000 species of protozoa have been described so far, of which more than half are represented in the fossil record. The repertoire of known living species (approximately 35,000) includes more than 10,000 that have been selected for life as parasites. Regardless of their lifestyle, all protozoans are eukaryotic single-cell organisms. Free-living species occupy every conceivable ecological niche, including marine trenches, rainforests, artesian and thermal springs, salt lakes, ice flows, glaciers, and many others, while parasitic protozoans infect a wide spectrum of vertebrate and invertebrate life.

Unlike the great majority of parasitic helminth species, protozoan parasites are able to replicate within a given host, often resulting in hundreds of thousands of new individuals within just a few days following initial infection. This single feature of their life cycle frequently has grave consequences for the host.

Parasitic protozoans have played a major role in the evolution of the human species, mainly due to lethal consequences of infection, or limiting where people can live by adversely affecting their livestock. These very same selection pressures continue to play out in many parts of the world today. For example, malaria in all its forms, African trypanosomiasis, and visceral leishmaniasis infect millions of people, and are responsible for untold numbers of deaths and debilitating chronic illnesses. Many others cause less severe disease (e.g., chronic diarrhea) that nonetheless results in lost time at work and school and loss of recreational activities we deem vital to living enriched, healthy, disease-free lives. This is due, in part, to the fact that some important species of parasitic protozoans are no longer susceptible to drugs that were once effective in limiting disease. There are no effective vaccines for the control of any protozoan infection in humans.

While the biology of parasitic protozoa varies widely from group to group, these organisms share many common features. A unit membrane that functions in a similar fashion to all other eukaryotic cells binds them. Nutrients may either be actively transported, phagocytized, or moved into the cell by pinocytosis. Digestion of particulate material is by lysosomal enzymes within the phagolysosome. Protozoans excrete wastes either by diffusion or by exocytosis. Mechanisms of motility take advantage of the presence of one of a variety of structures (e.g., cilia, flagella, pseudopod). All species of protozoans can divide asexually, usually by binary fission. In some instances the process is more complex, and includes multiple nuclear divisions followed by cytokinesis. Those capable of sexual reproduction do so within the definitive host, resulting in the formation of a zygote.

In addition, their cytoplasm may contain subcellular organelles, including Golgi apparatus, lysosomes, mitochondria, rough and smooth endoplasmic reticulum, and a wide variety of secretory granules of specialized function (e.g., the hydrogenosome of *Trichomonas vaginalis*, and the glycosome of kinetoplastidae). Collectively, these cytoplasmic inclusions enable the organism to respire, digest food, generate energy, grow, and reproduce.

Some species have evolved elaborate surface coats consisting of materials derived from the host, or secreted by the parasite that offer some protection from host immune responses, thereby extending their life within a given individual and resulting in great damage to the host as well.

The field of immunoparasitology, parasite genomics, and parasite proteomics has also matured over the past several years. New understanding regarding the role(s) of cytokines and interleukins in the pathogenesis of disease has led to new clinical approaches for several important protozoan diseases. In addition, the details of protective host mechanisms that counter the invasion process have been described, giving hope for the development of a new generation of drugs and perhaps even the first of many effective vaccines.

The following chapters are but a thumbnail sketch of some of the excitement generated in the field of protozoan parasitology. They are designed to present to the medical student and physician useful and practical information specific to the diagnosis, treatment, and management of infections caused by these pathogens.

1. *Giardia lamblia* (also known as *G. duodenalis* or *G. intestinalis*)
(Stiles 1915)

Introduction

Giardia lamblia (also known as *G. duodenalis* or *G. intestinalis*) is a flagellated protozoan that lacks a mitochondrion.[1] It is aerotolerant, but respires as an anaerobe, and lives in the small intestine. Other protozoa sharing this metabolic strategy include *Entamoeba histolytica*, and *Trichomonas vaginalis*. The species Giardia is divided into eight genetic groups, with groups A and B infecting humans.[2] *Giardia lamblia* produces a cyst stage that is environmentally resistant.[3] Infection is acquired through the fecal-oral route, most commonly via contaminated drinking water.[4] *G. lamblia* has a world-wide distribution, and is endemic in many regions.[5] Giardiasis frequently occurs in children, (especially those attending daycare centers), travelers, immunocompromised individuals (including HIV-infected individuals), and patients with genetic disorders such as cystic fibrosis.[6-11] *G. lamblia* is also a common infection in humans and domestic animals in the United States[12]. It is likely that many infected individuals remain undiagnosed and many more may harbor Giardia without obvious symptoms.[13] Beavers are major reservoir hosts that are often responsible for contaminating public drinking water supplies, and infection with *Giardia lamblia* is known in many parts of the country by the common name of *"beaver fever"*.[14, 15] Giardia is the subject of much intensive research, including a complete sequence analysis of its genome.[16] A survey of its genome has revealed the presence of genes for meiosis, although a sexual stage for this protozoan has not yet been described.[17] In 2001, an excellent review of the biology of *Giardia lamblia* was published by Adam, but much work has been added to this field since this comprehensive review was published.[18]

Historical Information

Antony Van Leeuwenhoek, the famous Dutch microscopist, in a letter written to Robert Hooke in 1681, described in detail the living trophozoite stage of *Giardia*, which he observed in a sample of his own stool: ". . . *animalcules a-moving very prettily. Their bodies were somewhat longer than broad, and their belly, which was flat-like, furnisht with sundry little paws. . . yet for all that they made but slow progress.*"[19] In 1859, Vilem Lambl described the main morphological features of the trophozoite stage that he obtained from the stools of various pediatric patients in Prague.[20] His elegant scientific drawings remain impressive, even in today's world of sophisticated, technologically advanced light microscopy. In 1921, C.E. Simon completed the description of its morphology.[21]

Life Cycle

Giardia lamblia exists in two forms: the trophozoite (Fig. 1.1) and the cyst (Fig. 1.2). The trophozoite is pear-shaped and motile, measuring 10-20 μm long and 7-10 μm. in diameter. It possesses eight flagella and is bi-nucleate. Both nuclei are transcriptionally active.[22] In addition, it contains two rigid structures, called median bodies, which

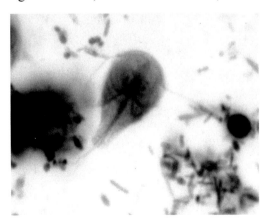

Figure 1.1. Trophozoite of *Giardia lamblia*. 15 μm.

Giardia lamblia

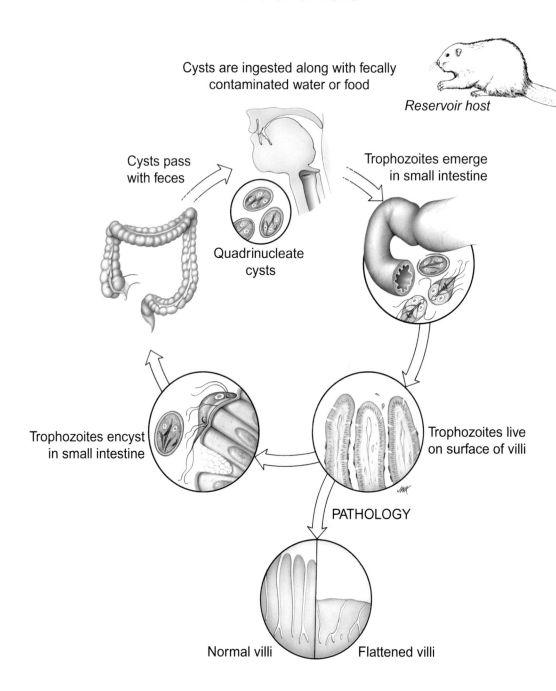

Cysts are ingested along with fecally contaminated water or food

Reservoir host

Cysts pass with feces

Quadrinucleate cysts

Trophozoites emerge in small intestine

Trophozoites encyst in small intestine

Trophozoites live on surface of villi

PATHOLOGY

Normal villi   Flattened villi

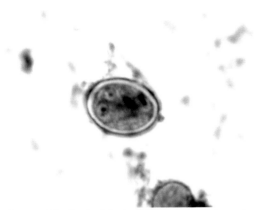

Figure 1.2. Cyst of *G. lamblia*. Two nuclei can be seen. 13 μm.

are now known to be part of the complex and unique cytoskeleton.[23] *G. lamblia* has no mitochondria, peroxisomes, hydrogenosomes, or related subcellular organelles that might be associated with energy metabolism, but does appear to use a homolog of the mitochondrial-like glycerol-3-phosphate dehydrogenase (GPDH) that is involved in glycolysis.[24] Some strains of the parasite carry double-stranded RNA viruses, known as *giardia*viruses, whose impact on virulence is still being explored.[25, 26] These viruses have facilitated the expression of foreign genes in Giardia, serving as shuttle vectors.[27]

Giardia lamblia's anterior ventral region has a disc-like organelle that it uses for attachment to the surface of epithelial cells. The integrity of the disk is maintained by tubulin and giardins.[28] The latter are members of the class III, low affinity, calcium binding annexins.[29] Its structure has been investigated using cryoelectron microscopy.[30]

Infection begins with ingestion of the quadrinucleate cyst, which must then excyst in response to a complex sequence of environmental cues received by the parasite.[31] Ingesting the trophozoite stage does not result in infection. As the cyst passes through the stomach and into the small intestine, it is sequentially exposed to HCl and then pancreatic enzymes.[32, 33] Excystation may be inhibited by ethanol and isopropanol-containing hand sanitizers.[34]

Each cyst produces two bi-nucleate trophozoites that then attach to epithelial cells by their ventral disks (Fig. 1.3). *G. lamblia* binds to the host cells using this specialized attachment organelle, the ventral disk, which appears to use an epsinR homolog (Glepsin) to bind both phosphatidylinositol (3,4,5)-triphosphate phospholipids without canonical domains for interaction with clathrin coat components.[35] Once attached to epithelial cells, the bi-nucleate trophozoites grow and divide by binary fission. Cysts are unable to replicate.

G. lamblia can be grown in vitro (Fig. 1.4). The full nutritional needs of the trophozoite have yet to be fully determined, but some of its biochemical energy pathways are known.[36, 37] Glucose and arginine appear to be its major sources of energy, and it may access a portion of its need for them through the breakdown of mucus.[38, 39] Giardia is unable to synthesize nucleic acid bases *de novo* and consequently employs salvage pathways.[40] Lipids are absorbed directly, likely facilitated by bile and bile salts, and perhaps by endocytosis of lipoproteins.[41, 42] *G. lamblia* is not considered an invasive or tissue parasite, but its ability to adhere closely to the columnar cells at the level of the microvilli, and its penchant for secreting proteins at the site, results in antibody production and, eventually, to protective immunity.[43] To exit the host and survive, trophozoites must encyst, and

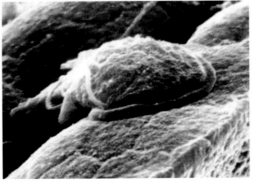

Figure 1.3. Scanning EM of a trophozoite of *G. muris* on epithelium of mouse small intestine. Courtesy R. Owen.

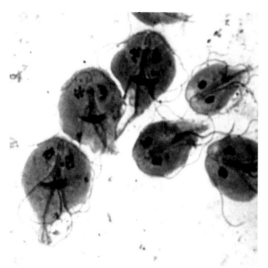

Figure 1.4. Trophozoites of *G. lamblia* in culture. Courtesy D. Lindmark.

pass into the large intestine. Bile salts seem to be involved in triggering this process.[3, 44, 45] Encystation *in vitro* is inducible by exposure of the trophozoite stage to bile and elevated pH, possibly by sequestering cholesterol.[46] Trophozoites take up and release conjugated bile salts.[45, 47] These conditions may be necessary for its survival in its essential niche (Fig. 1.3). Apparently, a novel transglutaminase is also required for encystment.[48] Encysted parasites can endure for long periods of time outside the host if they remain moist and the temperature is not elevated.[49] Both cysts and trophozoites pass out of the bowel with the fecal mass, but only the cyst stage survives. Cysts can withstand exposure to mild chemical treatments, such as chlorinated water for short periods of time at low temperatures.[50]

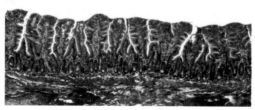

Figure 1.5. Flattened, fused villi of small intestine from a patient suffering from malabsorption syndrome due to *G. lamblia*.

Freezing, boiling, UV exposure or desiccation can destroy cysts.[51] Production of cysts occurs throughout the infection, but the number produced each day varies greatly, depending upon a wide variety of conditions, including the development of acquired protective immunity.[52] Protective immunity appears to be directed against both surface antigens[53] and antigens that are secreted.[54]

Cellular and Molecular Pathogenesis

Steatorrhea and malabsorption with flattening of the villi (Fig. 1.5), often accompanied by profound weight loss, are the dominant pathological consequences of chronic infection.[55, 56] Despite the fact that there are numerous related species of Giardia, and that they can be manipulated *in vivo* and *in vitro*, surprisingly little is known regarding their biological effect(s) on the physiology and biochemistry of the small intestine.[18] It appears that part of the diarrhea generated by *G. lamblia* is due to augmentation of peristalsis and alteration of host cell tight junctions.[57, 58]

Infection with *G. lamblia* induces numerous cellular and humoral responses, some of which are protective in nature.[59-61] Particularly important is secretory IgA. It has been shown for non-secretors that infection is easily established and not easily controlled.[62] Physiological changes experienced during symptomatic infection could relate to these host-based responses, and might even be induced by mechanisms related to allergies,[60] such as those observed in wheat-gluten-sensitive individuals.[61]

Antigenic variation of surface components of the trophozoite is typical in the early phase of infection,[53, 63] and most likely aids the parasite in avoiding elimination by humoral responses (e.g., IgA antibodies)[62] directed at trophozoite surface proteins.[64] Switching of cysteine-rich variant surface proteins (VSPs) also occurs when the parasite is about to excyst, allowing the parasite to evade immune elimination.[65] Severe combined immune deficiency (SCID) mice do not induce VSP switching, an indication that the overall process is under the control of B cell-mediated host responses. However, switching also occurs spontaneously or in response to physiological selection, but at a much slower pace than in immunocompetent hosts. Shuttle viral systems for transfecting *G. lamblia* have been developed.[66] Thus, genetic manipulation is now possible, which may lead to a more complete understanding of the molecular events governing pathogenesis.

Human breast milk is protective, because it contains antibodies of the IgA class.[67] Nonspecific defenses, such as lactoferrin or products of lipid hydrolysis of the milk in the normal digestive tract, may also play a role, as each is toxic to Giardia.[68-70] Nitric oxide, released luminally by intestinal epithelial cells in response to infection, inhibits parasite growth and differentiation, although Giardia might be able to disarm this potential defense mechanism by competitively consuming the arginine needed by the host cells for NO synthesis.[71] In summary, the duration and severity of infection depends upon both immune and nonimmune host defenses, as well as the parasite's ability to evade them.

Clinical Disease

It is estimated that a large portion of those who encounter *G. lamblia* and become infected fail to progress to a state of ill health.[72,73] Infected individuals may remain asymptomatic for long periods of time, even though they are still infected, and could become chronic carriers referred to as *cyst passers*. Of those who go on to develop disease, the most prominent symptom is protracted diarrhea.[39,74] The acute diarrhea of giardiasis is classically described as foul-smelling with flatulence, nausea, weight loss and abdominal cramps with bloating.[75] A minority of patients may describe systemic symptoms

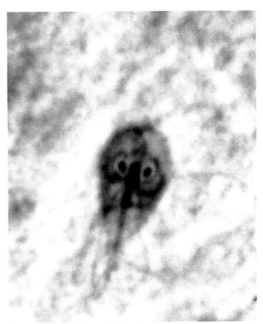

Figure 1.6a. *G. lamblia* trophozoite in stool sample.

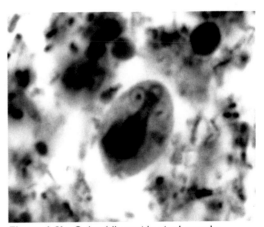

Figure 1.6b. *G. lamblia* cyst in stool sample.

such as fever.[75] Untreated, this type of diarrhea may last weeks or months, although it usually varies in intensity, affected children often fail to thrive.[76] Chronic infections are characterized by steatorrhea accompanied by malabsorption syndrome associated with rapid, substantial weight loss, general debility, and consequent fatigue.[39] In addition, some people may complain of epigastric discomfort, anorexia, and even pain.

Certain patient groups are at greater risk for acquiring giardiasis and for developing chronic infection. Patients suffering from immuno-compromising conditions (e.g., hypogammaglobulinemia, HIV/AIDS or cancer chemotherapies), cystic fibrosis and children with underlying malnutrition can have a protracted disease with more severe symptoms.[11, 77-79]

Diagnosis

The diagnosis of giardiasis has changed dramatically with the introduction of newer diagnostic modalities. Definitive diagnosis still depends upon direct, microscopic observation of trophozoites (Fig. 1.6a) or cysts (Fig. 1.6b) in concentrated stained stool.[80] Due to the challenges inherent in obtaining such specimens and the limited number of skilled laboratory personnel needed to examine these specimens, antigen-capture ELISA was introduced.[81] These stool antigen detection assays, particularly the direct fluorescent antibody test (DFA) have greater sensitivity than stool microscopy, faster turn around time, and only require a single stool collection.[82, 83] The string test, which involved swallowing a gelatin capsule attached to the end of a long string, is now relegated to a place in history as newer better-tolerated diagnostic techniques are becoming available.[84] Nucleic acid amplification tests (NAATs) are now available that are revolutionizing the diagnosis of infectious diarrhea. The BioFire, FilmArray, and the Luminex xTAG Gastrointestinal Pathogen Panel are among the commercially available NAAT tests that can detect with high sensitivity and specificity a broad number of viral, bacterial, and protozoan pathogens.[85-87]

Treatment

It is recommended that all symptomatic patients infected with Giardia be treated with antimicrobial therapy, as this has been shown to relieve symptoms with minimal side effects.[88] The nitroimidazoles, metronidazole and tinidazole, are the primary drugs used for treatment.[88, 89] Metronidazole, an inexpensive option, is usually given at a dose of 250 mg by mouth three times per day for 5-7 days for adults, while tinidazole can be given as a single oral dose of 2 grams with high efficacy. Another preferred drug option is nitazoxanide 500 mg by mouth twice a day for three days. Alternative antimicrobials include paromomycin (in pregnancy), furazolidone, quinacrine and albendazole.[88]

Recurrence or persistence of symptoms should be evaluated carefully, as persisting malabsorption and lactose intolerance can last for weeks to months following infection.[90] Prior to retreatment it is recommended that one re-evaluate the patient and confirm the presence of infection.[91] Resistant strains of Giardia are increasingly prevalent and many will retreat, but with a different class of antimicrobial therapy or a longer course of the original agent.[92-95] In some refractory cases combination antimicrobial therapy may be necessary.[96]

Prevention and Control

Giardia lamblia is primarily a waterborne infection, although food handlers and infected children in daycare centers no doubt play important roles in transmission.[4, 97] Prevention strategies include proper disposal of human waste, filtration of drinking water supplies, maintenance of buffer zones around watersheds when filtration is not practiced (e.g., in New York City), and maintaining the highest standards of hygiene in daycare centers and mental institutions, although this last recommendation is admittedly the most difficult one to achieve. A murine model for a protective giardia vaccine exists, however efforts to develop clinical candidate vaccines, including work on canine vaccines, are hampered by the lack of a well-articulated medical need for commitment of new resources in the setting of many effective therapeutic options.[98]

References

1. Roger, A. J.; Svärd, S. G.; Tovar, J.; Clark, C. G.; Smith, M. W.; Gillin, F. D.; Sogin, M. L., A mitochondrial-like chaperonin 60 gene in Giardia lamblia: evidence that diplomonads once harbored an endosymbiont related to the progenitor of mitochondria. *Proceedings of the National Academy of Sciences of the United States of America* **1998**, *95* (1), 229-34.
2. Vanni, I.; Caccio, S. M.; van Lith, L.; Lebbad, M.; Svard, S. G.; Pozio, E.; Tosini, F., Detection of Giardia duodenalis assemblages A and B in human feces by simple, assemblage-specific PCR assays. *PLoS Negl Trop Dis* **2012**, *6* (8), e1776.
3. Faso, C.; Bischof, S.; Hehl, A. B., The proteome landscape of Giardia lamblia encystation. *PLoS One* **2013**, *8* (12), e83207.
4. Levy, D. A.; Bens, M. S.; Craun, G. F.; Calderon, R. L.; Herwaldt, B. L., Surveillance for waterborne-disease outbreaks--United States, 1995-1996. *MMWR. CDC surveillance summaries : Morbidity and mortality weekly report. CDC surveillance summaries / Centers for Disease Control* **1998**, *47* (5), 1-34.
5. Feng, Y.; Xiao, L., Zoonotic potential and molecular epidemiology of Giardia species and giardiasis. *Clin Microbiol Rev* **2011**, *24* (1), 110-40.
6. Sagi, E. F.; Shapiro, M.; Deckelbaum, R.; J., Giardia lamblia: prevalance, influence on growth, and symptomatology in healthy nursery children. *Isr Sci* **1983**, *19* 815-817.
7. Pickering, L. K.; Woodward, W. E.; DuPont, H. L.; Sullivan, P., Occurrence of Giardia lamblia in children in day care centers. *The Journal of pediatrics* **1984**, *104* (4), 522-6.
8. Daszak, P., Giardia, HIV, and nature's horrifying beauty. *Ecohealth* **2014**, *11* (2), 277-8.
9. Cimino, A.; Ali, S. Z., Giardia intestinalis on anal PAP of an HIV-positive male. *Diagn Cytopathol* **2010**, *38* (11), 814-5.
10. Jelinek, T.; Loscher, T., Epidemiology of giardiasis in German travelers. *J Travel Med* **2000**, *7* (2), 70-3.
11. Roberts, D. M.; Craft, J. C.; Mather, F. J.; Davis, S. H.; Wright, J. A., Prevalence of giardiasis in patients with cystic fibrosis. *The Journal of pediatrics* **1988**, *112* (4), 555-9.
12. Mohamed, A. S.; Levine, M.; Camp, J. W., Jr.; Lund, E.; Yoder, J. S.; Glickman, L. T.; Moore, G. E., Temporal patterns of human and canine Giardia infection in the United States: 2003-2009. *Prev Vet Med* **2014**, *113* (2), 249-56.
13. Nash, T. E.; Herrington, D. A.; Losonsky, G. A.; Levine, M. M., Experimental human infections with Giardia lamblia. *J Infect Dis* **1987**, *156* (6), 974-84.
14. Carlson, D. W.; Finger, D. R., Beaver fever arthritis. *J Clin Rheumatol* **2004**, *10* (2), 86-8.
15. Taverne, J., Beaver fever and pinworm neuroses on the Net. *Parasitol Today* **1999**, *15* (9), 363-4.
16. Best, A. A.; Morrison, H. G.; McArthur, A. G.; Sogin, M. L.; Olsen, G. J., Evolution of eukaryotic transcription: insights from the genome of Giardia lamblia. *Genome research* **2004**, *14* (8), 1537-47.
17. Ramesh, M. A.; Malik, S.-B.; Logsdon, J. M., A phylogenomic inventory of meiotic genes; evidence for sex in Giardia and an early eukaryotic origin of meiosis. *Current biology : CB* **2005**, *15* (2), 185-91.
18. Adam, R. D., Biology of Giardia lamblia. *Clinical microbiology reviews* **2001**, *14* (3), 447-75.
19. Leenwenhoek, A.; Dobell, C., Van Cited by In Antony van Leeuwen-hoek and His "Little Animals". *Publications New Dover P* **1960**, *224*.
20. Lambi, V. D. F., Mikroskopische Untersuchungen der Darm-Excrete. *Beitrag zur Pathologie des Darms und zur Diagnostik am Krankenbette Vierteljahrschrift fur die Praktische Heilkunde Med Fac Prague* **1859**, *1*, 1-58.
21. Simon, C. E.; J., Giardia enterica, a parasitic intestinal flagellate of man. *Am* **1921**, *1*, 440-491.
22. Kabnick, K. S.; Peattie, D. A., In situ analyses reveal that the two nuclei of Giardia lamblia are equivalent. *Journal of cell science* **1990**, *95* (Pt 3), 353-60.
23. Piva, B.; Benchimol, M., The median body of Giardia lamblia: an ultrastructural study. *Biol Cell* **2004**, *96* (9), 735-46.
24. Lalle, M.; Camerini, S.; Cecchetti, S.; Finelli, R.; Sferra, G.; Muller, J.; Ricci, G.; Pozio, E., The

FAD-dependent glycerol-3-phosphate dehydrogenase of Giardia duodenalis: an unconventional enzyme that interacts with the g14-3-3 and it is a target of the antitumoral compound NBDHEX. *Front Microbiol* **2015,** *6,* 544.

25. Tai, J. H.; Chang, S. C.; Chou, C. F.; Ong, S. J., Separation and characterization of two related giardiaviruses in the parasitic protozoan Giardia lamblia. *Virology* **1996,** *216* (1), 124-32.

26. Janssen, M. E.; Takagi, Y.; Parent, K. N.; Cardone, G.; Nibert, M. L.; Baker, T. S., Three-dimensional structure of a protozoal double-stranded RNA virus that infects the enteric pathogen Giardia lamblia. *J Virol* **2015,** *89* (2), 1182-94.

27. Liu, Q.; Zhang, X.; Li, J.; Ying, J.; Chen, L.; Zhao, Y.; Wei, F.; Wu, T., Giardia lamblia: stable expression of green fluorescent protein mediated by giardiavirus. *Experimental parasitology* **2005,** *109* (3), 181-7.

28. Aggarwal, A.; Adam, R. D.; Nash, T. E., Characterization of a 29.4-kilodalton structural protein of Giardia lamblia and localization to the ventral disk [corrected]. *Infection and immunity* **1989,** *57* (4), 1305-10.

29. Bauer, B.; Engelbrecht, S.; Bakker-Grunwald, T.; Scholze, H., Functional identification of alpha 1-giardin as an annexin of Giardia lamblia. *FEMS microbiology letters* **1999,** *173* (1), 147-53.

30. Brown, J. R.; Schwartz, C. L.; Heumann, J. M.; Dawson, S. C.; Hoenger, A., A detailed look at the cytoskeletal architecture of the Giardia lamblia ventral disc. *J Struct Biol* **2016,** *194* (1), 38-48.

31. Hetsko, M. L.; McCaffery, J. M.; Svärd, S. G.; Meng, T. C.; Que, X.; Gillin, F. D., Cellular and transcriptional changes during excystation of Giardia lamblia in vitro. *Experimental parasitology* **1998,** *88* (3), 172-83.

32. Bingham, A. K.; Meyer, E. A., Giardia excystation can be induced in vitro in acidic solutions. *Nature* **1979,** *277* (5694), 301-2.

33. Rice, E. W.; Schaefer, F. W., Improved in vitro excystation procedure for Giardia lamblia cysts. *Journal of clinical microbiology* **1981,** *14* (6), 709-10.

34. Chatterjee, A.; Bandini, G.; Motari, E.; Samuelson, J., Ethanol and Isopropanol in Concentrations Present in Hand Sanitizers Sharply Reduce Excystation of Giardia and Entamoeba and Eliminate Oral Infectivity of Giardia Cysts in Gerbils. *Antimicrob Agents Chemother* **2015,** *59* (11), 6749-54.

35. Ebneter, J. A.; Hehl, A. B., The single epsin homolog in Giardia lamblia localizes to the ventral disk of trophozoites and is not associated with clathrin membrane coats. *Mol Biochem Parasitol* **2014,** *197* (1-2), 24-7.

36. Jarroll, E. L.; Manning, P.; Berrada, A.; Hare, D.; Lindmark, D. G., Biochemistry and metabolism of Giardia. *The Journal of protozoology* **1989,** *36* (2), 190-7.

37. Coombs, G. H.; Muller, M.; Marr, J. J., Energy Metabolism in Anaerobic Protozoa. 1995; p 109-131.

38. Edwards, M. R.; Schofield, P. J.; Sullivan, W. J.; Costello, M., Arginine metabolism during culture of Giardia intestinalis *Mol Biochem Parasitol* **1992,** *103,* 1-2.

39. Farthing, M. J. G.; Gorbach, S. L.; Bartlett, J. G.; Blacklow, N. R., Giardia lamblia. 1998; p 2399-2406.

40. Wang, C. C.; Aldritt, S., Purine salvage networks in Giardia lamblia. *The Journal of experimental medicine* **1983,** *158* (5), 1703-12.

41. Farthing, M. J.; Keusch, G. T.; Carey, M. C., Effects of bile and bile salts on growth and membrane lipid uptake by Giardia lamblia. Possible implications for pathogenesis of intestinal disease. *The Journal of clinical investigation* **1985,** *76* (5), 1727-32.

42. Lujan, H. D.; Mowatt, M. R.; Nash, T. E., Lipid requirements and lipid uptake by Giardia lamblia trophozoites in culture. *The Journal of eukaryotic microbiology* **1996,** *43* (3), 237-42.

43. Velazquez, C.; Beltran, M.; Ontiveros, N.; Rascon, L.; Figueroa, D. C.; Granados, A. J.; Hernandez-Martinez, J.; Hernandez, J.; Astiazaran-Garcia, H., Giardia lamblia infection induces different secretory and systemic antibody responses in mice. *Parasite Immunol* **2005,** *27* (9), 351-6.

44. Lujan, H. D.; Mowatt, M. R.; Nash, T. E., Mechanisms of Giardia lamblia differentiation into cysts *Microbio Mol Biol Rev* **1997,** *61* (3), 294-304.

45. Halliday, C. E.; Inge, P. M.; Farthing, M. J., Characterization of bile salt uptake by Giardia lamblia.

International journal for parasitology **1995**, *25* (9), 1089-97.

46.   Lujan, H. D.; Mowatt, M. R.; Byrd, L. G.; Nash, T. E., Cholesterol starvation induces differentiation of the intestinal parasite Giardia lamblia. *Proc Natl Acad* **1996**, *93* (15), 7628-33.

47.   Halliday, C. E.; Clark, C.; Farthing, M. J., Giardia-bile salt interactions in vitro and in vivo. *Transactions of the Royal Society of Tropical Medicine and Hygiene* **1988**, *82* (3), 428-32.

48.   Davids, B. J.; Mehta, K.; Fesus, L.; McCaffery, J. M.; Gillin, F. D., Dependence of Giardia lamblia encystation on novel transglutaminase activity. *Molecular and biochemical parasitology* **2004**, *136* (2), 173-80.

49.   Alum, A.; Absar, I. M.; Asaad, H.; Rubino, J. R.; Ijaz, M. K., Impact of environmental conditions on the survival of cryptosporidium and giardia on environmental surfaces. *Interdiscip Perspect Infect Dis* **2014**, *2014*, 210385.

50.   Jarroll, E. L.; Bingham, A. K.; Meyer, E. A., Effect of chlorine on Giardia lamblia cyst viability. *Appl Environ Microbiol* **1981**, *41* (2), 483-7.

51.   Einarsson, E.; Svard, S. G.; Troell, K., UV irradiation responses in Giardia intestinalis. *Exp Parasitol* **2015**, *154*, 25-32.

52.   Farthing, M. J.; Goka, A. J., Immunology of giardiasis. *Bailliere's clinical gastroenterology* **1987**, *1* (3), 589-603.

53.   Nash, T. E., Antigenic variation in Giardia lamblia and the host's immune response. *Philosophical transactions of the Royal Society of London. Series B, Biological sciences* **1997**, *352* (1359), 1369-75.

54.   Kaur, H.; Samra, H.; Ghosh, S.; Vinayak, V. K.; Ganguly, N. K., Immune effector responses to an excretory-secretory product of Giardia lamblia. *FEMS immunology and medical microbiology* **1999**, *23* (2), 93-105.

55.   Carroccio, A.; Montalto, G.; Iacono, G.; Ippolito, S.; Soresi, M.; Notarbartolo, A., Secondary impairment of pancreatic function as a cause of severe malabsorption in intestinal giardiasis: a case report. *The American journal of tropical medicine and hygiene* **1997**, *56* (6), 599-602.

56.   Gottstein, B.; Stocks, N. I.; Shearer, G. M.; Nash, T. E., Human cellular immune response to Giardia lamblia. *Infection* **1991**, *19* (6), 421-6.

57.   Buret, A. G.; Mitchell, K.; Muench, D. G.; Scott, K. G., Giardia lamblia disrupts tight junctional ZO-1 and increases permeability in non-transformed human small intestinal epithelial monolayers: effects of epidermal growth factor. *Parasitology* **2002**, *125* (Pt 1), 11-9.

58.   Troeger, H.; Epple, H. J.; Schneider, T.; Wahnschaffe, U.; Ullrich, R.; Burchard, G. D.; Jelinek, T.; Zeitz, M.; Fromm, M.; Schulzke, J. D., Effect of chronic Giardia lamblia infection on epithelial transport and barrier function in human duodenum. *Gut* **2007**, *56* (3), 328-35.

59.   Rosales-Borjas, D. M.; Díaz-Rivadeneyra, J.; Doña-Leyva, A.; Zambrano-Villa, S. A.; Mascaró, C.; Osuna, A.; Ortiz-Ortiz, L., Secretory immune response to membrane antigens during Giardia lamblia infection in humans. *Infection and immunity* **1998**, *66* (2), 756-9.

60.   Di Prisco, M. C.; Hagel, I.; Lynch, N. R.; Jiménez, J. C.; Rojas, R.; Gil, M.; Mata, E., Association between giardiasis and allergy. *Annals of allergy, asthma & immunology : official publication of the American College of Allergy, Asthma, & Immunology* **1998**, *81* (3), 261-5.

61.   Doe, W. F., An overview of intestinal immunity and malabsorption. *The American journal of medicine* **1979**, *67* (6), 1077-84.

62.   Eckmann, L., Mucosal defences against Giardia. *Parasite immunology* **2003**, *25* (5), 259-70.

63.   Nash, T. E., Surface antigenic variation in Giardia lamblia. *Molecular microbiology* **2002**, *45* (3), 585-90.

64.   Heyworth, M. F., Immunology of Giardia and Cryptosporidium infections. *The Journal of infectious diseases* **1992**, *166* (3), 465-72.

65.   Svard, S. G.; Meng, T. C.; Hetsko, M. L., Differentiation-associated surface antigen variation in the ancient eukaryote Giardia lamblia. *Molecular Microbiology* **1998**, *30* (5), 979-89.

66.   Singer, S. M.; Yee, J.; Nash, T. E., Episomal and integrated maintenance of foreign DNA in Giardia lamblia. *Molecular and biochemical parasitology* **1998**, *92* (1), 59-69.

67.   Nayak, N.; Ganguly, N. K.; Walia, B. N.; Wahi, V.; Kanwar, S. S.; Mahajan, R. C., Specific secretory IgA in the milk of Giardia lamblia-infected and uninfected women. *The Journal of*

infectious diseases **1987,** *155* (4), 724-7.

68.   Gillin, F. D.; Reiner, D. S.; Gault, M. J., Cholate-dependent killing of Giardia lamblia by human milk. *Infection and immunity* **1985,** *47* (3), 619-22.

69.   Hernell, O.; Ward, H.; Bläckberg, L.; Pereira, M. E., Killing of Giardia lamblia by human milk lipases: an effect mediated by lipolysis of milk lipids. *The Journal of infectious diseases* **1986,** *153* (4), 715-20.

70.   Reiner, D. S.; Wang, C. S.; Gillin, F. D., Human milk kills Giardia lamblia by generating toxic lipolytic products. *The Journal of infectious diseases* **1986,** *154* (5), 825-32.

71.   Eckmann, L.; Laurent, F.; Langford, T. D.; Hetsko, M. L.; Smith, J. R.; Kagnoff, M. F.; Gillin, F. D., Nitric oxide production by human intestinal epithelial cells and competition for arginine as potential determinants of host defense against the lumen-dwelling pathogen Giardia lamblia. *Journal of immunology (Baltimore, Md. : 1950)* **2000,** *164* (3), 1478-87.

72.   Ali, S. A.; Hill, D. R., Giardia intestinalis. *Current opinion in infectious diseases* **2003,** *16* (5), 453-60.

73.   Lopez, C. E.; Dykes, A. C.; Juranek, D. D.; Sinclair, S. P.; Conn, J. M.; Christie, R. W.; Lippy, E. C.; Schultz, M. G.; Mires, M. H., Waterborne giardiasis: a communitywide outbreak of disease and a high rate of asymptomatic infection. *Am J Epidemiol* **1980,** *112* (4), 495-507.

74.   Reinthaler, F. F.; Feierl, G.; Stünzner, D.; Marth, E., Diarrhea in returning Austrian tourists: epidemiology, etiology, and cost-analyses. *Journal of travel medicine* **1998,** *5* (2), 65-72.

75.   Hopkins, R. S.; Juranek, D. D., Acute giardiasis: an improved clinical case definition for epidemiologic studies. *Am J Epidemiol* **1991,** *133* (4), 402-7.

76.   Craft, J. C., Giardia and giardiasis in childhood. *Pediatric infectious disease* **1982,** *1* (3), 196-211.

77.   Moolasart, P., Giardia lamblia in AIDS patients with diarrhea. *Journal of the Medical Association of Thailand = Chotmaihet thangphaet* **1999,** *82* (7), 654-9.

78.   Bhaijee, F.; Subramony, C.; Tang, S. J.; Pepper, D. J., Human immunodeficiency virus-associated gastrointestinal disease: common endoscopic biopsy diagnoses. *Patholog Res Int* **2011,** *2011,* 247923.

79.   Sullivan, P. B.; Thomas, J. E.; Wight, D. G.; Neale, G.; Eastham, E. J.; Corrah, T.; Lloyd-Evans, N.; Greenwood, B. M., Helicobacter pylori in Gambian children with chronic diarrhoea and malnutrition. *Archives of disease in childhood* **1990,** *65* (2), 189-91.

80.   Kabani, A.; Cadrain, G.; Trevenen, C.; Jadavji, T.; Church, D. L., Practice guidelines for ordering stool ova and parasite testing in a pediatric population. The Alberta Children's Hospital. *American journal of clinical pathology* **1995,** *104* (3), 272-8.

81.   Boone, J. H.; Wilkins, T. D.; Nash, T. E.; Brandon, J. E.; Macias, E. A.; Jerris, R. C.; Lyerly, D. M., TechLab and alexon Giardia enzyme-linked immunosorbent assay kits detect cyst wall protein 1. *Journal of clinical microbiology* **1999,** *37* (3), 611-4.

82.   Weitzel, T.; Dittrich, S.; Mohl, I.; Adusu, E.; Jelinek, T., Evaluation of seven commercial antigen detection tests for Giardia and Cryptosporidium in stool samples. *Clin Microbiol Infect* **2006,** *12* (7), 656-9.

83.   Jahan, N.; Khatoon, R.; Ahmad, S., A Comparison of Microscopy and Enzyme Linked Immunosorbent Assay for Diagnosis of Giardia lamblia in Human Faecal Specimens. *J Clin Diagn Res* **2014,** *8* (11), DC04-6.

84.   Jones, J. E., String test for diagnosing giardiasis. *American family physician* **1986,** *34* (2), 123-6.

85.   Buss, S. N.; Leber, A.; Chapin, K.; Fey, P. D.; Bankowski, M. J.; Jones, M. K.; Rogatcheva, M.; Kanack, K. J.; Bourzac, K. M., Multicenter evaluation of the BioFire FilmArray gastrointestinal panel for etiologic diagnosis of infectious gastroenteritis. *J Clin Microbiol* **2015,** *53* (3), 915-25.

86.   Mengelle, C.; Mansuy, J. M.; Prere, M. F.; Grouteau, E.; Claudet, I.; Kamar, N.; Huynh, A.; Plat, G.; Benard, M.; Marty, N.; Valentin, A.; Berry, A.; Izopet, J., Simultaneous detection of gastrointestinal pathogens with a multiplex Luminex-based molecular assay in stool samples from diarrhoeic patients. *Clin Microbiol Infect* **2013,** *19* (10), E458-65.

87.   Claas, E. C.; Burnham, C. A.; Mazzulli, T.; Templeton, K.; Topin, F., Performance of the xTAG(R) gastrointestinal pathogen panel, a multiplex molecular assay for simultaneous detection of bacterial, viral, and parasitic causes of infectious gastroenteritis. *J Microbiol Biotechnol* **2013,** *23*

(7), 1041-5.

88. Granados, C. E.; Reveiz, L.; Uribe, L. G.; Criollo, C. P., Drugs for treating giardiasis. *Cochrane Database Syst Rev* **2012,** *12*, CD007787.

89. Freeman, C. D.; Klutman, N. E.; Lamp, K. C., Metronidazole. A therapeutic review and update. *Drugs* **1997,** *54* (5), 679-708.

90. Hanevik, K.; Dizdar, V.; Langeland, N.; Hausken, T., Development of functional gastrointestinal disorders after Giardia lamblia infection. *BMC Gastroenterol* **2009,** *9*, 27.

91. Gardner, T. B.; Hill, D. R., Treatment of giardiasis. *Clin Microbiol Rev* **2001,** *14* (1), 114-28.

92. Abboud, P.; Lemée, V.; Gargala, G.; Brasseur, P.; Ballet, J. J.; Borsa-Lebas, F.; Caron, F.; Favennec, L., Successful treatment of metronidazole- and albendazole-resistant giardiasis with nitazoxanide in a patient with acquired immunodeficiency syndrome. *Clinical infectious diseases : an official publication of the Infectious Diseases Society of America* **2001,** *32* (12), 1792-4.

93. Fox, L. M.; Saravolatz, L. D., Nitazoxanide: a new thiazolide antiparasitic agent. *Clinical infectious diseases : an official publication of the Infectious Diseases Society of America* **2005,** *40* (8), 1173-80.

94. Yereli, K.; Balcioğlu, I. C.; Ertan, P.; Limoncu, E.; Onağ, A., Albendazole as an alternative therapeutic agent for childhood giardiasis in Turkey. *Clinical microbiology and infection : the official publication of the European Society of Clinical Microbiology and Infectious Diseases* **2004,** *10* (6), 527-9.

95. Miyamoto, Y.; Eckmann, L., Drug Development Against the Major Diarrhea-Causing Parasites of the Small Intestine, Cryptosporidium and Giardia. *Front Microbiol* **2015,** *6*, 1208.

96. Lopez-Velez, R.; Batlle, C.; Jimenez, C.; Navarro, M.; Norman, F.; Perez-Molina, J., Short course combination therapy for giardiasis after nitroimidazole failure. *Am J Trop Med Hyg* **2010,** *83* (1), 171-3.

97. Steiner, T. S.; Thielman, N. M.; Guerrant, R. L., Protozoal agents: what are the dangers for the public water supply? *Annual review of medicine* **1997,** *48*, 329-40.

98. Jenikova, G.; Hruz, P.; Andersson, M. K.; Tejman-Yarden, N.; Ferreira, P. C.; Andersen, Y. S.; Davids, B. J.; Gillin, F. D.; Svard, S. G.; Curtiss, R., 3rd; Eckmann, L., Alpha1-giardin based live heterologous vaccine protects against Giardia lamblia infection in a murine model. *Vaccine* **2011,** *29* (51), 9529-37.

2. Introduction to the *Leishmania*

The genus *Leishmania* comprises a genetically diverse group of vector-borne haemoflagellate parasites.[1, 2] *Leishmania* spp. are transmitted from host to host by the bite of sand flies (Fig. 2.1). There are two genera of sand flies; *Phlebotomous* spp., vectors of Old World Leishmaniasis, and *Lutzomyia* spp. transmitting leishmaniasis throughout the Western Hemisphere.[3]

Leishmania spp. are primarily zoonotic in nature, infecting a wide range of vertebrates throughout the tropical and subtropical world.[4, 5] All *Leishmania* spp. possess a well-characterized kinetoplast and live as obligate intracellular parasites within macrophages and other phagocytic cells of the reticuloendothelial system. Infection of multiple cell types has been demonstrated including tissue resident macrophages, dendritic cells, lymph node fibroblasts and neutrophils.[6] All species of Leishmania share many features of their genetics, mode of transmission, biochemistry, molecular biology, immunobiology, and susceptibility to drugs. Differences at all the above levels exist between the cutaneous and visceralizing species of Leishmania.

Leishmania spp. are known to cause several different disease manifestations including visceral leishmaniasis, cutaneous leishmaniasis, mucocutaneous leishmaniasis, diffuse cutaneous leishmaniasis, and less commonly leishmaniasis recidivans.[7] The number of humans suffering from leishmaniasis is unknown, but it is estimated that there are 0.2 to 0.4 million cases of visceral leishmaniasis and 0.7-1.2 million cases of cutaneous leishmaniasis each year.[8] More than 350 million people live within an area of transmission.[8] Leishmaniasis occurs in 88 countries located in Southern Europe, Africa, Asia, South Asia, and South and Central America.[8] The subgenus Leishmania is distributed throughout the Old and the New World, whereas the subgenus Viannia is only found in the New World. In the Western Hemisphere, multiple species regularly infect people: *Leishmania (Leishmania) amazonensis, Leishmania (Viannia) braziliensis, L. (V.) peruviana, L. (V.) colombiensis, L. (L.) donovani, L. (L.) garnhami, L. (V.) guyanensis, L. (L.) infantum chagasi, L. (V.) lainsoni, L. (V.) lindenbergi, L. (L.) mexicana, L. (V.) naiffi, L. (V.) panamensis, L. (L.) pifanoi, L. (V.) shawi,* and *L. (L.) venezualensis*. In the Eastern Hemisphere, there are significantly fewer species that infect humans: *L. (L.) donovani, L. (L.) infantum, L. (L.) aethiopica, L. (L.) major,* and *L. (L.) tropica*.

As might be expected, clinical conditions caused by *Leishmania* spp. vary greatly, depending upon the species of leishmania and the immune status of the host. Disease can present as cutaneous lesions that resolve over time, or as systemic disease of the reticuloendothelial system often resulting in death of the host if left untreated. Fortunately, there are fewer clinical entities than the number of species of pathogens that cause them; cutaneous, muco-cutaneous, and visceral leishmaniasis, and less commonly disseminated cutaneous and recidivans.

This introductory chapter will summarize the biology and molecular biology of the entire group, with the tacit assumption that they all behave similarly in their intracellular environment and within their sand fly vectors. Exceptions will be presented whenever they relate to a disease process applicable only to that species. The Leishmania Genome Project is based on the genome of *Leishmania major* and in 2005 the full genomic sequence

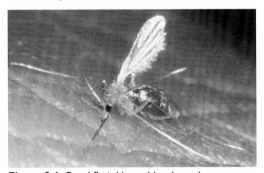

Figure 2.1. Sand fly taking a blood meal.

was completed.[9]

There are no commercially available vaccines as of yet, but infection with many of the species of leishmania results in permanent immunity to reinfection with the same species.[10] Perhaps data derived from the genome project will hasten the development of an effective, cheap, easy-to-administer vaccine against the most dangerous forms of leishmaniasis. The development of a vaccine for both animals and humans is an active area of research. [11]

Life Cycle

The sand fly

Infection of the sand fly begins when the insect obtains blood from an infected mammal. Both male and female sand flies suck blood and it is their sole source of nutrition. As it does so it injects saliva containing numerous well-characterized bioactive components, many of which are peptides or proteins.[12, 13] One such protein, maxadilan (a potent vasodilator), is a 7 kDa peptide believed essential to the taking of a blood meal by the fly.[14] Maxadilan's primary mode of action is to reduce intracellular calcium in the host at the site of the bite wound through a cAMP-dependent mechanism, causing arterial dilation.[15, 16] Blood can then easily be drawn up by the insect. The receptor for maxadilan is the pituitary adenylate cyclase-activating polypeptide, a membrane-bound protein found on many cell types in the body, including smooth muscle cells and macrophages.[15] During feeding, sand flies become maximally filled with blood and cannot regurgitate the excess, due to the inhibition of the emptying reflex by a parasite-specific peptide that interacts with myosin to prevent contraction of stomach muscle.[17] This enhances the chances for the sand fly to become infected and to remain so throughout the period that the parasite needs (i.e., 1-2 weeks) in order to develop into the infectious stage for a mammalian host.

The parasite undergoes a complex series of developmental changes inside the gut tract of the sand fly, and progresses to the flagellated metacyclic stage after about a week following ingestion.[2] The parasite first attaches to the wall of the gut tract by non-specific hydrophobic interactions between the surface of the parasite's flagella and the insect stomach cell membrane.[18] Attachment to other regions of the insect intestinal tract later on during the differentiation to the metacyclic promastigote stage is mediated, in part, by specific insect galectins (e.g., PpGalec), and the parasite cell surface multipurpose molecule, lipophosphoglycan.[19, 20] The release of infectious stage organisms, a necessary final step in their development, is mediated by arabinosyl capping of LPG scGal residues upon differentiation to the metacyclic stage.[21] The leptomonad stage (heretofore unrecognized) locates to the anterior region of the gut and secretes a gel-like substance that blocks the digestive tract of the sand fly, causing the infected insect to regurgitate its complement of infectious metacyclic promastigotes into the host's subcutaneous tissues during feeding.[2]

The mammalian host

The flagellated metacyclic promastigote stage (Fig. 2.2) resides in the anterior midgut and thorax and is injected into the host along with the dipteran's salivary secretions. In addition to aiding the parasite to establish infection in the sand fly, some of those same salivary proteins aid in leishmania's ability to colonize the mammalian host.[22, 23] Following injection of the metacyclic promastigote stage there is a rapid infiltration of neutrophils into the skin.[24] The promastigotes, however, are quickly taken up by several types of tissue resident phagocytic cells.[25] Maxadilan, produced by the parasite, induces negative effects on host immune cell function, including inhibition of the release of TNF-α, upregulation

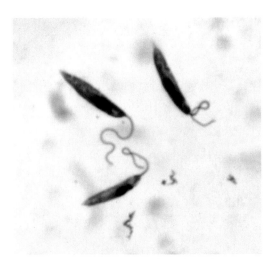

Figure 2.2. Promastigotes of *Leishmania* spp., as seen in culture.

of IL-6 synthesis in macrophages, increase in IL-10 production, and stimulation of prostaglandin E2 production.[26] This all leads to a down regulation of Th1-type cytokines and a shift to a Th2 response.[27]

The promastigotes deposited in the extracellular matrix at the site of the bite adhere there, aided by lipophosphoglycan and a surface membrane laminin receptor protein on their surface.[28] The promastigotes induce the production of antibodies and become opsonized. As a result, the C3 component of complement attaches to the parasite cell surface.[29] The promastigotes are then able to attach to red cells or platelets and become engulfed by dendritic cells or macrophages (Fig. 2.3).[30] Many would-be pathogens are unable to survive this step and are digested by inclusion into phagolysosomal vacuoles. In contrast, leishmania are able to avoid digestion and are free to differentiate into amastigotes to begin the intracellular phase of their life cycle due to their ability to inhibit phagolysosome maturation. The necessary inhibition of phagolysosome biogenesis is inhibited largely by the promastigote surface glycolipid lipophosphoglycan (LPG).[31] The mechanism of leishmania survival inside the macrophage involves alteration of the phagolysosome, and comes about as the result of host cell interaction

with lipophosphoglycan.[32] Infected phagocytes display abnormal maturation of the phagolysosome due to lipophosphoglycan's interference with F-actin, an essential component of the process of fusion of lysosomes with the phagocytic vacuole.[33] This lack of fusion, in part, enables the parasite to evade digestion.

It is at this point in the life cycle that differences between species of leishmania become apparent. Those that cause only cutaneous lesions remain at the site throughout the infection, while those that cause visceral or mucocutaneous lesions manage to find their way to the appropriate site in the body. The host and parasite factors resulting in these different infection strategies are still under investigation. For example, dendritic cells increase in number in the draining lymph nodes of experimentally infected mice infected with *L. (L.) tropica*, but infected dendritic cells do not appear to migrate to the lymph nodes.[34] How the parasites reach the draining lymphoid tissue remains to be demonstrated.

Amastigotes divide inside their host cells (Fig. 2.4) and can remain at the site of injection, resulting in the clinical condition known as cutaneous leishmaniasis. Alternatively, they can be carried by the phagocytes to mucocutaneous junctions, or to the reticuloendothelial tissues, resulting in mucocutaneous or visceral leishmaniasis, respectively.

Leishmania spp. have salvage pathways for nucleic acid synthesis.[33, 35] The enzymes

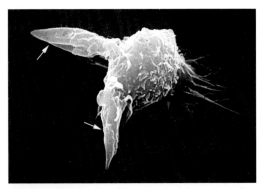

Figure 2.3. Scanning EM of macrophage ingesting two promastigotes (arrows). Courtesy K-P Chang.

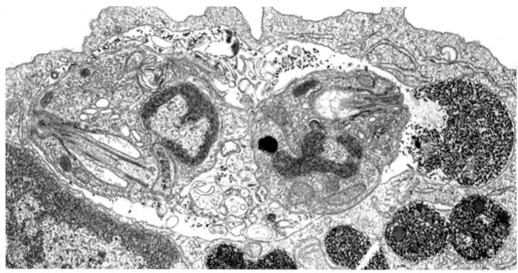

Figure 2.4. Electron micrograph of two amastigotes of *Leishmania* spp. Courtesy K-P Chang.

reside within the glycosome, a specialized organelle unique to the kinetoplastidae.[36] Cutaneous lesions form in most instances, allowing sand flies access to infected host cells at the raised margin. Circulating macrophages in blood-harboring amastigotes can also be taken up by the vector.

Cellular and Molecular Pathogenesis

Virulence factors and pathogenesis

The cell and molecular biology of *Leishmania* spp. and the complexity of its interaction with the host innate and adaptive immune system has been the subject of many extensive reviews which suggest that a better understanding of this interaction may lead to improved therapeutics.[6, 35, 37] Most of what is known regarding the biology of leishmania is derived from murine models and *in vitro* cell culture using various species of leishmania.[38] The following summary of pathogenic mechanisms is derived from both types of experimental approaches. The turning-on of heat shock genes, as well as cassettes of other developmentally regulated genes, occurs as the parasite makes the transition from an environment dependent upon ambient temperature (sand fly) to the homeothermic essential niche inside the mammalian host cell.[39, 40]

The amastigote downregulates IL-12, which delays the onset of cell-mediated protective immune responses.[41, 42] Amastigotes of *L. mexicana* interfere with antigen presentation by macrophages, employing cysteine protease B.[43] The amastigote stage also possesses potent cysteine protease inhibitors,[44] which it presumably uses to modify host cysteine protease activity during intracellular infection.

Replication of amastigotes is dependent upon host cyclophillins, since division is inhibited by cyclosporine A.[45, 46] The membrane of the promastigote contains a zinc protease, leishmanolysin, a 63 kDa glycoprotein whose crystalline structure has been determined.[47, 48] Current evidence favors a role for leishmanolysin in migration of parasites through the intracellular matrix by digestion of collagen type IV after their release from infected cells.[49] Induction of the chemokine MIP-1β by neutrophils harboring amastigotes attracts macrophages to the site of infection. Macrophages then engulf infected neutrophils, thus acquiring the infection.[50]

An exciting advance in understanding of the severity of certain forms of mucocutaneous disease was the discovery of an RNA virus that infects the *Leishmania Viannia* subgenus.[51] It appears that this leishmania *RNA virus-1* (LRV1) is recognized by host toll-like receptors and induces an inflammatory response that leads to a hyper-inflammatory immune response with resultant destructive lesions.[51]

Protective immune mechanism(s)

The mechanism(s) of protective immunity vary with clinical types of leishmania.[52] The cutaneous forms typically induce well-defined Th1 responses, which are T cell-mediated, and play a critical role in controlling and finally eliminating the organism.[53] Permanent immunity to reinfection with cutaneous leishmaniasis causing organisms is the rule, and depends upon inducing high levels of CD4[+] T-cell memory.[54] In addition, Langerhans cells are thought to play a major role in antigen presentation and in the induction of IL-12 and IL-27.[55-57] The main effector mechanism involves CD4[+] T cell-dependent macrophage activation and subsequent killing of amastigotes by nitric oxide.[58] Chemokines are also important for immunity,[59, 60] and include MIP-3β and INF-γ.[60] Antibodies appear to play no role in immunity to cuta-neous leishmaniasis, and probably aid the parasite in gaining entrance into the macrophage.[61]

Protective immune mechanisms induced by infection with visceral leishmaniasis (*L. (L.) donovani and L. (L.) infantum*), include IL-12 and INF-γ. Immunity is suppressed by IL-10 and TGF-β.[53]

To further complicate the clinical spectrum of diseases caused by leishmania, one has to be reminded of the fact that *Leishmania* spp. have been around a long time, and have, within the last 165 million years, begun to diverge evolutionarily due to continental drift. Organisms in the New World must, by necessity, behave somewhat differently from their ancestor species that still continue to infect mammals in the Old World. The same is true for its hosts, including humans. Thus, when considering the type of disease and the immune responses to them, there exist many exceptions to the above summaries. For an excellent review on this aspect of the biology of leishmania, see McMahon-Pratt and Alexander.[62]

References

1. Mauricio, I. L.; Howard, M. K.; Stothard, J. R.; Miles, M. A., Genomic diversity in the Leishmania donovani complex. *Parasitology* **1999**, *119 (Pt 3)*, 237-46.
2. Bates, P. A.; Rogers, M. E., New insights into the developmental biology and transmission mechanisms of Leishmania. *Current molecular medicine* **2004**, *4* (6), 601-9.
3. Bates, P. A., Transmission of Leishmania metacyclic promastigotes by phlebotomine sand flies. *Int J Parasitol* **2007**, *37* (10), 1097-106.
4. Ashford, R. W., The leishmaniases as model zoonoses. *Annals of tropical medicine and parasitology* **1997**, *91* (7), 693-701.
5. Quinnell, R. J.; Courtenay, O., Transmission, reservoir hosts and control of zoonotic visceral leishmaniasis. *Parasitology* **2009**, *136* (14), 1915-34.
6. Kaye, P.; Scott, P., Leishmaniasis: complexity at the host-pathogen interface. *Nat Rev Microbiol* **2011**, *9* (8), 604-15.
7. Marovich, M. A.; Lira, R.; Shepard, M.; Fuchs, G. H.; Kruetzer, R.; Nutman, T. B.; Neva, F. A., Leishmaniasis recidivans recurrence after 43 years: a clinical and immunologic report after successful treatment. *Clin Infect Dis* **2001**, *33* (7), 1076-9.
8. Alvar, J.; Velez, I. D.; Bern, C.; Herrero, M.; Desjeux, P.; Cano, J.; Jannin, J.; den Boer, M.; Team, W. H. O. L. C., Leishmaniasis worldwide and global estimates of its incidence. *PLoS One* **2012**, *7* (5), e35671.
9. Ivens, A. C.; Peacock, C. S.; Worthey, E. A.; Murphy, L.; Aggarwal, G.; Berriman, M.; Sisk, E.; Rajandream, M. A.; Adlem, E.; Aert, R.; Anupama, A.; Apostolou, Z.; Attipoe, P.; Bason, N.; Bauser, C.; Beck, A.; Beverley, S. M.; Bianchettin, G.; Borzym, K.; Bothe, G.; Bruschi, C. V.;

Collins, M.; Cadag, E.; Ciarloni, L.; Clayton, C.; Coulson, R. M.; Cronin, A.; Cruz, A. K.; Davies, R. M.; De Gaudenzi, J.; Dobson, D. E.; Duesterhoeft, A.; Fazelina, G.; Fosker, N.; Frasch, A. C.; Fraser, A.; Fuchs, M.; Gabel, C.; Goble, A.; Goffeau, A.; Harris, D.; Hertz-Fowler, C.; Hilbert, H.; Horn, D.; Huang, Y.; Klages, S.; Knights, A.; Kube, M.; Larke, N.; Litvin, L.; Lord, A.; Louie, T.; Marra, M.; Masuy, D.; Matthews, K.; Michaeli, S.; Mottram, J. C.; Muller-Auer, S.; Munden, H.; Nelson, S.; Norbertczak, H.; Oliver, K.; O'Neil, S.; Pentony, M.; Pohl, T. M.; Price, C.; Purnelle, B.; Quail, M. A.; Rabbinowitsch, E.; Reinhardt, R.; Rieger, M.; Rinta, J.; Robben, J.; Robertson, L.; Ruiz, J. C.; Rutter, S.; Saunders, D.; Schafer, M.; Schein, J.; Schwartz, D. C.; Seeger, K.; Seyler, A.; Sharp, S.; Shin, H.; Sivam, D.; Squares, R.; Squares, S.; Tosato, V.; Vogt, C.; Volckaert, G.; Wambutt, R.; Warren, T.; Wedler, H.; Woodward, J.; Zhou, S.; Zimmermann, W.; Smith, D. F.; Blackwell, J. M.; Stuart, K. D.; Barrell, B.; Myler, P. J., The genome of the kinetoplastid parasite, Leishmania major. *Science* **2005,** *309* (5733), 436-42.

10. Handman, E., Leishmaniasis: current status of vaccine development. *Clinical microbiology reviews* **2001,** *14* (2), 229-43.

11. Kumar, R.; Engwerda, C., Vaccines to prevent leishmaniasis. *Clin Transl Immunology* **2014,** *3* (3), e13.

12. Valenzuela, J. G.; Garfield, M.; Rowton, E. D.; Pham, V. M., Identification of the most abundant secreted proteins from the salivary glands of the sand fly Lutzomyia longipalpis, vector of Leishmania chagasi. *The Journal of experimental biology* **2004,** *207* (Pt 21), 3717-29.

13. Dominguez, M.; Moreno, I.; Aizpurua, C.; Torano, A., Early mechanisms of Leishmania infection in human blood. *Microbes Infect* **2003,** *5* 507-13.

14. Jackson, T. S.; Lerner, E.; Weisbrod, R. M.; Tajima, M.; Loscalzo, J.; Keaney, J. F., Vasodilatory properties of recombinant maxadilan. *The American journal of physiology* **1996,** *271* (3 Pt 2), H924-30.

15. Moro, O.; Lerner, E. A., Maxadilan, the vasodilator from sand flies, is a specific pituitary adenylate cyclase activating peptide type I receptor agonist. *The Journal of biological chemistry* **1997,** *272* (2), 966-70.

16. Uchida, D.; Tatsuno, I.; Tanaka, T.; Hirai, A.; Saito, Y.; Moro, O.; Tajima, M., Maxadilan is a specific agonist and its deleted peptide (M65) is a specific antagonist for PACAP type 1 receptor. *Annals of the New York Academy of Sciences* **1998,** *865*, 253-8.

17. Vaidyanathan, R., Isolation of a myoinhibitory peptide from Leishmania major (Kinetoplastida: Trypanosomatidae) and its function in the vector sand fly Phlebotomus papatasi (Diptera: Psychodidae). *Journal of medical entomology* **2005,** *42* (2), 142-52.

18. Wakid, M. H.; Bates, P. A., Flagellar attachment of Leishmania promastigotes to plastic film in vitro. *Experimental parasitology* **2004,** *106* (3-4), 173-8.

19. Kamhawi, S.; Ramalho-Ortigao, M.; Pham, V. M.; Kumar, S.; Lawyer, P. G.; Turco, S. J.; Barillas-Mury, C.; Sacks, D. L.; Valenzuela, J. G., A role for insect galectins in parasite survival. *Cell* **2004,** *119* (3), 329-41.

20. Beverley, S. M.; Dobson, D. E., Flypaper for parasites. *Cell* **2004,** *119* (3), 311-2.

21. Dobson, D. E.; Mengeling, B. J.; Cilmi, S.; Hickerson, S.; Turco, S. J.; Beverley, S. M., Identification of genes encoding arabinosyltransferases (SCA) mediating developmental modifications of lipophosphoglycan required for sand fly transmission of leishmania major. *The Journal of biological chemistry* **2003,** *278* (31), 28840-8.

22. Ribeiro, J. M., Blood-feeding arthropods: live syringes or invertebrate pharmacologists? *Infectious agents and disease* **1995,** *4* (3), 143-52.

23. Nuttall, P. A.; Paesen, G. C.; Lawrie, C. H.; Wang, H., Vector-host interactions in disease transmission. *Journal of molecular microbiology and biotechnology* **2000,** *2* (4), 381-6.

24. Peters, N. C.; Egen, J. G.; Secundino, N.; Debrabant, A.; Kimblin, N.; Kamhawi, S.; Lawyer, P.; Fay, M. P.; Germain, R. N.; Sacks, D., In vivo imaging reveals an essential role for neutrophils in leishmaniasis transmitted by sand flies. *Science* **2008,** *321* (5891), 970-4.

25. Ng, L. G.; Hsu, A.; Mandell, M. A.; Roediger, B.; Hoeller, C.; Mrass, P.; Iparraguirre, A.; Cavanagh, L. L.; Triccas, J. A.; Beverley, S. M.; Scott, P.; Weninger, W., Migratory dermal dendritic cells act as rapid sensors of protozoan parasites. *PLoS Pathog* **2008,** *4* (11), e1000222.

26. Soares, M. B.; Titus, R. G.; Shoemaker, C. B.; David, J. R.; Bozza, M., The vasoactive peptide maxadilan from sand fly saliva inhibits TNF-alpha and induces IL-6 by mouse macrophages through interaction with the pituitary adenylate cyclase-activating polypeptide (PACAP) receptor. *Journal of immunology (Baltimore, Md. : 1950)* **1998**, *160* (4), 1811-6.

27. Brodie, T. M.; Smith, M. C.; Morris, R. V.; Titus, R. G., Immunomodulatory effects of the Lutzomyia longipalpis salivary gland protein maxadilan on mouse macrophages. *Infect Immun* **2007**, *75* (5), 2359-65.

28. Ghosh, A.; Bandyopadhyay, K.; Kole, L.; Das, P. K., Isolation of a laminin-binding protein from the protozoan parasite Leishmania donovani that may mediate cell adhesion. *The Biochemical journal* **1999**, *337 (Pt 3)*, 551-8.

29. Antoine, J.-C.; Prina, E.; Courret, N.; Lang, T., Leishmania spp.: on the interactions they establish with antigen-presenting cells of their mammalian hosts. *Advances in parasitology* **2004**, *58*, 1-68.

30. Steigerwald, M.; Moll, H., Leishmania major modulates chemokine and chemokine receptor expression by dendritic cells and affects their migratory capacity. *Infection and immunity* **2005**, *73* (4), 2564-7.

31. Moradin, N.; Descoteaux, A., Leishmania promastigotes: building a safe niche within macrophages. *Front Cell Infect Microbiol* **2012**, *2*, 121.

32. Turco, S. J.; Descoteaux, A., The lipophosphoglycan of Leishmania parasites. *Annual review of microbiology* **1992**, *46*, 65-94.

33. Lodge, R.; Descoteaux, A., Modulation of phagolysosome biogenesis by the lipophosphoglycan of Leishmania. *Clinical immunology (Orlando, Fla.)* **2005**, *114* (3), 256-65.

34. Baldwin, T.; Henri, S.; Curtis, J.; O'Keeffe, M.; Vremec, D.; Shortman, K.; Handman, E., Dendritic cell populations in Leishmania major-infected skin and draining lymph nodes. *Infection and immunity* **2004**, *72* (4), 1991-2001.

35. Olivier, M.; Gregory, D. J.; Forget, G., Subversion mechanisms by which Leishmania parasites can escape the host immune response: a signaling point of view. *Clinical microbiology reviews* **2005**, *18* (2), 293-305.

36. Moyersoen, J.; Choe, J.; Fan, E.; Hol, W. G. J.; Michels, P. A. M., Biogenesis of peroxisomes and glycosomes: trypanosomatid glycosome assembly is a promising new drug target. *FEMS microbiology reviews* **2004**, *28* (5), 603-43.

37. Gull, K., The biology of kinetoplastid parasites: insights and challenges from genomics and post-genomics. *International journal for parasitology* **2001**, *31* (5-6), 443-52.

38. Debrabant, A.; Joshi, M. B.; Pimenta, P. F. P.; Dwyer, D. M., Generation of Leishmania donovani axenic amastigotes: their growth and biological characteristics. *International journal for parasitology* **2004**, *34* (2), 205-17.

39. Bente, M.; Harder, S.; Wiesgigl, M.; Heukeshoven, J.; Gelhaus, C.; Krause, E.; Clos, J.; Bruchhaus, I., Developmentally induced changes of the proteome in the protozoan parasite Leishmania donovani. *Proteomics* **2003**, *3* (9), 1811-29.

40. Duncan, R. C.; Salotra, P.; Goyal, N.; Akopyants, N. S.; Beverley, S. M.; Nakhasi, H. L., The application of gene expression microarray technology to kinetoplastid research. *Current molecular medicine* **2004**, *4* (6), 611-21.

41. Sutterwala, F. S.; Mosser, D. M., The taming of IL-12: suppressing the production of proinflammatory cytokines. *Journal of leukocyte biology* **1999**, *65* (5), 543-51.

42. McDowell, M. A.; Sacks, D. L., Inhibition of host cell signal transduction by Leishmania: observations relevant to the selective impairment of IL-12 responses. *Current opinion in microbiology* **1999**, *2* (4), 438-43.

43. Buxbaum, L. U.; Denise, H.; Coombs, G. H.; Alexander, J.; Mottram, J. C.; Scott, P., Cysteine protease B of Leishmania mexicana inhibits host Th1 responses and protective immunity. *Journal of immunology (Baltimore, Md. : 1950)* **2003**, *171* (7), 3711-7.

44. Besteiro, S.; Coombs, G. H.; Mottram, J. C., A potential role for ICP, a Leishmanial inhibitor of cysteine peptidases, in the interaction between host and parasite. *Molecular microbiology* **2004**, *54* (5), 1224-36.

45. Hoerauf, A.; Rascher, C.; Bang, R.; Pahl, A.; Solbach, W.; Brune, K.; Röllinghoff, M.; Bang, H.,

Host-cell cyclophilin is important for the intracellular replication of Leishmania major. *Molecular microbiology* **1997**, *24* (2), 421-9.

46. Meissner, U.; Juttner, S.; Rollinghoff, M.; Gessner, A.; Cyclosporin, A., mediated killing of Leishmania major by macrophages is independent of reactive nitrogen and endogenous TNF-alpha and is not inhibited by IL-10 and 13. *Parasitol Res* **2002**, *89*, 221-7.

47. Chaudhuri, G.; Chaudhuri, M.; Pan, A.; Chang, K. P., Surface acid proteinase (gp63) of Leishmania mexicana. A metalloenzyme capable of protecting liposome-encapsulated proteins from phagolysosomal degradation by macrophages. *The Journal of biological chemistry* **1989**, *264* (13), 7483-9.

48. Schlagenhauf, E.; Etges, R.; Metcalf, P., The crystal structure of the Leishmania major surface proteinase leishmanolysin (gp63). *Structure (London, England : 1993)* **1998**, *6* (8), 1035-46.

49. McGwire, B. S.; Chang, K.-P.; Engman, D. M., Migration through the extracellular matrix by the parasitic protozoan Leishmania is enhanced by surface metalloprotease gp63. *Infection and immunity* **2003**, *71* (2), 1008-10.

50. van Zandbergen, G.; Klinger, M.; Mueller, A.; Dannenberg, S.; Gebert, A.; Solbach, W.; Laskay, T., Cutting edge: neutrophil granulocyte serves as a vector for Leishmania entry into macrophages. *Journal of immunology (Baltimore, Md. : 1950)* **2004**, *173* (11), 6521-5.

51. Ives, A.; Ronet, C.; Prevel, F.; Ruzzante, G.; Fuertes-Marraco, S.; Schutz, F.; Zangger, H.; Revaz-Breton, M.; Lye, L. F.; Hickerson, S. M.; Beverley, S. M.; Acha-Orbea, H.; Launois, P.; Fasel, N.; Masina, S., Leishmania RNA virus controls the severity of mucocutaneous leishmaniasis. *Science* **2011**, *331* (6018), 775-8.

52. Wilson, M. E.; Jeronimo, S. M. B.; Pearson, R. D., Immunopathogenesis of infection with the visceralizing Leishmania species. *Microbial pathogenesis* **2005**, *38* (4), 147-60.

53. Scott, P.; Artis, D.; Uzonna, J.; Zaph, C., The development of effector and memory T cells in cutaneous leishmaniasis: the implications for vaccine development. *Immunological reviews* **2004**, *201*, 318-38.

54. Gabaglia, C. R.; Sercarz, E. E.; Diaz-De-Durana, Y.; Hitt, M.; Graham, F. L.; Gauldie, J.; Braciak, T. A., Life-long systemic protection in mice vaccinated with L. major and adenovirus IL-12 vector requires active infection, macrophages and intact lymph nodes. *Vaccine* **2004**, *23* (2), 247-57.

55. Oliveira, M. A. P.; Tadokoro, C. E.; Lima, G. M. C. A.; Mosca, T.; Vieira, L. Q.; Leenen, P. J. M.; Abrahamsohn, I. A., Macrophages at intermediate stage of maturation produce high levels of IL-12 p40 upon stimulation with Leishmania. *Microbes and infection / Institut Pasteur* **2005**, *7* (2), 213-23.

56. Simin, M.; Shahriar, D., A quantitative study of epidermal Langerhans cells in cutaneous Leishmaniasis caused by Leishmania tropica. *International Journal of Dermatology* **2004**, *43*, 819-823.

57. Hunter, C. A.; Villarino, A.; Artis, D.; Scott, P., The role of IL-27 in the development of T-cell responses during parasitic infections. *Immunological reviews* **2004**, *202*, 106-14.

58. Awasthi, A.; Mathur, R. K.; Saha, B., Immune response to Leishmania infection. *The Indian journal of medical research* **2004**, *119* (6), 238-58.

59. Roychoudhury, K.; Roy, S., Role of chemokines in Leishmania infection. *Current molecular medicine* **2004**, *4* (6), 691-6.

60. Mitra, R.; Dharajiya, N.; Kumari, L.; Varalakshmi, C.; Khar, A., Migration of antigen presenting cells from periphery to the peritoneum during an inflammatory response: role of chemokines and cytokines. *FASEB journal : official publication of the Federation of American Societies for Experimental Biology* **2004**, *18* (14), 1764-6.

61. Miles, S. A.; Conrad, S. M.; Alves, R. G.; Jeronimo, S. M. B.; Mosser, D. M., A role for IgG immune complexes during infection with the intracellular pathogen Leishmania. *The Journal of experimental medicine* **2005**, *201* (5), 747-54.

62. McMahon-Pratt, D.; Alexander, J., Does the Leishmania major paradigm of pathogenesis and protection hold for New World cutaneous leishmaniases or the visceral disease? *Immunological reviews* **2004**, *201*, 206-24.

3. Cutaneous Leishmaniasis

Leishmania (L) major
(Yakimov and Schockov 1915)

Leishmania (L) tropica
(Wright 1903)

Leishmania (L) mexicana
(Biagi 1953)

Introduction

Cutaneous leishmaniasis (CL) is a complicated disease to understand because of the large numbers of different species and clinical variants. Roughly speaking we consider CL divided along the lines of Old World CL, meaning it's found predominantly in the Middle East and North Africa (MENA) region, East Africa, South Asia and Central Asia, and New World CL in the Americas. Each of these species varies with respect to its geographic distribution, clinical manifestations, sand fly intermediate host, and whether or not it is zoonotic, meaning transmission requires a significant animal reservoir such as dogs or rodents (e.g., *Leishmania major*), or is anthroponotic meaning that the disease cycles only or predominantly between humans and sand flies (e.g. *Leishmania tropica*).

Old World CL is caused by four species in the Old World: *Leishmania (Leishmania) aethiopica, L. (L.) major, L. (L.) tropica,* and *L. (L.) infantum*. Their vectors include sand flies of the following species; *Phlebotomous papatasi, P. sergenti, P. longipes, P. argentipes,* and *P. ariasi*. At least 15 species of leishmania in the New World cause similar types of disease: *Leishmania (Leishmania) amazonensis, L. (V.) braziliensis, L. (L.) colombiensis, L. (L.) garnhami, L. (V.) guyanensis, L. (L.) infantum chagasi, L. (V.) lainsoni, L. (L.) lindenbergi, L. (L.) mexicana, L. (V.) naiffi, L. (V.) panamensis, L. (V.) peruviana, L. (L.)* *pifanoi, L. (L.) shawi, L. (L.) venezuelensis.* The principal vector species are *Lutzomyia olmeca olmeca, Lu. flaviscutellata,* and *Lu. trapidoi.* In some locales and in some populations, *L. (L.) tropica* visceralizes, as was seen in soldiers returning from Operation Desert Storm (1990-1991) suggesting that another strain of this species exists with quite different characteristics from the one that only causes cutaneous lesions or more likely that host factors such as genetic backgrounds or immune history may influence the type of disease that manifests.[1,2]

Although accurate statistics regarding incidence rates and prevalence are not available, it is estimated that there are 0.7-1.2 million cases of cutaneous leishmaniasis each year.[3] Rodents are a primary reservoir for human infection caused by *L. (L.) major*, while domestic dogs serve as reservoirs in many parts of the world for other species of leishmania.[4] Within the last five years there has been an explosion of old world CL cases linked to the breakdown in public health infrastructure resulting from the conflicts in Islamic State of Iraq and the Levant (ISIL)-

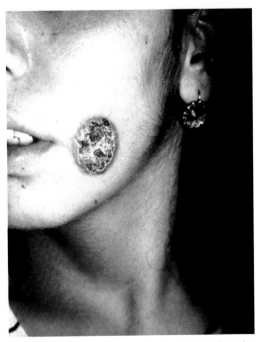

Figure 3.1. Old lesion on face due to *Leishmania major*.

Leishmania tropica

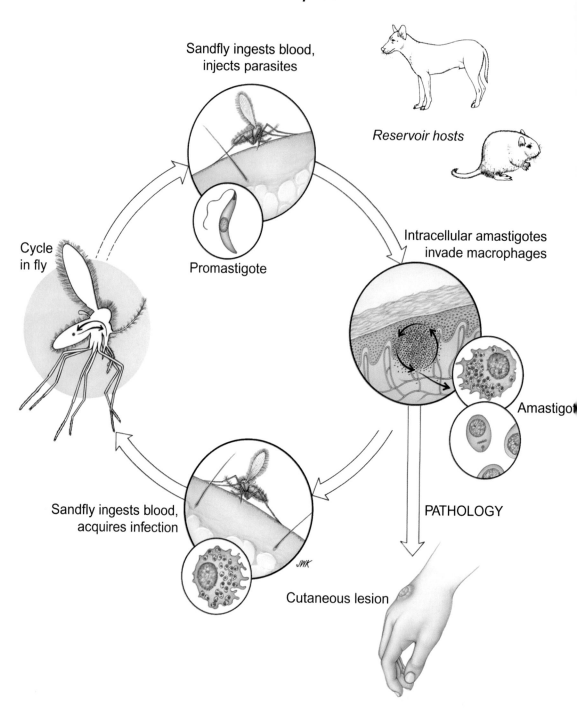

Sandfly ingests blood, injects parasites

Reservoir hosts

Promastigote

Cycle in fly

Intracellular amastigotes invade macrophages

Amastigote

Sandfly ingests blood, acquires infection

PATHOLOGY

Cutaneous lesion

occupied areas of Syria, Iraq, and Libya.[5] Estimates are difficult to come by due to the absence of public health surveillance in these regions, but it is believed that the numbers could be in the hundreds of thousands. New world CL is also linked to conflict and human migrations including cases connected with guerilla movements, narcotrafficking in South America, and a Cuban diaspora through the Darien jungle of Panama.[6, 7]

Historical Information

In 1856, Alexander Russell described the clinical aspects of CL.[8] In 1885, David Cunningham, while working in India, accurately described the leishmania organism he saw in a fixed histological section of a skin lesion.[9] In 1921, Edouard Sergent and Etienne Sergent demonstrated that sand flies were the vectors responsible for transmitting leishmania to humans; one species bears his name. Cosme Bueno, much earlier (1764) suspected the same was true for "uta," a cutaneous lesion, later shown to be caused by infection with leishmania.[10]

"Oriental sore" is common among people living in endemic areas of the Middle East, India, and Africa. A rudimentary kind of immunization referred to as "leishmanization" was practiced in the Middle East, where it was known that infection results in permanent immunity to reinfection.[11] Uninfected individuals were deliberately inoculated in areas other than the face with scrapings containing organisms from the margins of active lesions. This controlled the region of the body on which the scar developed.[12] Unfortunately a significant number of individuals would develop chronic lesions that did not heal as a result of these inoculations, and much effort is being put into alternative approaches.[13]

Life Cycle

Infection begins with the bite of an

infected sand fly. The promastigotes are introduced into the subcutaneous tissue, attach to the extracellular matrix and are then taken up by dendritic cells and macrophages. The promastigotes transform into the amastigote stage and begin to replicate. Infection progresses at the site of the bite only. Eventually, a large, painless craterform ulcer forms as the result of extensive cell death.[14] Sand flies acquire the infection by feeding on blood taken up at the margin of the ulcer. [15]

Clinical Disease

Cutaneous leishmaniasis (CL) is first recognized as a small red papule at the site of the bite wound approximately 2-8 weeks after injection of metacyclic promastigotes. The lesion progresses from a painless nodule, measuring approximately 1 cm in diameter, into a much larger one by the formation of satellite papules (Fig. 3.1). The area around the bite wound eventually ulcerates due to intense destruction of cells, and becomes depressed, then heals through scarring (Fig. 3.2). Organisms are found only in the living tissue at the raised margin, regardless of the age of the lesion (Fig. 3.3). Occasionally, more than one lesion is present (Fig. 3.4).

After the ulcer heals, which may take weeks to months, immunity to reinfection is often permanent, and is also effective against

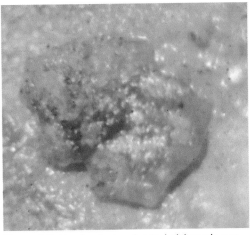

Figure 3.2. Healing lesion due to *Leishmania* spp.

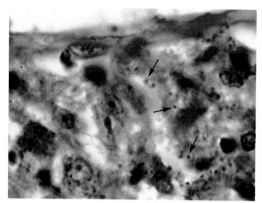

Figure 3.3. Histologic section of skin showing amastigotes (arrows) of *Leishmania* spp. in dendritic cells and macrophages.

other leishmania species that cause only cutaneous lesions.[12] In experimental infections in rodents, exposure to *L. (V.) braziliensis* confers protection against challenge with *L. (L.) major*, suggesting that shared, cross-reacting antigens might be good candidates for a CL vaccine.[16, 17]

Regardless of which species causes the lesion, it may vary in size and shape, sometimes confounding even the most experienced clinician. CL should always be suspected in travelers, or patients from endemic areas when any lesion that fails to heal is encountered.[18] This is particularly true for CL in the western hemisphere.[19] Prolonged infection is the rule in a subset of patients that have an altered pattern of immunity.[20] Chiclero's ulcer, on the pinna of the ear (Fig. 3.5), is a good example of this exception.[21]

Infection due to *L. (L.) aethiopica* is restricted to Ethiopia and Kenya, and causes a wide spectrum of disease, including diffuse cutaneous leishmaniasis (DCL), characterized by involvement of the entire surface of the skin.[22-24] Other species of leishmania (e.g., *L. (V.) braziliensis, L. (L.) amazonensis*) have also been diagnosed in patients suffering from DCL.[25] DCL begins as a single nodule on an exposed part of the skin, then starts to grow and spread, eventually involving vast areas of the skin. Patients can resemble those suffering from various forms of leprosy.[26]

Similarly, *L. (L.) mexicana, L (L.) amazonensis and L. (L.) venezuelensis* occasionally cause anergic disseminated cutaneous leishmaniasis (ADCL), which is similar to DCL.[27] Nodules and large patches of involved skin, in which abundant amastigote-infected cells can be found, are typical and may remain so for many years. Chemotherapy is of little consequence to the outcome, which includes extensive scarring of all involved areas. However, patients may benefit from newer treatment approaches.[28-30]

Leishmania (L.) infantum can cause cutaneous lesions, but is more commonly associated with visceral disease in children throughout the Mediterranean basin. [14]

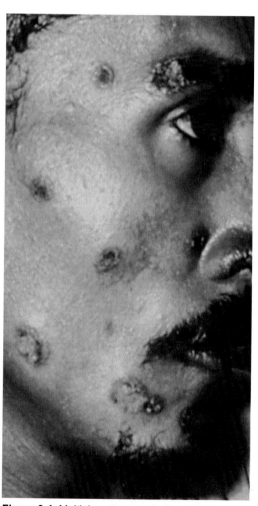

Figure 3.4. Multiple cutaneous lesions due to *Leishmania panamanensis*.

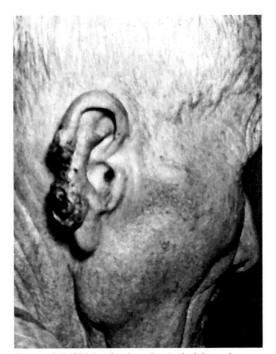

Figure 3.5. Chiclero's ulcer due to *Leishmania* spp.

Patients with HIV/AIDS may present with cutaneous lesions only, or the infection can visceralize.[19] Co-infection with leishmania and HIV are not common in the New World, but this lack of association is not due to the low number of individuals harboring either group of infectious agents.[31]

Diagnosis

The typical lesion seen in cutaneous leishmaniasis is a nodule that enlarges into a painless ulcer with an indurated border. Although most cutaneous lesions caused by leishmania look similar (i.e., craterform with a raised edge), there are many other dermatological conditions that might be mistaken for CL. Diagnosis of all forms of CL due to leishmania is best done with isolation of the organism or PCR. Samples for culture, microscopy or nucleic acid amplification testing (NAAT) should be taken from the margin of an active ulcer that is not obviously superinfected.[32] The edge can be scraped gently with a scalpel to obtain material, an aspiration can be performed, or a full thickness biopsy can be obtained and the ulcer edge and a touch prep can be performed prior to sending specimens off for histology, culture, microscopy, and NAAT.[32] NAAT techniques have high sensitivities and also offer the advantage of species identification.[33-37] Species identification can be critical in determining whether the infecting species has the potential to progress to mucocutaneous disease.[38] Histopathological examination of biopsy tissue has less sensitivity than NAAT techniques and requires recognition of the characteristic amastigote tissue form of the parasite with the nucleus and kinetoplast (the *dot and dash*).[39] Culture of needle aspiration samples, scrapings and biopsy specimens is a viable alternative to PCR, but takes much longer (several days), due to the slow growth of the promastigotes at 20^0 C. Laboratories. with the most experience in parasite culture generally have the highest rates of success.[40-42]

Serology is not routinely used in the diagnosis of cutaneous leishmaniasis, but in some instances, antibody testing has been used in the evaluation of patients from non-endemic areas.[43] The leishmaniasis skin test is used in certain parts of the world and involves injecting killed promastigotes intradermally and is read at 48 to 72 hours, much like the PPD skin test for tuberculosis infection.[44] An IFN-γ release assay (IGRA) is also being developed for leismaniasis.[45]

Treatment

Treatment of cutaneous leishmaniasis is dictated by the severity of the lesion, its location, and the species involved. Uncomplicated infections that do not involve species that are associated with mucosal disease may be treated with local therapy, as many resolve clinically without treatment. It is important to note that the goal of therapy is clinical cure and not complete clearance of parasites, as some parasites will persist even with successful therapy.[46, 47] In the majority of cases spontaneous healing will occur with proper hygiene and wound care.[48, 49] Cryotherapy using liquid nitrogen has been successfully employed.[50-52] Treatment with thermotherapy delivered by radiofrequency, superficial heat at 50^0 C, or application of heated prongs can result in clinical cure but must be used with caution to avoid nerve damage and burns.[53, 54] Topical paromomycin and intra-lesional sodium stibogluconate (pentavalent antimony) are alternative but less studied approaches. Intra-lesional injections of pentavalent antimony are not approved in the United States, and are associated with significant pain.[55-57]

Several systemic therapies are in use for the treatment of cutaneous leishmaniasis including; pentavalent antimonials (sodium stibogluconate or meglumine antimoniate), amphotericin, miltefosine, pentamidine, and azole drugs.[58] Systemic therapy is recommended if the there is concern that the infecting species has the ability to cause mucosal disease based on species identification or acquisition of the infection in what is referred to as the mucosal belt (Brazil, Bolivia, and portions of Peru).[59] Sodium stibogluconate, an antimony-containing drug with many serious side effects, including rash, headache, arthralgias and myalgias, pancreatitis, transaminitis, and hematologic suppression, is the drug of choice in many parts of the world, in part due to its relatively low cost, but increasing rates of resistance has already limited its use.[60] Amphotericin B and its liposomal form are other highly effective options for treatment.[61] In the developed world liposomal amphotericin B is a frequent choice of therapy but its cost is prohibitive in many areas of the world where this disease is endemic. Miltefosine is an effective but expensive option that allows for systemic therapy with oral dosing that is currently FDA approved in the United States for treatment of leishmaniaisis.[29, 62-65] Pentamidine is a little-used therapy owing to concerning side effects and limited data on its efficacy.[66] Azoles such as, ketoconazole, fluconazole, intraconazole, and posaconazole are alternative therapies, but ones that show variable efficacy compared to other options based on the particular species of leishmania parasite involved.[55, 67-73]

Prevention and Control

Since humans are a dead-end host in most cases, treatment of infected humans is not expected to have a significant impact on disease transmission.[74] Although dogs have been identified as a significant reservoir, infection in multiple mammals, both wild and domesticated, is not appreciated.[75] Eradication of sand fly breeding sites near suburban and urban centers, attaching pyrethroid-impregnated collars to domestic dogs, and sleeping under insecticide-impregnated bed netting are cost-effective control measures.[55] Sand flies only bite at certain times of the day in what is termed a crepuscular/nocturnal pattern; in the morning, late in the evening and at night.[76] Although avoidance of outdoor activities during these times reduces the chance of being bitten, this can be difficult advice for travelers to endemic areas, who may have limited time to accomplish what they have on their itinerary and perhaps impossible for long term residents who do not have the luxury to adjust their schedule. Additional and perhaps more viable approaches to avoid sand fly bites that are in use by travelers and workers in high risk areas are the use of insect repellents and insecticide-treated clothing that covers most of the body.[77, 78]

Vaccines, employing combinations of proven protection-inducing parasite proteins, offer hope that a standard vaccine for use against CL and VL forms of leishmaniasis may eventually be available, but no human vaccine is currently available.[17, 79] A recent health economic study confirmed the cost effectiveness of a CL vaccine.[80]

References

1. Berman, J., Recent Developments in Leishmaniasis: Epidemiology, Diagnosis, and Treatment. *Current infectious disease reports* **2005**, *7* (1), 33-38.
2. Magill, A. J.; Grogl, M.; Gasser, R. A., Jr.; Sun, W.; Oster, C. N., Visceral infection caused by Leishmania tropica in veterans of Operation Desert Storm. *N Engl J Med* **1993**, *328* (19), 1383-7.
3. Alvar, J.; Velez, I. D.; Bern, C.; Herrero, M.; Desjeux, P.; Cano, J.; Jannin, J.; den Boer, M.; Team, W. H. O. L. C., Leishmaniasis worldwide and global estimates of its incidence. *PLoS One* **2012**, *7* (5), e35671.
4. Rassi, Y.; Gassemi, M. M.; Javadian, E.; Rafizadeh, S.; Motazedian, H.; Vatandoost, H., Vectors and reservoirs of cutaneous leishmaniasis in Marvdasht district, southern Islamic Republic of Iran. *East Mediterr Health J* **2007**, *13* (3), 686-93.
5. Hotez, P. J., Vaccine Science Diplomacy: Expanding Capacity to Prevent Emerging and Neglected Tropical Diseases Arising from Islamic State (IS)--Held Territories. *PLoS Negl Trop Dis* **2015**, *9* (9), e0003852.
6. Beyrer, C.; Villar, J. C.; Suwanvanichkij, V.; Singh, S.; Baral, S. D.; Mills, E. J., Neglected diseases, civil conflicts, and the right to health. *Lancet* **2007**, *370* (9587), 619-27.
7. Barry, M. A.; Koshelev, M. V.; Sun, G. S.; Grekin, S. J.; Stager, C. E.; Diwan, A. H.; Wasko, C. A.; Murray, K. O.; Woc-Colburn, L., Cutaneous leishmaniasis in Cuban immigrants to Texas who traveled through the Darien Jungle, Panama. *Am J Trop Med Hyg* **2014**, *91* (2), 345-7.
8. Russell, A.; Millar, A., Natural History of Aleppo and Parts Adjacent. 1856; p 262-266.
9. Cunningham, D. D., On the presence of peculiar parasitic organisms in the tissue of a specimen of Delhi boil. *Sci Mem Med Officers Army India* **1885**, *1* 21-31.
10. Theodorides, J., Note historique sur la decouverte de la transmission de la leishmaniose cutanee par les phlebotomes. *Bull Soc Pathol Exot* **1997**, *90*, 177-180.
11. Handman, E., Leishmaniasis: current status of vaccine development. *Clinical microbiology reviews* **2001**, *14* (2), 229-43.
12. McCall, L. I.; Zhang, W. W.; Ranasinghe, S.; Matlashewski, G., Leishmanization revisited: immunization with a naturally attenuated cutaneous Leishmania donovani isolate from Sri Lanka protects against visceral leishmaniasis. *Vaccine* **2013**, *31* (10), 1420-5.
13. Greenblatt, C. L., The present and future of vaccination for cutaneous leishmaniasis. *Prog Clin Biol Res* **1980**, *47*, 259-85.
14. del Giudice, P.; Marty, P.; Lacour, J. P.; Perrin, C.; Pratlong, F.; Haas, H.; Dellamonica, P.; Le Fichoux, Y., Cutaneous leishmaniasis due to Leishmania infantum. Case reports and literature review. *Archives of dermatology* **1998**, *134* (2), 193-8.
15. Bates, P. A., Transmission of Leishmania metacyclic promastigotes by phlebotomine sand flies. *Int J Parasitol* **2007**, *37* (10), 1097-106.
16. Lima, H. C.; DeKrey, G. K.; Titus, R. G., Resolution of an infection with Leishmania braziliensis confers complete protection to a subsequent challenge with Leishmania major in BALB/c mice. *Memorias do Instituto Oswaldo Cruz* **1999**, *94* (1), 71-6.
17. Coler, R. N.; Reed, S. G., Second-generation vaccines against leishmaniasis. *Trends in parasitology* **2005**, *21* (5), 244-9.
18. Mansueto, P.; Seidita, A.; Vitale, G.; Cascio, A., Leishmaniasis in travelers: a literature review. *Travel Med Infect Dis* **2014**, *12* (6 Pt A), 563-81.
19. Lainson, R.; Shaw, J. J.; Collier, L.; Balows, A.; Sussman, M.; Cox, F. E. G.; Despommier, D. D.; Kreier, J. P.; Wakelin, D., New World Leishmaniasis-The Neotropical Leishmania Species. 2005.
20. van Griensven, J.; Carrillo, E.; Lopez-Velez, R.; Lynen, L.; Moreno, J., Leishmaniasis in immunosuppressed individuals. *Clin Microbiol Infect* **2014**, *20* (4), 286-99.
21. Lianson, R.; Strangeways-Dixon, J., Leishmania mexicana: The epidemiology of dermal Leishmaniasis in British Honduras. *Trasn Roy Soc Trop Med Hyg* **1963**, *57*, 242-265.
22. Hailu, A., The use of direct agglutination test (DAT) in serological diagnosis of Ethiopian cutaneous leishmaniasis. *Diagnostic microbiology and infectious disease* **2002**, *42* (4), 251-6.
23. Akuffo, H.; Maasho, K.; Blostedt, M.; Höjeberg, B.; Britton, S.; Bakhiet, M., Leishmania

aethiopica derived from diffuse leishmaniasis patients preferentially induce mRNA for interleukin-10 while those from localized leishmaniasis patients induce interferon-gamma. *The Journal of infectious diseases* **1997,** *175* (3), 737-41.

24. Bryceson, A. D., Diffuse cutaneous leishmaniasis in Ethiopia. I. The clinical and histological features of the disease. *Transactions of the Royal Society of Tropical Medicine and Hygiene* **1969,** *63* (6), 708-37.

25. Turetz, M. L.; Machado, P. R.; Ko, A. I.; Alves, F.; Bittencourt, A.; Almeida, R. P.; Mobashery, N.; Johnson, W. D.; Carvalho, E. M., Disseminated leishmaniasis: a new and emerging form of leishmaniasis observed in northeastern Brazil. *The Journal of infectious diseases* **2002,** *186* (12), 1829-34.

26. Dassoni, F.; Abebe, Z.; Naafs, B.; Morrone, A., Cutaneous and mucocutaneous leishmaniasis resembling borderline-tuberculoid leprosy: a new clinical presentation? *Acta Derm Venereol* **2013,** *93* (1), 74-7.

27. Bonfante-Garrido, R.; Barroeta, S.; de Alejos, M. A.; Meléndez, E.; Torrealba, J.; Valdivia, O.; Momen, H.; Grimaldi Júnior, G., Disseminated American cutaneous leishmaniasis. *International journal of dermatology* **1996,** *35* (8), 561-5.

28. Sharquie, K. E.; Najim, R. A., Disseminated cutaneous leishmaniasis. *Saudi medical journal* **2004,** *25* (7), 951-4.

29. Machado, P. R.; Penna, G., Miltefosine and cutaneous leishmaniasis. *Curr Opin Infect Dis* **2012,** *25* (2), 141-4.

30. Ordaz-Farias, A.; Munoz-Garza, F. Z.; Sevilla-Gonzalez, F. K.; Arana-Guajardo, A.; Ocampo-Candiani, J.; Trevino-Garza, N.; Becker, I.; Camacho-Ortiz, A., Case report: Transient success using prolonged treatment with miltefosine for a patient with diffuse cutaneous leishmaniasis infected with Leishmania mexicana mexicana. *Am J Trop Med Hyg* **2013,** *88* (1), 153-6.

31. Postigo, C.; Llamas, R.; Zarco, C.; Rubio, R.; Pulido, F.; Costa, J. R.; Iglesias, L., Cutaneous lesions in patients with visceral leishmaniasis and HIV infection. *The Journal of infection* **1997,** *35* (3), 265-8.

32. Handler, M. Z.; Patel, P. A.; Kapila, R.; Al-Qubati, Y.; Schwartz, R. A., Cutaneous and mucocutaneous leishmaniasis: Differential diagnosis, diagnosis, histopathology, and management. *J Am Acad Dermatol* **2015,** *73* (6), 911-26.

33. Mimori, T.; Sasaki, J.; Nakata, M.; Gomez, E. A.; Uezato, H.; Nonaka, S.; Hashiguchi, Y.; Furuya, M.; Saya, H., Rapid identification of Leishmania species from formalin-fixed biopsy samples by polymorphism-specific polymerase chain reaction. *Gene* **1998,** *210* (2), 179-86.

34. Gangneux, J.-P.; Menotti, J.; Lorenzo, F.; Sarfati, C.; Blanche, H.; Bui, H.; Pratlong, F.; Garin, Y.-J.-F.; Derouin, F., Prospective value of PCR amplification and sequencing for diagnosis and typing of old world Leishmania infections in an area of nonendemicity. *Journal of clinical microbiology* **2003,** *41* (4), 1419-22.

35. Mouttaki, T.; Morales-Yuste, M.; Merino-Espinosa, G.; Chiheb, S.; Fellah, H.; Martin-Sanchez, J.; Riyad, M., Molecular diagnosis of cutaneous leishmaniasis and identification of the causative Leishmania species in Morocco by using three PCR-based assays. *Parasit Vectors* **2014,** *7,* 420.

36. Nzelu, C. O.; Caceres, A. G.; Guerrero-Quincho, S.; Tineo-Villafuerte, E.; Rodriquez-Delfin, L.; Mimori, T.; Uezato, H.; Katakura, K.; Gomez, E. A.; Guevara, A. G.; Hashiguchi, Y.; Kato, H., A rapid molecular diagnosis of cutaneous leishmaniasis by colorimetric malachite green-loop-mediated isothermal amplification (LAMP) combined with an FTA card as a direct sampling tool. *Acta Trop* **2016,** *153,* 116-9.

37. Yehia, L.; Adib-Houreih, M.; Raslan, W. F.; Kibbi, A. G.; Loya, A.; Firooz, A.; Satti, M.; El-Sabban, M.; Khalifeh, I., Molecular diagnosis of cutaneous leishmaniasis and species identification: analysis of 122 biopsies with varied parasite index. *J Cutan Pathol* **2012,** *39* (3), 347-55.

38. Palumbo, E., Treatment strategies for mucocutaneous leishmaniasis. *J Glob Infect Dis* **2010,** *2* (2), 147-50.

39. Faber, W. R.; Oskam, L.; van Gool, T.; Kroon, N. C. M.; Knegt-Junk, K. J.; Hofwegen, H.; van der Wal, A. C.; Kager, P. A., Value of diagnostic techniques for cutaneous leishmaniasis. *Journal of the American Academy of Dermatology* **2003,** *49* (1), 70-4.

40.   Dey, T.; Afrin, F.; Anam, K.; Ali, N., Infectivity and virulence of Leishmania donovani promastigotes: a role for media, source, and strain of parasite. *The Journal of eukaryotic microbiology* **2002**, *49* (4), 270-4.

41.   Luz, Z. M.; Silva, A. R.; Silva Fde, O.; Caligiorne, R. B.; Oliveira, E.; Rabello, A., Lesion aspirate culture for the diagnosis and isolation of Leishmania spp. from patients with cutaneous leishmaniasis. *Mem Inst Oswaldo Cruz* **2009**, *104* (1), 62-6.

42.   Castelli, G.; Galante, A.; Lo Verde, V.; Migliazzo, A.; Reale, S.; Lupo, T.; Piazza, M.; Vitale, F.; Bruno, F., Evaluation of two modified culture media for Leishmania infantum cultivation versus different culture media. *J Parasitol* **2014**, *100* (2), 228-30.

43.   Szargiki, R.; Castro, E. A.; Luz, E.; Kowalthuk, W.; Machado, A. M.; Thomaz-Soccol, V., Comparison of serological and parasitological methods for cutaneous leishmaniasis diagnosis in the state of Parana, Brazil. *Braz J Infect Dis* **2009**, *13* (1), 47-52.

44.   Skraba, C. M.; de Mello, T. F.; Pedroso, R. B.; Ferreira, E. C.; Demarchi, I. G.; Aristides, S. M.; Lonardoni, M. V.; Silveira, T. G., Evaluation of the reference value for the Montenegro skin test. *Rev Soc Bras Med Trop* **2015**, *48* (4), 437-44.

45.   Turgay, N.; Balcioglu, I. C.; Toz, S. O.; Ozbel, Y.; Jones, S. L., Quantiferon-Leishmania as an epidemiological tool for evaluating the exposure to Leishmania infection. *Am J Trop Med Hyg* **2010**, *83* (4), 822-4.

46.   Bogdan, C.; Gessner, A.; Solbach, W.; Rollinghoff, M., Invasion, control and persistence of Leishmania parasites. *Curr Opin Immunol* **1996**, *8* (4), 517-25.

47.   Mendonca, M. G.; de Brito, M. E.; Rodrigues, E. H.; Bandeira, V.; Jardim, M. L.; Abath, F. G., Persistence of leishmania parasites in scars after clinical cure of American cutaneous leishmaniasis: is there a sterile cure? *J Infect Dis* **2004**, *189* (6), 1018-23.

48.   Willard, R. J.; Jeffcoat, A. M.; Benson, P. M.; Walsh, D. S., Cutaneous leishmaniasis in soldiers from Fort Campbell, Kentucky returning from Operation Iraqi Freedom highlights diagnostic and therapeutic options. *J Am Acad Dermatol* **2005**, *52* (6), 977-87.

49.   Morizot, G.; Kendjo, E.; Mouri, O.; Thellier, M.; Perignon, A.; Foulet, F.; Cordoliani, F.; Bourrat, E.; Laffitte, E.; Alcaraz, I.; Bodak, N.; Ravel, C.; Vray, M.; Grogl, M.; Mazier, D.; Caumes, E.; Lachaud, L.; Buffet, P. A.; Cutaneous Leishmaniasis French Study, G., Travelers with cutaneous leishmaniasis cured without systemic therapy. *Clin Infect Dis* **2013**, *57* (3), 370-80.

50.   al-Majali, O.; Routh, H. B.; Abuloham, O.; Bhowmik, K. R.; Muhsen, M.; Hebeheba, H., A 2-year study of liquid nitrogen therapy in cutaneous leishmaniasis. *Int J Dermatol* **1997**, *36* (6), 460-2.

51.   Dobrev, H. P.; Nocheva, D. G.; Vuchev, D. I.; Grancharova, R. D., Cutaneous Leishmaniasis - Dermoscopic Findings And Cryotherapy. *Folia Med (Plovdiv)* **2015**, *57* (1), 65-8.

52.   Farajzadeh, S.; Esfandiarpour, I.; Haghdoost, A. A.; Mohammadi, S.; Mohebbi, A.; Mohebbi, E.; Mostafavi, M., Comparison between Combination Therapy of Oral Terbinafine and Cryotherapy versus Systemic Meglumine Antimoniate and Cryotherapy in Cutaneous Leishmaniasis: A Randomized Clinical Trial. *Iran J Parasitol* **2015**, *10* (1), 1-8.

53.   Pizinger, K.; Cetkovska, P.; Kacerovska, D.; Kumpova, M., Successful treatment of cutaneous leishmaniasis by photodynamic therapy and cryotherapy. *Eur J Dermatol* **2009**, *19* (2), 172-3.

54.   Sbeghen, M. R.; Voltarelli, E. M.; Campois, T. G.; Kimura, E.; Aristides, S. M.; Hernandes, L.; Caetano, W.; Hioka, N.; Lonardoni, M. V.; Silveira, T. G., Topical and Intradermal Efficacy of Photodynamic Therapy with Methylene Blue and Light-Emitting Diode in the Treatment of Cutaneous Leishmaniasis Caused by Leishmania braziliensis. *J Lasers Med Sci* **2015**, *6* (3), 106-11.

55.   Shazad, B.; Abbaszadeh, B.; Khamesipour, A., Comparison of topical paromomycin sulfate (twice/day) with intralesional meglumine antimoniate for the treatment of cutaneous leishmaniasis caused by L. major. *European journal of dermatology : EJD* **2005**, *15* (2), 85-7.

56.   Soto, J.; Rojas, E.; Guzman, M.; Verduguez, A.; Nena, W.; Maldonado, M.; Cruz, M.; Gracia, L.; Villarroel, D.; Alavi, I.; Toledo, J.; Berman, J., Intralesional antimony for single lesions of bolivian cutaneous leishmaniasis. *Clin Infect Dis* **2013**, *56* (9), 1255-60.

57.   Shin, J. Y.; Lee, Y. B.; Cho, B. K.; Park, H. J., New world cutaneous leishmaniasis treated with intralesional injection of pentavalent antimony. *Ann Dermatol* **2013**, *25* (1), 80-3.

58.   Singh, N.; Kumar, M.; Singh, R. K., Leishmaniasis: current status of available drugs and new

potential drug targets. *Asian Pac J Trop Med* **2012,** *5* (6), 485-97.

59. Hodiamont, C. J.; Kager, P. A.; Bart, A.; de Vries, H. J.; van Thiel, P. P.; Leenstra, T.; de Vries, P. J.; van Vugt, M.; Grobusch, M. P.; van Gool, T., Species-directed therapy for leishmaniasis in returning travellers: a comprehensive guide. *PLoS Negl Trop Dis* **2014,** *8* (5), e2832.

60. Aronson, N. E.; Wortmann, G. W.; Johnson, S. C.; Jackson, J. E.; Gasser, R. A.; Magill, A. J.; Endy, T. P.; Coyne, P. E.; Grogl, M.; Benson, P. M.; Beard, J. S.; Tally, J. D.; Gambel, J. M.; Kreutzer, R. D.; Oster, C. N., Safety and efficacy of intravenous sodium stibogluconate in the treatment of leishmaniasis: recent U.S. military experience. *Clinical infectious diseases : an official publication of the Infectious Diseases Society of America* **1998,** *27* (6), 1457-64.

61. Sundar, S.; Chakravarty, J., Liposomal amphotericin B and leishmaniasis: dose and response. *J Glob Infect Dis* **2010,** *2* (2), 159-66.

62. Madke, B.; Kharkar, V.; Chikhalkar, S.; Mahajan, S.; Khopkar, U., Successful treatment of multifocal cutaneous leishmaniasis with miltefosine. *Indian J Dermatol* **2011,** *56* (5), 587-90.

63. Rubiano, L. C.; Miranda, M. C.; Muvdi Arenas, S.; Montero, L. M.; Rodriguez-Barraquer, I.; Garcerant, D.; Prager, M.; Osorio, L.; Rojas, M. X.; Perez, M.; Nicholls, R. S.; Gore Saravia, N., Noninferiority of miltefosine versus meglumine antimoniate for cutaneous leishmaniasis in children. *The Journal of infectious diseases* **2012,** *205* (4), 684-92.

64. Monge-Maillo, B.; Lopez-Velez, R., Miltefosine for visceral and cutaneous leishmaniasis: drug characteristics and evidence-based treatment recommendations. *Clinical infectious diseases : an official publication of the Infectious Diseases Society of America* **2015,** *60* (9), 1398-404.

65. Dorlo, T. P.; van Thiel, P. P.; Schoone, G. J.; Stienstra, Y.; van Vugt, M.; Beijnen, J. H.; de Vries, P. J., Dynamics of parasite clearance in cutaneous leishmaniasis patients treated with miltefosine. *PLoS neglected tropical diseases* **2011,** *5* (12), e1436.

66. Jaureguiberry, S.; Graby, G.; Caumes, E., Efficacy of short-course intramuscular pentamidine isethionate treatment on Old World localized cutaneous leishmaniasis in 2 patients. *Clin Infect Dis* **2006,** *42* (12), 1812-3.

67. Laffitte, E.; Genton, B.; Panizzon, R. G., Cutaneous leishmaniasis caused by Leishmania tropica: treatment with oral fluconazole. *Dermatology (Basel, Switzerland)* **2005,** *210* (3), 249-51.

68. Morizot, G.; Delgiudice, P.; Caumes, E.; Laffitte, E.; Marty, P.; Dupuy, A.; Sarfati, C.; Hadj-Rabia, S.; Darie, H.; AS, L. E. G.; Salah, A. B.; Pratlong, F.; Dedet, J. P.; Grogl, M.; Buffet, P. A., Healing of Old World cutaneous leishmaniasis in travelers treated with fluconazole: drug effect or spontaneous evolution? *The American journal of tropical medicine and hygiene* **2007,** *76* (1), 48-52.

69. Saenz, R. E.; Paz, H.; Berman, J. D., Efficacy of ketoconazole against Leishmania braziliensis panamensis cutaneous leishmaniasis. *The American journal of medicine* **1990,** *89* (2), 147-55.

70. Firooz, A.; Khatami, A.; Dowlati, Y., Itraconazole in the treatment of cutaneous leishmaniasis. *International journal of dermatology* **2006,** *45* (12), 1446-7.

71. Baroni, A.; Aiello, F. S.; Vozza, A.; Vozza, G.; Faccenda, F.; Brasiello, M.; Ruocco, E., Cutaneous leishmaniasis treated with itraconazole. *Dermatol Ther* **2009,** *22 Suppl 1*, S27-9.

72. Saleem, K.; Rahman, A., Comparison of oral itraconazole and intramuscular meglumine antimoniate in the treatment of cutaneous leishmaniasis. *J Coll Physicians Surg Pak* **2007,** *17* (12), 713-6.

73. Paniz Mondolfi, A. E.; Stavropoulos, C.; Gelanew, T.; Loucas, E.; Perez Alvarez, A. M.; Benaim, G.; Polsky, B.; Schoenian, G.; Sordillo, E. M., Successful treatment of Old World cutaneous leishmaniasis caused by Leishmania infantum with posaconazole. *Antimicrob Agents Chemother* **2011,** *55* (4), 1774-6.

74. Maroli, M.; Khoury, C., [Prevention and control of leishmaniasis vectors: current approaches]. *Parassitologia* **2004,** *46* (1-2), 211-5.

75. Quinnell, R. J.; Courtenay, O., Transmission, reservoir hosts and control of zoonotic visceral leishmaniasis. *Parasitology* **2009,** *136* (14), 1915-34.

76. Rivas, G. B.; de Souza, N. A.; Peixoto, A. A.; Bruno, R. V., Effects of temperature and photoperiod on daily activity rhythms of Lutzomyia longipalpis (Diptera: Psychodidae). *Parasites & vectors* **2014,** *7*, 278.

77.   Banks, S. D.; Murray, N.; Wilder-Smith, A.; Logan, J. G., Insecticide-treated clothes for the control of vector-borne diseases: a review on effectiveness and safety. *Med Vet Entomol* **2014,** *28 Suppl 1,* 14-25.

78.   Moore, S. J.; Mordue Luntz, A. J.; Logan, J. G., Insect bite prevention. *Infect Dis Clin North Am* **2012,** *26* (3), 655-73.

79.   Kumar, R.; Engwerda, C., Vaccines to prevent leishmaniasis. *Clin Transl Immunology* **2014,** *3* (3), e13.

80.   Bacon, K. M.; Hotez, P. J.; Kruchten, S. D.; Kamhawi, S.; Bottazzi, M. E.; Valenzuela, J. G.; Lee, B. Y., The potential economic value of a cutaneous leishmaniasis vaccine in seven endemic countries in the Americas. *Vaccine* **2013,** *31* (3), 480-6.

4. Mucocutaneous Leishmaniasis

Leishmania (V) braziliensis
(Vianna 1911)

Introduction

There are currently approximately twenty species of leishmania that are capable of causing mucocutaneous disease (MCL; also known as espundia), with the majority of subspecies classified in the L. Vianna subgenus.[1] *L. (V.) braziliensis* is mainly responsible for MCL, perhaps due to its ability to trigger a T cell hypersensitivity response.[2] Mucocutaneous disease has been observed to develop in 2-10% of patients initially infected with these subspecies, but the risk appears to depend on a patient's gender, age, and nutritional status.[3] Usually following primary infection, but at times coincident with cutaneous disease, the parasites metastasize to mucocutaneous junctions (oral cavity, urogenital, and anal areas), where they erode the soft tissues.[4] This is often a disfiguring condition as it can affect the face and lead to extensive destruction.[5, 6] Since MCL is in general restricted to the New World, sand flies of the genus *Lutzomyia* are considered to be the vector.[7] MCL is mainly concentrated in Ecuador, Bolivia, and North-

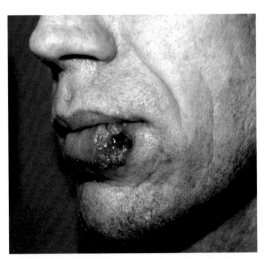

Figure 4.1. Cutaneous lesion on lower lip due to *Leishmania braziliensis*.

ern Brazil.[8] A number of the clinical cases of MCL involve leishmania parasites that are infected with a double-stranded RNA virus (leishmaniavirus), which appears to correlate with disease severity.[9-11]

Historical Information

In 1911, Antonio Carini identified patients suffering from mucocutaneous lesions as being different from those only demonstrating cutaneous lesions, thereby establishing MCL as a separate clinical entity.[12] In the following year, Gaspar Vianna identified and named *L. (V.) braziliensis* as the causative agent.[13] Israel Kligler, in 1916, and Hadeyo Noguchi, in 1929, using serological and culture methods, succeeded in characterizing this parasite as a distinct species, despite the lack of modern laboratory equipment.[14, 15]

Life Cycle

This disease starts the same as cutaneous leishmaniasis with an infected sand fly taking a blood meal. Metacyclic promastigotes are injected into the subcutaneous tissue and adhere to the extracellular matrix. A primary lesion forms at the bite site as the result of infection in dendritic cells and macrophages (Fig. 2.3). The lesion evolves into an ulcer (Fig. 4.1), which is indistinguishable from that induced by any number of other species causing cutaneous leishmaniasis. Amastigotes are transported to the mucocutaneous junction early on during infection, although lesions at this site are slow to appear, even if the patient goes on to develop MCL.[4] At these distant mucocutaneous sites, the amastigotes divide within resident macrophages and tissue erosion begins to develop. It is likely that this destruction is attributable more to an exuberant host response driven by an exaggerated T cell response than any factors intrinsic to the parasite.[2] Perhaps the presence of an RNA virus infecting the responsible leishma-

Leishmania braziliensis

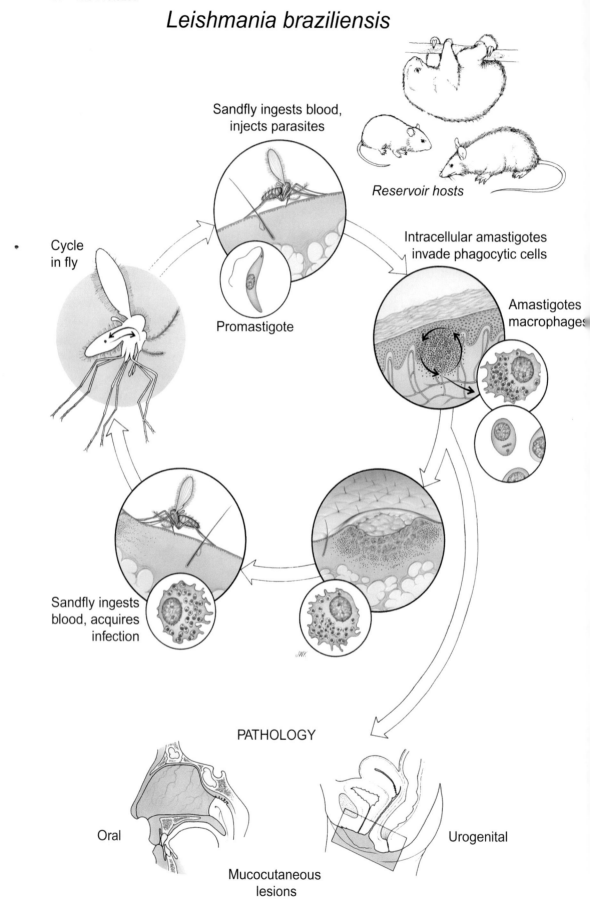

Sandfly ingests blood, injects parasites

Reservoir hosts

Cycle in fly

Promastigote

Intracellular amastigotes invade phagocytic cells

Amastigotes macrophages

Sandfly ingests blood, acquires infection

PATHOLOGY

Oral

Mucocutaneous lesions

Urogenital

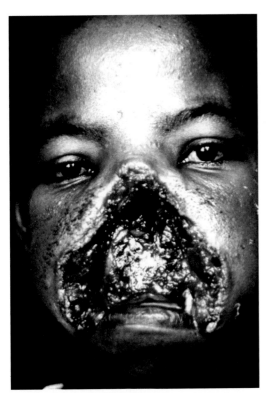

Figure 4.2. Espundia. This lesion resulted in the erosion of the soft palette. Most lesions do not advance this far before medical intervention.

nia parasites plays a role in augmenting this immune response and driving this hypersensitivity response.[11] Infections typically "smolder" for long periods of time, usually months to years.

Person-to-person transmission probably does not occur. Rather, reservoir hosts (domestic dogs, rodents, and various rainforest mammals) serve as the source of infection.[16]

Clinical Disease

MCL lesions developing in the nasal passage (the most common mucocutaneous site) are characterized by a necrotizing inflammation of mixed cell types (plasma cells, lymphocytes).[5] Skin, mucous membranes, and cartilage can also be involved.[17] Lesions of the oral cavity eventually result in the destruction of the soft palate and nasal septum, as well as invasion of the larynx.[18] When this

occurs, the patient may die from infection that spreads to the lungs.[4] MCL is a pauciparasitic disease, and parasites are seldom demonstrated in lesions, although they can be revealed by PCR.[19] The ulcers are replaced by fibrous granulomas that heal slowly, scar, and deform the tissues. The most advanced cases are known as "espundia" (Fig. 4.2).[20] Unlike cutaneous leishmaniasis, MCL does not usually heal spontaneously.[8, 17]

Multiple cutaneous lesions, as well as extensive mucocutaneous involvement have been described in patients co-infected with HIV-1.[21-23] Due to enormous genetic variation among strains of *Leishmania* spp. causing MCL, the patterns of disease in rarely occurring MCL infections in HIV-1 patients presents as an exceedingly complex and difficult clinical picture.[24, 25]

Diagnosis

Definitive diagnosis is by PCR.[26] Organisms are difficult to find in biopsy of infected palate and soft tissues of the oral cavity, so microscopy of histological sections is not an option for diagnosis. Culture of biopsy material is a possibility (see diagnosis for CL), but growth of promastigotes at room temperature is slow.

Treatment

As a general rule systemic therapies are used for the treatment of mucocutaneous leishmaniais including; pentavalent antimony, amphotericin B, miltefosine, pentamidine, or azole drugs.[8, 27] Sodium stibogluconate, an antimony-containing drug with many serious side effects, including rash, headache, arthralgias and myalgias, pancreatitis, transaminitis, and hematologic suppression, is the drug of choice in many parts of the world, in part due to its relatively low cost.[28] Amphotericin B and its liposomal form are highly effective options for treatment and many now consider the liposomal form the drug of choice for mucocutaneous as well as visceral leishmaniasis. In the developing world, standard amphotericin is often employed for the treatment of mucocutaneous leishmaniasis if antimonial therapy fails. Miltefosine is an effective but expensive option that allows for systemic therapy with oral dosing that is currently FDA approved in the United States for treatment of leishmaniaisis.[29-33] Pentamidine is another option that has demonstrated efficacy for the treatment of MCL.[34, 35] Azoles such as, ketoconazole, fluconazole, intraconazole, and posaconazole are alternative oral therapies with variable efficacy compared to other options based on the particular species of leishmania parasite involved.[36-43]

None of the above therapies is 100% effective at eliminating all parasites in all patients. Persistence of infection beyond the treatment period has been recorded in longstanding infections, as judged by PCR on experimentally infected monkeys and in follow up of some patients.[44]

Prevention and Control

Transmission of *L. (V.) braziliensis* and related species capable of causing MCL occurs through close contact of human populations with reservoir hosts (wild and domestic mammals). Deforestation of vast regions of rainforest for agriculture, mining, oil exploration, all of which leads to increased urbanization in South and Central America, has allowed large numbers of people access to the edges of the rainforest. Edges of natural systems are special ecologically defined areas termed ecotones.[34, 45] These zones constitute the borders between ecosystems, and are further characterized by ecological stress on all plant and animal species in that zone due to intra and inter-specific competition for resources. Distribution of sand fly species is determined by the availability of natural habitat and of that created by human encroachment. Some species favor unaltered forest, while others thrive in ecologically disturbed situations.[34] It is unfortunately beyond the scope of this text to illustrate this concept with specific examples, but many could be given that would serve to reinforce the idea that when ecological change due to human settlement occurs, those living there are at greater risk from acquiring zoonotic infectious diseases (e.g., Yellow Fever virus, Ebola virus, Marburg virus, Lassa fever virus).[45] The number of new species of leishmania now known to infect humans throughout South America alone has increased dramatically [4]

Avoidance of contact with vectors of MCL is too naive a recommendation to actually work, given the lack of awareness of their presence on the part of those living in close proximity to them. For those traveling to endemic areas wishing to avoid the bites of sand flies altogether, the following advice may be helpful. Sand flies only bite at certain times of the day in what is termed a crepuscular/nocturnal pattern; in the morning, late in the evening and at night.[7] Although avoidance of outdoor activities during these times reduces the chance of being bitten this can be difficult advice for travelers to endemic areas, who may have limited time to accomplish what they have on their itinerary and perhaps impossible for long term residents who do not have the luxury to adjust their schedule. Additional and perhaps more viable approaches to avoid sand fly bites that are in use by travelers and workers in high risk areas are the use of insect repellents and insecticide-treated clothing that covers most of the body.[46, 47] Growing rates of insecticide resistance in sand fly populations are already limiting the utility of this approach in many parts of the world. Some species of sand fly bite only during the rainy season.[48]

The use of insecticide-impregnated clothing and bed netting has helped reduce disease transmission for malaria, particularly in Africa, and has now been proven effective in the reduction in transmission of leishmania, as well. Maintaining wide buffer zones between settlements and the surrounding native forest appears to be the best environmentally based long-term solution to controlling the incidence of infection in endemic transmission zones, a recommendation originally made to those wishing to avoid becoming infected with the Yellow Fever virus. Curtailing this human imperative has, so far, been all but impossible to enforce.

Vaccines, using protection-inducing parasite proteins, offer hope that a vaccine for use against CL and VL forms of leishmaniasis may eventually be available, but no human vaccine is currently available, despite continued efforts.[49, 50]

References

1. Herwaldt, B. L., Leishmaniasis. *Lancet* **1999**, *354* (9185), 1191-9.
2. Silveira, F. T.; Lainson, R.; De Castro Gomes, C. M.; Laurenti, M. D.; Corbett, C. E., Immunopathogenic competences of Leishmania (V.) braziliensis and L. (L.) amazonensis in American cutaneous leishmaniasis. *Parasite Immunol* **2009**, *31* (8), 423-31.
3. Machado-Coelho, G. L.; Caiaffa, W. T.; Genaro, O.; Magalhaes, P. A.; Mayrink, W., Risk factors for mucosal manifestation of American cutaneous leishmaniasis. *Trans R Soc Trop Med Hyg* **2005**, *99* (1), 55-61.
4. Lainson, R.; Shaw, J. J.; Collier, L.; Balows, A.; Sussman, M.; Cox, F. E. G.; Despommier, D. D.; Kreier, J. P.; Wakelin, D., New World Leishmaniasis-The Neotropical Leishmania Species. 2005.
5. Crovetto-Martinez, R.; Aguirre-Urizar, J. M.; Orte-Aldea, C.; Araluce-Iturbe, I.; Whyte-Orozco, J.; Crovetto-De la Torre, M. A., Mucocutaneous leishmaniasis must be included in the differential diagnosis of midline destructive disease: two case reports. *Oral Surg Oral Med Oral Pathol Oral Radiol* **2015**, *119* (1), e20-6.
6. Garcia, A. L.; Kindt, A.; Quispe-Tintaya, K. W.; Bermudez, H.; Llanos, A.; Arevalo, J.; Bañuls, A. L.; De Doncker, S.; Le Ray, D.; Dujardin, J. C., American tegumentary leishmaniasis: antigen-gene polymorphism, taxonomy and clinical pleomorphism. *Infection, genetics and evolution : journal of molecular epidemiology and evolutionary genetics in infectious diseases* **2005**, *5* (2), 109-16.
7. Rivas, G. B.; de Souza, N. A.; Peixoto, A. A.; Bruno, R. V., Effects of temperature and photoperiod on daily activity rhythms of Lutzomyia longipalpis (Diptera: Psychodidae). *Parasites & vectors* **2014**, *7*, 278.
8. Palumbo, E., Treatment strategies for mucocutaneous leishmaniasis. *J Glob Infect Dis* **2010**, *2* (2), 147-50.
9. Chung, I. K.; Armstrong, T. C.; Scheffter, S. M.; Lee, J. H.; Kim, Y. M.; Patterson, J. L., Generation of the short RNA transcript in Leishmaniavirus correlates with the growth of its parasite host, Leishmania. *Molecules and cells* **1998**, *8* (1), 54-61.
10. Ogg, M. M.; Carrion, R.; Botelho, A. C. d. C.; Mayrink, W.; Correa-Oliveira, R.; Patterson, J. L., Short report: quantification of leishmaniavirus RNA in clinical samples and its possible role in pathogenesis. *The American journal of tropical medicine and hygiene* **2003**, *69* (3), 309-13.
11. Ives, A.; Ronet, C.; Prevel, F.; Ruzzante, G.; Fuertes-Marraco, S.; Schutz, F.; Zangger, H.; Revaz-Breton, M.; Lye, L. F.; Hickerson, S. M.; Beverley, S. M.; Acha-Orbea, H.; Launois, P.; Fasel, N.; Masina, S., Leishmania RNA virus controls the severity of mucocutaneous leishmaniasis. *Science* **2011**, *331* (6018), 775-8.
12. Carini, A., Leishmaniose de Ia muqucuse rhinobuccopharyngee. *Bull Soc Pathol Exot* **1911**, *4* 289-291.
13. Vianna, G., Tratamento da leishmaniose tegumentar por injecoes intravenososas de tartaro emetico. *Ann Congress Brasil Med Cirur* **1912**, *4* 426-428.
14. Kligler, I. J., Some Regulating Factors in Bacterial Metabolism. *Journal of bacteriology* **1916**, *1* (6), 663-71.

15.   Noguchi, H.; S., Comparative studies on herpetomonads and Leishmaniasis. *II Differentiation of the organisms by serological reactions and fermentation tests Med* **1929**, *44*, 305-314.

16.   Alexander, B.; Lozano, C.; Barker, D. C.; McCann, S. H.; Adler, G. H., Detection of Leishmania (Viannia) braziliensis complex in wild mammals from Colombian coffee plantations by PCR and DNA hybridization. *Acta tropica* **1998**, *69* (1), 41-50.

17.   Ahluwalia, S.; Lawn, S. D.; Kanagalingam, J.; Grant, H.; Lockwood, D. N., Mucocutaneous leishmaniasis: an imported infection among travellers to central and South America. *Bmj* **2004**, *329* (7470), 842-4.

18.   Lohuis, P. J.; Lipovsky, M. M.; Hoepelman, A. I.; Hordijk, G. J.; Huizing, E. H., Leishmania braziliensis presenting as a granulomatous lesion of the nasal septum mucosa. *The Journal of laryngology and otology* **1997**, *111* (10), 973-5.

19.   Belli, A.; Rodriguez, B.; Aviles, H.; Harris, E., Simplified polymerase chain reaction detection of new world Leishmania in clinical specimens of cutaneous leishmaniasis. *The American journal of tropical medicine and hygiene* **1998**, *58* (1), 102-9.

20.   Marsden, P. D., Mucosal leishmaniasis ("espundia" Escomel, 1911). *Transactions of the Royal Society of Tropical Medicine and Hygiene* **1986**, *80* (6), 859-76.

21.   Machado, E. S.; Braga, M. d. P.; Da Cruz, A. M.; Coutinho, S. G.; Vieira, A. R.; Rutowitsch, M. S.; Cuzzi-Maya, T.; Grimaldi júnior, G.; Menezes, J. A., Disseminated American muco-cutaneous leishmaniasis caused by Leishmania braziliensis braziliensis in a patient with AIDS: a case report. *Memorias do Instituto Oswaldo Cruz* **1992**, *87* (4), 487-92.

22.   Mattos, M.; Caiza, A.; Fernandes, O.; Gonçalves, A. J.; Pirmez, C.; Souza, C. S.; Oliveira-Neto, M. P., American cutaneous leishmaniasis associated with HIV infection: report of four cases. *Journal of the European Academy of Dermatology and Venereology : JEADV* **1998**, *10* (3), 218-25.

23.   Torrico, F.; Parrado, R.; Castro, R.; Marquez, C. J.; Torrico, M. C.; Solano, M.; Reithinger, R.; Garcia, A. L., Co-Infection of Leishmania (Viannia) braziliensis and HIV: report of a case of mucosal leishmaniasis in Cochabamba, Bolivia. *The American journal of tropical medicine and hygiene* **2009**, *81* (4), 555-8.

24.   Da-Cruz, A. M.; Filgueiras, D. V.; Coutinho, Z.; Mayrink, W.; Grimaldi, G.; De Luca, P. M.; Mendonca, S. C.; Coutinho, S. G., Atypical mucocutaneous leishmaniasis caused by Leishmania braziliensis in an acquired immunodeficiency syndrome patient: T-cell responses and remission of lesions associated with antigen immunotherapy. *Memorias do Instituto Oswaldo Cruz* **1999**, *94* (4), 537-42.

25.   Chouicha, N.; Lanotte, G., Phylogenetic taxonomy of Leishmania (Viannia) braziliensis based on isoenzymatic study of 137 isolates. *Parasitology* **1998**, *115*, 343-8.

26.   Olivier, M.; Gregory, D. J.; Forget, G., Subversion mechanisms by which Leishmania parasites can escape the host immune response: a signaling point of view. *Clinical microbiology reviews* **2005**, *18* (2), 293-305.

27.   Singh, N.; Kumar, M.; Singh, R. K., Leishmaniasis: current status of available drugs and new potential drug targets. *Asian Pac J Trop Med* **2012**, *5* (6), 485-97.

28.   Aronson, N. E.; Wortmann, G. W.; Johnson, S. C.; Jackson, J. E.; Gasser, R. A.; Magill, A. J.; Endy, T. P.; Coyne, P. E.; Grogl, M.; Benson, P. M.; Beard, J. S.; Tally, J. D.; Gambel, J. M.; Kreutzer, R. D.; Oster, C. N., Safety and efficacy of intravenous sodium stibogluconate in the treatment of leishmaniasis: recent U.S. military experience. *Clinical infectious diseases : an official publication of the Infectious Diseases Society of America* **1998**, *27* (6), 1457-64.

29.   Madke, B.; Kharkar, V.; Chikhalkar, S.; Mahajan, S.; Khopkar, U., Successful treatment of multifocal cutaneous leishmaniasis with miltefosine. *Indian J Dermatol* **2011**, *56* (5), 587-90.

30.   Rubiano, L. C.; Miranda, M. C.; Muvdi Arenas, S.; Montero, L. M.; Rodriguez-Barraquer, I.; Garcerant, D.; Prager, M.; Osorio, L.; Rojas, M. X.; Perez, M.; Nicholls, R. S.; Gore Saravia, N., Noninferiority of miltefosine versus meglumine antimoniate for cutaneous leishmaniasis in children. *The Journal of infectious diseases* **2012**, *205* (4), 684-92.

31.   Monge-Maillo, B.; Lopez-Velez, R., Miltefosine for visceral and cutaneous leishmaniasis: drug characteristics and evidence-based treatment recommendations. *Clinical infectious diseases : an official publication of the Infectious Diseases Society of America* **2015**, *60* (9), 1398-404.

32.   Machado, P. R.; Penna, G., Miltefosine and cutaneous leishmaniasis. *Curr Opin Infect Dis* **2012**,

25 (2), 141-4.

33. Dorlo, T. P.; van Thiel, P. P.; Schoone, G. J.; Stienstra, Y.; van Vugt, M.; Beijnen, J. H.; de Vries, P. J., Dynamics of parasite clearance in cutaneous leishmaniasis patients treated with miltefosine. *PLoS neglected tropical diseases* **2011,** *5* (12), e1436.

34. Salomon, O. D.; Rossi, G. C.; Spinelli, G. R., Ecological aspects of phebotomine (Diptera, Psychodidae) in an endemic area of tegumentary leishmaniasis in the northeastern Argentina, 1993-1998. *Memorias do Instituto Oswaldo Cruz* **2002,** *97* (2), 163-8.

35. Jaureguiberry, S.; Graby, G.; Caumes, E., Efficacy of short-course intramuscular pentamidine isethionate treatment on Old World localized cutaneous leishmaniasis in 2 patients. *Clin Infect Dis* **2006,** *42* (12), 1812-3.

36. Laffitte, E.; Genton, B.; Panizzon, R. G., Cutaneous leishmaniasis caused by Leishmania tropica: treatment with oral fluconazole. *Dermatology (Basel, Switzerland)* **2005,** *210* (3), 249-51.

37. Shazad, B.; Abbaszadeh, B.; Khamesipour, A., Comparison of topical paromomycin sulfate (twice/day) with intralesional meglumine antimoniate for the treatment of cutaneous leishmaniasis caused by L. major. *European journal of dermatology : EJD* **2005,** *15* (2), 85-7.

38. Morizot, G.; Delgiudice, P.; Caumes, E.; Laffitte, E.; Marty, P.; Dupuy, A.; Sarfati, C.; Hadj-Rabia, S.; Darie, H.; AS, L. E. G.; Salah, A. B.; Pratlong, F.; Dedet, J. P.; Grogl, M.; Buffet, P. A., Healing of Old World cutaneous leishmaniasis in travelers treated with fluconazole: drug effect or spontaneous evolution? *The American journal of tropical medicine and hygiene* **2007,** *76* (1), 48-52.

39. Saenz, R. E.; Paz, H.; Berman, J. D., Efficacy of ketoconazole against Leishmania braziliensis panamensis cutaneous leishmaniasis. *The American journal of medicine* **1990,** *89* (2), 147-55.

40. Firooz, A.; Khatami, A.; Dowlati, Y., Itraconazole in the treatment of cutaneous leishmaniasis. *International journal of dermatology* **2006,** *45* (12), 1446-7.

41. Baroni, A.; Aiello, F. S.; Vozza, A.; Vozza, G.; Faccenda, F.; Brasiello, M.; Ruocco, E., Cutaneous leishmaniasis treated with itraconazole. *Dermatol Ther* **2009,** *22 Suppl 1,* S27-9.

42. Saleem, K.; Rahman, A., Comparison of oral itraconazole and intramuscular meglumine antimoniate in the treatment of cutaneous leishmaniasis. *J Coll Physicians Surg Pak* **2007,** *17* (12), 713-6.

43. Paniz Mondolfi, A. E.; Stavropoulos, C.; Gelanew, T.; Loucas, E.; Perez Alvarez, A. M.; Benaim, G.; Polsky, B.; Schoenian, G.; Sordillo, E. M., Successful treatment of Old World cutaneous leishmaniasis caused by Leishmania infantum with posaconazole. *Antimicrob Agents Chemother* **2011,** *55* (4), 1774-6.

44. Osman, O. F.; Oskam, L.; Zijlstra, E. E.; el-Hassan, A. M.; el-Naeim, D. A.; Kager, P. A., Use of the polymerase chain reaction to assess the success of visceral leishmaniasis treatment. *Transactions of the Royal Society of Tropical Medicine and Hygiene* **1998,** *92* (4), 397-400.

45. Despommier, D.; Ellis, B. R.; Wilcox, B. A., The role of ecotones in emerging infectious diseases. *Ecohealth* **2006.**

46. Banks, S. D.; Murray, N.; Wilder-Smith, A.; Logan, J. G., Insecticide-treated clothes for the control of vector-borne diseases: a review on effectiveness and safety. *Med Vet Entomol* **2014,** *28 Suppl 1,* 14-25.

47. Moore, S. J.; Mordue Luntz, A. J.; Logan, J. G., Insect bite prevention. *Infect Dis Clin North Am* **2012,** *26* (3), 655-73.

48. Souza, N. A.; Andrade-Coelho, C. A.; Vilela, M. L.; Peixoto, A. A.; Rangel, E. F., Seasonality of Lutzomyia intermedia and Lutzomyia whitmani (Diptera: Psychodidae: Phlebotominae), occurring sympatrically in area of cutaneous leishmaniasis in the State of Rio de Janeiro, Brazil. *Memorias do Instituto Oswaldo Cruz* **2002,** *97* (6), 759-65.

49. Coler, R. N.; Reed, S. G., Second-generation vaccines against leishmaniasis. *Trends in parasitology* **2005,** *21* (5), 244-9.

50. Kumar, R.; Engwerda, C., Vaccines to prevent leishmaniasis. *Clin Transl Immunology* **2014,** *3* (3), e13.

5. Visceral Leishmaniasis

Leishmania (L) donovani
(Ross 1903)

Leishmania (L) infantum
(Cunha and Chagas 1937)

Introduction

Compared to the many species of leishmania that cause cutaneous disease, visceral leishmaniasis is primarily caused by only two species within the *Leishmania donovani* complex; *Leishmania donovani* and *Leishmania infantum*.[1] Previously a third species of leishmania, *Leishmania chagasi* was identified but this organism is considered to be the same species as *Leishmania infantum*.[2, 3] In Europe, Africa, and Asia, both species, *Leishmania donovani* and *Leishmania infantum,* are found in fairly well-defined geographical distributions, while most New World visceral leishmaniasis (VL) is caused by *Leishmania infantum*.[4] In this invasive form of leishmaniasis, leishmania promastigotes infect macrophages, transform into amastigotes and infect multiple cells in which they multiply causing a series of often-fatal diseases collectively referred to as visceral leishmaniasis (VL). A few other species such as *Leishmania tropica, Leishmania amazonensis, and Leishmania mexicana* can also rarely visceralize.[5-9] The illness is characterized by hepatosplenomegaly and high fever. VL is especially prevalent in children.[10, 11] It is currently estimated that each year there are 400,000 new cases and 40,000 deaths due to visceral leishmaniasis.[4, 12] The majority of disease occurs in a concentrated area in Northern India, Nepal, and Bangladesh.[13] As with all other species of leishmania, the vectors of VL are numerous species of sand flies. Humans are the primary source of *L. (L.) donovani* infection, although domestic dogs are sometimes infected as well. In Northern India, Nepal, and Bangladesh the cycle is almost entirely anthroponotic, while in other areas such as East Africa there are significant roles for a wide variety of reservoir hosts, including the domestic dog and numerous rodent species.

With regard to the presence of VL in the New World, one hypothesis favors *L. infantum* as being introduced into the New World at least several million years ago, since it is found in a fox species native to the remote inner Amazon River basin and causes no disease in that host.[14] This latter point is taken as evidence for its adaptation to that fox host species at reduced virulence. Another view favors its introduction by the Spanish some 500 years ago during the time of the their colonization.[15, 16] In either case, it is found in peridomestic habitats, infecting domestic dogs and humans. In addition, it occurs in a broad range of natural environments, where it infects a wide variety of wild mammals in dense forest areas, providing ample biological opportunities for eventual radiation into numerous new varieties and perhaps even new species. *L. donovani* does not appear to

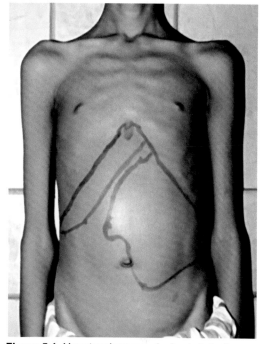

Figure 5.1. Hepatosplenomegaly due to infection with *Leishmania donovani*.

Leishmania donovani

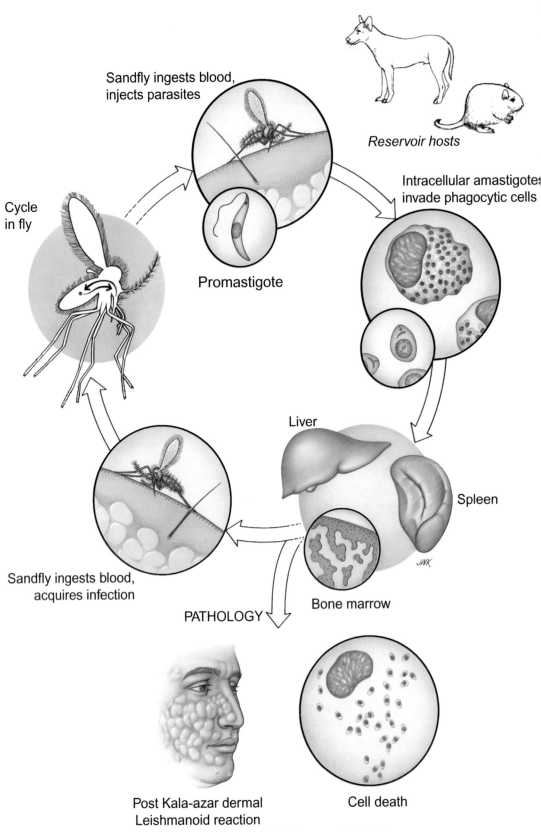

Sandfly ingests blood, injects parasites

Reservoir hosts

Cycle in fly

Promastigote

Intracellular amastigotes invade phagocytic cells

Liver

Spleen

Bone marrow

Sandfly ingests blood, acquires infection

PATHOLOGY

Post Kala-azar dermal Leishmanoid reaction

Cell death

be closely related to any western hemisphere species of leishmania, despite the fact that its mini circle DNA shows strong homology with New World species.[17]

Historical Information

Leishmania donovani was described in 1903 by two physicians, William Leishman and Charles Donovan, while they were working in separate locations in India.[18, 19] Leishman was an officer in the British Army, and Donovan served as a physician in the Indian Medical Service. Ronald Ross, then the editor of the British Medical Journal, reviewed their separate manuscript submissions, recognized that they had observed the same disease, and named the genus and species after them in recognition of their landmark discovery. In 1908, Charles Nicolle discovered that other mammals, particularly the dog, could also become infected.[20] C. S. Swaminath and colleagues, working in India in 1942, using human volunteers, showed that the infection was transmitted by sand flies of the genus *Phlebotomus*.[21]

A single case, of what was most probably American visceral leishmaniasis (AVL), was described by Lewis.E. Migone in a patient in Paraguay in 1913. A.M. Cunha and Carlos Chagas classified it and named it *Leishmania chagasi* in 1937.[22]

Life Cycle

Infection begins with the bite of an infected sand fly (Fig. 2.1). The promastigotes enter the subcutaneous tissues, attach to the extracellular matrix, and are eventually taken up by dendritic cells and macrophages (Fig. 2.3).[23] The parasites transform into amastigotes and divide, eventually killing the host cell. The released amastigotes circulate or are carried by infected cells to new areas of the body, where macrophages again become infected. The ability of some

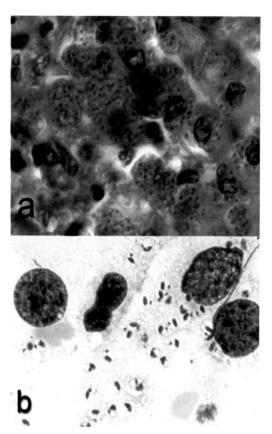

Figure 5.2a. Biopsy of liver positive for amastigotes of *L. donovani.*

Figure 5.2b. Bone marrow aspirate positive for amastigotes of *L. donovani.*

Leishmania spp. to visceralize, in contrast to those species restricted to the skin, may relate to the VL type's survival at higher body temperatures.[24] In some mouse models, dendritic cells increase in lymphoid tissue and eventually become heavily infected, but do appear to be involved in transporting the organisms away from the site of the bite.[23]

The entire reticuloendothelial system eventually becomes involved, compromising the ability of the host to mount an effective immune attack against other invading microbes. The spleen, liver, and bone marrow are the most seriously affected organs (Fig. 5.1). Amastigotes have been observed in peripheral blood in greater densities at night than during daylight hours, a biological phenomenon similar to that found in periodic filariasis.[25] Since sand flies bite more frequently at night, this diurnal rhythm makes the acquisition of parasites by the vector more likely.

The cycle is completed when an infected human is bitten by an uninfected sand fly, which ingests macrophages containing the amastigotes. The duration of the cycle within the fly is approximately 10 days. Rarely, *L. donovani* has been transmitted by organ transplantation.[26]

Immunity is dependent upon Th1 responses and loss of or decreased Th1 response to leishmania may be critical to development of VL.[27] T cells producing INF-γ, TNF-α, and IL-2 activate macrophages that kill intracellular parasites by nitric oxide synthesis.[28] Despite high levels of IgG and IgE being generated during infection, there is no evidence that these are functional or playing any significant role in protection.[29]

Clinical Disease

Kala-azar (Old World VL)

Although not directly translatable from modern standardized Hindi, the term "Kala-azar" appears to have derived originally from the Hindustani (Assamese) word 'kala' referring to black and 'azar' referring to fever or sickness.[30] Kala-azar is roughly translated as "black fever", because of the appearance of the febrile patient's skin at the height of the infection. Most cases of Kala-azar have an incubation period of 3-6 months.[30] A large number of patients who are infected remain asymptomatic with variable frequency that may be due to parasite virulence, host genetics, nutritional status, and age of infected host.[31-34] When disease does manifest, the onset can be gradual or sudden.[30] In the former, the initial symptoms can be nonspecific, often relating to splenomegaly, which may eventually occupy most of the left side of the abdomen. The clinical diagnosis is often missed, or is discovered by accident when patients present with other acute illnesses, such as a respiratory or gastrointestinal infection.[35]

Onset of disease is accompanied by high fever, which may be irregular, often giving rise to a characteristic double daily spike. Fever is intermittent, subsiding for days or weeks only to return, and resembles the pattern seen in patients suffering from undulant fever.

The infected individual, though weak, does not necessarily feel ill, and is able to endure bouts of fever without complaint, distinguishing them from individuals with typhoid fever, tuberculosis, or malaria. Diagnosing the disease can require a high index of suspicion as many presentations are similar to the other febrile diseases common in the areas where VL is endemic.[36] Generalized lymphadenopathy, and later, hepatomegaly eventually develop. In different areas where VL is seen, the classic darkening of the skin associated with this disease is seen at variable frequencies.[37]

VL is progressive and the individual eventually suffers the consequences of a compromised immune system. Many people die with Kala-azar rather than from it because of the acquisition of intercurrent infections. HIV-1 infection is notable in accelerating the overall immune dysfunction when co-infection is present.[38]

As VL progresses patients may develop anemia, low platelet levels (thrombocytopenia), hepatosplenomegaly, and a drop in Hgb.[36] High concentrations of serum protein, approaching 10 g/dl, is due almost exclusively to a rise in non-protective IgG resulting from a polyclonal activation of B cells.[29,39] Patients infected with HIV/AIDS and VL due to *L. (L.) donovani* and *L. (L.) infantum* sometimes present with cutaneous lesions in which organisms can be demonstrated, in addition to involvement of the reticuloendothelial system.[40,41]

Congenital Kala-azar

Infants born to mothers with Kala-azar

can acquire the infection in utero.[42] Organisms are brought to the developing fetus by infected macrophages. The pathology and clinical presentation of congenital visceral leishmaniasis in newborns is similar to the adult form.[43]

Post-Kala-azar Dermal Leishmaniasis

A number of treated patients develop a skin rash six months to several years after the initial presentation of VL.[12] This condition, known as post-Kala-azar dermal leishmaniasis (PKDL), is characterized by a hypopigmented or erythematous macular rash that eventually becomes papular and nodular.[44] The rash and associated lesions are particularly prominent on the face and the upper parts of the body, resembling lesions of lepromatous leprosy. The lesions are filled with histocytes containing amastigotes and serve as sources of infection for sand flies. There may be neurological damage.[45] Among African patients, only 2% of those who recover develop such skin lesions. Involvement of the eye is also common.[46] PKDL is strongly associated with an IL-10-driven (Th2) cytokine pattern.[47-49] Individuals with PKDL are a significant concern in areas where anthroponotic transmission is significant, as these individuals are felt to be highly efficient spreaders of disease.[12]

Atypical cutaneous leishmaniasis has also been described for infections caused by *L. infantum*; it may either be a form of PKDL following a subclinical infection, or a form of Kala-azar that presents with solely cutaneous manifestations.[50]

Diagnosis

Definitive diagnosis of VL depends upon isolation of the organism or using nucleic acid amplification tests (NAAT).[51-53] PKDL can also be diagnosed by NAAT.[54] Specimens for testing can be obtained from either bone marrow or splenic aspiration. The higher risk procedure of splenic aspiration is used less often, since similar results can be achieved with large volume bone marrow aspirations and NAAT testing, Samples of bone marrow or splenic aspiration can be sent for culture, microscopic evaluation, and NAAT.[55-58] Culture of bone marrow aspirates is effective at revealing the organisms, but it is takes three to four days for the parasites to grow to significant numbers. Parasites can also be seen on microscopy of sectioned or biopsied material (Figs. 5.2a, 5.2b). Additional tests, such as serum antibody, urine antigen, and the leishmanin test (LST), are no longer routinely used. In their place, the highly sensitive and highly specific rK39 antigen ELISA is now widely available and used in many settings.[59, 60] A simple point of care lateral flow rK39 assay is now often utilized in many endemic areas.[61]

Treatment

The treatment of choice for VL is systemic therapy. Liposomal amphotericin B is currently the drug of choice for VL in India due to its safety profile, high efficacy, and the development of resistance to other therapies.[62] The liposomal form of amphotericin is better tolerated, has a better safety profile, improved bioavailability compared to amphotericin, and is taken up by the phagocytic cells that are infected by the leishmania amastigotes.[63]

Sodium stibogluconate is preferred for use in East Africa for Kala-azar patients, but resistance limits its use as an alternative in India and must be monitored elsewhere.[64, 65] Continued use of antimonials currently depends on regional resistance rates (high in India), and access to alternative therapies.[62] Miltefosine is an oral agent available as a secondary choice for systemic treatment of VL, and further studies will help define its role in treatment of childhood VL.[66, 67] Miltefosine may be an important part of short course combination treatment with liposomal amphotericin B, but more studies are needed.[68] Pentamidine and sitamaquine (another oral agent) are alternatives that may end up having a role in therapy of VL.[62] Response to any therapy is generally assessed clinically with resolution of fever, reduced splenic size, and weight gain.

Prevention and Control

Infection due to *L. donovani* and *L. infantum* differ from one another regarding the source or reservoir of infection. Transmission of *L. donovani*, is largely anthroponotic while mammals such as the domestic dog are a major source of infection for *L. infantum*. A Cochrane review evaluated the evidence as weak for the effectiveness of sand flies or reservoir control emphasizing the neglected nature of these diseases. India has had limited success in controlling visceral leishmaniasis despite progress against other neglected diseases, such as Yaws which has been eliminated.[69, 70] Political unrest, forced migration due to wars (primarily in Africa and Afghanistan), and prolonged periods of drought (primarily in India) have triggered recent large epidemics of Kala-azar.[5, 71] These situations concentrate people into areas that favor high transmission rates. The unavailability of insecticides, insect repellents, and bed netting, as well as the general lack of proper attention to health care needs during

times of high stress, often allow vector-borne diseases to "have their way" with refugees, and *Leishmania spp.* are no exception.

Attempts to control *L. infantum* transmission by controlling its spread in domestic dogs throughout the Mediterranean basin have met with a singular lack of success, as is also the case throughout South and Central America. Leishmaniasis in domestic and wild dogs has been recently described in the United States, due to *L. infantum*.[72] No human cases have been reported from this area of the world yet, but the proper vector species of sand flies are present, and perhaps it is just a matter of time before a human outbreak occurs.

Research to develop a human leishmania vaccine are longstanding yet confounded by host status, multiple species and our lack of understanding of what constitutes immune protection.[73] A canine vaccine exists and given recent advances in novel adjuvant development together with improved antigen preparations, this may provide hope for progress toward a human vaccine.[74] Remote sensing efforts have identified rainfall and altitude as the two most important environmental variables in predicting outbreaks of VL in certain parts of the world.[75] It is hoped that future studies using this powerful new technology will result in even greater application of satellite data to the control of leishmaniasis in other parts of the world as well.

References

1. Chappuis, F.; Sundar, S.; Hailu, A.; Ghalib, H.; Rijal, S.; Peeling, R. W.; Alvar, J.; Boelaert, M., Visceral leishmaniasis: what are the needs for diagnosis, treatment and control? *Nat Rev Microbiol* **2007,** *5* (11), 873-82.
2. Dantas-Torres, F., Leishmania infantum versus Leishmania chagasi: do not forget the law of priority. *Mem Inst Oswaldo Cruz* **2006,** *101* (1), 117-8; discussion 118.
3. Dantas-Torres, F., Final comments on an interesting taxonomic dilemma: Leishmania infantum versus Leishmania infantum chagasi. *Mem Inst Oswaldo Cruz* **2006,** *101* (8), 929-30.
4. Ready, P. D., Epidemiology of visceral leishmaniasis. *Clin Epidemiol* **2014,** *6,* 147-54.
5. Berman, J., Recent Developments in Leishmaniasis: Epidemiology, Diagnosis, and Treatment. *Current infectious disease reports* **2005,** *7* (1), 33-38.

6.   Pastor-Santiago, J. A.; Chavez-Lopez, S.; Guzman-Bracho, C.; Flisser, A.; Olivo-Diaz, A., American visceral leishmaniasis in Chiapas, Mexico. *The American journal of tropical medicine and hygiene* **2012**, *86* (1), 108-14.

7.   Monroy-Ostria, A.; Hernandez-Montes, O.; Barker, D. C., Aetiology of visceral leishmaniasis in Mexico. *Acta tropica* **2000**, *75* (2), 155-61.

8.   Magill, A. J.; Grogl, M.; Gasser, R. A., Jr.; Sun, W.; Oster, C. N., Visceral infection caused by Leishmania tropica in veterans of Operation Desert Storm. *N Engl J Med* **1993**, *328* (19), 1383-7.

9.   Magill, A. J.; Grögl, M.; Gasser, R. A.; Sun, W.; Oster, C. N., Visceral infection caused by Leishmania tropica in veterans of Operation Desert Storm. *The New England journal of medicine* **1993**, *328* (19), 1383-7.

10. Maltezou, H. C.; Siafas, C.; Mavrikou, M.; Spyridis, P.; Stavrinadis, C.; Karpathios, T.; Kafetzis, D. A., Visceral leishmaniasis during childhood in southern Greece. *Clinical infectious diseases : an official publication of the Infectious Diseases Society of America* **2000**, *31* (5), 1139-43.

11. Haidar, N. A.; Diab, A. B.; El-Sheik, A. M., Visceral Leishmaniasis in children in the Yemen. *Saudi medical journal* **2001**, *22* (6), 516-9.

12. Desjeux, P.; Ghosh, R. S.; Dhalaria, P.; Strub-Wourgaft, N.; Zijlstra, E. E., Report of the Post Kala-azar Dermal Leishmaniasis (PKDL) Consortium Meeting, New Delhi, India, 27-29 June 2012. *Parasit Vectors* **2013**, *6*, 196.

13. Alvar, J.; Velez, I. D.; Bern, C.; Herrero, M.; Desjeux, P.; Cano, J.; Jannin, J.; den Boer, M.; Team, W. H. O. L. C., Leishmaniasis worldwide and global estimates of its incidence. *PLoS One* **2012**, *7* (5), e35671.

14. Lainson, R.; Shaw, J. J.; Collier, L.; Balows, A.; Sussman, M.; Cox, F. E. G.; Despommier, D. D.; Kreier, J. P.; Wakelin, D., New World Leishmaniasis-The Neotropical Leishmania Species. 2005.

15. Mauricio, I. L.; Howard, M. K.; Stothard, J. R.; Miles, M. A., Genomic diversity in the Leishmania donovani complex. *Parasitology* **1999**, *119 (Pt 3)*, 237-46.

16. I., J. M. A. M.; Mauricio, I. L., The strange case of Leishmania chagasi. *Parasitol Today* **2000**, *16*, 188-189.

17. Singh, N.; Curran, M. D.; Middleton, D.; Rastogi, A. K., Characterization of kinetoplast DNA minicircles of an Indian isolate of Leishmania donovani. *Acta tropica* **1999**, *73* (3), 313-9.

18. Leishman, W. B., On the possibility of occurrence of trypanosomiasis in India. *BMJ* **1903**, *1*, 1252-1254.

19. Donovan, C., On the possibility of occurrence of trypanosomiasis in India. *BMJ 79* **1903**, *2*

20. Nicolle, C., Nouvelles acquisitions sur kala-azar: cultures: inoculation au chien: etiologie. . *Hebdom Sci* **1908**, *146*, 498-499.

21. Swaminath, C. S.; Shortt, H. E.; Anderson, L. A. P.; J., Transmission of Indian kala-azar to man by the bites of Phlebotomus argentipes. *Ann Brun Indian Res* **1942**, *30*, 473-477.

22. Cunha, A. M.; Chagas, E., Nova especie de protozoario do genero Leishmania pathogenico para o homen. *Leishmania chagasi n spp Nota PreviaHospital Rio de Janerio* **1937**, *11* 3-9.

23. Baldwin, T.; Henri, S.; Curtis, J.; O'Keeffe, M.; Vremec, D.; Shortman, K.; Handman, E., Dendritic cell populations in Leishmania major-infected skin and draining lymph nodes. *Infection and immunity* **2004**, *72* (4), 1991-2001.

24. Callahan, H. L.; Portal, I. F.; Bensinger, S. J.; Grogl, M., Leishmania spp: temperature sensitivity of promastigotes in vitro as a model for tropism in vivo. *Experimental parasitology* **1996**, *84* (3), 400-9.

25. Saran, R.; Sharma, M. C.; Gupta, A. K.; Sinha, S. P.; Kar, S. K., Diurnal periodicity of Leishmania amastigotes in peripheral blood of Indian Kala-azar patients. *Acta tropica* **1997**, *68* (3), 357-60.

26. Hernandez-Perez, J.; Yebra-Bango, M., Visceral Leishmaniasis (kala-azar) in solid organ transplantation: report of five cases and review. *Clin Infect Dis* **1999**, *29*, 918-21.

27. Bern, C.; Amann, J.; Haque, R.; Chowdhury, R.; Ali, M.; Kurkjian, K. M.; Vaz, L.; Wagatsuma, Y.; Breiman, R. F.; Secor, W. E.; Maguire, J. H., Loss of leishmanin skin test antigen sensitivity and potency in a longitudinal study of visceral leishmaniasis in Bangladesh. *Am J Trop Med Hyg* **2006**, *75* (4), 744-8.

28. Arora, S. K.; Pal, N. S.; Mujtaba, S., Leishmania donovani: identification of novel vaccine

candidates using human reactive sera and cell lines. *Experimental parasitology* **2005,** *109* (3), 163-70.

29.   Ravindran, R.; Anam, K.; Bairagi, B. C.; Saha, B.; Pramanik, N.; Guha, S. K.; Goswami, R. P.; Banerjee, D.; Ali, N., Characterization of immunoglobulin G and its subclass response to Indian kala-azar infection before and after chemotherapy. *Infection and immunity* **2004,** *72* (2), 863-70.

30.   Herwaldt, B. L., Leishmaniasis. *Lancet (London, England)* **1999,** *354* (9185), 1191-9.

31.   Singh, O. P.; Hasker, E.; Sacks, D.; Boelaert, M.; Sundar, S., Asymptomatic Leishmania infection: a new challenge for Leishmania control. *Clin Infect Dis* **2014,** *58* (10), 1424-9.

32.   Das, S.; Matlashewski, G.; Bhunia, G. S.; Kesari, S.; Das, P., Asymptomatic Leishmania infections in northern India: a threat for the elimination programme? *Trans R Soc Trop Med Hyg* **2014,** *108* (11), 679-84.

33.   Clemente, W. T.; Rabello, A.; Faria, L. C.; Peruhype-Magalhaes, V.; Gomes, L. I.; da Silva, T. A.; Nunes, R. V.; Iodith, J. B.; Protil, K. Z.; Fernandes, H. R.; Cortes, J. R.; Lima, S. S.; Lima, A. S.; Romanelli, R. M., High prevalence of asymptomatic Leishmania spp. infection among liver transplant recipients and donors from an endemic area of Brazil. *Am J Transplant* **2014,** *14* (1), 96-101.

34.   Picado, A.; Ostyn, B.; Singh, S. P.; Uranw, S.; Hasker, E.; Rijal, S.; Sundar, S.; Boelaert, M.; Chappuis, F., Risk factors for visceral leishmaniasis and asymptomatic Leishmania donovani infection in India and Nepal. *PLoS One* **2014,** *9* (1), e87641.

35.   Badaro, R.; Jones, T. C.; Carvalho, E. M.; Sampaio, D.; Reed, S. G.; Barral, A.; Teixeira, R.; Johnson, W. D., New perspectives on a subclinical form of visceral leishmaniasis. *The Journal of infectious diseases* **1986,** *154* (6), 1003-11.

36.   Tanoli, Z. M.; Rai, M. E.; Gandapur, A. S., Clinical presentation and management of visceral leishmaniasis. *J Ayub Med Coll Abbottabad* **2005,** *17* (4), 51-3.

37.   Seaman, J.; Mercer, A. J.; Sondorp, H. E.; Herwaldt, B. L., Epidemic visceral leishmaniasis in southern Sudan: treatment of severely debilitated patients under wartime conditions and with limited resources. *Ann Intern Med* **1996,** *124* (7), 664-72.

38.   Ritmeijer, K.; Veeken, H.; Melaku, Y.; Leal, G.; Amsalu, R.; Seaman, J.; Davidson, R. N., Ethiopian visceral leishmaniasis: generic and proprietary sodium stibogluconate are equivalent; HIV co-infected patients have a poor outcome. *Transactions of the Royal Society of Tropical Medicine and Hygiene* **2001,** *95* (6), 668-72.

39.   Galvao-Castro, B.; Sa Ferreira, J. A.; Marzochi, K. F.; Marzochi, M. C.; Coutinho, S. G.; Lambert, P. H., Polyclonal B cell activation, circulating immune complexes and autoimmunity in human american visceral leishmaniasis. *Clin Exp Immunol* **1984,** *56* (1), 58-66.

40.   Alvar, J.; Cañavate, C.; Gutiérrez-Solar, B.; Jiménez, M.; Laguna, F.; López-Vélez, R.; Molina, R.; Moreno, J., Leishmania and human immunodeficiency virus coinfection: the first 10 years. *Clinical microbiology reviews* **1997,** *10* (2), 298-319.

41.   Agostoni, C.; Dorigoni, N.; Malfitano, A.; Caggese, L.; Marchetti, G.; Corona, S.; Gatti, S.; Scaglia, M., Mediterranean leishmaniasis in HIV-infected patients: epidemiological, clinical, and diagnostic features of 22 cases. *Infection* **1998,** *26* (2), 93-9.

42.   Eltoum, I. A.; Zijlstra, E. E.; Ali, M. S.; Ghalib, H. W.; Satti, M. M.; Eltoum, B.; el-Hassan, A. M., Congenital kala-azar and leishmaniasis in the placenta. *The American journal of tropical medicine and hygiene* **1992,** *46* (1), 57-62.

43.   Meinecke, C. K.; Schottelius, J.; Oskam, L.; Fleischer, B., Congenital transmission of visceral leishmaniasis (Kala Azar) from an asymptomatic mother to her child. *Pediatrics* **1999,** *104* (5), e65.

44.   Beena, K. R.; Ramesh, V.; Mukherjee, A., Identification of parasite antigen, correlation of parasite density and inflammation in skin lesions of post kala-azar dermal leishmaniasis. *Journal of cutaneous pathology* **2003,** *30* (10), 616-20.

45.   Khandpur, S.; Ramam, M.; Sharma, V. K.; Salotra, P.; Singh, M. K.; Malhotra, A., Nerve involvement in Indian post kala-azar dermal leishmaniasis. *Acta dermato-venereologica* **2004,** *84* (3), 245-6.

46.   el Hassan, A. M.; Khalil, E. A.; el Sheikh, E. A.; Zijlstra, E. E.; Osman, A.; Ibrahim, M. E., Post

kala-azar ocular leishmaniasis. *Transactions of the Royal Society of Tropical Medicine and Hygiene* **1998,** *92* (2), 177-9.

47.   Gasim, S.; Elhassan, A. M.; Khalil, E. A.; Ismail, A.; Kadaru, A. M.; Kharazmi, A.; Theander, T. G., High levels of plasma IL-10 and expression of IL-10 by keratinocytes during visceral leishmaniasis predict subsequent development of post-kala-azar dermal leishmaniasis. *Clinical and experimental immunology* **1998,** *111* (1), 64-9.

48.   Kharazmi, A.; Kemp, K.; Ismail, A.; Gasim, S.; Gaafar, A.; Kurtzhals, J. A.; El Hassan, A. M.; Theander, T. G.; Kemp, M., T-cell response in human leishmaniasis. *Immunology letters* **1999,** *65* (1-2), 105-8.

49.   Atta, A. M.; D'Oliveira; Correa, J.; Atta, M. L.; Almeida, R. P.; Carvalho, E. M., Anti-leishmanial IgE antibodies: a marker of active disease in visceral leishmaniasis. *The American journal of tropical medicine and hygiene* **1998,** *59* (3), 426-30.

50.   Ponec, J.; Földes, O.; Lichardus, B., Failure to demonstrate natriuretic activity in the posterior pituitary after immunoneutralization of the vasopressin content. *Hormone and metabolic research = Hormon- und Stoffwechselforschung = Hormones et metabolisme* **1991,** *23* (10), 473-5.

51.   Andresen, K.; Gasim, S.; Elhassan, A. M.; Khalil, E. A.; Barker, D. C.; Theander, T. G.; Kharazmi, A., Diagnosis of visceral leishmaniasis by the polymerase chain reaction using blood, bone marrow and lymph node samples from patients from the Sudan. *Tropical medicine & international health : TM & IH* **1997,** *2* (5), 440-4.

52.   Minodier, P.; Piarroux, R.; Garnier, J. M.; Unal, D.; Perrimond, H.; Dumon, H., Pediatric visceral leishmaniasis in southern France. *The Pediatric infectious disease journal* **1998,** *17* (8), 701-4.

53.   Sinha, P. K.; Pandey, K.; Bhattacharya, S. K., Diagnosis & management of leishmania/HIV co-infection. *The Indian journal of medical research* **2005,** *121* (4), 407-14.

54.   Osman, O. F.; Oskam, L.; Kroon, N. C.; Schoone, G. J.; Khalil, E. T.; El-Hassan, A. M.; Zijlstra, E. E.; Kager, P. A., Use of PCR for diagnosis of post-kala-azar dermal leishmaniasis. *Journal of clinical microbiology* **1998,** *36* (6), 1621-4.

55.   da Silva, M. R.; Stewart, J. M.; Costa, C. H., Sensitivity of bone marrow aspirates in the diagnosis of visceral leishmaniasis. *Am J Trop Med Hyg* **2005,** *72* (6), 811-4.

56.   Lightner, L. K.; Chulay, J. D.; Bryceson, A. D., Comparison of microscopy and culture in the detection of Leishmania donovani from splenic aspirates. *Am J Trop Med Hyg* **1983,** *32* (2), 296-9.

57.   Chulay, J. D.; Bryceson, A. D., Quantitation of amastigotes of Leishmania donovani in smears of splenic aspirates from patients with visceral leishmaniasis. *Am J Trop Med Hyg* **1983,** *32* (3), 475-9.

58.   Mbui, J.; Wasunna, M.; Martin, K., A simple and inexpensive medium for culture of splenic aspirates in visceral leishmaniasis. *East Afr Med J* **1999,** *76* (6), 358.

59.   Quinnell, R. J.; Carson, C.; Reithinger, R.; Garcez, L. M.; Courtenay, O., Evaluation of rK39 rapid diagnostic tests for canine visceral leishmaniasis: longitudinal study and meta-analysis. *PLoS Negl Trop Dis* **2013,** *7* (1), e1992.

60.   Cunningham, J.; Hasker, E.; Das, P.; El Safi, S.; Goto, H.; Mondal, D.; Mbuchi, M.; Mukhtar, M.; Rabello, A.; Rijal, S.; Sundar, S.; Wasunna, M.; Adams, E.; Menten, J.; Peeling, R.; Boelaert, M.; Network, W. T. V. L. L., A global comparative evaluation of commercial immunochromatographic rapid diagnostic tests for visceral leishmaniasis. *Clin Infect Dis* **2012,** *55* (10), 1312-9.

61.   Boelaert, M.; Verdonck, K.; Menten, J.; Sunyoto, T.; van Griensven, J.; Chappuis, F.; Rijal, S., Rapid tests for the diagnosis of visceral leishmaniasis in patients with suspected disease. *Cochrane Database Syst Rev* **2014,** *6*, CD009135.

62.   Freitas-Junior, L. H.; Chatelain, E.; Kim, H. A.; Siqueira-Neto, J. L., Visceral leishmaniasis treatment: What do we have, what we need and how to deliver it? *Int J Parasitol Drugs Drug Resist* **2012,** *2*, 11-9.

63.   Torchilin, V. P., Recent advances with liposomes as pharmaceutical carriers. *Nat Rev Drug Discov* **2005,** *4* (2), 145-60.

64.   Karki, P.; Koirala, S.; Parija, S. C.; Hansdak, S. G.; Das, M. L., A thirty day course of sodium stibogluconate for treatment of Kala-azar in Nepal. *The Southeast Asian journal of tropical medicine and public health* **1998,** *29* (1), 154-8.

65.   Lira, R.; Sundar, S.; Makharia, A.; Kenney, R.; Gam, A.; Saraiva, E.; Sacks, D., Evidence that the high incidence of treatment failures in Indian kala-azar is due to the emergence of antimony-resistant strains of Leishmania donovani. *The Journal of infectious diseases* **1999,** *180* (2), 564-7.

66.   World Health, O., Control of the leishmaniases. *World Health Organ Tech Rep Ser* **2010,** (949), xii-xiii, 1-186, back cover.

67.   Bhattacharya, S. K.; Jha, T. K.; Sundar, S.; Thakur, C. P.; Engel, J.; Sindermann, H.; Junge, K.; Karbwang, J.; Bryceson, A. D. M.; Berman, J. D., Efficacy and tolerability of miltefosine for childhood visceral leishmaniasis in India. *Clinical infectious diseases : an official publication of the Infectious Diseases Society of America* **2004,** *38* (2), 217-21.

68.   Omollo, R.; Alexander, N.; Edwards, T.; Khalil, E. A.; Younis, B. M.; Abuzaid, A. A.; Wasunna, M.; Njoroge, N.; Kinoti, D.; Kirigi, G.; Dorlo, T. P.; Ellis, S.; Balasegaram, M.; Musa, A. M., Safety and efficacy of miltefosine alone and in combination with sodium stibogluconate and liposomal amphotericin B for the treatment of primary visceral leishmaniasis in East Africa: study protocol for a randomized controlled trial. *Trials* **2011,** *12,* 166.

69.   Gonzalez, U.; Pinart, M.; Sinclair, D.; Firooz, A.; Enk, C.; Velez, I. D.; Esterhuizen, T. M.; Tristan, M.; Alvar, J., Vector and reservoir control for preventing leishmaniasis. *Cochrane Database Syst Rev* **2015,** *8,* CD008736.

70.   Gurunath, U.; Joshi, R.; Agrawal, A.; Shah, V., An overview of visceral leishmaniasis elimination program in India: a picture imperfect. *Expert Rev Anti Infect Ther* **2014,** *12* (8), 929-35.

71.   WHO: http://www.who.int/csr/don/_05_22/en/index.html. 2002.

72.   Alvar, J.; Cañavate, C.; Molina, R.; Moreno, J.; Nieto, J., Canine leishmaniasis. *Advances in parasitology* **2004,** *57,* 1-88.

73.   Coler, R. N.; Reed, S. G., Second-generation vaccines against leishmaniasis. *Trends in parasitology* **2005,** *21* (5), 244-9.

74.   Jain, K.; Jain, N. K., Vaccines for visceral leishmaniasis: A review. *J Immunol Methods* **2015,** *422,* 1-12.

75.   Elnaiem, D.-E. A.; Schorscher, J.; Bendall, A.; Obsomer, V.; Osman, M. E.; Mekkawi, A. M.; Connor, S. J.; Ashford, R. W.; Thomson, M. C., Risk mapping of visceral leishmaniasis: the role of local variation in rainfall and altitude on the presence and incidence of kala-azar in eastern Sudan. *The American journal of tropical medicine and hygiene* **2003,** *68* (1), 10-7.

6. African trypanosomiasis

Trypanosoma brucei gambiense
(Dutton 1902)

Trypanosoma brucei rhodesiense
(Stephens and Fantham 1910)

Introduction

Human African sleeping sickness or human African trypanosomiasis (HAT) are two similar but distinct diseases caused by the two vector-borne flagellated protozoans, *Trypanosoma brucei gambiense* (West African trypanosomiasis) and *T. b. rhodesiense* (East African trypanosomiasis) that are able to live in the blood of mammals. Both types of human African trypanosomiasis are spread by the bite of the tsetse fly. West African and East African sleeping sickness are restricted to Africa. Some 60 million people are at risk for human African trypanosomiasis based on the range of the tsetse fly vectors.[1, 2] There have been several major outbreaks due mainly to extensive forced migration caused by civil turmoil leading to the breakdown of control measures against the vector, but the total number of cases each year does seem to be decreasing with the implementation of effective vector control programs.[3] *T. brucei* and related species are part of a larger group of organisms characterized by the presence of a kinetoplast (a primitive mitochondrion), and are members of the kinetoplastidae (e.g., *Leishmania* spp., *Trypanosoma. cruzi*).

Tsetse flies of the genus *Glossina* transmit trypanosomes throughout a broad region of equatorial Africa, ecologically restricted to the boundaries of the Sahara desert to the north and the dryer temperate regions south of the equator. *T. b. gambiense* is found mainly in the western and central African countries of Cameroon, Benin, Central African Republic, Gabon, Ghana, Guinea, Ivory Coast, Liberia, Nigeria, Senegal, The Gambia, Uganda, and the Democratic Republic of Congo. *T. b. rhodesiense* occurs mainly in Burundi, Botswana, Congo, Ethiopia, Kenya, Mozambique, Rwanda, Sudan, Tanzania, Uganda, Zambia, and Zimbabwe. In general, *T. b. gambiense* and *T. b. rhodesiense* are found in different geographical areas except in Uganda where both forms are present.[3]

In West Africa, the domestic pig is considered the most important reservoir host for *T. b. gambiense*.[4] In contrast, many species of wild animals and domestic cattle of East Africa are reservoirs for *T. b. rhodesiense*. Cases of East African sleeping sickness have occurred in travelers who entered game parks in these areas to view large wild animals.[5, 6] Trypanosomiasis is also a serious problem in domestic animals imported to Africa from Europe. In addition, many species of the trypanosomes related to those infecting humans cause severe disease in cattle.[7, 8] The genome of *Trypanosoma brucei* has been determined.[9, 10]

Historical Information

Sleeping sickness was known in Europe since the 1700s, when John Atkins published his observations of the disease.[11] In 1895,

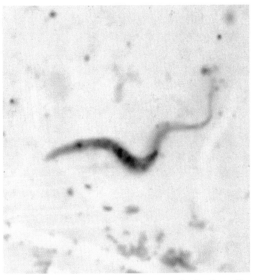

Figure 6.1. Metacyclic trypanomastigote from the tsetse fly. 20 µm. Courtesy I. Cunningham.

Trypanosoma brucei gambiense and *T. b. rhodesiense*

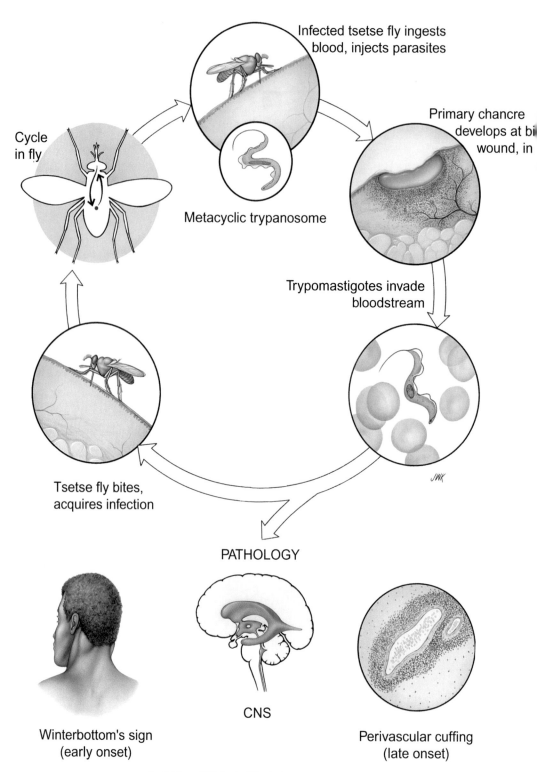

Infected tsetse fly ingests blood, injects parasites

Metacyclic trypanosome

Cycle in fly

Primary chancre develops at bi wound, in

Trypomastigotes invade bloodstream

Tsetse fly bites, acquires infection

PATHOLOGY

CNS

Winterbottom's sign (early onset)

Perivascular cuffing (late onset)

David Bruce described the disease and its causative agent by showing that *nagana*, a disease of cattle, was caused by trypanosomes, and that tsetse flies were the vectors.[12] In 1902, Robert Forde, working in West Africa, described a clinical condition in humans similar to that in cattle caused by *T. b. gambiense*.[13] In 1910, John Stephens and Harold Fantham isolated and described *T. b. rhodesiense* from human cases in East Africa.[14] The two organisms are morphologically identical. Allan Kinghorn and Warrington Yorke, in 1912, demonstrated that *T. b. rhodesiense* could be transmitted from humans to animals by tsetse flies.[15] They also concluded that game animals, such as waterbuck, hartebeest, impala, and warthog, could serve as reservoir hosts for the East African trypanosome.

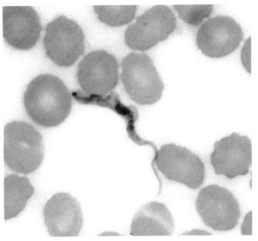

Figure 6.3. Bloodstream trypanomastigote. 15 µm.

Life Cycle

Biological characteristics of the two subspecies are very similar. African trypanosomes live extracellularly, both in the mammalian and insect host.[16] The bloodstream form measures 15-40 µm in length (Fig. 6.1).

The human host acquires the organism when the metacyclic stage is injected intradermally by the bite of an infected tsetse fly (Fig. 6.2). The organisms immediately transform into bloodstream form trypomastigotes (long, slender forms) (Fig. 6.3), and divide by binary fission in the interstitial spaces at the site of the bite. As the result of repeated replication cycles, buildup of metabolic wastes and cell debris occurs, leading to extensive

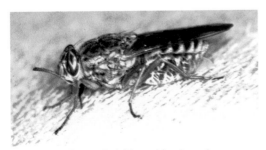

Figure 6.2. Tsetse fly taking a blood meal.

necrosis and the formation of a soft, painless chancre at the site of the tsetse fly bite that is dependent on a host T-cell response.[17] Replication continues in the blood, resulting in millions of new trypomastigotes. During this time, they behave like anaerobes, processing glucose. Trypanosomes have several intracellular inclusions; the kinetoplast-mitochondrion,[18] the glycosome,[19-21] and a multi-protein aggregate termed the editosome.[22] One of its unusual features is that all the DNA of the mitochondrion, which can be up to 25% of the total cellular DNA, is localized in the kinetoplast, adjacent to the flagellar pocket. Kinetoplast DNA or kDNA exists in two forms; mini circles and maxi circles. Mini circle DNA encodes guide RNAs that direct extensive editing of RNA transcripts post transcriptionally.[23-25] Maxi circle DNA contains sequences that, when edited, direct the translation of mitochondrial proteins.[26, 27]

In the vertebrate host, trypanosomes depend entirely upon glucose for energy and are highly aerobic, despite the fact that the kinetoplast-mitochondrion completely lacks cytochromes. Instead, mitochondrial oxygen consumption is based on an alternative oxidase that does not produce ATP. The parasite develops a conventional cytochrome chain and TCA cycle in the vector.[28]

The surface of the trypanosome has numerous membrane-associated transport proteins for obtaining nucleic acid bases, glucose, and other small molecular weight nutrients.[29,] [30] [31] These essential proteins are shielded by allosteric interference provided by the variant surface glycoprotein (VSG) coat proteins.[32]

The trypomastigote enters the bloodstream through the lymphatics and divides further, producing a patent parasitemia. The number of parasites in the blood varies with stage of disease and whether the infection is with *Trypanosoma brucei gambiense* (West African Trypanosomiasis) or *T. b. rhodesiense* (East African Trypanosomiasis). Early in infection with *T. b. rhodesiense* there can be enough parasites in the blood that they can be detected on thick blood smears. Blood smears are usually negative in all stages of infection with *T. b. gambiense* due to a lower level of parasites in the blood. At some point, trypanosomes enter the central nervous system, but remain extracellular, with serious pathological consequences for humans. Some parasites transform into the non-dividing short, stumpy form, which has a biochemistry similar to those of the long, slender form and the form found in the insect vector.[33]

Both male and female tsetse flies become infected by ingesting a blood meal from an infected host.[34] These short, stumpy forms are pre-adapted to the vector, having a well-developed mitochondrion with a partial TCA cycle. Meiosis occurs in the parasites immediately after they are ingested by the vector.[35] The trypanosomes then develop into procyclic trypomastigotes in the midgut of the fly, and continue to divide for approximately 10 days. Here they gain a fully functional cytochrome system and TCA cycle. When the division cycles are completed, the organisms migrate to the salivary glands, and transform into epimastigotes. This form, in turn, divides and transforms further into the metacyclic trypanosome stage, and is infective for humans and reservoir hosts. The cycle in the insect takes 25-50 days, depending upon the species

of tsetse, the strain of the trypanosome, and the ambient temperature.[34] If tsetse flies ingest more than one strain of trypanosome, there is the possibility of genetic exchange between the two strains, generating an increase in genetic diversity.[36]

The vector remains infected for life (2-3 months for females). Tsetse flies inject over 40,000 metacyclic trypanosomes each time they feed. The minimum infective dose for most hosts is 300-500 organisms, although experimental animals have been infected with a single organism.

Infection can also be acquired by eating raw meat from an infected animal.[37] In East Africa, this mode of transmission may be important in maintaining the cycle in some reservoir hosts, such as lions, cheetahs, leopards, hyenas, and wild dogs.

Cellular and Molecular Pathogenesis

African trypanosomes have lived a balanced coexistence between themselves and non-human hosts, since none of the wild animals native to East Africa appear to be severely affected by this parasite (Fig. 6.4).In contrast, humans and the numerous mammals introduced into Africa from Europe, such as non-African breeds of cattle, all suffer, all suffer the pathological consequences of infection from this group of hemoflagellates. African trypanosomes have

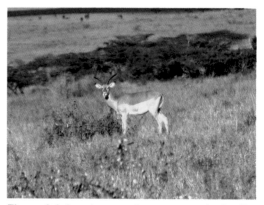

Figure 6.4. Impala, one of many reservoirs for *Trypanosoma brucei rhodesiense*.

evolved several molecular strategies enabling them to avoid elimination from the mammalian host; varying the antigenicity of its surface protein coat, destruction of complement, and the ability to survive in elevated levels of IFN-γ.[38, 39] All infected mammals produce antibodies against a membrane-associated antigen of the trypanosome referred to as the variant surface glycoprotein (VSG).[40] Specific IgG antibodies destroy all clonal organisms sharing the same surface protein (e.g., VSG-1) by agglutination and lysis. However, a few trypanosomes can produce a second variety of surface protein (e.g., VSG-2), with a completely different antigenic signature, in addition to the original one. If some of these organisms shed VSG-1 prior to encountering antibody against it, and continue to synthesize VSG-2 exclusively, they escape lysis, and replace those that were destroyed.[41, 42] A second IgG antibody with specificity to VSG-2 arises, killing all VSG-2 parasites but selecting for VSG-3 organisms, and so on. This antigen-antibody battle between parasite and host continues, until the infected individual is overcome by exhaustion due to glucose depletion and the buildup of metabolic wastes from the parasite (Fig. 6.5).

Antigenic variation depends upon trans-splicing of mRNAs encoded by genes that have been rearranged, duplicated, and expressed at a unique site in the genome.[43, 44] In experimental animal models, the rep-

ertoire of antigenic variants of the bloodstream trypomastigotes is large, numbering in the hundreds. In human disease, the maximum number of VSGs that can be produced remains unknown, although the genome codes for about 1000. Antigenic variation is one reason why vaccine development against this pathogen has not progressed.[45]

In addition to antigenic variation, certain genotypes of trypanosomes have the ability to survive in the presence of high levels of IFN-γ while other genotypes have the ability to avoid complement-mediated destruction.[38] In some cases, patients are infected with multiple genotypes that display multiple mechanisms of immune evasion.[46]

Neuropathology

Trypanosomes remain in the bloodstream and lymph nodes throughout the infection period, which can last weeks to years, depending upon the subspecies of parasite and the immune capabilities of the infected individual. All nodes become enlarged, but enlargement of the posterior cervical nodes is the most noticeable.[47] This cervical lymph node enlargement is known as "Winterbottom's sign". The invasion of the central nervous system induces a lethargic condition, leading eventually to coma and death.[48] Organisms enter the central nervous system much earlier in the infection with *T. b. rhodesiense* than with *T. b. gambiense*. Replication of the parasite in the CSF results in leptomeningitis, cerebral edema, and encephalopathy.[49] Dysregulated inflammation is the chief pathological correlate, with perivascular cuffing consisting of infiltrates of glial cells, lymphocytes, and plasma cells (Fig. 6.6). Astrocytes are induced to release prostaglandin D2 (PGD2), a sleep-regulating molecule.[50] Anti-inflammatory interleukins (IL-10 and TGF-β) are produced early on in the infection, but loose their effectiveness during the chronic and late phase.[51]

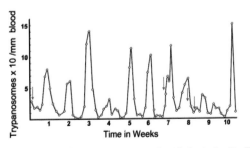

Figure 6.5. Parasitemia in a patient infected with *T. b. rhodesiense*. Each peak of parasitemia represents a new antigenic variant. Arrows indicate attempts at chemotherapy. Ultimately, the patient died of overwhelming infection.

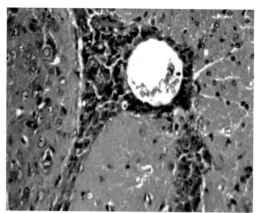

Figure 6.6. Perivascular cuffing around vein in brain of patient who died of sleeping sickness.

Clinical Disease

The disease caused by the two species of trypanosomes, although both called African sleeping sickness, are very different in many ways. Infection rapidly progresses on to disease with *T. b. rhodesiense*, with an incubation period of only 2-3 weeks, and a course of several weeks. Central nervous system involvement occurs some 3-4 weeks after infection. In contrast, *T. b. gambiense* has an incubation period of several weeks to months, and may not involve the brain for months or even years. Europeans exposed to *T. b. gambiense* tend to present with a more rapidly progressive course indicating some degree of tolerance in African populations.[52] Both forms of sleeping sickness are characterized by two defined stages. The early stage is known as the hemolymphatic stage and a late stage is known as the CNS stage. During the early stage there is intermittent fever, malaise, and joint pain that probably correlates with waves of parasitemia. It is during this time that generalized enlargement of the lymph nodes occurs and hepatosplenomegaly may occur.[53] This early stage lasts on average for 3 years with *T. b. gambiense* and for months with *T. b. rhodesiense*.[54]

A large, painless chancre (Fig. 6.7) containing the dividing organisms usually develops at the site of the bite within 2-5 days, and subsequently heals.[17] The chancre is more often described in *T. b. gambiense* than in *T. b. rhodesiense,* but there may be recall bias based on time to diagnosis or a difference in the reaction at the site of the tsetse fly bite due to the differences in host response triggered by the two trypanosomes. Intermittent fever coincides with the organisms entering the bloodstream. Some patients develop rash, generalized pruritus, weight loss, and facial swelling.[55] Winterbottom's sign is characteristic but not always present.[47] Dr. Thomas Masterman Winterbottom was an English physician and abolitionist who travelled to the colony of the Sierra Leone Company and spent 4 years in Africa. Upon returning to England to take over his father's medical practice, Dr. Winterbottom published a description of diseases he had seen including West African trypanosomiasis and noted that the slave traders would avoid taking slaves with this physical finding.[56]

When trypanosomes invade the central nervous system, patients experience severe headache, stiff neck, periods of sleeplessness, and depression. Focal seizures, tremors, and palsies are also common. Coma eventually develops, and the patient dies, usually of associated causes such as pneumonia, or sepsis.

Anemia is a complication of infection

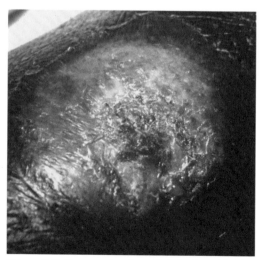

Figure 6.7. Chancre due to early infection with *T. b. gambiense*. Courtesy WHO.

with *T. b. rhodesiense*, but is not always seen due to the fulminating nature of this form of sleeping sickness.

Diagnosis

Definitive diagnosis depends upon finding the organisms in Wright's or Giemsa-stained blood smears, lymph node aspirates, cerebrospinal fluid (CSF), or from aspirates taken at the edge of chancres (Fig. 6.3). Cultures are more sensitive than smears, since thick blood smears miss a large percentage of infections.[57] A number of screening programs in endemic areas rely on an initial serological screening test performed using a card agglutination test for trypanosomiasis (CATT).[58, 59] Antigen detection testing is currently not routinely employed due to concerns about specificity with currently available tests.[60] Molecular testing is another approach that has been developed, but this approach is still not widely used in endemic areas.[61, 62] Since parasites often are present at only low concentrations, even in a patient dying of the disease, techniques to improve the sensitivity of diagnosis such as buffy coat examination and centrifuging sediment of the CSF have been employed.[63]

Examination of CSF is mandatory in the diagnostic evaluation of trypanosomiasis and a WBC ≥5 cells/uL is considered indicative of CNS involvement.[64, 65] Large plasma cells containing eosinophilic inclusions, Mott cells, are uncommon but characteristic and likely represent cells with large amounts of IgM that they are unable to secrete.[66, 67] The determination of CNS involvement is important, as this will guide the choice of appropriate therapy.

History of travel in to endemic area, recalling a painful fly bite, and the presence of a chancre can lead the clinician to the diagnosis. The differential diagnosis includes syphilis, leishmaniasis, and malaria. Finding malarial parasites in the

blood of a patient with trypanosomiasis may occur given the geographic overlap of the two parasites, however this should not mislead the clinician, diverting their attention from the diagnosis of trypanosomiasis.

Treatment

The treatment of sleeping sickness is dependent on the type of trypanosome involved and the stage of the disease.[68] Critical for selection of appropriate treatment for both East African and West African trypanosomiasis is the determination of the clinical stage of disease; early or hemolymphatic stage, versus late or encephalitic stage, and the species of trypanosome.[69]

For treatment of West African sleeping sickness, infection with *T. brucei gambiense*, currently recommended therapy for early stage infection is with IV or IM pentamidine.[70] Suramin as also first line therapy for early stage East African sleeping sickness An alternative therapy for early hemolymphatic stage infection with *T. brucei gambiense* is suramin, which is equal in efficacy to pentamidine.[70] Suramin has been associ-

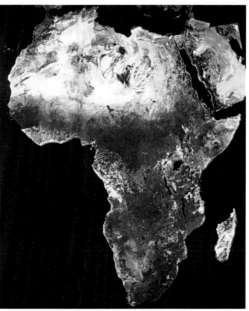

Figure 6.8. Landsat photograph of African continent, colorized to show vegetation (in brown). Photo, NASA.

ated with a hypersensitivity reaction so a test dose should be given before starting treatment with this agent.[71] In early hemolymphatic stage infection suramin is the preferred therapeutic agent.[72, 73] Suramin can be used only for the early stages of the infection as it does not cross the blood-brain barrier.[68]

There is significantly more difference in recommendations for therapy of late or encephalitic stage infection for these two protozoan parasites. For West African trypanosomiasis, infection with *T. brucei gambiense*, combination therapy with eflornithine and nifurtimox or monotherapy with eflornithine is recommended.[74] For East African trypanosomiasis, infection with *T. brucei rhodesiense*, melarsoprol is the treatment of choice. Unfortunately, melarsoprol is the only effective drug for treatment of *T. brucei rhodesiense* with CNS involvement, and this toxic drug is associated with encephalopathy in about 3% of cases.[75] Eflornithine, although effective therapy for late stage with *T. brucei gambiense* infection, is not an effective therapy for infection with *T. brucei rhodesiense*.[76]

Prevention and Control

Previously, periods of political upheaval in different parts of Africa have resulted in dramatic increases in human cases of sleeping sickness.[77] A 2005 WHO report indicated at least 450,000 new cases that year, alone, while prior to 1995, the estimate was fewer than 70,000.[2] Military action and civil unrest in the Sudan, Ethiopia, Sierra Leone, Congo, and Liberia have been responsible for forced migration of millions of individuals, placing them at high risk from a number of parasitic infections. Tsetse fly control programs are also compromised in these same regions due to political and economic instability, exacerbating an already intractable situation. *T. brucei gambiense* may not depend completely on tsetse fly bites and are emerging that a latent human reservoir and reactivation exists under these conditions of stress, which may play a role in outbreaks.[78] In addition to all this turmoil, HIV/AIDS has complicated the picture, adding new, dimensions to the general problem of disease control. Limited resources in countries bordering conflicted areas cannot keep up with the need for vector control, due to large influxes of refugees. Tsetse flies and mosquitoes do not obey political boundaries, and thrive in certain disturbed environments.[79]

Work on vaccines based on VSG antigens has not progressed, however there are a number of active investigations into further understanding the immune response and what constitutes protection from trypanosomiasis.[80-82] Other protein antigens, particularly transporters on the membrane of the flagellar pocket and tubulin offer promise.[83] Diagnostic tests, other than microscopy, would help in earlier patient diagnosis and control efforts particularly when there are low parasite numbers and in latent infections.

References

1.   Simarro, P. P.; Cecchi, G.; Paone, M.; Franco, J. R.; Diarra, A.; Ruiz, J. A.; Fevre, E. M.; Courtin, F.; Mattioli, R. C.; Jannin, J. G., The Atlas of human African trypanosomiasis: a contribution to global mapping of neglected tropical diseases. *Int J Health Geogr* **2010,** *9,* 57.

2.   World Health Organization estimates for 2005. http://www.who.org. **2005**.

3.   Simarro, P. P.; Diarra, A.; Ruiz Postigo, J. A.; Franco, J. R.; Jannin, J. G., The human African trypanosomiasis control and surveillance programme of the World Health Organization 2000-2009: the way forward. *PLoS Negl Trop Dis* **2011,** *5* (2), e1007.

4.   Schares, G.; Mehlitz, D., Sleeping sickness in Zaire: a nested polymerase chain reaction improves the identification of Trypanosoma (Trypanozoon) brucei gambiense by specific kinetoplast DNA probes. *Tropical medicine & international health : TM & IH* **1996,** *1* (1), 59-70.

5.   Migchelsen, S. J.; Buscher, P.; Hoepelman, A. I.; Schallig, H. D.; Adams, E. R., Human African trypanosomiasis: a review of non-endemic cases in the past 20 years. *Int J Infect Dis* **2011,** *15* (8), e517-24.

6.   Sinha, A.; Grace, C.; Alston, W. K.; Westenfeld, F.; Maguire, J. H., African trypanosomiasis in two travelers from the United States. *Clin Infect Dis* **1999,** *29* (4), 840-4.

7.   Leak, S. G.; Peregrine, A. S.; Mulatu, W.; Rowlands, G. J.; D'Ieteren, G., Use of insecticide-impregnated targets for the control of tsetse flies (Glossina spp.) and trypanosomiasis occurring in cattle in an area of south-west Ethiopia with a high prevalence of drug-resistant trypanosomes. *Tropical medicine & international health : TM & IH* **1996,** *1* (5), 599-609.

8.   Katakura, K.; Lubinga, C.; Chitambo, H.; Tada, Y., Detection of Trypanosoma congolense and T. brucei subspecies in cattle in Zambia by polymerase chain reaction from blood collected on a filter paper. *Parasitology research* **1997,** *83* (3), 241-5.

9.   Ghedin, E.; Bringaud, F.; Peterson, J.; Myler, P.; Berriman, M.; Ivens, A.; Andersson, B.; Bontempi, E.; Eisen, J.; Angiuoli, S.; Wanless, D.; Von Arx, A.; Murphy, L.; Lennard, N.; Salzberg, S.; Adams, M. D.; White, O.; Hall, N.; Stuart, K.; Fraser, C. M.; El-Sayed, N. M. A., Gene synteny and evolution of genome architecture in trypanosomatids. *Molecular and biochemical parasitology* **2004,** *134* (2), 183-91.

10. Berriman, M.; Ghedin, E.; Hertz-Fowler, C.; Blandin, G.; Renauld, H.; Bartholomeu, D. C.; Lennard, N. J.; Caler, E.; Hamlin, N. E.; Haas, B.; Bohme, U.; Hannick, L.; Aslett, M. A.; Shallom, J.; Marcello, L.; Hou, L.; Wickstead, B.; Alsmark, U. C.; Arrowsmith, C.; Atkin, R. J.; Barron, A. J.; Bringaud, F.; Brooks, K.; Carrington, M.; Cherevach, I.; Chillingworth, T. J.; Churcher, C.; Clark, L. N.; Corton, C. H.; Cronin, A.; Davies, R. M.; Doggett, J.; Djikeng, A.; Feldblyum, T.; Field, M. C.; Fraser, A.; Goodhead, I.; Hance, Z.; Harper, D.; Harris, B. R.; Hauser, H.; Hostetler, J.; Ivens, A.; Jagels, K.; Johnson, D.; Johnson, J.; Jones, K.; Kerhornou, A. X.; Koo, H.; Larke, N.; Landfear, S.; Larkin, C.; Leech, V.; Line, A.; Lord, A.; Macleod, A.; Mooney, P. J.; Moule, S.; Martin, D. M.; Morgan, G. W.; Mungall, K.; Norbertczak, H.; Ormond, D.; Pai, G.; Peacock, C. S.; Peterson, J.; Quail, M. A.; Rabbinowitsch, E.; Rajandream, M. A.; Reitter, C.; Salzberg, S. L.; Sanders, M.; Schobel, S.; Sharp, S.; Simmonds, M.; Simpson, A. J.; Tallon, L.; Turner, C. M.; Tait, A.; Tivey, A. R.; Van Aken, S.; Walker, D.; Wanless, D.; Wang, S.; White, B.; White, O.; Whitehead, S.; Woodward, J.; Wortman, J.; Adams, M. D.; Embley, T. M.; Gull, K.; Ullu, E.; Barry, J. D.; Fairlamb, A. H.; Opperdoes, F.; Barrell, B. G.; Donelson, J. E.; Hall, N.; Fraser, C. M.; Melville, S. E.; El-Sayed, N. M., The genome of the African trypanosome Trypanosoma brucei. *Science* **2005,** *309* (5733), 416-22.

11. Atkins, J.; J., The Navy Surgeon, or Practical System of Surgery with a Dissertation on Cold and Hot Mineral Springs and Physical Observations on the Coast of Guinea. *London 1742.*

12. Bruce, D., Preliminary Report of the Tsetse Fly Disease or Nagana in Zululand. *Bennet Davis Durban* **1895**.

13. Forde, R. M.; J., Some clinical notes on a European patient in whose blood a trypanosome was observed. *Med* **1902,** *5* 261-263.

14. Stephens, J. W. W.; Fantham, H. B.; R., On the peculiar morphology of a trypanosome from a case of sleeping sickness and the possibility of its being a new species (T. rhodesiense). . *Proc Lond [Biol]* **1910,** *83,* 23-33.

15. Kinghorn, A.; Yorke, W., On the transmission of human trypanosomes by Glossina morsitans, and on the occurrence of human trypanosomes in game. *Ann Trop Med Parasitol* **1912,** *6* 1-23.

16. Gull, K., The cell biology of parasitism in Trypanosoma brucei: insights and drug targets from genomic approaches? *Current pharmaceutical design* **2002,** *8* (4), 241-56.

17. Naessens, J.; Mwangi, D. M.; Buza, J.; Moloo, S. K., Local skin reaction (chancre) induced following inoculation of metacyclic trypanosomes in cattle by tsetse flies is dependent on CD4 T lymphocytes. *Parasite Immunol* **2003,** *25* (8-9), 413-9.

18. Shlomai, J., The structure and replication of kinetoplast DNA. *Current molecular medicine* **2004,** *4* (6), 623-47.

19. Opperdoes, F. R.; Borst, P., Localization of nine glycolytic enzymes in a microbody-like organelle in Trypanosoma brucei: the glycosome. *FEBS letters* **1977,** *80* (2), 360-4.

20. Verlinde, C. L.; Hannaert, V.; Blonski, C.; Willson, M.; Périé, J. J.; Fothergill-Gilmore, L. A.; Opperdoes, F. R.; Gelb, M. H.; Hol, W. G.; Michels, P. A., Glycolysis as a target for the design of new anti-trypanosome drugs. *Drug resistance updates : reviews and commentaries in antimicrobial and anticancer chemotherapy* **2001,** *4* (1), 50-65.

21. Parsons, M., Glycosomes: parasites and the divergence of peroxisomal purpose. *Molecular microbiology* **2004,** *53* (3), 717-24.

22. Panigrahi, A. K.; Schnaufer, A.; Ernst, N. L.; Wang, B.; Carmean, N.; Salavati, R.; Stuart, K., Identification of novel components of Trypanosoma brucei editosomes. *RNA (New York, N.Y.)* **2003,** *9* (4), 484-92.

23. Feagin, J. E.; Stuart, K., Differential expression of mitochondrial genes between life cycle stages of Trypanosoma brucei. *Proceedings of the National Academy of Sciences of the United States of America* **1985,** *82* (10), 3380-4.

24. Stuart, K.; Kable, M. L.; Allen, T. E.; Lawson, S., Investigating the mechanism and machinery of RNA editing. *Methods (San Diego, Calif.)* **1998,** *15* (1), 3-14.

25. Simpson, L.; Aphasizhev, R.; Gao, G.; Kang, X., Mitochondrial proteins and complexes in Leishmania and Trypanosoma involved in U-insertion/deletion RNA editing. *RNA (New York, N.Y.)* **2004,** *10* (2), 159-70.

26. Stuart, K., Mitochondrial DNA of an African trypanosome. *J Cell Biochem* **1983,** *23* (1-4), 13-26.

27. Shapiro, T. A., Kinetoplast DNA maxicircles: networks within networks. *Proceedings of the National Academy of Sciences of the United States of America* **1993,** *90* (16), 7809-13.

28. Walker, R.; Saha, L.; Hill, G. C.; Chaudhuri, M., The effect of over-expression of the alternative oxidase in the procyclic forms of Trypanosoma brucei. *Mol Biochem Parasitol* **2005,** *139* 153-62.

29. Borst, P.; Fairlamb, A. H., Surface receptors and transporters of Trypanosoma brucei. *Annual review of microbiology* **1998,** *52,* 745-78.

30. Sanchez, M. A.; Ullman, B.; Landfear, S. M.; Carter, N. S., Cloning and functional expression of a gene encoding a P1 type nucleoside transporter from Trypanosoma brucei. *The Journal of biological chemistry* **1999,** *274* (42), 30244-9.

31. Natto, M. J.; Wallace, L. J. M.; Candlish, D.; Al-Salabi, M. I.; Coutts, S. E.; de Koning, H. P., Trypanosoma brucei: expression of multiple purine transporters prevents the development of allopurinol resistance. *Experimental parasitology* **2005,** *109* (2), 80-6.

32. Donelson, J. E., Antigenic variation and the African trypanosome genome. *Acta tropica* **2003,** *85* (3), 391-404.

33. Kioy, D.; Jannin, J.; Mattock, N., Human African trypanosomiasis. *Nature reviews. Microbiology* **2004,** *2* (3), 186-7.

34. Vickerman, K.; Tetley, L.; Hendry, K. A.; Turner, C. M., Biology of African trypanosomes in the tsetse fly. *Biology of the cell / under the auspices of the European Cell Biology Organization* **1988,** *64* (2), 109-19.

35. Peacock, L.; Bailey, M.; Carrington, M.; Gibson, W., Meiosis and haploid gametes in the pathogen Trypanosoma brucei. *Curr Biol* **2014,** *24* (2), 181-6.

36. Gibson, W., Genetic exchange in trypanosomes. *Bulletin et memoires de l'Academie royale de medecine de Belgique* **1996,** *151* (2), 203-10.

37. Betram, B. C. R., Sleeping sickness survey in the Serengeti area (Tanzania) . III. Discussion of the relevance of the trypanosome survey to the biology of large mammals in the Serengeti. *Acta Trop Basel* **1973,** *30,* 36-48.

38. Donelson, J. E.; Hill, K. L.; El-Sayed, N. M., Multiple mechanisms of immune evasion by African trypanosomes. *Molecular and biochemical parasitology* **1998,** *91* (1), 51-66.

39. Barry, J. D.; McCulloch, R., Antigenic variation in trypanosomes: enhanced phenotypic variation in a eukaryotic parasite. *Advances in parasitology* **2001,** *49,* 1-70.

40. Cross, G. A., Identification, purification and properties of clone-specific glycoprotein antigens constituting the surface coat of Trypanosoma brucei. *Parasitology* **1975,** *71* (3), 393-417.

41. Pays, E.; Vanhamme, L.; Berberof, M., Genetic controls for the expression of surface antigens in African trypanosomes. *Annual review of microbiology* **1994,** *48,* 25-52.

42. McCulloch, R., Antigenic variation in African trypanosomes: monitoring progress. *Trends in*

parasitology **2004,** *20* (3), 117-21.

43.   Gray, A. R., Antigenic variation in a strain of Trypanosoma brucei transmitted by Glossina morsitans and G. palpalis. *Journal of general microbiology* **1965,** *41* (2), 195-214.

44.   Borst, P.; Bitter, W.; Blundell, P. A.; Chaves, I.; Cross, M.; Gerrits, H.; van Leeuwen, F.; McCulloch, R.; Taylor, M.; Rudenko, G., Control of VSG gene expression sites in Trypanosoma brucei. *Molecular and biochemical parasitology* **1998,** *91* (1), 67-76.

45.   Barbour, A. G.; Restrepo, B. I., Antigenic variation in vector-borne pathogens. *Emerging infectious diseases* **2000,** *6* (5), 449-57.

46.   Truc, P.; Ravel, S.; Jamonneau, V.; N'Guessan, P.; Cuny, G., Genetic variability within Trypanosoma brucei gambiense: evidence for the circulation of different genotypes in human African trypanosomiasis patients in Cote d'Ivoire. *Trans R Soc Trop Med Hyg* **2002,** *96* (1), 52-5.

47.   Winterbottom, T. M., An Account of the Native Africans in the Neighborhood of Sierra Leone. 1803; Vol. 2.

48.   Mhlanga, J. D.; Bentivoglio, M.; Kristensson, K., Neurobiology of cerebral malaria and African sleeping sickness. *Brain research bulletin* **1997,** *44* (5), 579-89.

49.   Odiit, M.; Kansiime, F.; Enyaru, J. C., Duration of symptoms and case fatality of sleeping sickness caused by Trypanosoma brucei rhodesiense in Tororo, Uganda. *East African medical journal* **1997,** *74* (12), 792-5.

50.   Pentreath, V. W.; Rees, K.; Owolabi, O. A.; Philip, K. A.; Doua, F., The somnogenic T lymphocyte suppressor prostaglandin D2 is selectively elevated in cerebrospinal fluid of advanced sleeping sickness patients. *Transactions of the Royal Society of Tropical Medicine and Hygiene* **1990,** *84* (6), 795-9.

51.   Sternberg, J. M., Human African trypanosomiasis: clinical presentation and immune response. *Parasite immunology* **2004,** *26* (11-12), 469-76.

52.   Blum, J. A.; Neumayr, A. L.; Hatz, C. F., Human African trypanosomiasis in endemic populations and travellers. *Eur J Clin Microbiol Infect Dis* **2012,** *31* (6), 905-13.

53.   Boatin, B. A.; Wyatt, G. B.; Wurapa, F. K.; Bulsara, M. K., Use of symptoms and signs for diagnosis of Trypanosoma brucei rhodesiense trypanosomiasis by rural health personnel. *Bull World Health Organ* **1986,** *64* (3), 389-95.

54.   Malvy, D.; Chappuis, F., Sleeping sickness. *Clin Microbiol Infect* **2011,** *17* (7), 986-95.

55.   Uslan, D. Z.; Jacobson, K. M.; Kumar, N.; Berbari, E. F.; Orenstein, R., A woman with fever and rash after African safari. *Clin Infect Dis* **2006,** *43* (5), 609, 661-2.

56.   Texas Southern University. Library.; Heartman Negro Collection., Catalog, Heartman Negro Collection. Library Staff, Texas Southern University: Houston, Texas, 1956; p 325 p.

57.   Robays, J.; Bilengue, M. M.; Van der Stuyft, P.; Boelaert, M., The effectiveness of active population screening and treatment for sleeping sickness control in the Democratic Republic of Congo. *Trop Med Int Health* **2004,** *9* (5), 542-50.

58.   Chappuis, F.; Stivanello, E.; Adams, K.; Kidane, S.; Pittet, A.; Bovier, P. A., Card agglutination test for trypanosomiasis (CATT) end-dilution titer and cerebrospinal fluid cell count as predictors of human African Trypanosomiasis (Trypanosoma brucei gambiense) among serologically suspected individuals in southern Sudan. *Am J Trop Med Hyg* **2004,** *71* (3), 313-7.

59.   Inojosa, W. O.; Augusto, I.; Bisoffi, Z.; Josenado, T.; Abel, P. M.; Stich, A.; Whitty, C. J., Diagnosing human African trypanosomiasis in Angola using a card agglutination test: observational study of active and passive case finding strategies. *BMJ* **2006,** *332* (7556), 1479.

60.   Asonganyi, T.; Doua, F.; Kibona, S. N.; Nyasulu, Y. M.; Masake, R.; Kuzoe, F., A multi-centre evaluation of the card indirect agglutination test for trypanosomiasis (TrypTect CIATT). *Ann Trop Med Parasitol* **1998,** *92* (8), 837-44.

61.   Deborggraeve, S.; Lejon, V.; Ekangu, R. A.; Mumba Ngoyi, D.; Pati Pyana, P.; Ilunga, M.; Mulunda, J. P.; Buscher, P., Diagnostic accuracy of PCR in gambiense sleeping sickness diagnosis, staging and post-treatment follow-up: a 2-year longitudinal study. *PLoS Negl Trop Dis* **2011,** *5* (2), e972.

62.   Becker, S.; Franco, J. R.; Simarro, P. P.; Stich, A.; Abel, P. M.; Steverding, D., Real-time PCR for detection of Trypanosoma brucei in human blood samples. *Diagnostic microbiology and infectious*

disease **2004,** *50* (3), 193-9.

63. Bailey, J. W.; Smith, D. H., The use of the acridine orange QBC technique in the diagnosis of African trypanosomiasis. *Trans R Soc Trop Med Hyg* **1992,** *86* (6), 630.

64. Kennedy, P. G., Human African trypanosomiasis of the CNS: current issues and challenges. *J Clin Invest* **2004,** *113* (4), 496-504.

65. Rodgers, J., Human African trypanosomiasis, chemotherapy and CNS disease. *J Neuroimmunol* **2009,** *211* (1-2), 16-22.

66. Bain, B. J., Russell bodies and Mott cells. *Am J Hematol* **2009,** *84* (8), 516.

67. Weinstein, T.; Mittelman, M.; Djaldetti, M., Electron microscopy study of Mott and Russell bodies in myeloma cells. *J Submicrosc Cytol* **1987,** *19* (1), 155-9.

68. Jannin, J.; Cattand, P., Treatment and control of human African trypanosomiasis. *Current opinion in infectious diseases* **2004,** *17* (6), 565-71.

69. Kennedy, P. G., The continuing problem of human African trypanosomiasis (sleeping sickness). *Ann Neurol* **2008,** *64* (2), 116-26.

70. Barrett, M. P.; Boykin, D. W.; Brun, R.; Tidwell, R. R., Human African trypanosomiasis: pharmacological re-engagement with a neglected disease. *Br J Pharmacol* **2007,** *152* (8), 1155-71.

71. Thibault, A.; Figg, W. D.; Cooper, M. R.; Prindiville, S. A.; Sartor, A. O.; Headlee, D. J.; Myers, C. E., Anaphylactoid reaction with suramin. *Pharmacotherapy* **1993,** *13* (6), 656-7.

72. Woo, P.; Soltys, M. A., The effect of suramin on blood and tissue forms of Trypanosoma brucei and Trypanosoma rhodesiense. *Ann Trop Med Parasitol* **1971,** *65* (4), 465-9.

73. Arroz, J.; Djedje, M., Suramin and metronidazole in the treatment of Trypanosoma brucei rhodesiense. *Trans R Soc Trop Med Hyg* **1988,** *82* (3), 421.

74. Kennedy, P. G., Clinical features, diagnosis, and treatment of human African trypanosomiasis (sleeping sickness). *Lancet Neurol* **2013,** *12* (2), 186-94.

75. Legros, D.; Fournier, C.; Gastellu Etchegorry, M.; Maiso, F.; Szumilin, E., [Therapeutic failure of melarsoprol among patients treated for late stage T.b. gambiense human African trypanosomiasis in Uganda]. *Bulletin de la Societe de pathologie exotique (1990)* **1999,** *92* (3), 171-2.

76. Bacchi, C. J.; McCann, P. P.; Pegg, A. E.; Sjoerdsma, A., Parasitic protozoa and polyamines. 1987; p 317-44.

77. Chretien, J.-P.; Smoak, B. L., African Trypanosomiasis: Changing Epidemiology and Consequences. *Current infectious disease reports* **2005,** *7* (1), 54-60.

78. Welburn, S. C.; Molyneux, D. H.; Maudlin, I., Beyond Tsetse - Implications for Research and Control of Human African Trypanosomiasis Epidemics. *Trends Parasitol* **2016,** *32* (3), 230-41.

79. Molyneux, D. H., Vector-borne parasitic diseases--an overview of recent changes. *International journal for parasitology* **1998,** *28* (6), 927-34.

80. Silva, M. S.; Prazeres, D. M.; Lanca, A.; Atouguia, J.; Monteiro, G. A., Trans-sialidase from Trypanosoma brucei as a potential target for DNA vaccine development against African trypanosomiasis. *Parasitol Res* **2009,** *105* (5), 1223-9.

81. La Greca, F.; Magez, S., Vaccination against trypanosomiasis: can it be done or is the trypanosome truly the ultimate immune destroyer and escape artist? *Hum Vaccin* **2011,** *7* (11), 1225-33.

82. Magez, S.; Caljon, G.; Tran, T.; Stijlemans, B.; Radwanska, M., Current status of vaccination against African trypanosomiasis. *Parasitology* **2010,** *137* (14), 2017-27.

83. Lubega, G. W.; Byarugaba, D. K.; Prichard, R. K., Immunization with a tubulin-rich preparation from Trypanosoma brucei confers broad protection against African trypanosomosis. *Experimental parasitology* **2002,** *102* (1), 9-22.

7. American Trypanosomiasis

Trypanosoma cruzi
(Chagas 1909)

Introduction

Trypanosoma cruzi is the causative agent of American trypanosomiasis, also known as Chagas Disease. It is an intracellular parasite for the majority of its life, in contrast to its relatives, the African trypanosomes, that live in the blood and lymph.[1] *T. cruzi* infects many species of mammals native to South and Central America and is vector-borne.[2-5] Insects in the order Hemiptera (true bugs), called "kissing bugs," are the only known vectors (see Figs. 7.1, 38.29).[6] Chronic infection with this parasite often leads to life-threatening disease. Chagas disease is one of the world's leading causes of cardiomyopathy.[7-9] *T. cruzi* is found throughout Central and South America, where according to the Global Burden of Disease study it infects approximately 9-10 million people.[10-12] A recent health economic assessment indicates that Chagas disease results in over $7 billion in economic losses annually.[13]

According to the World Health Organization, the largest number of people living with Chagas disease is in Argentina, followed by Brazil and Mexico, but Bolivia has the world's highest prevalence rate.[14] It is estimated that there are currently more than 300,000 individuals living in the United States infected with Chagas disease.[15] In Texas, there is strong evidence that transmission occurs within the state, where a high percentage of dogs is also infected.[16] Through globalization, Chagas disease cases are also now found in Southern Europe (especially Spain and Portugal), and even Australia and Japan, although there is no disease transmission in these areas.[17] As demonstrated by a prevalence study in Brazil, the incidence of this disease varies based on location and can be as low as 0% to above 25%.[18] Control of Chagas disease requires constant vigilance and has now re-emerged in countries that previously reported that they had eliminated transmission of the disease.[19] Despite concerted efforts at the clinical level to lower the mortality rate of chronic Chagas Disease, acute Chagas disease can have a case fatality rate as high as 5%.[20] In individuals who already exhibt signs and symptoms of heart disease, the five year mortality has been estimated at around 17%.[21]

In addition to spread by the kissing bug (Triatomine), infection can be transmitted through blood transfusion, bone marrow transplants, organ transplants, transplacentally, and ingestion of contaminated beverages.[22-27] Oral transmission to humans of American trypanosomiasis has transformed this disease from one restricted to certain geographic hot spots to one seen in urban outbreaks.[28] Oral transmission is likely the most frequent mechanism in non-human mammals, and is now linked to several outbreaks with guava juice, sugar cane juice, food, water, soup, and fruit juices.[28-30] Still another transmission route of increasing importance is vertical transmission of *T. cruzi* infection from mother to child.[31]

Rats, dogs, sloths, bats, and various non-human primates are important reservoir hosts, depending upon the region.[32-37] Transmission takes place in both rural and urban

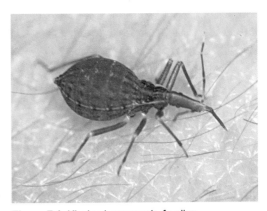

Figure 7.1. Kissing bug nymph, feeding.

settings. Incidence is highest in children, with the notable exceptions of Brazil and Chile.[38]

Historical Information

In 1909, Carlos Chagas observed the infective stage of *T. cruzi* by chance while conducting a survey for vectors of malaria.[39, 40] Carlos Chagas inoculated many species of mammals with the new agent and showed that they all became infected. He correctly speculated that humans were likely to be infected as well. He identified infected people in rural areas of Brazil. He also described the major clinical features of the disease and the morphology of the trypomastigote stage of the parasite. All this work was accomplished within months after his initial discovery. He named the organism after his beloved teacher and close friend, Oswaldo Cruz. Chagas went on to describe the essentials of the life cycle as well. Alexandre Brumpt, in 1912, completed the description of the life cycle of *T. cruzi*, while Gaspar Vianna, in 1916, published the details of the pathological consequences of infection with this important pathogenic protozoan.[41, 42]

Life Cycle

The biology, molecular biology, and epidemiology of American trypanosmiasis are starting to be revealed at the genetic level.[43-45] Organisms (metacyclic trypomastigote stage) are present in the fecal droppings of the infected reduviid bug. (Fig. 7.1) Transmission occurs usually by a person rubbing the organisms into a mucous membrane or bite wound, although oral ingestion is a well-described means of transmission. Triatomid bugs are large, robust insects, and characteristically feed at night, biting the victim near the mouth or eyes while they are asleep. The reduviid bug is often called the "kissing" bug because the bite is painless and it usually bites around the mouth or eyes.[46] The bug's saliva contains antigens that induce intense pruritis.[47]

The vector ingests a large quantity of blood, and in order to make room for the new meal, it simultaneously defecates the remains of the last one, depositing it adjacent to the bite wound. The salivary secretions of the bug induce itching, causing the victim to rub the bug feces, laden with parasites, into the wound, or mucus membranes.[6]

The infection can also occur without direct contact with the vector. Thatched roofs of rural houses can harbor large numbers of the bugs (Fig. 7.2), and their feces have the opportunity to fall onto people while they are sleeping. Simply rubbing the parasites into their mucous membranes of the eye or oral cavity can lead to infection. The probability of infection by this route is high, because kissing bugs feed on many mammals, and rural peoples live in close proximity to their livestock and pets. Infection by transfusion, organ transplantation, or congenital transmission introduces the parasite directly into the host. For a somewhat gory account of what it's like to wake up covered with well-fed kissing bugs, see Charles Darwin's description in his famous journal, *Voyage of The Beagle*. Because of this encounter, much speculation has centered around the possibility that Darwin actually contracted and suffered from chronic Chagas disease. In fact, he most likely suffered from lactose intolerance masquerading as Chagas disease![48]

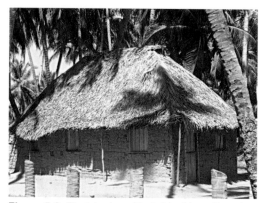

Figure 7.2. Thatched roof hut. Ideal breeding sites for kissing bugs.

Trypanosoma cruzi

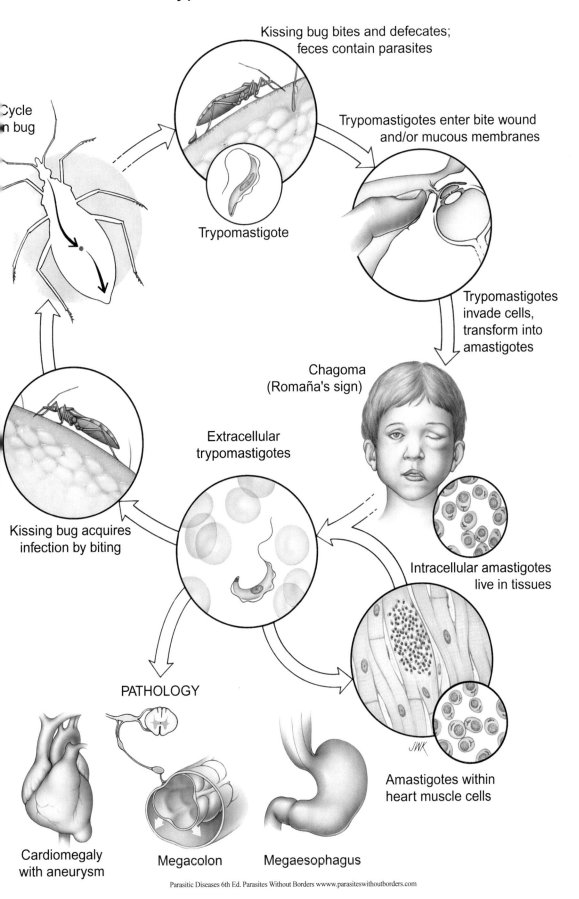

Kissing bug bites and defecates; feces contain parasites

Cycle in bug

Trypomastigote

Trypomastigotes enter bite wound and/or mucous membranes

Trypomastigotes invade cells, transform into amastigotes

Chagoma (Romaña's sign)

Extracellular trypomastigotes

Intracellular amastigotes live in tissues

Kissing bug acquires infection by biting

PATHOLOGY

Amastigotes within heart muscle cells

Cardiomegaly with aneurysm

Megacolon

Megaesophagus

JWK

Attachment is mediated through galectin-3 on the surface of host cells.[49] The parasite protein that binds to galactin-3 has yet to be identified. The trypomastigote can penetrate a wide variety of cells, and the process is mediated by calcium ions and at least two parasite membrane proteins; a neuraminidase/trans-sialidase, which binds to sialic acid, and penetrin, which binds to heparin sulfate.[50, 51] Another protein, gp82 might also be necessary for penetration into gastric epithelium if the metacyclic trypomastigote stage is swallowed.[52] Just such an outbreak occurred in Santa Catarina, Brazil involving the ingestion of sugar cane juice contaminated with at least one infected kissing bug. Animals can become infected by ingesting infected kissing bugs, and this might be the usual way for them to acquire the infection.[53]

After entering the parasitophorous vacuole, the trypomastigote enlists several escape mechanisms to aid in its survival there. It begins by neutralizing the pH of that intracellular space, thereby escaping the potentially damaging effects of exposure to the active forms of lysosomal enzymes.[51] The organism also produces a number of proteins that offer it additional advantages once inside the host cell. Chagasin is a cysteine protease inhibitor and is apparently necessary for avoiding lysosomal-derived cysteine protease activity and insures that the parasite has the time needed to differentiate into the amastigote stage.[54] Cruzipain is thought to play a major role in helping the parasite avoid being digested once inside the parasitophorous vacuole. Cruzipain also induces the upregulation of host-derived arginase-2, a known inhibitor of apoptosis.[55] The parasite may be engineering the longevity of its host cell, while at the same time, avoiding the ravages of lysosomal digestion.

The parasite then rapidly penetrates into the cytosol and differentiates into the amastigote stage. This is the dividing form of *T. cruzi* and the one that inflicts cell damage on the host. After several division cycles, some of the parasites transform back into trypomastigotes. The affected cells die, releasing the parasites that can now enter the bloodstream and become distributed throughout the body. They infect cells in many types of tissues, including the central nervous system, heart muscle, the myenteric plexus, the urogenital tract, and the reticuloendothelial system.

Triatomines become infected by taking a blood meal from an infected individual.[56] The trypomastigote migrates to the midgut of the insect, where it transforms into the epimastigote, and then undergoes many divisions. Thousands of organisms are produced within one insect without apparently affecting it. The triatomines remain infected for life (~1-2 years). Epimastigotes maintain their place in the gut of the insect by specific receptor-ligand interactions involving at least one parasite surface glycoprotein and a carbohydrate lectin on the gut cells of the insect.[57] Ultimately, epimastigotes transform into metacyclic trypomastigotes and migrate to the hindgut, and from there they are excreted with feces following the taking of a blood meal.

Cellular and Molecular Pathogenesis

Infection with *Trypanosoma cruzi* results in partial immunosuppression that further aids the parasite in remaining inside the host cell for extended periods of time.[58, 59] For example, *in vitro* culture of human dendritic cells infected with *T. cruzi* resulted in a dramatic down regulation of synthesis of IL-6, IL-12, TNF-α, HLA-DR, and CD-40, and inhibited their maturation into antigen processing cells.[60] Parasite-derived calreticulin may also be important for amastigote survival in the intracellular environment, implicating a central role for calcium trafficking and storage in the life of the parasite.[61]

Release of trypomastigotes into the bloodstream seemingly places them at risk for immune attack, since serum antibodies against them can be demonstrated at this time in the infected host. However, *T. cruzi* has an answer for this defense strategy. The surface coat of the free-swimming trypomastigote contains a specific complement regulatory protein that binds the C3b and C4b components, inhibiting the alternate pathway.[62]

Host protection can develop, despite these highly evolved parasite evasion mechanisms. Immunity depends on CD1d antigen presentation and the upregulation of IL-12 for the production of natural killer cells, the protective arm of the immune system most effective against the amastigotes in the tissues.[63] Parasites are killed by way of induction of nitric oxide synthase and the production of nitric oxide.[64] CD8[+] T cells with specificities for parasite antigen are thought to be essential in maintaining some control of the infection throughout the chronic phase.[65]

Chagas disease manifests in many organs. Infected individuals remain infected for life and most of the pathological consequences result from cell death (Fig. 7.3). Myenteric plexus damage results in loss of muscle tone and enlargement of the organ, particularly the digestive tract. It is thought that most of the damage to the myenteric plexus is directly resultant on damage that occurs early in infection and is not thought to be prevented by treatment of chronic Chagas.[66] Megacolon and megaesophagus are late onset sequelae to chronic infection. Heart damage is almost invariably associated with Chagas disease in

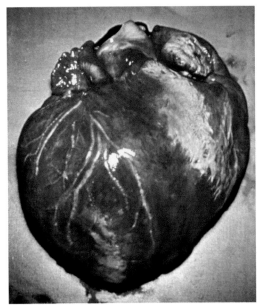

Figure 7.4. Enlarged heart of a patient who died of chronic Chagas' disease.

some regions of Central and South America[67], and is detectable early on in infection.[68] Erosion of heart tissue is typical, and in many cases results in aneurysm and heart failure (Figs. 7.4, 7.5).

Current thinking regarding a dominant role for auto-antibodies inducing cardiomyopathy plays down this mechanism to account for heart damage during chronic infection.[68] This is because PCR has been able to demonstrate the presence of *T. cruzi* in heart tissue, even at times when biopsy material used in conventional histological mode could not reveal the presence of the parasite, and disease pro-

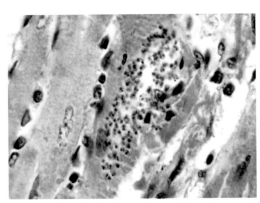

Figure 7.3. Histologic section of heart muscle infected with *Trypanosoma cruzi* amastigotes.

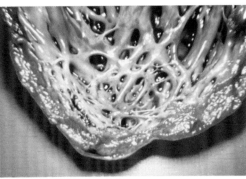

Figure 7.5. Portion of enlarged heart of a patient who died of chronic Chagas' disease. Note thin wall of ventricle.

gresses rapidly when parasites are abundant and not as fast when they are hard to demonstrate on biopsy.[68, 69] Thus parasite persistence leading to fibrosis and damage to the heart (including the cardiac conduction system) has emerged as the dominant theme to explain the pathogenesis of Chagas cardiomyopathy.[70] Nonetheless, autoantibodies have been detected in many individuals suffering from long-term infection with *T. cruzi*.[71, 72] Meningoencephalitis can occur during the acute phase and is characterized by infiltrates of CD8+ T cells.[73] Meningoencephalitis can also occur in patients with underlying HIV/AIDS.[74]

Clinical Disease

Acute Chagas Disease

The incubation period of Chagas disease varies based on means of transmission. In acute Chagas disease acquired from the kissing bug, the incubation period is from a few days to two weeks before the onset of symptoms.[75] With disease acquired through other means such as transfusion or transplant, the incubation period may be as long as four months.[76] Acute disease can range from mild nonspecific symptoms such as malaise and fever to severe manifestations. Some patients are asymptomatic. Severe acute manifestations are estimated to develop in approximately 1% of cases and may involve acute myocarditis, pericardial effusion, and in some cases meningoencephalitis.[77, 78] The risk of severe disease and mortality during the acute disease tends to be the highest with orally acquired infection.[79] In a few patients, but clearly only the minority, a characteristic hemi-facial edema or swelling called a chagoma develops at the site of the bite or inoculation within 2-4 days. If organisms are introduced into the body through mucous membranes by rubbing them into the eye, then the swelling associated with the chagoma is known as Romaña's sign.[80, 81] It occurs mostly as a unilateral swelling. The swollen eyelid is firm to the touch, and there may be associated conjunctivitis. If the bite occurs elsewhere, the adjacent area is erythematous, brawny, and firm to the touch. When the chagoma disappears after several weeks, it leaves an area of depigmentation. An associated neuropathy develops, and then disappears when the patient enters the chronic phase of the infection.

Chronic Chagas Disease

Most patients survive the acute phase and become asymptomatic. Patients at this point enter the chronic phase and although they may remain symptomatic they are capable of transmitting parasites to the insect vector. During the chronic phase of Chagas disease individuals enter an indeterminant or latent stage, which may continue for the life of most (70-80%) affected individuals, or which may later manifest with injury to the heart or gastrointestinal system. Unfortunately, in as many as a third of patients, there is a progression of the disease that usually manifests as cardiac or gastrointestinal disease.[82, 83] There continues to be much controversy over the exact mechanism that leads to this delayed appearance of symptoms, but there is evidence that parasite persistence may be involved in the development of cardiac manifestations.[82] Another factor is genetics of the parasite. There are six different genetic 'demes' or strains of *T. cruzi*, and certain ones are more prone to cause heart disease versus gastrointestinal disease. Ultrastructural studies showed that vinculin costameres in cardiomyocytes become disrupted during intracellular infection with the amastiogote stage, and this is thought to make a major contribution to the cardiomyopathy so typically seen in the chronic infection.[84]

Clinically, the patient experiences extrasystoles, right ventricular enlargement, and eventually heart failure. Right bundle branch block is typically the earliest disturbance evident on ECG, and eventually progression of cardiac disease may lead to death.[85] Some investigators believe that it is the conduction system disturbances that represent the most common cause of death from Chagasic heart disease, rather than the dramatic cardiomyopathy and heart failure seen in some patients.

Gastrointestinal involvement mainly manifests with the development of megaesophagus, characterized by dysphagia and regurgitation, and megacolon, leading to constipation and fecal retention.[86] The pathogenesis of gastrointestinal disease involves denervation due to destruction and fibrosis of the submucosal and myenteric nerve plexuses.[87] The development of gastrointestinal manifestations versus cardiac manifestations may be related to strain differences in the parasite, as the various manifestations differ based on the locales where the infection is acquired with more gastrointestinal disease seen in individuals acquiring disease in South America rather than Latin America.[88]

Disease is not limited to the heart and gut. Rarely it also leads to megaureters, megabladder, megagallbladder, and bronchiectasis. Adult patients may experience reduced night vision.[89]

A reactivation of Chagas disease is now described in patients who become immunocompromised through infection with certain pathogens, such as HIV-1, or through immunosuppressive medications. Patients suffering from HIV/AIDS exhibit signs and symptoms of the acute phase of infection, and if left untreated, usually die from overwhelming infection due to *T. cruzi* or neurologic involvement.[74, 90] Patients in the chronic phase of infection that acquire HIV can experience a reactivation of *T. cruzi* resembling the acute phase of the disease.[91]

Congenital Chagas Disease

Congenital Chagas disease mostly occurs if infants are born to infected mothers with acute Chagas disease. It is estimated that 1-10% of infants born to an infected mother will acquire congenital Chagas disease.[92] More recent estimates place the vertical transmission rate at around 5%.[31] Unfortunately transmission can also occur during chronic Chagas disease, as was documented in the United States in August of 2010.[93] Congenital infection can lead to acute disease or may progress to chronic disease in the absence of treatment.[94]

Diagnosis

The approach to diagnosis is based on the stage of disease. In acute disease the level of parasites in the blood is high enough that trypomastigotes can be detected on examination of Giemsa-stained blood smears, and both a thin and thick smear should be ordered (Fig. 7.3).[95] The use of PCR has greatly facilitated diagnosis in patients, as it becomes positive earlier in the disease and has improved sensitivity over microscopic evaluation of blood smears.[95-97]

For chronic disease the diagnosis is usually based on the detection of serum IgG.[98] Since no currently available tests for Chagas serology have the required specificity, a diagnosis is based on two positive diagnostic serology tests.[99] It is of note that many patients present to their physician after a positive screening test result when they are donating blood. This screening test is not a diagnostic test and

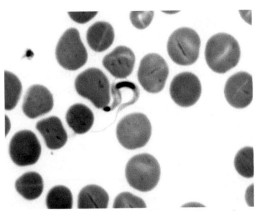

Figure 7.6. Trypomastigote of *T. cruzi*. 20μm x 3μm.

would not count as one of the two diagnostic test results. PCR tests are not routinely employed to diagnose chronic disease. Parasites can also be identified microscopically from biopsy samples of infected tissue. Inoculating blood from suspected individuals into susceptible animals can reveal the organism, but this approach presents too much impracticality for most diagnostic facilities. Xenodiagnosis, employing uninfected kissing bugs, allowing them to feed on the patient, then dissecting the bugs some days later, can also reveal the presence of parasites in chronically infected individuals, but it is a special test requiring extensive laboratory infrastructure and technical assistance. Currently xenodiagnosis is rarely used.

Treatment

The only drugs with proven efficacy against T. *cruzi* are nifurtimox and benznidazole.[99-101] Both drugs are associated with high toxicity and incomplete cure rates in adults, especially when they are used to treat the chronic phase of the infection.[101] Benznidazole has been recommended for use in children who have either just acquired the disease (i.e., congenitally), or who are in the chronic phase of their infection.[102] Nifurtimox disrupts T. cruzi metabolism of carbohydrates, while benznidazole may promote lethal double stranded DNA breaks in T. *cruzi*.[103, 104] Both drugs can cause severe side effects including skin rashes, and hematologic disturbances just to name a few. Also prolonged treatments are required lasting 1-2 months, and many patients (as many as one in five) cannot tolerate full treatment courses. Additional new and sobering information indicates that once heart involvement begins, it may be too late for the drugs to have a clinical impact.[105] There is an urgent need to develop improved drugs and clinical algorithms. Newer drugs are being developed, some of which take advantage of known metabolic pathways.[106, 107] Another approach involves the development of a therapeutic vaccine to treat patients in their indeterminant phase in order to prevent or delay the onset of Chagas cardiomyopathy.[108] Such a vaccine is believed to be both cost-effective and cost-saving.[109]

Heart transplantation as a treatment modality for the cardiomyopathic aspects of Chagas disease has been in vogue for as long as heart transplantation has been tried in humans.[110, 111] In fact, the fourth recipient ever to receive a heart transplant suffered from chronic T. *cruzi* infection. Fortunately current immunosuppressive regimens have allowed for successful transplantation in a large number of patients that had developed cardiac manifestations of Chagas disease.[110, 111]

Despite a paucity of well controlled trials on the efficacy of treatment for acute Chagas disease, there is a general consensus that treatment should be given for both acute and congenitally acquired disease.[112] Treatment decisions for chronic Chagas are based on patient's age and overall health. It is generally recommended that patients with indeterminant stage Chagas who are under the age of 50 undergo treatment. Treatment for patients over the age of 50 should be individualized based on risks and benefits. Treatment for patients with advanced cardiomyopathy or gastrointestinal manifestations is currently not recommended. Unfortunately these recommendations for treatment of chronic disease are not based on well-controlled trials and a study treating patients with established cardiomyopathy did not show any positive impact on disease progression.[105]

Prevention and Control

Control of Chagas disease depends upon interfering with two major routes of transmission; vector-borne and transfusion. Control of vectors, by prudent use of insecticides (pyrethroids), has significantly reduced transmission of *T. cruzi* in Brazil and Chile.[113, 114] Unfortunately, this trend has been slow to spread to neighboring countries and there is now evidence of insecticide resistance.[115] Prevalence remains high throughout Central and South America. Transfusion-induced infection is a problem, especially in countries where *T. cruzi* is not vector-borne, complicating the control of disease.[116] Blood bank screening for *T. cruzi* should be mandatory in all countries experiencing high rates of immigration from South and Central America. In the US there is currently selective screening of blood using serological testing to reduce the chance of transfusion related transmission of Chagas disease.[117] It is recommended that paid blood donors be banned in all countries in which Chagas disease is endemic.[116] A more permanent solution, and one that interfaces well with the concepts of medical ecology, is building better housing for the poor.[118, 119]

Houses constructed without a thatched roof, the slat board wood siding, or rough textured wall surfaces inside the house are relatively safe from kissing bug colonization. Keeping pet dogs and pigs out of the house further reduces the chances of acquiring Chagas disease.[120]

The risk to travelers is thought to be low, although there have been documented cases in travelers to endemic areas.[121] It is recommended that travellers sleep under insecticide-treated bednets and avoid sleeping in dwellings that provide habitats favoring the survival and reproduction of kissing bugs.[122] Consuming sugar cane juice or fruit drinks while on vacation on the beaches of Brazil, Central America or other parts of South America are likely low risk activities despite the occasional outbreaks reported.[28-30]

References

1. de Souza, W.; de Carvalho, T. M.; Barrias, E. S., Review on Trypanosoma cruzi: Host Cell Interaction. *Int J Cell Biol* **2010**, *2010*.

2. De Araujo, V. A.; Boite, M. C.; Cupolillo, E.; Jansen, A. M.; Roque, A. L., Mixed infection in the anteater Tamandua tetradactyla (Mammalia: Pilosa) from Para State, Brazil: Trypanosoma cruzi, T. rangeli and Leishmania infantum. *Parasitology* **2013**, *140* (4), 455-60.

3. Rocha, F. L.; Roque, A. L.; Arrais, R. C.; Santos, J. P.; Lima Vdos, S.; Xavier, S. C.; Cordeir-Estrela, P.; D'Andrea, P. S.; Jansen, A. M., Trypanosoma cruzi TcI and TcII transmission among wild carnivores, small mammals and dogs in a conservation unit and surrounding areas, Brazil. *Parasitology* **2013**, *140* (2), 160-70.

4. Rocha, F. L.; Roque, A. L.; de Lima, J. S.; Cheida, C. C.; Lemos, F. G.; de Azevedo, F. C.; Arrais, R. C.; Bilac, D.; Herrera, H. M.; Mourao, G.; Jansen, A. M., Trypanosoma cruzi infection in neotropical wild carnivores (Mammalia: Carnivora): at the top of the T. cruzi transmission chain. *PLoS One* **2013**, *8* (7), e67463.

5. Roque, A. L.; Xavier, S. C.; Gerhardt, M.; Silva, M. F.; Lima, V. S.; D'Andrea, P. S.; Jansen, A. M., Trypanosoma cruzi among wild and domestic mammals in different areas of the Abaetetuba municipality (Para State, Brazil), an endemic Chagas disease transmission area. *Vet Parasitol* **2013**, *193* (1-3), 71-7.

6. Klotz, S. A.; Dorn, P. L.; Mosbacher, M.; Schmidt, J. O., Kissing bugs in the United States: risk for vector-borne disease in humans. *Environ Health Insights* **2014**, *8* (Suppl 2), 49-59.

7. Bocchi, E. A., Heart failure in South America. *Curr Cardiol Rev* **2013**, *9* (2), 147-56.

8. Dokainish, H.; Teo, K.; Zhu, J.; Roy, A.; AlHabib, K. F.; ElSayed, A.; Palileo-Villaneuva, L.; Lopez-Jaramillo, P.; Karaye, K.; Yusoff, K.; Orlandini, A.; Sliwa, K.; Mondo, C.; Lanas, F.; Prabhakaran, D.; Badr, A.; Elmaghawry, M.; Damasceno, A.; Tibazarwa, K.; Belley-Cote, E.; Balasubramanian, K.; Yacoub, M. H.; Huffman, M. D.; Harkness, K.; Grinvalds, A.; McKelvie, R.; Yusuf, S.; Investigators, I.-C., Heart Failure in Africa, Asia, the Middle East and South America:

The INTER-CHF study. *Int J Cardiol* **2015**, *204*, 133-141.

9.   Bocchi, E. A.; Guimaraes, G.; Tarasoutshi, F.; Spina, G.; Mangini, S.; Bacal, F., Cardiomyopathy, adult valve disease and heart failure in South America. *Heart* **2009**, *95* (3), 181-9.

10. Schiffier, R. I.; Mansur, G. P., Indigenous Chagas' disease (American trypanosomiasis) in California. *JAMA* **1984**, *251* 2983-2984.

11. Woody, N. C.; Woody, H. B., American trypanosomiasis (Chagas' disease): first indigenous case in the USA. *JAMA* **1955**, *159*.

12. Global Burden of Disease Study, C., Global, regional, and national incidence, prevalence, and years lived with disability for 301 acute and chronic diseases and injuries in 188 countries, 1990-2013: a systematic analysis for the Global Burden of Disease Study 2013. *Lancet* **2015**, *386* (9995), 743-800.

13. Lee, B. Y.; Bacon, K. M.; Bottazzi, M. E.; Hotez, P. J., Global economic burden of Chagas disease: a computational simulation model. *Lancet Infect Dis* **2013**, *13* (4), 342-8.

14. http://www.who.int/wer/2015/wer9006.pdf.

15. Hotez, P. J.; Dumonteil, E.; Betancourt Cravioto, M.; Bottazzi, M. E.; Tapia-Conyer, R.; Meymandi, S.; Karunakara, U.; Ribeiro, I.; Cohen, R. M.; Pecoul, B., An unfolding tragedy of Chagas disease in North America. *PLoS neglected tropical diseases* **2013**, *7* (10), e2300.

16. Garcia, M. N.; Aguilar, D.; Gorchakov, R.; Rossmann, S. N.; Montgomery, S. P.; Rivera, H.; Woc-Colburn, L.; Hotez, P. J.; Murray, K. O., Evidence of autochthonous Chagas disease in southeastern Texas. *Am J Trop Med Hyg* **2015**, *92* (2), 325-30.

17. Schmunis, G. A.; Yadon, Z. E., Chagas disease: a Latin American health problem becoming a world health problem. *Acta Trop* **2010**, *115* (1-2), 14-21.

18. Martins-Melo, F. R.; Ramos, A. N., Jr.; Alencar, C. H.; Heukelbach, J., Prevalence of Chagas disease in Brazil: a systematic review and meta-analysis. *Acta tropica* **2014**, *130*, 167-74.

19. Reiche, E. M.; Inouye, M. M.; Pontello, R.; Morimoto, H. K.; Itow Jankevicius, S.; Matsuo, T.; Jankevicius, J. V., Seropositivity for anti-trypanosoma cruzi antibodies among blood donors of the "Hospital Universitário Regional do Norte do Paraná", Londrina, Brazil. *Revista do Instituto de Medicina Tropical de Sao Paulo* **1996**, *38* (3), 233-40.

20. Koberle, F., Chagas' disease and Chagas' syndromes: pathology of American trypanosomiasis. *Adv Parasitol* **1968**, *6*, 63-116.

21. Pecoul, B.; Batista, C.; Stobbaerts, E.; Ribeiro, I.; Vilasanjuan, R.; Gascon, J.; Pinazo, M. J.; Moriana, S.; Gold, S.; Pereiro, A.; Navarro, M.; Torrico, F.; Bottazzi, M. E.; Hotez, P. J., The BENEFIT Trial: Where Do We Go from Here? *PLoS Negl Trop Dis* **2016**, *10* (2), e0004343.

22. Wendel, S., Transfusion-transmitted Chagas' disease. *Current opinion in hematology* **1998**, *5* (6), 406-11.

23. Blejer, J. L.; Saguier, M. C.; Dinapoli, R. A.; Salamone, H. J., [Prevalence of Trypanosoma cruzi antibodies in blood donors]. *Medicina* **1999**, *59* (2), 129-32.

24. Dictar, M.; Sinagra, A.; Verón, M. T.; Luna, C.; Dengra, C.; De Rissio, A.; Bayo, R.; Ceraso, D.; Segura, E.; Koziner, B.; Riarte, A., Recipients and donors of bone marrow transplants suffering from Chagas' disease: management and preemptive therapy of parasitemia. *Bone marrow transplantation* **1998**, *21* (4), 391-3.

25. Carvalho, M. F.; de Franco, M. F.; Soares, V. A., Amastigotes forms of Trypanosoma cruzi detected in a renal allograft. *Revista do Instituto de Medicina Tropical de Sao Paulo* **1997**, *39* (4), 223-6.

26. Altclas, J.; Jaimovich, G.; Milovic, V.; Klein, F.; Feldman, L., Chagas' disease after bone marrow transplantation. *Bone marrow transplantation* **1996**, *18* (2), 447-8.

27. Russomando, G.; de Tomassone, M. M.; de Guillen, I.; Acosta, N.; Vera, N.; Almiron, M.; Candia, N.; Calcena, M. F.; Figueredo, A., Treatment of congenital Chagas' disease diagnosed and followed up by the polymerase chain reaction. *The American journal of tropical medicine and hygiene* **1998**, *59* (3), 487-91.

28. Shikanai-Yasuda, M. A.; Carvalho, N. B., Oral transmission of Chagas disease. *Clinical infectious diseases : an official publication of the Infectious Diseases Society of America* **2012**, *54* (6), 845-52.

29. Benitez, J. A.; Araujo, B.; Contreras, K.; Rivas, M.; Ramirez, P.; Guerra, W.; Calderon, N.; Ascaso

Terren, C.; Barrera, R.; Rodriguez-Morales, A. J., Urban outbreak of acute orally acquired Chagas disease in Tachira, Venezuela. *J Infect Dev Ctries* **2013**, *7* (8), 638-41.

30. Alarcon de Noya, B.; Diaz-Bello, Z.; Colmenares, C.; Ruiz-Guevara, R.; Mauriello, L.; Zavala-Jaspe, R.; Suarez, J. A.; Abate, T.; Naranjo, L.; Paiva, M.; Rivas, L.; Castro, J.; Marques, J.; Mendoza, I.; Acquatella, H.; Torres, J.; Noya, O., Large urban outbreak of orally acquired acute Chagas disease at a school in Caracas, Venezuela. *The Journal of infectious diseases* **2010**, *201* (9), 1308-15.

31. Gebrekristos, H. T.; Buekens, P., Mother-to-Child Transmission of Trypanosoma cruzi. *J Pediatric Infect Dis Soc* **2014**, *3 Suppl 1*, S36-40.

32. Steindel, M.; Kramer Pacheco, L.; Scholl, D.; Soares, M.; de Moraes, M. H.; Eger, I.; Kosmann, C.; Sincero, T. C.; Stoco, P. H.; Murta, S. M.; de Carvalho-Pinto, C. J.; Grisard, E. C., Characterization of Trypanosoma cruzi isolated from humans, vectors, and animal reservoirs following an outbreak of acute human Chagas disease in Santa Catarina State, Brazil. *Diagnostic microbiology and infectious disease* **2008**, *60* (1), 25-32.

33. Yabsley, M. J.; Brown, E. L.; Roellig, D. M., Evaluation of the Chagas Stat-Pak assay for detection of Trypanosoma cruzi antibodies in wildlife reservoirs. *The Journal of parasitology* **2009**, *95* (3), 775-7.

34. Peterson, A. T.; Sanchez-Cordero, V.; Beard, C. B.; Ramsey, J. M., Ecologic niche modeling and potential reservoirs for Chagas disease, Mexico. *Emerging infectious diseases* **2002**, *8* (7), 662-7.

35. Lima, M. M.; Sarquis, O.; de Oliveira, T. G.; Gomes, T. F.; Coutinho, C.; Daflon-Teixeira, N. F.; Toma, H. K.; Britto, C.; Teixeira, B. R.; D'Andrea, P. S.; Jansen, A. M.; Boia, M. N.; Carvalho-Costa, F. A., Investigation of Chagas disease in four periurban areas in northeastern Brazil: epidemiologic survey in man, vectors, non-human hosts and reservoirs. *Trans R Soc Trop Med Hyg* **2012**, *106* (3), 143-9.

36. Olsen, P. F.; Shoemaker, J. P.; Turner, H. F.; Hays, K. L., Incidence of Trypanosoma Cruzi (Chagas) in Wild Vectors and Reservoirs in East-Central Alabama. *The Journal of parasitology* **1964**, *50*, 599-603.

37. Zeledon, R.; Solano, G.; Saenz, G.; Swartzwelder, J. C., Wild reservoirs of Trypanosoma cruzi with special mention of the opossum, Didelphis marsupialis, and its role in the epidemiology of Chagas' disease in an endemic area of Costa Rica. *The Journal of parasitology* **1970**, *56* (1), 38.

38. Chile and Brazil to be certified free of transmission of Chagas' Disease. Tropical Diseases Research News (WHO publication). No. 59 June. **1999**.

39. Chagas, C., Nova trypanozomiaze humana: estudos sobre a morfolojia e o ciclo evolutivo do Schizotrypanum cruzi n. *gen n spec ajente etiolojico de nova entidade morbida de homem Mem Inst Oswaldo Cruz* **1909**, *1 SRC - GoogleScholar*, 159-218.

40. Perleth, M., The discovery of Chagas' disease and the formation of the early Chagas' disease concept. *History and philosophy of the life sciences* **1997**, *19* (2), 211-36.

41. Brumpt, A. J. E., Le Trypanosoma cruzi evolue chez Conorhinus megistus. *Cimex ectularius Cimex boueti et Ornithodorus moubata cycle evolutif de ce parasite Bull Soc Pathol Exot* **1912**, *5*, 360-364.

42. Vianna, G., Contribuicao para o estudo da anatomia patolojica da anatomia patolojica 'moletia de Carlos Chagas" (esquizotripanoze humana ou tireodite parazitaria). . *Mem Inst Oswaldo Cruz* **1916**, *3*, 276-294.

43. Gull, K., The biology of kinetoplastid parasites: insights and challenges from genomics and post-genomics. *International journal for parasitology* **2001**, *31* (5-6), 443-52.

44. Miles, M. A.; Feliciangeli, M. D.; de Arias, A. R., American trypanosomiasis (Chagas' disease) and the role of molecular epidemiology in guiding control strategies. *BMJ (Clinical research ed.)* **2003**, *326* (7404), 1444-8.

45. Mortara, R. A.; Andreoli, W. K.; Taniwaki, N. N.; Fernandes, A. B.; Silva, C. V. d.; Fernandes, M. C. D. C.; L'Abbate, C.; Silva, S. d., Mammalian cell invasion and intracellular trafficking by Trypanosoma cruzi infective forms. *Anais da Academia Brasileira de Ciencias* **2005**, *77* (1), 77-94.

46. Senior, K., Chagas disease: moving towards global elimination. *Lancet Infect Dis* **2007**, *7* (9), 572.

47. Nichols, N.; Green, T. W., Allergic reactions to "kissing bug" bites. *Calif Med* **1963,** *98,* 267-8.

48. Campbell, A. K.; Matthews, S. B., Darwin's illness revealed. *Postgraduate medical journal* **2005,** *81* (954), 248-51.

49. Kleshchenko, Y. Y.; Moody, T. N.; Furtak, V. A.; Ochieng, J.; Lima, M. F.; Villalta, F., Human galectin-3 promotes Trypanosoma cruzi adhesion to human coronary artery smooth muscle cells. *Infection and immunity* **2004,** *72* (11), 6717-21.

50. Ortega-Barria, E.; Pereira, M. E., Entry of Trypanosoma cruzi into eukaryotic cells. *Infectious agents and disease* **1992,** *1* (3), 136-45.

51. Herrera, E. M.; Ming, M.; Ortega-Barria, E.; Pereira, M. E., Mediation of Trypanosoma cruzi invasion by heparan sulfate receptors on host cells and penetrin counter-receptors on the trypanosomes. *Molecular and biochemical parasitology* **1994,** *65* (1), 73-83.

52. Neira, I.; Silva, F. A.; Cortez, M.; Yoshida, N., Involvement of Trypanosoma cruzi metacyclic trypomastigote surface molecule gp82 in adhesion to gastric mucin and invasion of epithelial cells. *Infection and immunity* **2003,** *71* (1), 557-61.

53. Calvo Mendez, M. L.; Torres, B.; Aguilar, R., Calvo Nogueda Alejandre The oral route: an access port for Trypanosoma cruzi. *Rev Latinoam Microbiol* **1992,** *34,* 39-42.

54. Santos, C. C.; Sant'anna, C.; Terres, A.; Cunha-e-Silva, N. L.; Scharfstein, J.; de A Lima, A. P. C., Chagasin, the endogenous cysteine-protease inhibitor of Trypanosoma cruzi, modulates parasite differentiation and invasion of mammalian cells. *Journal of cell science* **2005,** *118* (Pt 5), 901-15.

55. Aoki, M. P.; Guinazu, N. L.; J., Cruzipain, a major Trypanosoma cruzi antigen, promotes arginase-2 expression and survival of neonatal mouse cardiomyocytes. *Am Cell Physiol* **2003,** *286,* C206-12.

56. Garcia, E. S.; Azambuja, P., Development and interactions of Trypanosoma cruzi within the insect vector. *Parasitology today (Personal ed.)* **1991,** *7* (9), 240-4.

57. Pereira, M. E.; Loures, M. A.; Villalta, F.; Andrade, A. F., Lectin receptors as markers for Trypanosoma cruzi. Developmental stages and a study of the interaction of wheat germ agglutinin with sialic acid residues on epimastigote cells. *The Journal of experimental medicine* **1980,** *152* (5), 1375-92.

58. Sher, A.; Snary, D., Specific inhibition of the morphogenesis of Trypanosoma cruzi by a monoclonal antibody. *Nature London* **1985,** *300,* 639-640.

59. Majumder, S.; Kierszenbaum, F., Mechanisms of Trypanosoma cruzi-induced down-regulation of lymphocyte function. Inhibition of transcription and expression of IL-2 receptor gamma (p64IL-2R) and beta (p70IL-2R) chain molecules in activated normal human lymphocytes. *Journal of immunology (Baltimore, Md. : 1950)* **1996,** *156* (10), 3866-74.

60. Van Overtvelt, L.; Vanderheyde, N.; Verhasselt, V.; Ismaili, J.; De Vos, L.; Goldman, M.; Willems, F.; Vray, B., Trypanosoma cruzi infects human dendritic cells and prevents their maturation: inhibition of cytokines, HLA-DR, and costimulatory molecules. *Infection and immunity* **1999,** *67* (8), 4033-40.

61. Ferreira, V.; Molina, M. C.; Valck, C.; Rojas, A.; Aguilar, L.; Ramírez, G.; Schwaeble, W.; Ferreira, A., Role of calreticulin from parasites in its interaction with vertebrate hosts. *Molecular immunology* **2004,** *40* (17), 1279-91.

62. Beucher, M.; Meira, W. S. F.; Zegarra, V.; Galvão, L. M. C.; Chiari, E.; Norris, K. A., Expression and purification of functional, recombinant Trypanosoma cruzi complement regulatory protein. *Protein expression and purification* **2003,** *27* (1), 19-26.

63. Duthie, M. S.; Kahn, M.; White, M.; Kapur, R. P.; Kahn, S. J., Both CD1d antigen presentation and interleukin-12 are required to activate natural killer T cells during Trypanosoma cruzi infection. *Infection and immunity* **2005,** *73* (3), 1890-4.

64. Vespa, G. N.; Cunha, F. Q.; Silva, J. S., Nitric oxide is involved in control of Trypanosoma cruzi-induced parasitemia and directly kills the parasite in vitro. *Infection and immunity* **1994,** *62* (11), 5177-82.

65. Martin, D. L.; Tarleton, R. L., Antigen-specific T cells maintain an effector memory phenotype during persistent Trypanosoma cruzi infection. *Journal of immunology (Baltimore, Md. : 1950)* **2005,** *174* (3), 1594-601.

66. Bern, C., Antitrypanosomal therapy for chronic Chagas' disease. *N Engl J Med* **2011,** *364* (26), 2527-34.
67. Parada, H.; Carrasco, H. A.; Añez, N.; Fuenmayor, C.; Inglessis, I., Cardiac involvement is a constant finding in acute Chagas' disease: a clinical, parasitological and histopathological study. *International journal of cardiology* **1997,** *60* (1), 49-54.
68. de Andrade, A. L.; Zicker, F.; Rassi, A.; Rassi, A. G.; Oliveira, R. M.; Silva, S. A.; de Andrade, S. S.; Martelli, C. M., Early electrocardiographic abnormalities in Trypanosoma cruzi-seropositive children. *The American journal of tropical medicine and hygiene* **1998,** *59* (4), 530-4.
69. Tarleton, R. L., Chagas disease: a role for autoimmunity? *Trends in parasitology* **2003,** *19* (10), 447-51.
70. Machado, F. S.; Tyler, K. M.; Brant, F.; Esper, L.; Teixeira, M. M.; Tanowitz, H. B., Pathogenesis of Chagas disease: time to move on. *Front Biosci (Elite Ed)* **2012,** *4*, 1743-58.
71. Vermelho, A. B.; de Meirelles, M. d. N.; Pereira, M. C.; Pohlentz, G.; Barreto-Bergter, E., Heart muscle cells share common neutral glycosphingolipids with Trypanosoma cruzi. *Acta tropica* **1997,** *64* (3-4), 131-43.
72. Cunha-Neto, E.; Coelho, V.; Guilherme, L.; Fiorelli, A.; Stolf, N.; Kalil, J., Autoimmunity in Chagas' disease. Identification of cardiac myosin-B13 Trypanosoma cruzi protein crossreactive T cell clones in heart lesions of a chronic Chagas' cardiomyopathy patient. *The Journal of clinical investigation* **1996,** *98* (8), 1709-12.
73. Roffe, E.; Silva, A. A.; J., Essential role of VLA-4/VCAM-1 pathway in the establishment of CD8+ T-cell-mediated Trypanosoma cruzi-elicited meningoencephalitis. **2003,** *142* 17-30.
74. Yasukawa, K.; Patel, S. M.; Flash, C. A.; Stager, C. E.; Goodman, J. C.; Woc-Colburn, L., Trypanosoma cruzi meningoencephalitis in a patient with acquired immunodeficiency syndrome. *Am J Trop Med Hyg* **2014,** *91* (1), 84-5.
75. Anez, N.; Crisante, G.; Rojas, A., Update on Chagas' Disease in Venezuela-a review. *Mem Inst Oswaldo Cruz* **2004,** *99*, 781-7.
76. Kun, H.; Moore, A.; Mascola, L.; Steurer, F.; Lawrence, G.; Kubak, B.; Radhakrishna, S.; Leiby, D.; Herron, R.; Mone, T.; Hunter, R.; Kuehnert, M.; Chagas Disease in Transplant Recipients Investigation, T., Transmission of Trypanosoma cruzi by heart transplantation. *Clin Infect Dis* **2009,** *48* (11), 1534-40.
77. Tanowitz, H. B.; Machado, F. S.; Jelicks, L. A.; Shirani, J.; de Carvalho, A. C.; Spray, D. C.; Factor, S. M.; Kirchhoff, L. V.; Weiss, L. M., Perspectives on Trypanosoma cruzi-induced heart disease (Chagas disease). *Prog Cardiovasc Dis* **2009,** *51* (6), 524-39.
78. Andrade, D. V.; Gollob, K. J.; Dutra, W. O., Acute chagas disease: new global challenges for an old neglected disease. *PLoS Negl Trop Dis* **2014,** *8* (7), e3010.
79. Beltrao Hde, B.; Cerroni Mde, P.; Freitas, D. R.; Pinto, A. Y.; Valente Vda, C.; Valente, S. A.; Costa Ede, G.; Sobel, J., Investigation of two outbreaks of suspected oral transmission of acute Chagas disease in the Amazon region, Para State, Brazil, in 2007. *Trop Doct* **2009,** *39* (4), 231-2.
80. Dias, J. C., [Cecilio Romana, Romana's sign and Chagas' disease]. *Rev Soc Bras Med Trop* **1997,** *30* (5), 407-13.
81. Delaporte, F., Romana's sign. *J Hist Biol* **1997,** *30* (3), 357-66.
82. Gutierrez, F. R.; Guedes, P. M.; Gazzinelli, R. T.; Silva, J. S., The role of parasite persistence in pathogenesis of Chagas heart disease. *Parasite Immunol* **2009,** *31* (11), 673-85.
83. Engman, D. M.; Leon, J. S., Pathogenesis of Chagas heart disease: role of autoimmunity. *Acta Trop* **2002,** *81* (2), 123-32.
84. Melo, T. G.; Almeida, D. S.; de Meirelles, M. d. N. S. L.; Pereira, M. C., Trypanosoma cruzi infection disrupts vinculin costameres in cardiomyocytes. *European journal of cell biology* **2004,** *83* (10), 531-40.
85. Jorge, M. T.; Macedo, T. A. A.; Janones, R. S.; Carizzi, D. P.; Heredia, R. A. G.; Achá, R. E. S., Types of arrhythmia among cases of American trypanosomiasis, compared with those in other cardiology patients. *Annals of tropical medicine and parasitology* **2003,** *97* (2), 139-48.
86. Meneghelli, U. G., Chagasic enteropathy. *Revista da Sociedade Brasileira de Medicina Tropical* **2004,** *37* (3), 252-60.

87. Jabari, S.; de Oliveira, E. C.; Brehmer, A.; da Silveira, A. B., Chagasic megacolon: enteric neurons and related structures. *Histochem Cell Biol* **2014**, *142* (3), 235-44.

88. Pinazo, M. J.; Lacima, G.; Elizalde, J. I.; Posada, E. J.; Gimeno, F.; Aldasoro, E.; Valls, M. E.; Gascon, J., Characterization of digestive involvement in patients with chronic T. cruzi infection in Barcelona, Spain. *PLoS Negl Trop Dis* **2014**, *8* (8), e3105.

89. Matsumoto, S. C.; Labovsky, V.; Roncoroni, M.; Guida, M. C.; Giménez, L.; Mitelman, J.; Gori, H.; Jurgelevicius, R.; Grillo, A.; Manfredi, P.; Levin, M. J.; Paveto, C., Retinal dysfunction in patients with chronic Chagas' disease is associated to anti-Trypanosoma cruzi antibodies that cross-react with rhodopsin. *FASEB journal : official publication of the Federation of American Societies for Experimental Biology* **2006**, *20* (3), 550-2.

90. Antunes, A. C. M.; Cecchini, F. M. d. L.; Bolli, F. v. B.; Oliveira, P. P. d.; Reboucas, R. G.; Monte, T. L.; Fricke, D., Cerebral trypanosomiasis and AIDS. *Arquivos de neuro-psiquiatria* **2002**, *60* (3-B), 730-3.

91. Harms, G.; Feldmeier, H., The impact of HIV infection on tropical diseases. *Infectious disease clinics of North America* **2005**, *19* (1), 121-35, ix.

92. Yadon, Z. E.; Schmunis, G. A., Congenital Chagas disease: estimating the potential risk in the United States. *Am J Trop Med Hyg* **2009**, *81* (6), 927-33.

93. Centers for Disease, C.; Prevention, Congenital transmission of Chagas disease - Virginia, 2010. *MMWR Morb Mortal Wkly Rep* **2012**, *61* (26), 477-9.

94. Carlier, Y.; Torrico, F.; Sosa-Estani, S.; Russomando, G.; Luquetti, A.; Freilij, H.; Albajar Vinas, P., Congenital Chagas disease: recommendations for diagnosis, treatment and control of newborns, siblings and pregnant women. *PLoS Negl Trop Dis* **2011**, *5* (10), e1250.

95. Rosenblatt, J. E., Laboratory diagnosis of infections due to blood and tissue parasites. *Clin Infect Dis* **2009**, *49* (7), 1103-8.

96. Britto, C.; Cardoso, M. A.; Vanni, C. M.; Hasslocher-Moreno, A.; Xavier, S. S.; Oelemann, W.; Santoro, A.; Pirmez, C.; Morel, C. M.; Wincker, P., Polymerase chain reaction detection of Trypanosoma cruzi in human blood samples as a tool for diagnosis and treatment evaluation. *Parasitology* **1995**, *110 (Pt 3)*, 241-7.

97. Junqueira, A. C.; Chiari, E.; Wincker, P., Comparison of the polymerase chain reaction with two classical parasitological methods for the diagnosis of Chagas disease in an endemic region of north-eastern Brazil. *Transactions of the Royal Society of Tropical Medicine and Hygiene* **1996**, *90* (2), 129-32.

98. Almeida, I. C.; Covas, D. T.; Soussumi, L. M.; Travassos, L. R., A highly sensitive and specific chemiluminescent enzyme-linked immunosorbent assay for diagnosis of active Trypanosoma cruzi infection. *Transfusion* **1997**, *37* (8), 850-7.

99. Bern, C., Chagas' Disease. *N Engl J Med* **2015**, *373* (5), 456-66.

100. Kirchhoff, L. V., Changing Epidemiology and Approaches to Therapy for Chagas Disease. *Current infectious disease reports* **2003**, *5* (1), 59-65.

101. Cerecetto, H.; González, M., Chemotherapy of Chagas' disease: status and new developments. *Current topics in medicinal chemistry* **2002**, *2* (11), 1187-213.

102. Schenone, H.; Contreras, M.; Solari, A.; García, A.; Rojas, A.; Lorca, M., [Nifurtimox treatment of chronic Chagasic infection in children]. *Revista medica de Chile* **2003**, *131* (9), 1089-90.

103. Diaz, E. G.; Montalto de Mecca, M.; Castro, J. A., Reactions of nifurtimox with critical sulfhydryl-containing biomolecules: their potential toxicological relevance. *Toxicol* **2004**, *24*, 189-95.

104. Rajao, M. A.; Furtado, C.; Alves, C. L.; Passos-Silva, D. G.; de Moura, M. B.; Schamber-Reis, B. L.; Kunrath-Lima, M.; Zuma, A. A.; Vieira-da-Rocha, J. P.; Garcia, J. B.; Mendes, I. C.; Pena, S. D.; Macedo, A. M.; Franco, G. R.; de Souza-Pinto, N. C.; de Medeiros, M. H.; Cruz, A. K.; Motta, M. C.; Teixeira, S. M.; Machado, C. R., Unveiling benznidazole's mechanism of action through overexpression of DNA repair proteins in Trypanosoma cruzi. *Environ Mol Mutagen* **2014**, *55* (4), 309-21.

105. Morillo, C. A.; Marin-Neto, J. A.; Avezum, A.; Sosa-Estani, S.; Rassi, A., Jr.; Rosas, F.; Villena, E.; Quiroz, R.; Bonilla, R.; Britto, C.; Guhl, F.; Velazquez, E.; Bonilla, L.; Meeks, B.; Rao-Melacini, P.; Pogue, J.; Mattos, A.; Lazdins, J.; Rassi, A.; Connolly, S. J.; Yusuf, S.; Investigators, B.,

Randomized Trial of Benznidazole for Chronic Chagas' Cardiomyopathy. *N Engl J Med* **2015**, *373* (14), 1295-306.

106. Engel, J. C.; Doyle, P. S.; Hsieh, I.; McKerrow, J. H., Cysteine protease inhibitors cure an experimental Trypanosoma cruzi infection. *The Journal of experimental medicine* **1998**, *188* (4), 725-34.

107. Choe, Y.; Brinen, L. S.; Price, M. S.; Engel, J. C.; Lange, M.; Grisostomi, C.; Weston, S. G.; Pallai, P. V.; Cheng, H.; Hardy, L. W.; Hartsough, D. S.; McMakin, M.; Tilton, R. F.; Baldino, C. M.; Craik, C. S., Development of alpha-keto-based inhibitors of cruzain, a cysteine protease implicated in Chagas disease. *Bioorganic & medicinal chemistry* **2005**, *13* (6), 2141-56.

108. Dumonteil, E.; Bottazzi, M. E.; Zhan, B.; Heffernan, M. J.; Jones, K.; Valenzuela, J. G.; Kamhawi, S.; Ortega, J.; Rosales, S. P.; Lee, B. Y.; Bacon, K. M.; Fleischer, B.; Slingsby, B. T.; Cravioto, M. B.; Tapia-Conyer, R.; Hotez, P. J., Accelerating the development of a therapeutic vaccine for human Chagas disease: rationale and prospects. *Expert Rev Vaccines* **2012**, *11* (9), 1043-55.

109. Lee, B. Y.; Bacon, K. M.; Wateska, A. R.; Bottazzi, M. E.; Dumonteil, E.; Hotez, P. J., Modeling the economic value of a Chagas' disease therapeutic vaccine. *Hum Vaccin Immunother* **2012**, *8* (9), 1293-301.

110. de Carvalho, V. B.; Sousa, E. F.; Vila, J. H.; da Silva, J. P.; Caiado, M. R.; Araujo, S. R.; Macruz, R.; Zerbini, E. J., Heart transplantation in Chagas' disease. 10 years after the initial experience. *Circulation* **1996**, *94* (8), 1815-7.

111. Bocchi, E. A.; Bellotti, G.; Mocelin, A. O.; Uip, D.; Bacal, F.; Higuchi, M. L.; Amato-Neto, V.; Fiorelli, A.; Stolf, N. A.; Jatene, A. D.; Pileggi, F., Heart transplantation for chronic Chagas' heart disease. *The Annals of thoracic surgery* **1996**, *61* (6), 1727-33.

112. Rodriques Coura, J.; de Castro, S. L., A critical review on Chagas disease chemotherapy. *Mem Inst Oswaldo Cruz* **2002**, *97* (1), 3-24.

113. Schofield, C. J.; Diaz, J. C. P.; Baker, J. R.; Muller, R.; Rollinson, D., Advances in Parasitology. 1999; p 2-30.

114. Moncayo, A., Chagas disease: current epidemiological trends after the interruption of vectorial and transfusional transmission in the Southern Cone countries. *Memorias do Instituto Oswaldo Cruz* **2003**, *98* (5), 577-91.

115. Zerba, E. N., Susceptibility and resistance to insecticides of Chagas disease vectors. *Medicina (B Aires)* **1999**, *59 Suppl 2*, 41-6.

116. Schmunis, G. A.; Cruz, J. R., Safety of the blood supply in Latin America. *Clinical microbiology reviews* **2005**, *18* (1), 12-29.

117. Agapova, M.; Busch, M. P.; Custer, B., Cost-effectiveness of screening the US blood supply for Trypanosoma cruzi. *Transfusion* **2010**, *50* (10), 2220-32.

118. Chaudhuri, N., Interventions to improve children's health by improving the housing environment. *Reviews on environmental health* **2004**, *19* (3-4), 197-222.

119. Cecere, M. C.; Gürtler, R. E.; Canale, D. M.; Chuit, R.; Cohen, J. E., Effects of partial housing improvement and insecticide spraying on the reinfestation dynamics of Triatoma infestans in rural northwestern Argentina. *Acta tropica* **2002**, *84* (2), 101-16.

120. Cohen, J. E.; Gürtler, R. E., Modeling household transmission of American trypanosomiasis. *Science (New York, N.Y.)* **2001**, *293* (5530), 694-8.

121. Carter, Y. L.; Juliano, J. J.; Montgomery, S. P.; Qvarnstrom, Y., Acute Chagas disease in a returning traveler. *Am J Trop Med Hyg* **2012**, *87* (6), 1038-40.

122. Kroeger, A.; Villegas, E.; Ordonez-Gonzalez, J.; Pabon, E.; Scorza, J. V., Prevention of the transmission of Chagas' disease with pyrethroid-impregnated materials. *Am J Trop Med Hyg* **2003**, *68* (3), 307-11.

8. *Trichomonas vaginalis*
(Donné 1836)

Introduction

Trichomonas vaginalis is a flagellated, microaerophilic protozoan that is mainly transmitted from person to person by sexual contact.[1, 2] Although non-sexual transmission has been described, it is likely rare.[3] Its distribution is worldwide, with high incidence in areas with limited access to healthcare. Prevalence is over 25% in some sexually transmitted infection (STI) clinics in the United States.[4-6] *T. vaginalis* infects both males and females. In males, infection can be asymptomatic and typically lasts 10 days. Most infected females are also asymptomatic, but infection can induce clinical disease that includes vaginal itching, inflammation, and purulent discharge with infection lasting for years if untreated.[7] Women infected with *T. vaginalis* typically experience periods of discomfort, and untreated infection may lead to infertility, pelvic inflammatory disease, cervical neoplasia, and increased susceptibility to HIV-1 infection.[8-12] *T. vaginalis* can also infect the newborn during their passage through the birth canal of an infected woman.[13] Infants may experience ectopic infection in the respiratory tract and other sites, as well. There are no reservoir hosts and exposure does not lead to permanent immunity, so reinfection after treatment is common. Although drug-resistant *T. vaginalis* exists, most treatment failures result from noncompliance with therapy.[14] The genome of *T. vaginalis* was sequenced in 2007, and it is very large with approximately 60,000 protein-coding genes organized into 6 chromosomes.[15]

Historical Information

In 1837, Alfred Donné described the organism in purulent secretions from women but not the clinical aspects of infection, citing Dujardin's unpublished morphologic description of this flagellate.[16] Proof that *T. vaginalis* is indeed a pathogen came much later, in 1940, when John Kessel and co-workers inoculated healthy volunteers with *T. vaginalis*. Many of these individuals developed the signs and symptoms of the disease. The investigators were then able to match these symptoms with patients who were naturally infected.[17] This study also provided an accurate description of the pathologic findings of trichomoniasis.

Life Cycle

T. vaginalis exists mainly in the trophozoite stage measuring 10-25 μm by 7-8 μm (Fig. 8.1). *T. vaginalis* has no true cyst form, but a pseudocyst form has been recognized that may play a role in cervical neoplasia.[18, 19] The trophozoite is motile, and possesses four flagella projecting from the anterior portion, an undulating membrane formed by a posterior extending flagellum, and a rigid axostyle.[20] The axostyle is a sheet of microtubules believed to be involved in motility and mitosis.[21, 22] *T. vaginalis* has a simple, direct life cycle. The organism is acquired during

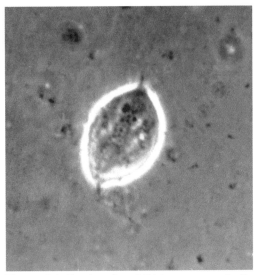

Figure 8.1. Trophozoite of *Trichomonas vaginalis*. Phase contrast. 20 μm x 10 μm.

Trichomonas vaginalis

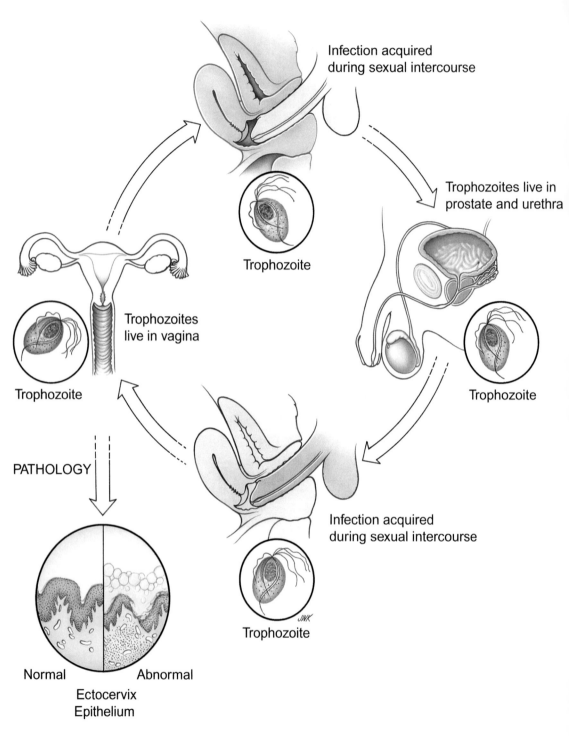

Infection acquired during sexual intercourse

Trophozoites live in prostate and urethra

Trophozoite

Trophozoite

Trophozoites live in vagina

Trophozoite

Infection acquired during sexual intercourse

PATHOLOGY

Trophozoite

Normal

Abnormal

Ectocervix Epithelium

sexual intercourse with an infected person. *T. vaginalis* then takes up residence in the female urethra, vagina, or endocervix, but can spread into the endometrium, adnexa and Bartholin glands. In men, *T. vaginalis* tends to infect the urethra and prostate. In order to cause infection, the trophozoites must be able to adhere to epithelial cells, and this is facilitated by adhesins and specific ligand-carbohydrate interactions.[23] Mannose and N-acetyl-glucosamine are two parasite membrane-associated sugar residues that are used for attachment.[24, 25] Secretion of lysosomal hydrolases, such as acid phosphatase, occurs at the host cell-parasite interface immediately following attachment.[26] These parasite enzymes are cytotoxic, causing the target cells to lyse, releasing their contents.[27] The cell debris is then ingested by the parasite. *T. vaginalis* phagocytize epithelial cells, erythrocytes, and bacteria. The parasite's main energy source is carbohydrates. *T. vaginalis* uses carbohydrases, including N-acetyl glucosaminidase, and α-mannosidase, to detach itself from the target cell membrane, and move on to the next cell.[28]

T. vaginalis reproduces by binary fission, and there is recent evidence for a sexual cycle, although no morphologically identifiable stage has been described.[29] Trophozoites secrete molecular hydrogen as a by-product of energy metabolism. Despite its ability to induce clinical disease, *T. vaginalis* is quite fragile and has a limited period of viability even in moist environments.

Cellular and Molecular Pathogenesis

T. vaginalis possesses an unusual organelle, the hydrogenosome (Figs. 8.2, 8.3), a subcellular organelle derived from an ancient mitochondrion, but which functions in anaerobic metabolism.[30-34] The hydrogenosome contains some of the necessary enzymes for processing glucose to acetate to molecular hydrogen, and putrescine biosynthesis.[35, 36]

The rest of the glycolytic cycle is cytosolic. Putrescine biosynthesis is essential for parasite growth. Inhibition of putrescine synthesis by analogues of putrescine kills the trophozoite.[37] Iron plays an important role in the attachment process.[23] Because *T. vaginalis* secretes proteases at the site of attachment, cell death is the usual outcome.[26] It is not known whether or not the release of molecular hydrogen into the vaginal tract has any pathological consequence other than producing foul-smelling exudates. Isolates of *T. vaginalis* from patients suffering clinical manifestations showed different capabilities with regards to their ability to induce damage in a mouse model, but the molecular basis for this variation is not fully understood.[38] *T. vaginalis* has been divided into two types, type 1 and type 2, based on pathogenicity that may be enhanced by the presence of *Trichomonas-virus*, a double-stranded RNA viruses (Toti-

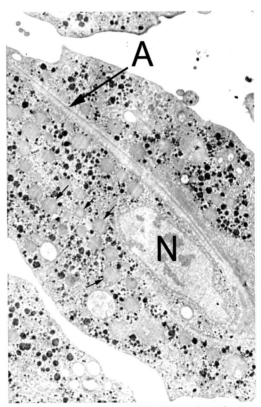

Figure 8.2. Transmission EM of a portion of a trophozoite of *T. vaginalis*. N=nucleus, A=axostyle. Arrows indicate hydrogenosomes. Courtesy H. Shio.

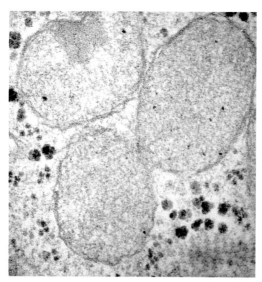

Figure 8.3. Higher magnification EM of hydrogenosomes. Courtesy H. Shio.

viridae), as well as *Mycoplasma hominis*. In some areas, the majority of isolates show co-infection with these organisms.[39, 40] The relevance of these co-infections is currently the subject of active investigation.

Clinical Disease

Approximately 20% of women infected are asymptomatic. Common clinical symptoms include; mild vaginal discomfort and dyspareunia, vaginal itching, burning on urination associated with thick, yellow, blood-tinged discharge and rarely incapacitating illness.[41, 42] Rarely, urticaria is a complication of heavy infection.[43] Infection with *T. vaginalis* typically raises the vaginal pH from 4.5 to greater than 5.[44]

On physical examination, women frequently present with *colpitis macularis* ("strawberry cervix") and vaginal and vulvar erythema.[45] All of these signs and symptoms are exacerbated during menstruation.

Symptomatic disease in males can involve the urethra as well as the prostate. When the prostate becomes infected, pain in the groin and dysuria may be reported.[46] Infection increases the chances of transmission of HIV-1, in part due to disruption of the vaginal wall.[47, 48]

Infants born of mothers harboring the infection often acquire infection upon passing through the birth canal.[13] Clinical consequences of infection in newborns include urinary tract infection (females only), and rare involvement of the lung, resulting in a pneumonia-like syndrome.[49, 50]

Diagnosis

The majority of men and women infected with *T. vaginalis* are asymptomatic with 85% of infected females and 77% of infected males reporting no symptoms.[51, 52]   Due to the high prevalence of asymptomatic infection, it is important to screen patients rather than rely on symptoms, as the majority of *T. vaginalis* infections would be missed. Diagnosis can be made by identifying the organism by microscopic observation, positive culture, rapid antigen testing, nucleic acid probe test, or by use of nucleic acid amplification testing (NAAT)[53] (Fig. C.5). If direct microscopy of wet mount preparations is to be employed this should be done immediately, as organisms only remain motile for approximately 10 minutes. The sensitivity of this approach is approximately 65% sensitivity but decreases when there is delay.[54] Culture offers higher sensitivity than wet mount but takes time, limiting its use as a point of care test. Rapid antigen testing offers a point of care option and currently these tests are commercially available, but may have variable degrees of sensitivity depending on the test selected.[55] Nucleic acid probe testing is a highly sensitive option for diagnosis that has demonstrated efficacy for testing of vaginal swabs or urine.[55] Diagnosis by NAAT is by far more sensitive than any other method, and is now the preferred method in most hospital parasitology diagnostic laboratories.[53]

Treatment

Metronidazole continues to be the drug of choice.[1] It can be given orally as a single 2 gram dose but is often given as a 7-day course at 500mg twice a day. Metronidazole is also available as a vaginal gel. Its use as an intra-vaginal suppository did poorly in a number of clinical trials.[45] The drug is typically well tolerated, but metallic taste, antabuse-like side effects with alcohol consumption and longer term treatment could have other toxicities.[56] Metronidazole is converted to active intermediates by hydrogenosome-associated pyruvate ferredoxin oxidoreductase and hydrogenase under anaerobic conditions. The parasite is inhibited from growing by exposure to those intermediates, but the precise biochemical mechanisms of the process are unknown. Resistant strains (approximately 2-5% of all infected infections) have inactive forms of pyruvate ferridoxin oxidoreductase and hydrogenase, deriving all their energy from glucose by alternate pathways.[57] Tinida-zole, an alternate drug for treating infection, is now available and may be better tolerated as a single dose option, but is more costly.[1] Reinfection is likely if the infected sexual partner is not treated concurrently. Treatment of the partner [expedited partner therapy (EPT)] results in a significant reduction in reinfection but in high prevalence settings reinfection is still seen.[58] Recurrence may represent reinfection rather than treatment failure but in refractory cases where drug resistance is suspected therapeutic options are available and drug sensitivity testing can be performed.

Prevention and Control

Use of a condom during sexual intercourse and limiting the number of sexual partners should reduce the risk of infection. Treating all sexual partners with metronidazole can be effective in some cases, particularly when the number of new sexual partners is low. Active screening is essential with the high rate of asymptomatic infections.

References

1. Schwebke, J. R.; Burgess, D., Trichomoniasis. *Clinical microbiology reviews* **2004**, *17* (4), 794-803, table of contents.
2. Lehker, M. W.; Alderete, J. F., Biology of trichomonosis. *Current opinion in infectious diseases* **2000**, *13* (1), 37-45.
3. Crucitti, T.; Jespers, V.; Mulenga, C.; Khondowe, S.; Vandepitte, J.; Buve, A., Non-sexual transmission of Trichomonas vaginalis in adolescent girls attending school in Ndola, Zambia. *PLoS One* **2011**, *6* (1), e16310.
4. Meites, E.; Llata, E.; Braxton, J.; Schwebke, J. R.; Bernstein, K. T.; Pathela, P.; Asbel, L. E.; Kerani, R. P.; Mettenbrink, C. J.; Weinstock, H. S., Trichomonas vaginalis in selected U.S. sexually transmitted disease clinics: testing, screening, and prevalence. *Sex Transm Dis* **2013**, *40* (11), 865-9.
5. Johnston, V. J.; Mabey, D. C., Global epidemiology and control of Trichomonas vaginalis. *Curr Opin Infect Dis* **2008**, *21* (1), 56-64.
6. Leitsch, D., Recent Advances in the Trichomonas vaginalis Field. *F1000Res* **2016**, *5*.
7. Krieger, J. N., Trichomoniasis in men: old issues and new data. *Sex Transm Dis* **1995**, *22* (2), 83-96.
8. Sayed el-Ahl, S. A.; el-Wakil, H. S.; Kamel, N. M.; Mahmoud, M. S., A preliminary study on the relationship between Trichomonas vaginalis and cervical cancer in Egyptian women. *J Egypt Soc Parasitol* **2002**, *32* (1), 167-78.
9. Moodley, P.; Wilkinson, D.; Connolly, C.; Moodley, J.; Sturm, A. W., Trichomonas vaginalis is associated with pelvic inflammatory disease in women infected with human immunodeficiency virus. *Clinical infectious diseases : an official publication of the Infectious Diseases Society of*

America **2002,** *34* (4), 519-22.

10.   El-Shazly, A. M.; El-Naggar, H. M.; Soliman, M.; El-Negeri, M.; El-Nemr, H. E.; Handousa, A. E.; Morsy, T. A., A study on Trichomoniasis vaginalis and female infertility. *J Egypt Soc Parasitol* **2001,** *31* (2), 545-53.

11.   Kissinger, P.; Adamski, A., Trichomoniasis and HIV interactions: a review. *Sex Transm Infect* **2013,** *89* (6), 426-33.

12.   Chesson, H. W.; Blandford, J. M.; Pinkerton, S. D., Estimates of the annual number and cost of new HIV infections among women attributable to trichomoniasis in the United States. *Sex Transm Dis* **2004,** *31* (9), 547-51.

13.   Smith, L. M.; Wang, M.; Zangwill, K.; Yeh, S., Trichomonas vaginalis infection in a premature newborn. *Journal of perinatology : official journal of the California Perinatal Association* **2002,** *22* (6), 502-3.

14.   Kulda, J., Trichomonads, hydrogenosomes and drug resistance. *International journal for parasitology* **1999,** *29* (2), 199-212.

15.   Carlton, J. M.; Hirt, R. P.; Silva, J. C.; Delcher, A. L.; Schatz, M.; Zhao, Q.; Wortman, J. R.; Bidwell, S. L.; Alsmark, U. C.; Besteiro, S.; Sicheritz-Ponten, T.; Noel, C. J.; Dacks, J. B.; Foster, P. G.; Simillion, C.; Van de Peer, Y.; Miranda-Saavedra, D.; Barton, G. J.; Westrop, G. D.; Muller, S.; Dessi, D.; Fiori, P. L.; Ren, Q.; Paulsen, I.; Zhang, H.; Bastida-Corcuera, F. D.; Simoes-Barbosa, A.; Brown, M. T.; Hayes, R. D.; Mukherjee, M.; Okumura, C. Y.; Schneider, R.; Smith, A. J.; Vanacova, S.; Villalvazo, M.; Haas, B. J.; Pertea, M.; Feldblyum, T. V.; Utterback, T. R.; Shu, C. L.; Osoegawa, K.; de Jong, P. J.; Hrdy, I.; Horvathova, L.; Zubacova, Z.; Dolezal, P.; Malik, S. B.; Logsdon, J. M., Jr.; Henze, K.; Gupta, A.; Wang, C. C.; Dunne, R. L.; Upcroft, J. A.; Upcroft, P.; White, O.; Salzberg, S. L.; Tang, P.; Chiu, C. H.; Lee, Y. S.; Embley, T. M.; Coombs, G. H.; Mottram, J. C.; Tachezy, J.; Fraser-Liggett, C. M.; Johnson, P. J., Draft genome sequence of the sexually transmitted pathogen Trichomonas vaginalis. *Science* **2007,** *315* (5809), 207-12.

16.   Donne, A.; R., C., Animalcules observes dans la matieres purulentes et le produit des secretions des or-ganes genitaux de l'homme et da Ia femme. *Seanc Acad Sci* **1837,** *3,* 385-386.

17.   Kessel, I. F.; Gafford, J. A.; J., Observations on the pathology of Trichomonas vaginitis and on vaginal implants with Trichomonas vaginalis and Trichomonas intestinalis. *Am Gynecol* **1940,** *39,* 1005-1014.

18.   Pereira-Neves, A.; Ribeiro, K. C.; Benchimol, M., Pseudocysts in trichomonads--new insights. *Protist* **2003,** *154* (3-4), 313-29.

19.   Afzan, M. Y.; Suresh, K., Pseudocyst forms of Trichomonas vaginalis from cervical neoplasia. *Parasitol Res* **2012,** *111* (1), 371-81.

20.   Kissinger, P., Trichomonas vaginalis: a review of epidemiologic, clinical and treatment issues. *BMC Infect Dis* **2015,** *15,* 307.

21.   Benchimol, M.; Diniz, J. A.; Ribeiro, K., The fine structure of the axostyle and its associations with organelles in Trichomonads. *Tissue Cell* **2000,** *32* (2), 178-87.

22.   Ribeiro, K. C.; Monteiro-Leal, L. H.; Benchimol, M., Contributions of the axostyle and flagella to closed mitosis in the protists Tritrichomonas foetus and Trichomonas vaginalis. *J Eukaryot Microbiol* **2000,** *47* (5), 481-92.

23.   Garcia, A. F.; Chang, T.-H.; Benchimol, M.; Klumpp, D. J.; Lehker, M. W.; Alderete, J. F., Iron and contact with host cells induce expression of adhesins on surface of Trichomonas vaginalis. *Molecular microbiology* **2003,** *47* (5), 1207-24.

24.   Mirhaghani, A.; Warton, A., Involvement of Trichomonas vaginalis surface-associated glycoconjugates in the parasite/target cell interaction. A quantitative electron microscopy study. *Parasitology research* **1998,** *84* (5), 374-81.

25.   Singh, B. N.; Lucas, J. J.; Beach, D. H.; Shin, S. T.; Gilbert, R. O., Adhesion of Tritrichomonas foetus to bovine vaginal epithelial cells. *Infection and immunity* **1999,** *67* (8), 3847-54.

26.   Lockwood, B. C.; North, M. J.; Coombs, G. H., The release of hydrolases from Trichomonas vaginalis and Tritrichomonas foetus. *Molecular and biochemical parasitology* **1988,** *30* (2), 135-42.

27.   Chen, W.; Cai, H.; Chen, J.; Zhong, X.; Chen, L., Study on ultrastructural cytochemistry and

pathogenic mechanism of Trichomonas vaginalis. *Chinese medical journal* **1996,** *109* (9), 695-9.

28. Savoia, D.; Martinotti, M. G., Secretory hydrolases of Trichomonas vaginalis. *Microbiologica* **1989,** *12* (2), 133-8.

29. Conrad, M. D.; Gorman, A. W.; Schillinger, J. A.; Fiori, P. L.; Arroyo, R.; Malla, N.; Dubey, M. L.; Gonzalez, J.; Blank, S.; Secor, W. E.; Carlton, J. M., Extensive genetic diversity, unique population structure and evidence of genetic exchange in the sexually transmitted parasite Trichomonas vaginalis. *PLoS Negl Trop Dis* **2012,** *6* (3), e1573.

30. Embley, T. M.; R., Giezen. M. Hydrogenosomes and mitochondria are two forms of the same fundamental organelle. *Phil Trans Lond* **2002,** *358,* 191-201.

31. Vanacova, S.; Liston, D. R.; Tachezy, J.; Johnson, P. J., Molecular biology of the amitochondriate parasites, Giardia intestinalis, Entamoeba histolytica and Trichomonas vaginalis. *International journal for parasitology* **2003,** *33* (3), 235-55.

32. PrDiaz, J. A.; Souza, W., De Purification and biochemical characterization of the hydrogenosomes of the flagellate protozoan Tritrichomonas foetus. *Eur J Cell Biol* **1997,** *74* (1), 85-91.

33. Williams, B. A. P.; Keeling, P. J., Cryptic organelles in parasitic protists and fungi. *Advances in parasitology* **2003,** *54,* 9-68.

34. Lindmark, D. G.; Muller, M., Hydrogenosome, a cytoplasmic organelle of the anaerobic flagellate Tritrichomonas foetus, and its role in pyruvate metabolism. *J Biol Chem* **1973,** *248* (22), 7724-8.

35. Wu, G.; Müller, M., Glycogen phosphorylase sequences from the amitochondriate protists, Trichomonas vaginalis, Mastigamoeba balamuthi, Entamoeba histolytica and Giardia intestinalis. *The Journal of eukaryotic microbiology* **2003,** *50* (5), 366-72.

36. North, M. J.; Lockwood, B. C.; Bremner, A. F.; Coombs, G. H., Polyamine biosynthesis in trichomonads. *Molecular and biochemical parasitology* **1986,** *19* (3), 241-9.

37. Reis, I. A.; Martinez, M. P.; Yarlett, N.; Johnson, P. J.; Silva-Filho, F. C.; Vannier-Santos, M. A., Inhibition of polyamine synthesis arrests trichomonad growth and induces destruction of hydrogenosomes. *Antimicrobial agents and chemotherapy* **1999,** *43* (8), 1919-23.

38. Hussien, E. M.; El-Sayed, H. Z.; Shaban, M. M.; Salm, A. M.; Rashwan, M., Biological variability of Trichomonas vaginalis clinical isolates from symptomatic and asymptomatic patients. *Journal of the Egyptian Society of Parasitology* **2004,** *34* (3), 979-88.

39. da Luz Becker, D.; dos Santos, O.; Frasson, A. P.; de Vargas Rigo, G.; Macedo, A. J.; Tasca, T., High rates of double-stranded RNA viruses and Mycoplasma hominis in Trichomonas vaginalis clinical isolates in South Brazil. *Infect Genet Evol* **2015,** *34,* 181-7.

40. Goodman, R. P.; Freret, T. S.; Kula, T.; Geller, A. M.; Talkington, M. W.; Tang-Fernandez, V.; Suciu, O.; Demidenko, A. A.; Ghabrial, S. A.; Beach, D. H.; Singh, B. N.; Fichorova, R. N.; Nibert, M. L., Clinical isolates of Trichomonas vaginalis concurrently infected by strains of up to four Trichomonasvirus species (Family Totiviridae). *J Virol* **2011,** *85* (9), 4258-70.

41. Deligeoroglou, E.; Salakos, N.; Makrakis, E.; Chassiakos, D.; Hassan, E. A.; Christopoulos, P., Infections of the lower female genital tract during childhood and adolescence. *Clinical and experimental obstetrics & gynecology* **2004,** *31* (3), 175-8.

42. Petrin, D.; Delgaty, K.; Bhatt, R.; Garber, G., Clinical and microbiological aspects of Trichomonas vaginalis. *Clinical microbiology reviews* **1998,** *11* (2), 300-17.

43. Purello-D'Ambrosio, F.; Gangemi, S., Urticaria from Trichomonas vaginalis infection. *Allergol Clin Immunol* **1999,** *9* (2), 123-5.

44. Petrin, D.; Delgaty, K.; Bhatt, R.; Garber, G., Clinical and microbiological aspects of Trichomonas vaginalis. *Clinical microbiology reviews* **1998,** *11* (2), 300-17.

45. Wolner-Hanssen, P.; Krieger, J. N.; Stevens, C. E., Clinical manifestations of vaginal trichomoniasis. *JAMA* **1989,** *26,* 571-576.

46. Krieger, J. N.; Riley, D. E., Chronic prostatitis: Charlottesville to Seattle. *The Journal of urology* **2004,** *172* (6 Pt 2), 2557-60.

47. Mason, P. R.; Fiori, P. L.; Cappuccinelli, P.; Rappelli, P.; Gregson, S., Seroepidemiology of Trichomonas vaginalis in rural women in Zimbabwe and patterns of association with HIV infection. *Epidemiology and infection* **2005,** *133* (2), 315-23.

48. Moodley, P.; Wilkinson, D.; Connolly, C.; Moodley, J.; Sturm, A. W., Trichomonas vaginalis is

associated with pelvic inflammatory disease in women infected with human immunodeficiency virus. *Clinical infectious diseases : an official publication of the Infectious Diseases Society of America* **2002,** *34* (4), 519-22.

49. Hoffman, D. J.; Brown, G. D.; Wirth, F. H.; Gebert, B. S.; Bailey, C. L.; Anday, E. K., Urinary tract infection with Trichomonas vaginalis in a premature newborn infant and the development of chronic lung disease. *Journal of perinatology : official journal of the California Perinatal Association* **2003,** *23* (1), 59-61.

50. Szarka, K.; Temesvári, P.; Kerekes, A.; Tege, A.; Repkény, A., Neonatal pneumonia caused by Trichomonas vaginalis. *Acta microbiologica et immunologica Hungarica* **2002,** *49* (1), 15-9.

51. Sutton, M.; Sternberg, M.; Koumans, E. H.; McQuillan, G.; Berman, S.; Markowitz, L., The prevalence of Trichomonas vaginalis infection among reproductive-age women in the United States, 2001-2004. *Clinical infectious diseases : an official publication of the Infectious Diseases Society of America* **2007,** *45* (10), 1319-26.

52. Sena, A. C.; Miller, W. C.; Hobbs, M. M.; Schwebke, J. R.; Leone, P. A.; Swygard, H.; Atashili, J.; Cohen, M. S., Trichomonas vaginalis infection in male sexual partners: implications for diagnosis, treatment, and prevention. *Clinical infectious diseases : an official publication of the Infectious Diseases Society of America* **2007,** *44* (1), 13-22.

53. Negm, A. Y.; el-Haleem, D. A., Detection of trichomoniasis in vaginal specimens by both conventional and modern molecular tools. *Journal of the Egyptian Society of Parasitology* **2004,** *34* (2), 589-600.

54. Krieger, J. N.; Tam, M. R.; Stevens, C. E.; Nielsen, I. O.; Hale, J.; Kiviat, N. B.; Holmes, K. K., Diagnosis of trichomoniasis. Comparison of conventional wet-mount examination with cytologic studies, cultures, and monoclonal antibody staining of direct specimens. *JAMA : the journal of the American Medical Association* **1988,** *259* (8), 1223-7.

55. Andrea, S. B.; Chapin, K. C., Comparison of Aptima Trichomonas vaginalis transcription-mediated amplification assay and BD affirm VPIII for detection of T. vaginalis in symptomatic women: performance parameters and epidemiological implications. *Journal of clinical microbiology* **2011,** *49* (3), 866-9.

56. Freeman, C. D.; Klutman, N. E.; Lamp, K. C., Metronidazole. A therapeutic review and update. *Drugs* **1997,** *54* (5), 679-708.

57. Muller, M.; Lossick, J. G., in vitro susceptibility of Trichomonas vaginalis to metronidazole and treatment outcome in vaginal trichomoniasis. *Sex Trans Dis* **1988,** *15* 17-24.

58. Lyng, J.; Christensen, J., A double-blind study of the value of treatment with a single dose tinidazole of partners to females with trichomoniasis. *Acta Obstet Gynecol Scand* **1981,** *60* (2), 199-201.

9. The Malarias

Plasmodium falciparum
(Welch 1898)

Plasmodium vivax
(Grassi and Filetti 1889)

Plasmodium ovale
(Stephens 1922)

Plasmodium malariae
(Laveran 1880)

Plasmodium knowlesi
(Knowles and Das Gupta 1932)

Introduction

Malaria is a mosquito-borne (Fig. 9.1) infection caused by protozoa of the genus *Plasmodium*. Humans are commonly infected by four species of the parasite*: P. falciparum, P. vivax, P. ovale*, and *P. malariae*. A fifth species, *P. knowlesi*, has been added to this list of human malaria. Malaria remains the most important parasitic infection and one of the most prevalent infectious diseases. For much of human history malaria has been a major cause of human morbidity and mortality with over 200 million cases and over 400,000 deaths in 2015.[1-3] Most of these deaths were among children living in sub-Saharan Africa.

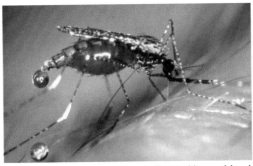

Figure 9.1. Adult *Anopheles dirus* taking a blood meal from one of the authors (RWG).

Global morbidity and mortality from malaria are on the decline and WHO released a document in 2015 titled: Global Technical Strategy for Malaria 2016-2030, that together with other publications, begins the process for considering technical and financial requirements critical to considering elimination of malaria as a leading cause of childhood deaths.[3-5] Although formerly found throughout much of the world, with seasonal outbreaks extending well into temperate zones, malaria is now generally restricted to tropical and subtropical regions. Travel and persistence of mosquito vectors in areas of the world that no longer have the malaria parasites continue to pose the threat of reintroduction into non-immune populations.

Historical Information

Malaria afflicted humankind's ancestors as evidenced by its genetic footprint on the human genome.[6-8] The earliest medical writers in China, Assyria, and India described malaria-like intermittent fevers, which they attributed to evil spirits. By the fifth century BCE, Hippocrates was able to differentiate quotidian, tertian, and quartan fevers and the clinical symptoms of the disease.[9] At that time it was assumed that vapors and mists arising from swamps and marshes caused the disease. These theories persisted for more than 2,000 years and were reinforced by repeated observations that the draining of swamps led to a reduction in the number of cases of malaria. Indeed, the names for this disease, malaria (mal, bad; aria, air) and paludism (palus, marsh) reflect these beliefs.

All concepts of malaria changed within 20 years after Charles Laveran's 1880 description of the crescent-shaped sexual stage of *P. falciparum,* and his observation of the dramatic release of the parasite's highly motile microgametes in the fresh blood of an infected soldier.[10] In 1898, Ronald Ross, using a species of bird malaria, and Giovanni

Grassi and colleagues, working with human malaria, showed that the parasite developed in the mosquito and was transmitted by the bite of that insect.[11] Ultimately, Ross and Laveran were awarded Nobel prizes for their contributions.[12, 13]

Although most of the basic features of the life cycle of the malarial parasite were understood by 1900, it was not until 1947 that Henry Shortt and Cyril Garnham demonstrated in avian malaria that a phase in the liver preceded the parasite cycles in the blood.[14] While Miles Markus suggested in 1976 that a dormant stage of *Plasmodium* might exist and suggested the term 'hypnozoite', Wojciech Krotoski, an American physician, is credited with describing the dormant liver phase for *P. vivax* in 1980.[15-18]

Early strategies to control malaria mainly sought to reduce the number of mosquitoes and to treat those infected. Chemotherapy of malaria preceded the description of the parasite by nearly 300 years. The Peruvian bark of cinchona, or "fever tree", was first used during the early part of the seventeenth century, but the details of its discovery and its introduction into Europe are still controversial.[19-22] In 1820, Pierre-Joseph Pelletier and Joseph-Bienaimé Caventou isolated the alkaloids of the cinchona tree, quinine and cinchonine. Synthetic anti-malarial compounds effective against various stages of the parasite were later developed in Germany (pamaquine in 1924, mepacrine in 1930, chloroquine in 1934), in Britain (proguanil in 1944), and in the United States (pyrimethamine and primaquine in 1952).[22]

The Greeks and Romans practiced the earliest forms of malaria control, albeit inadvertently, by draining swamps and marshes. Their primary purpose was reclamation of land. These techniques were continued for centuries before the role of the mosquito as vector was discovered. Almost immediately after the discovery of the mosquito as the vector for malaria, malarial control became

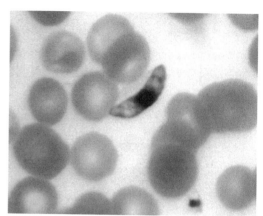

Figure 9.2. Gametocyte of *Plasmodium falciparum*.

synonymous with the control of mosquitoes. Destruction of breeding places by drainage and filling the swamps, killing the larvae by placing crude oil on the waters, and later adding the larvicide Paris green, were typical early attempts. With the development of DDT, a residual insecticide, large-scale control programs became possible. They culminated in 1957 when the World Health Organization launched a worldwide eradication program.

Plasmodium falciparum

Infection caused by *P. falciparum* (Figs. 9.2, 9.16) produces a form of malaria historically referred to as aestivoautumnal, malignant tertian, or simply falciparum malaria. It is the most pathogenic of the human malarias, and accounts for most of the mortality from the illness. *P. falciparum* is the most prevalent of the human malarial infections, and is mostly confined to tropical and subtropical regions. It is the primary cause of malaria in sub-Saharan Africa.

Identification of *P. falciparum* is usually based on the presence of small ring-stage parasites on blood smears (Fig. 9.3). Infected erythrocytes are not enlarged, and multiple infections of single erythrocytes are common. The rings often show two distinct chromatin dots. As trophozoites mature, they become sequestered in the capillaries of internal organs, such as the heart, brain, spleen, skeletal muscles, and placenta, where

Mosquito Cycle (Sporogony)

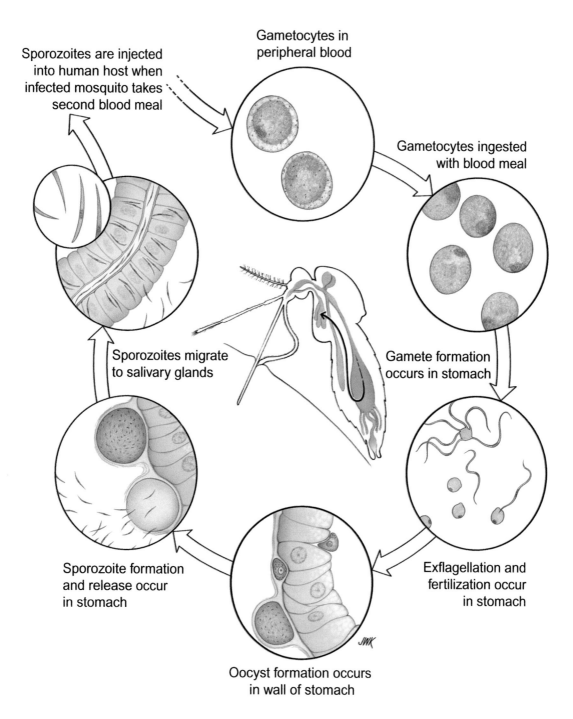

Sporozoites are injected into human host when infected mosquito takes second blood meal

Gametocytes in peripheral blood

Gametocytes ingested with blood meal

Gamete formation occurs in stomach

Sporozoites migrate to salivary glands

Exflagellation and fertilization occur in stomach

Sporozoite formation and release occur in stomach

Oocyst formation occurs in wall of stomach

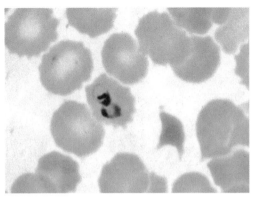

Figure 9.3. Signet ring stage of *Plasmodium* spp.

they complete their development. As a result of sequestration, maturing parasites usually are not present in the peripheral circulation. The appearance of the mature asexual stages (larger trophozoites and schizonts) in the peripheral circulation indicates the increasing severity of the disease.

Gametocytogenesis also proceeds in sequestered erythrocytes and requires approximately ten days. The falciparum gametocytes are characteristically crescentic, or banana-shaped (Fig. 9.2). They remain infectious for mosquitoes for as long as four days.

Falciparum malaria does not relapse because there is no persistent liver stage (see *P. vivax* and *P. ovale* that do produce hypnozoites). Once parasites have developed to the erythrocytic stage and exit from the hepatocytes, they are unable to re-infect the liver. Recrudescence (reappearance of infected erythrocytes from the deep tissues into the peripheral blood) is common, and can recur for about two years.

Plasmodium vivax

Plasmodium vivax infection is called benign tertian or vivax malaria. Red blood cells infected with *P. vivax* (Fig. 9.4, 9.17) are enlarged and, when properly stained with Giemsa, often show stippling on the erythrocyte membrane, known as Schüffner's dots. All stages of the parasite are present in the peripheral circulation. Single infections of invaded erythrocytes are characteristic. Ga-

metocytes appear simultaneously with the first asexual parasites. The duration of the viability of the sexual stages appears to be less than 12 hours. *Plasmodium vivax* produces the classic relapsing malaria, initiated from hypnozoites in the liver that have resumed development after a period of latency. Relapses can occur at periods ranging from every few weeks to a few months for up to five years after the initial infection. The specific periodicity of the relapses is a characteristic of the geographic strain of the parasite. Vivax malaria also recrudescences due to persistent low numbers of circulating infected erythrocytes.

Plasmodium ovale

Plasmodium ovale (Figs. 9.5, 19.19) is limited to tropical Africa and to discrete areas of the Western Pacific. Ovale malaria produces a tertian fever clinically similar to that of vivax malaria but somewhat less severe. It exhibits relapses for the same duration as vivax malaria.

Plasmodium malariae

The disease caused by *P. malariae* is known as quartan malaria. *P. malariae* has a wide but spotty distribution throughout the world. Development in the mosquito is slow, and infection in humans is not as intense as those caused by the other *Plasmodium* spe-

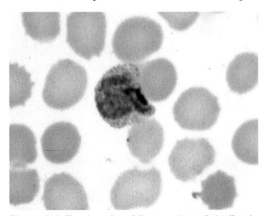

Figure 9.4. Trophozoite of *P. vivax*. Note Schüffner's dots in the parasite, and surrounding red cells that are smaller than the infected one.

Plasmodium falciparum

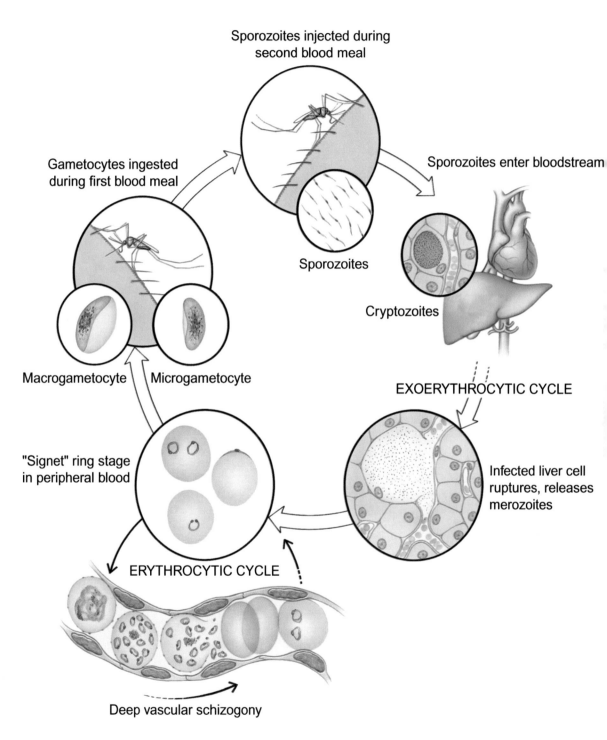

Sporozoites injected during second blood meal

Gametocytes ingested during first blood meal

Sporozoites enter bloodstream

Sporozoites

Cryptozoites

Macrogametocyte   Microgametocyte

EXOERYTHROCYTIC CYCLE

"Signet" ring stage in peripheral blood

Infected liver cell ruptures, releases merozoites

ERYTHROCYTIC CYCLE

Deep vascular schizogony

Parasitic Diseases 6th Ed. Parasites Without Borders www.parasiteswithoutborders.com

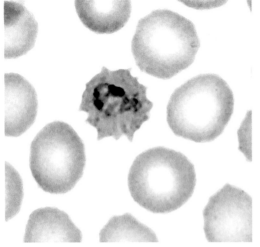

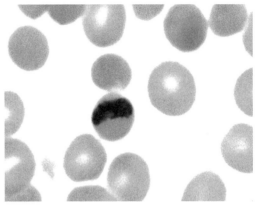

Figure 9.7. *Plasmodium malariae* trophozoite.

Figure 9.5. Trophozoite of *P. ovale*. Note "crenated" appearance of infected red cell. Courtesy M. Guelpe.

cies. Most current evidence indicates that *P. malariae* does not relapse. It does recrudescence due to chronic low-level parasitemia that may persist for decades.[23, 24] Erythrocytes infected with *P. malariae* remain the same size throughout schizogony (Figs. 9.6, 9.7, 9.18).

Plasmodium knowlesi

Some species of *Plasmodium* that are parasites of chimpanzees, orangutans, and monkeys occasionally infect humans.[13] In 1932, Knowles and Das Gupta described the experimental transmission of *P. knowlesi* to humans.[25] It later became established as the

fifth human malaria.[26, 27] The disease it causes can range from mild to severe. Most notable is the quotidian fever (24-hour cycle). Although certain other simian malarias such as *P. cynomolgi, P. brasilianum, P. eylesi, P. inui, P. schwetzi* and *P. simium* may be transmissible to humans through the bite of a mosquito, the vivax-like malaria caused by *P. cynomolgi* is the only other naturally acquired malaria documented.[28, 29] Recognition of human infection with *P. knowlesi* is becoming more common, but this may be due in part to our ability to differentiate otherwise morphologically similar human and simian parasites at the molecular level.[30-32]

Life Cycles

The biology of all *Plasmodium* species is generally similar, and consists of two discrete phases: asexual and sexual. The asexual stages develop in humans; first in the liver and then in the circulating erythrocytes. The sexual stages develop in the mosquito.

Asexual Stages

When the infected female anopheles mosquito takes a blood meal (Fig. 9.1), she injects salivary fluids into the wound. These fluids contain sporozoites (Fig. 9.8), small (10-15 µm long), spindle-shaped, motile forms of the parasite, which initiate the infection. They are cleared from the circulation within an hour,

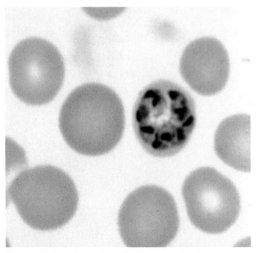

Figure 9.6. Schizont of *P. malariae*. Note red cells are the same size as the infected cell.

Plasmodium vivax

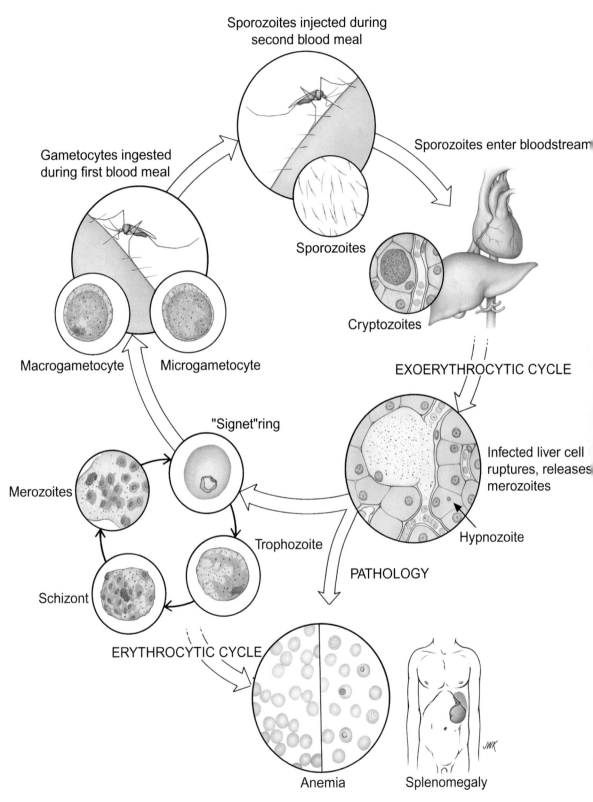

Sporozoites injected during second blood meal

Gametocytes ingested during first blood meal

Sporozoites enter bloodstream

Sporozoites

Cryptozoites

Macrogametocyte

Microgametocyte

EXOERYTHROCYTIC CYCLE

"Signet"ring

Infected liver cell ruptures, releases merozoites

Merozoites

Trophozoite

Hypnozoite

Schizont

PATHOLOGY

ERYTHROCYTIC CYCLE

Anemia

Splenomegaly

JWK

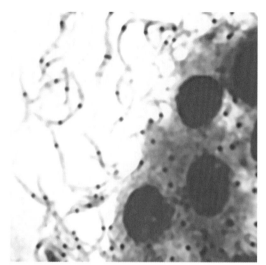

Figure 9.8. Sporozoites of malaria in infected mosquito stomach preparation.

and eventually reach parenchymal cells of the liver. How sporozoites traffic to and enter the liver has been a subject of much investigation.[33-35] Evidence suggests that sporozoites bind to CD68 on the surface of Küpffer cells facilitating entry into hepatocytes.[36] Once inside the liver cell, the parasites undergo asexual division (exoerythrocytic schizogony) (Fig. 9.9). A prescribed number of merozoites are produced over a period of days to weeks, depending upon the species. *P. vivax* matures within 6-8 days, and each sporozoite produces about 10,000 daughter parasites. For *P. ovale*, these values are 9 days and 15,000 merozoites; for *P. malariae*, 12-16 days and 2000 merozoites; and for *P. falciparum*, 5-7 days and 40,000 merozoites.[37]

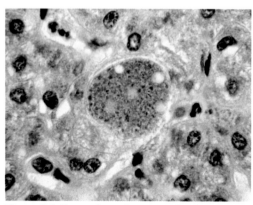

Figure 9.9. Exoerythrocytic stages of malaria in liver parenchymal cell.

The phenomenon of relapse in certain malarias (*P. vivax, P. ovale, P. cynomolgi*) is because each of these species produces hypnozoites. By definition, a parasitologic malarial relapse is the reappearance of parasitemia in peripheral blood in a sporozoite-induced infection, following adequate blood schizonticidal therapy.[38] It had been long accepted that the exoerythrocytic forms of relapsing malaria persist in the liver as a result of cyclic development (rupture of infected cells and invasion of new cells).[39] However, experimental evidence has lent support to a different hypothesis for the mechanism of relapse. It holds that some sporozoites fail to initiate immediate exoerythrocytic development in the liver, and remain latent as the so-called hypnozoites capable of delayed development and initiation of relapse.[40] Several patterns of relapse have been described, often related to the geographic origin of the parasite. Temperate strains of *P. vivax* may show delayed primary attacks and relapses, whereas more tropical forms emerge from the liver within weeks of infection. In vivax and ovale malarias, eradication of parasites from the peripheral circulation with drugs aborts the acute infection. Subsequently, a fresh wave of exoerythrocytic merozoites from the liver can reinitiate the infection. The dormant parasites, or hypnozoites can remain quiescent in the liver for as long as five years.[24, 41-43] To achieve radical cure, it is necessary to destroy not only the circulating parasites but also the hypnozoites.[44]

Plasmodium falciparum and *P. malariae* do not develop hypnozoites, and therefore lack the capacity to relapse. Untreated *P. falciparum* can recrudesce for 1-2 years through the continuation of the erythrocytic cycle, which for periods of time remains at a subclinical, asymptomatic level. *Plasmodium malariae* can do so for 30 years or more.[23] For infections with *P. falciparum* and *P. malariae*, drugs that only eradicate parasites in the peripheral circulation are sufficient to achieve cure.

Erythrocytic Phase

When merozoites are released from the liver, they invade red blood cells (Fig. 9.10) and initiate the erythrocytic phase of infection. Invasion of the erythrocytes consists of a complex sequence of events, beginning with contact between a free-floating merozoite and the red blood cell.[45] Attachment of the merozoite to the erythrocyte membrane involves interaction with specific receptors on the surface of erythrocytes.[46] Thereafter the erythrocyte undergoes rapid and marked deformation. The parasite enters by a localized endocytic invagination of the red blood cell membrane, utilizing a moving junction between the parasite and the host cell membrane.[47]

Once within the cell, the parasite begins to grow, first forming the ring-like early trophozoite, and eventually enlarging to fill the cell. The organism then undergoes asexual division and becomes a schizont composed of merozoites. The parasites are nourished by the hemoglobin within the erythrocytes, and produce a characteristic pigmented waste product called hemozoin. The erythrocytic cycle is completed when the red blood cell ruptures and releases merozoites that are then free to invade other erythrocytes.[35]

The asexual cycle is characteristically synchronous and periodic. *Plasmodium falciparum, P. vivax*, and *P. ovale* complete the development from invasion by merozoites to rupture of the erythrocyte within 48 hours, exhibiting "tertian" periodicity. *Plasmodium malariae*, which produces "quartan" malaria, requires 72 hours for completion of the cycle. Counting the days is such that the first day is day one and 48 hours later on day three of the tertian day fever is seen in *Plasmodium falciparum, P. vivax*, and *P. ovale*. When counting for *Plasmodium malariae*, day one is the first day and 72 hours, or three days later, is the fourth day and thus the term quartan fever is applied.[48]

Infection with erythrocytic phase merozoites can also occur as a result of blood transfusion from an infected donor, or via a contaminated needle shared among drug users. Malaria acquired in this manner is referred to as "induced" malaria.[49] Congenital malaria as a result of transplacental infection is perhaps more common than originally suspected due

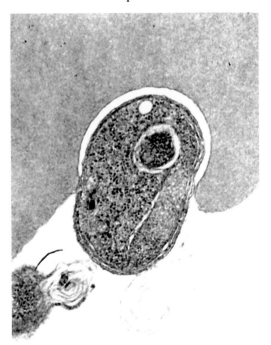

Figure 9.10. Transmission EM of a merozoite entering a red cell. Note points of attachment. Courtesy S. Langreth.

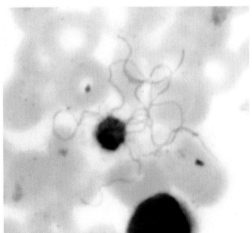

Figure 9.11. Exflagellation of the microgametocyte of a malaria parasite. Each "flagella" is actually a male gamete.

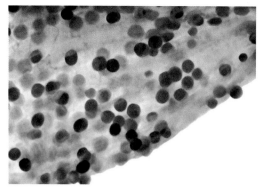

Figure 9.12. Portion of an infected mosquito stomach. Note numerous oocysts on outer wall.

to its high rate of spontaneous clearance, but appears to be increased in the context of HIV infection.[50-54]

Sexual Stages

Not all merozoites develop asexually. Some differentiate into the sexual forms – macrogametocytes (female) and microgametocytes (males) – which can complete their development only within the gut of an appropriate mosquito vector. On ingestion by the mosquito in the blood meal, the gametocytes shed their protective erythrocyte membrane in the gut. Male gametocytes initiate exflagellation (Fig. 9.11), a rapid process that produces up to eight active, sperm-like microgametes, each of which can eventually fertilize the macrogametes. The resulting zygotes elongate into diploid vermiform ookinetes, which penetrate the gut wall and come to lie under

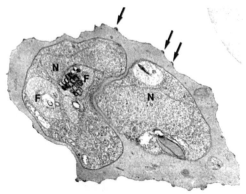

Figure 9.13. Transmission EM of red cell infected with *P. falciparum*. Arrows indicate points of attachment to host endothelial cells. N=nucleus, F=food vacuole. Courtesy S. Langreth.

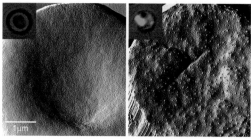

Figure 9.14. Atomic force microscopy of normal (left) and *Plasmodium falciparum* infected (right) red cells. Courtesy J. Dvorak.

the basement membrane (Fig. 9.12). The parasites then transform into oocysts within 24 hours of ingestion of the blood meal. Development of sporozoites follows, leading to the production of more than 1,000 of these now-haploid forms in each oocyst. They mature within 10–14 days, escape from the oocyst, and invade the salivary glands. When the mosquito bites another human host, a new cycle begins.

Although the different species have marked physiologic differences and some major differences in the pathologic course they pursue, they are most simply differentiated on the basis of their morphology. The blood smear, typically fixed and stained with

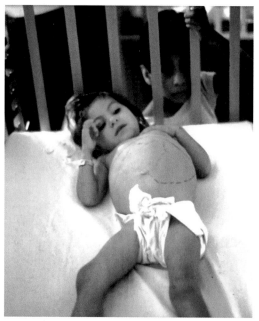

Figure 9.15. Child infected with malaria, probably *P. malariae*. Note enlarged spleen.

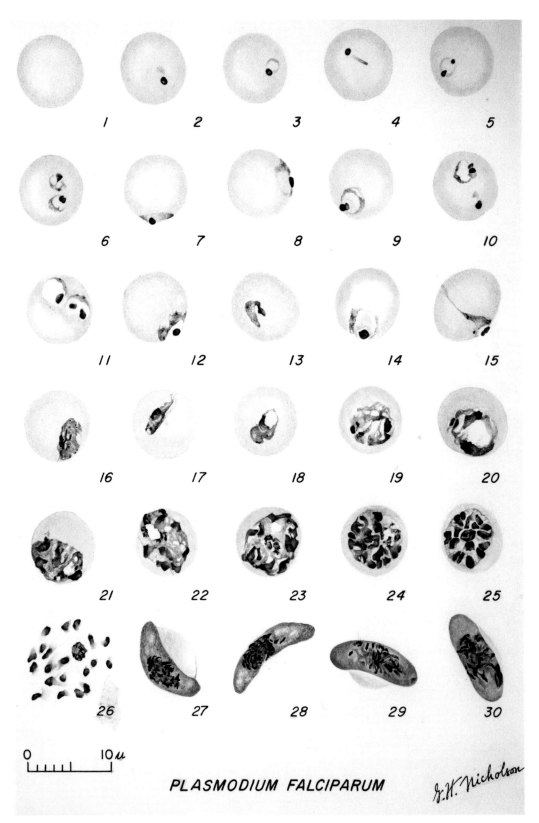

Figure 9.16.

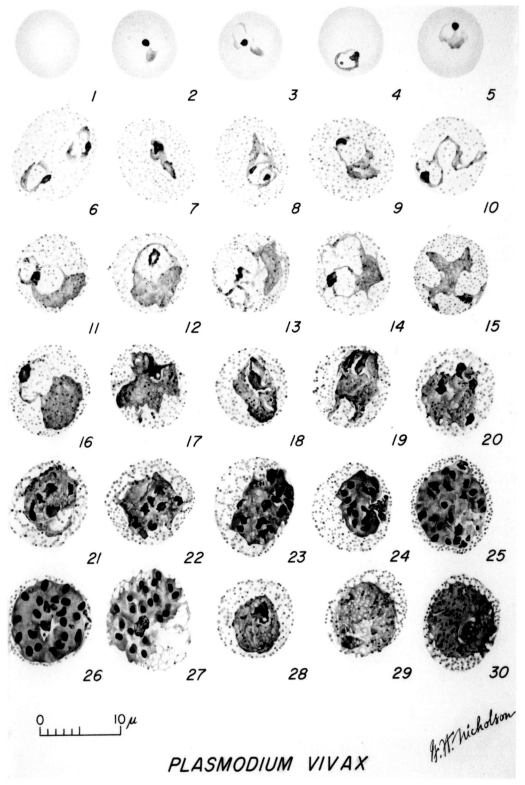

PLASMODIUM VIVAX

Figure 9.17.

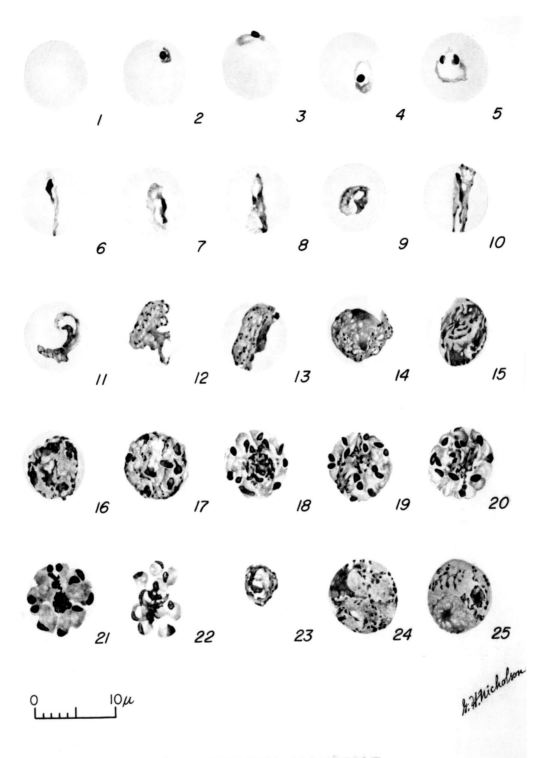

PLASMODIUM MALARIAE

Figure 9.18.

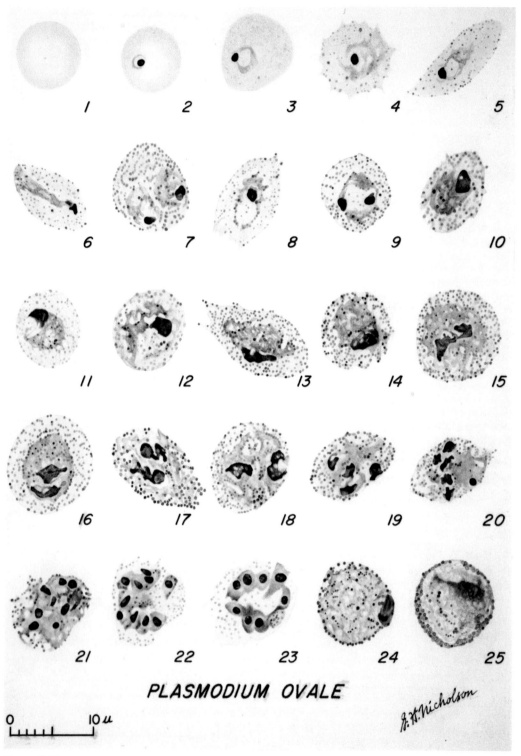

PLASMODIUM OVALE

0 [   ] 10 μ

Figure 9.19.

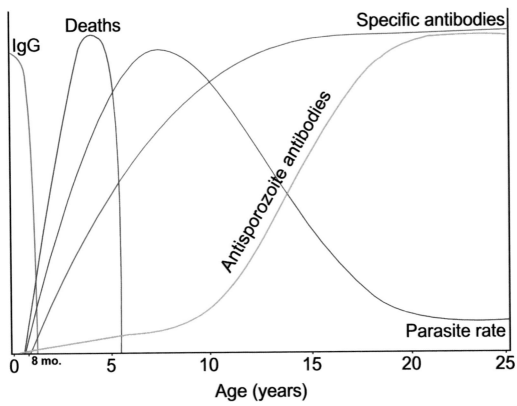

Figure 9.20. Graph indicating relationships between age of patient, susceptibility to infection, production of antibodies against different stages of parasite, and lethality of infection.

Giemsa or Wright solution, is the basis of the fundamental diagnostic test, although alternatives are now available. Commercially available methods for malaria parasite detection and characterization are becoming increasingly sensitive, and are supplanting microscopy in more advanced laboratories (see Diagnosis).[55]

Cellular and Molecular Pathogenesis

The release of cytokines following rupture of infected erythrocytes is accompanied by fever and the consequent chills and sweating associated with malaria.[56] The pathogenesis of general malaise, myalgia, and headache appears related to the release of certain cytokines and their levels correlate with disease severity.[57] The characteristic periodicity of the fever, based on synchronous infections, is not invariable; the early phases of infections are often not synchronous. Some infections may be due to two or more broods of parasites, with the periodicity of one independent of that of the others.

Cerebral malaria is the most devastating manifestation of severe falciparum infection.[58] It is caused by blockage of the cerebral capillaries with infected erythrocytes, which adhere to the endothelium.[59, 60] The mechanism of cytoadherence is thought to be related to the presence of histidine-rich "knobs" on the surface of the infected red blood cells that express strain-specific adhesive proteins (PfEMP1), and the subsequent attachment to appropriate receptors on the host endothelium (Figs. 9.13, 9.14).[61, 62] Although not essential for cytoadherence, the knobs seem to enhance binding.[63] These knobs are induced by the parasite and facilitate endothelial cell binding by the infected erythrocytes to a number of endothelial targets.[64, 65] Binding to endothelial cells involves several host cell receptors, including CD36, intercellular adhesion molecule 1 (ICAM1), and chondroitin sulfate A (CSA). In the brain ICAM1 is likely the most important while CD36 is likely the most important in other organs.[37] Cytoadherence in the placentae of women in their first pregnancies involves parasite binding to chondroitin sulfate A (CSA).[66, 67] Sequestration of malaria parasites in the placentae of primagravid females is a major cause of death, fetal mortality, fetal wastage and low birth weight.[67-69] With falciparum malaria, anemia caused by hemolysis can be severe. Damage to the erythrocytes by intravascular hemolysis can exceed that caused by rupture of the infected cells alone. Even uninfected cells have an increased osmotic fragility. Also present is bone marrow depression, which contributes to the anemia. Disseminated intravascular coagulopathy occurs in severely infected individuals.

The spleen plays a major role in host defense against malaria (Fig. 9.15). Parasitized cells accumulate in its capillaries and sinusoids, causing general congestion. Malarial pigment becomes concentrated in the spleen and is responsible for the darkening of this organ. Chronic infection, particularly with P. malariae, often causes persistent splenomegaly and is responsible for "big spleen disease," or tropical splenomegaly syndrome, consisting of hepatomegaly, portal hypertension, anemia, leukopenia, and thrombocytopenia.[70] With vivax malaria, the spleen can become acutely enlarged and is susceptible to rupture. A significant portion of the anemia seen in vivax malaria is driven by splenic clearance of non-infected erythrocytes.[71] The liver is darkened by the accumulated malarial pigment and shows degeneration and necrosis of the centrilobular regions. The gastrointestinal tract is also affected. There are focal hemorrhages, edema, and consequent malabsorption. The kidneys, particularly with severe falciparum malaria, show punc-

tate hemorrhages and even tubular necrosis. Accumulation of hemoglobin in the tubules is responsible for hemoglobinuria, or blackwater fever, which occurs after repeated attacks of falciparum malaria and is complicated by therapy with quinine.[72] Blackwater fever is a consequence of severe hemolysis exacerbated by the host immune response against the intracellular parasites.

Chronic infections with P. malariae can lead to nephrotic syndrome, characterized by focal hyalinization of the tufts of glomeruli, and by endothelial proliferation, apparently caused by the deposition of immune complexes.[48] This process can lead to endocapillary cell proliferation and reduplication of the basement membrane.

Congenital malaria can develop with any of the species of Plasmodia, although the incidence of this complication is relatively low. The mechanism by which the fetus becomes infected is uncertain. Some investigators have postulated damage to the placenta as a prerequisite to congenital malaria, but it is also possible that the parasites can infect the fetus through an intact placenta or at the time of birth.[53] Malarial infections tend to suppress cell-mediated immune responses. It has been suggested that Burkitt's lymphoma is caused by infection with the Epstein-Barr virus under the influence of immunosuppression by chronic falciparum malaria, but the competing hypothesis is that it is the chronic immune activation that drives Burkitt's lymphoma.[73-75]

HIV and Malaria

The relationship between infection with malaria and the human immunodeficiency virus is a subject of great interest and intense scrutiny.[76] In Africa, these two agents overlap in their geographic ranges and the populations they infect. While the focus is often on how HIV infection predisposes to an increase in malaria severity there is evidence that malaria infection increases T cell activation and causes both a decrease in CD4[+] T cell counts and increases in viral loads.[77-79] There is also evidence to suggest a relationship between HIV-induced reduction of CD4[+] T cell counts and a rise in incidence of malaria.[79-83] HIV does confer an increased susceptibility to symptomatic malaria.[84, 85] There is conflicting information regarding the severity of clinical malaria when it manifests in HIV-infected individuals, but most evidence suggests that they experience higher levels of parasitemia and an increased risk for severe malaria.[86, 87]

Clinical Disease

The most pronounced clinical manifestations of adult-onset malaria are periodic chills and fever, usually accompanied by frontal headache, fatigue, abdominal discomfort, and myalgia.[37, 55] Fever may persist for several days before the typical periodicity develops. In contrast, young children often present with non-specific symptoms, including fever, cough, vomiting, and diarrhea. Symptoms of malaria usually first appear 10-15 days after the bite of the infected mosquito, although delays of several months in the onset of symptoms and the appearance of parasites in peripheral blood are common, particularly for some strains of *P. vivax* found in temperate zones. Patients undergoing chemoprophylaxis may not develop any symptoms until they stop taking the drug. The classic pattern of clinical disease consists of paroxysms of chills and fever, reaching 41°C and lasting six hours, followed by sweating and defervescence.

Vomiting can also develop and may be intense. Difficulty breathing is seen in up to 25% of adults with severe malaria, and in approximately 40% of children with severe malaria.[88] Initially, there can be mild anemia with an elevation of the reticulocyte count. The leukocyte count tends to be normal or even low; there is no eosinophilia.

All forms of untreated malaria tend to become chronic, including those without a hypnozoite stage. Repeated attacks are caused by recrudescence or relapses. The development of immunity eventually leads to spontaneous cure of falciparum malaria within two years and of vivax and ovale malarias within five years, although individuals are susceptible to reinfection during and after this period (Fig. 9.20). Infection with the quartan parasite can persist 30 years or more. Untreated falciparum malaria can be fatal during the initial attack, an unfortunately frequent event in young children (Fig. 9.20).

Unexplained fever in patients who have received transfusions, or who are i.v. drug users may signal the presence of induced malaria. An infant who develops fever during the neonatal period should be suspected of malaria if the mother had been exposed to this infection. Diagnostic tests for induced or congenital malaria are the same as for the conventional forms of the infection. It must be emphasized that neither induced nor congenital malaria has an exoerythrocytic cycle in the liver, and therapy directed against the liver cycle is not required. Innate resistance to malaria is mediated by factors other than immune mechanisms. *Plasmodium vivax* and *P. ovale* preferentially invade reticulocytes. Usually only about 2% of red blood cells are parasitized with *P. vivax* and *P. ovale* infections. Clinical disease is typically mild. *P. malariae* tends to invade older erythrocytes, again limiting maximum parasitemia. In contrast, *P. falciparum* attacks erythrocytes of all ages, permitting high levels of parasitemia.

There are a number of genetic factors in human populations that confer varying levels of susceptibility to malaria.[35, 89, 90] Individuals carrying the gene for sickle-cell hemoglobin receive some advantage against falciparum malaria. Those with sickle-cell trait (A and S hemoglobins) have a selective advantage over those with the hemoglobin AA genotype because the heterozygotes limit the severity of malaria. The hemoglobin SS individuals are also at an advantage, but their sickle-cell disease leads to early death.[89-91] In areas of Africa with the highest frequency of this gene, it is estimated that the death rate due to malaria required to fix this gene frequency may have exceeded 25% and is an excellent example of a balanced polymorphism.[92]

In 2011, a group of researchers demonstrated that sickle hemoglobin provides protection against malaria through induction of the expression of heme oxygenase-1 (HO-1).[93] HO-1 prevents accumulation of circulating heme, and is particularly protective against cerebral malaria. Sickle hemoglobin is also able to inhibit the activation and expansion of cytotoxic CD8$^+$ T cells resulting in lower cellular activation and higher cellular reactivity in response to malarial antigens.[93-95] Hemoglobin C mutations appear to provide similar protection against falciparum malaria in certain ethnic groups.[96, 97]

Glucose-6-phosphate dehydrogenase (G6PD) deficiency, β-thalassemia, and ovalocytosis, the latter common in Southeast Asia, have been implicated as mediators of innate resistance against *P. falciparum* infection.[98] It has been suggested that the protective effect of thalassemia may be related to enhanced immune recognition and clearance of parasitized erythrocytes.[99] Evidence also supports the idea that certain of these hemoglobinopathies reduce the intraerythrocyte multiplication of plasmodium species.[100]

Duffy blood type determinants are associated with receptor sites for *P. vivax* merozoites on the erythrocytes. While it is doubtful that the blood group carbohydrate itself is the actual receptor, most West Africans are negative for the Duffy blood type and have decreased susceptibility to infection with *P. vivax*.[92, 101] Instead, they have a higher than normal incidence of infection with *P. ovale*.[102]

Acquired immunity to malaria develops after long exposure and is characterized by low levels of parasitemia. Immune individuals have intermittent parasitemia with only mild symptoms. This clinical state has been referred to as premunition, in contrast with classic immunity, which prevents any degree of infection. Unfortunately, premunition does not last for life and individuals returning to endemic areas after even only one year away often have lost this protective immunity.[103-105]

Diagnosis

For over a century a definitive diagnosis of malaria depended on the microscopic identification of the parasite on Giemsa-stained blood smears. This procedure permits not only the confirmation of the presence of the parasite, but makes possible the identification of the species of malaria and an indication of the level of parasitemia in the infected host.[106] Under normal conditions, both thick and thin smears should be examined. When malaria is suspected, the clinician should take a thorough travel history. Should the initial blood smears prove to be negative, new specimens should be examined at 6-hour intervals.

Identification of malaria on thick and thin blood smears requires an experienced microscopist who is well trained in parasite morphology. A British study indicated that at least 10% of positive slides are not identified.[107] Antibody-based rapid diagnostic tests that are simple, specific and do not require a highly trained microscopist have been introduced and are now widely available.[108] These rapid tests detect PfHRP2, which is present in all plasmodium species, and then allow species level discrimination by using lactate dehydrogenase (LDH) or aldolase antigens that are species-specific.[109-111] A number of molecular tests have been developed that have been employed in research and epidemiological studies.[112] The introduction of loop mediated isothermal amplification (LAMP) assays may allow molecular testing to move from the research setting to field diagnosis.[113-115]

The identification of parasite genes conferring resistance to antimalarial drugs has permitted the development of mutation-specific PCR primers that can readily identify resistant parasites. Such detection systems are available and in use in the field for pyrimethamine, sulfadoxine, cycloguanil, chloroquine, and artemisinin.[116-120] Epidemiologic studies requiring information on sporozoite inoculation rates by mosquito vectors have been facilitated by ELISA systems using species-specific monoclonal antibodies directed against the predominant surface antigens of the sporozoites.[121] The capacity for rapidly determining the proportion of mosquito populations coming to feed that have infectious sporozoites in their salivary glands allows accurate prediction of risk of infection or assessment of the effects of intervention strategies for the control of malaria.

Treatment

The long reliance on chloroquine to treat *P. falciparum* is no longer tenable, due to the worldwide spread of drug resistance.[122] The two major choices for treatment of severe malaria are the cinchona alkaloids (quinine and quinidine) and the artemisinin derivatives (artesunate, artemether, and artemotil). Parenteral artesunate is the most rapidly acting of the artemisinin compounds, and is associated with more rapid clearance of parasitemia than treatment with the cinchona alkaloid quinine.[123, 124] Artesunate treatment has demonstrated a significant reduction in mortality in both adults and children compared to treatment with quinine.[123, 124] While artemisinin-based therapy was initially recommended as primary therapy in areas of high drug resistance, it is now first line therapy in most cases of severe malaria.[125, 126] A significant and striking exception to this worldwide recommendation is malaria treatment in the United States. For parts of the world where artesunate is not available, quinine and quinidine are alternative therapies. In 1991, parenteral quinine was no longer stocked by the Centers for Disease Control (CDC), when they concluded that parenteral quinidine gluconate could serve as an alternative.[127] Quinidine gluconate remains the only currently approved therapy by the US Food and Drug Administration (FDA) for the parenteral therapy of severe malaria, although many hospital pharmacies do not routinely stock this medicine. Intravenous artesunate is only available in the United States under an investigational protocol through the CDC for select patients and should be considered early in therapy given the favorable comparative data.[128] In addition to artesunate, quinine, or quinidine, a second long-acting medication is required, such as doxycycline, tetracycline, or clindamycin, for successful treatment.

When treating severe malaria infections with quinidine, care must include, monitoring patients with standard cardiac monitors, careful tracking of blood glucose, cautious fluid management, and delayed initiation of enteral feeding; factors critical to successful treatment outcomes.[37] Seizures may need to be managed with anti-seizure medications or benzodiazepines, and protection of the airway may be required in severe cases. Broad-spectrum intravenous antibiotics may be indicated in certain cases due to the high rate of bacterial sepsis that can occur in severe malaria.[129]

Exchange transfusions, once felt to be essential in management of severe malaria, are no longer recommended by the CDC, since a meta-analysis of previous studies revealed no significant survival advantage.[130] Blood transfusions for patients have been recommended, based on the results of small randomized trials and a few large observational trials, if hemoglobin levels are below 4 g/dl or if hemoglobin levels below 6 g/dl and there is parasitemia greater than 20%, or other concerning clinical features.[131, 132]

In contrast to severe or complicated malaria, non-complicated malaria is defined as symptomatic malaria with lower levels of parasitemia, ability to take oral medicine, and no evidence of vital organ dysfunction. For the treatment of uncomplicated malaria, if a patient has *P. falciparum* infection acquired from a region without chloroquine resistance, such as the Carribean and Central America west of the Panama Canal, chloroquine can be used, as there is little resistance to the drug in this region.[133] In the rest of the world, resistance to chloroquine is so frequently reported that every patient must be assumed to have a resistant form of *P. falciparum*. If the origin of infection is unknown, as may be the case with induced malaria, one must treat the infection as if the organisms were resistant. Currently artemisinin combination therapy (ACT) is the recommended first line therapy for all human malaria.[134] There are several available forms of ACT with no one choice clearly superior over the other.[134] Alternative drugs may be selected on a region-by-region basis with knowledge of local resistance rates.[135] Fansidar, a pyrimethamine-sulfadoxine combination, lost effectiveness as a replacement for chloroquine in East African countries, but still may have a role as part of intermittent preventive therapy in pregnancy.[136-138] Mefloquine can be given as part of combination therapy with a second agent such as doxycycline, with cure rates estimated to be greater than 90% in areas without resistance.[139] Malarone (atovaquone-proguanil) is an effective option that has demonstrated superior efficacy over mefloquine treatment and may have a better safety profile.[140, 141] The Sentinel sites in the International Centers of Excellence for Malaria Research (ICEMRs) provide essential data to monitor the emergence of drug resistance globally and the underlying mechanisms to further understand the impact.[142]

When the infecting strain is *P. vivax* or *P. ovale*, successful treatment may leave untreated hypnozoites that must be cleared to prevent relapses. Relapses due to *P. vivax* or *P. ovale* infections can be prevented by a course of primaquine to eradicate the hypnozoite liver stage. It need not be started immediately but can be deferred until the patient has recovered from the acute attack. Primaquine tends to cause hemolysis in individuals with glucose-6-phosphate dehydrogenase (G6PD) deficiency. The drug should not be administered until the proper test for this enzyme has been performed.

Chemoprophylaxis for Malaria

In areas without chloroquine resistance, such as the Carribean and Central America west of the Panama Canal, chloroquinine can be used for chemoprophylaxis, as there is little resistance to the drug in this region.[133] Mefloquine is an inexpensive option with weekly dosing that can be used in most of the world, except for localized areas where resistance has been reported. Many are hesitant to prescribe or take mefloquine due to concerns regarding its potential to induce psychosis.[143] Malarone (atovaquone-proguanil) is a prophylactic drug for travelers to areas where *P. falciparum* is resistant to other medications, but requires once daily dosing and is often very expensive. Daily doxycycline is another alternative, but patients should be cautioned about the associated photosensitivity. In some regions of the world, primaquine is used as a form of chemoprophylaxis, but the efficacy of this approach may be inferior to other chemoprophylaxis regimen. G6PD testing should be performed prior to using primaquine.[144]

Prevention and Control

There are more than 300 species of *Anopheles* mosquitoes, but only about 60 species are considered important vectors of malaria. Some of the factors that influence the efficiency of the insect are their feeding habits (most importantly, a preference for human blood), longevity, susceptibility to infection with the malarial parasite, and the size of the mosquito population (seasonal variability). The variability of the parasite plays an important role in the pathogenicity of the disease. For example, geographic strains of *P. vivax* show markedly different incubation periods and patterns of relapses, and *P. falciparum* shows considerable variability in its responses to anti-malarial drugs. The susceptibility of geographic strains of vector mosquitoes may be highly variable.

Malaria in the United States, since the 1960s, has been of the imported variety. The wars in Korea and Vietnam increased the numbers of these imported cases because of the returning infected service personnel. Refugees or immigrants from endemic areas constitute the largest number of imported cases. In addition, there is a steady incidence of malaria among travelers returning from endemic areas. Autochthonous infections are rare in the United States, despite large, persistent populations of the anopheline vectors, *An. quadrimaculatus* in the East and *An. freeborni* in the West. Outbreaks of *P. vivax* in southern California have been associated with the vector species, *An. hermsi*.[145] There are rare reports of malaria transmission in the U.S., usually limited to one or two cases transmitted by local anopheline mosquitoes.

In addition to chemoprophylaxis when indicated, travelers should avoid or minimize contact with mosquitoes. Since most anophelines bite at night, sleeping under insecticide treated bed netting and, if possible, in rooms fitted with window screens is effective, but not without issues of proper use.[146] Clothing that covers much of the skin and insect repellents, particularly those containing diethyltoluamide (DEET), are useful adjuncts to transmission prevention.

Controlling the mosquito vector remains the most practical method for wide-scale control of malaria. A reduction in the number of mosquitoes through drainage or modification of breeding sites has been accomplished in some areas. Insecticides still offer the best but increasingly less-acceptable method for reducing populations of mosquitoes, or of interrupting transmission by targeting only those infected mosquitoes coming to feed in houses. However, the rising costs of these insecticides and the development of resistance by the insects have severely limited their application and usefulness. Insecticide-impregnated bed nets have been shown to have a significant impact on the morbidity and mortality of infection due to *P. falciparum* and *P. vivax* in China, and to *P. falciparum* in Africa.[147, 148] Malaria control schemes based on genetic modification of the capacity of vector mosquitoes to transmit the parasite have been suggested.[149] In addition, the development of more efficient methods for introducing advantageous genes into the mosquito genome are being investigated, as well as methods for replacing vector populations in the field with populations of mosquitoes unable to transmit the parasite.[150, 151]

A malaria vaccine remains the "holy grail" of control strategies. For over 50 years, researchers have been attempting to find antigens that could induce protective immunity. After years of sporadic advances, vaccine research was reinvigorated by the demonstration that animals could develop immunity to infection with sporozoites, and stimulated by the development of methods for the *in vitro* cultivation of the asexual and sexual stages of *P. falciparum* by Trager and Jensen.[152] The revolution of molecular biology made possible the identification of specific genes coding for specific antigens and sub-unit vaccines became possible.[153]

There are three phases of the malaria life cycle that have been targeted by the vaccine hunters.[154, 155] Vaccines directed against the pre-erythrocytic stages of the parasite are intended to prevent infection by blocking the invasion or development of sporozoites freshly injected by a feeding mosquito or the development of the parasite in the liver. Secondarily it has been suggested that even partial efficacy (the blockage of most pre-erythrocytic development) could reduce the intensity of the primary infection and be useful in concert with antigens directed against other stages. Because such vaccines may have short-term efficacy, the target population for pre-erythrocytic stage vaccines has usually been considered to be non-immune individuals moving through malarious areas, including tourists and military personnel. Even with a short life, such vaccines could be useful in areas of low transmission, or in children and pregnant women in areas of high transmission.[156]

Vaccines directed against the erythrocytic (blood) stages of the parasite are not expected to induce sterile immunity and totally prevent infection. Rather, it is expected that a successful vaccine could reduce the parasite burden, eliminate most deaths and reduce morbidity. The primary target for blood stage vaccines are children and pregnant women in areas of

intense transmission.[35]

Vaccines directed against the mosquito (sexual) stages of the parasite are designed to block the development of the parasite in the mosquito vector. An effective vaccine could interrupt transmission to additional victims. In combination with other antigens, a transmission-blocking component could prevent the spread of parasites resistant to other vaccines. A transmission-blocking vaccine could be used in an eradication scheme or to prevent epidemics in areas of unstable malaria transmission.[35] The investigational malaria vaccines are listed by stage of clinical development at The Malaria Vaccine Initiative website.[157] The most advanced candidate provided modest protection in children hence the need to continue to evaluate the earlier stage vaccines in the pipeline.[158]

References

1. Greenwood, B. M.; Bojang, K.; Whitty, C. J. M.; Targett, G. A. T., Malaria. *Lancet (London, England)* **2005**, *365* (9469), 1487-98.
2. Carter, R.; Mendis, K. N., Evolutionary and historical aspects of the burden of malaria. *Clinical microbiology reviews* **2002**, *15* (4), 564-94.
3. WHO, World Malaria Report 2015. *Geneva, World Health Organization* **2015**.
4. WHO, http://www.who.int/malaria/areas/global_technical_strategy/en/ (accessed May 2016). **2016**.
5. Newby, G.; Bennett, A.; Larson, E.; Cotter, C.; Shretta, R.; Phillips, A. A.; Feachem, R. G., The path to eradication: a progress report on the malaria-eliminating countries. *Lancet* **2016**, *387* (10029), 1775-84.
6. Cholera, R.; Brittain, N. J.; Gillrie, M. R.; Lopera-Mesa, T. M.; Diakite, S. A.; Arie, T.; Krause, M. A.; Guindo, A.; Tubman, A.; Fujioka, H.; Diallo, D. A.; Doumbo, O. K.; Ho, M.; Wellems, T. E.; Fairhurst, R. M., Impaired cytoadherence of Plasmodium falciparum-infected erythrocytes containing sickle hemoglobin. *Proc Natl Acad Sci U S A* **2008**, *105* (3), 991-6.
7. Taylor, S. M.; Parobek, C. M.; Fairhurst, R. M., Haemoglobinopathies and the clinical epidemiology of malaria: a systematic review and meta-analysis. *Lancet Infect Dis* **2012**, *12* (6), 457-68.
8. Cyrklaff, M.; Sanchez, C. P.; Kilian, N.; Bisseye, C.; Simpore, J.; Frischknecht, F.; Lanzer, M., Hemoglobins S and C interfere with actin remodeling in Plasmodium falciparum-infected erythrocytes. *Science* **2011**, *334* (6060), 1283-6.
9. Adams, H. C., The Genuine Works of Hippocrates. **1886**, The Epidemics Book 1.
10. Laveran, A., Note sur un nouveau parasite trouve´ dans le sang de plusieurs malades atteints de fie`vre palustre. *Bull. Acad. Med* **1880**, *8*, 1235-1236.
11. Kean, B. H.; Mott, K. E.; Russell, A. J., Tropical medicine and parasitology: classic investigations. *Cornell University Press, Ithaca, NY* **1978**.
12. Harrison, G., Mosquitoes, Malaria, and Man. **1978**.
13. Bruce-Chwat, L. J.; Wernsdorfer, W. H.; McGregor, S. I., History of malaria from pre-history to eradication. *In Malaria Principles and Practice of Malariology eds Churchill Livingstone*

Edinburgh pp **1988**, 1-59.

14. Shortt, H. E.; Garnham, P. C., Pre-erythrocytic stage in mammalian malaria parasites. *Nature* **1948,** *161* (4082), 126.

15. Krotoski, W. A.; Krotoski, D. M.; Garnham, P. C.; Bray, R. S.; Killick-Kendrick, R.; Draper, C. C.; Targett, G. A.; Guy, M. W., Relapses in primate malaria: discovery of two populations of exoerythrocytic stages. Preliminary note. *Br Med J* **1980,** *280* (6208), 153-4.

16. Krotoski, W. A.; Collins, W. E.; Bray, R. S.; Garnham, P. C.; Cogswell, F. B.; Gwadz, R. W.; Killick-Kendrick, R.; Wolf, R.; Sinden, R.; Koontz, L. C.; Stanfill, P. S., Demonstration of hypnozoites in sporozoite-transmitted Plasmodium vivax infection. *Am J Trop Med Hyg* **1982,** *31* (6), 1291-3.

17. Markus, M. B., Possible support for the sporozoite hypothesis of relapse and latency in malaria. *Trans R Soc Trop Med Hyg* **1976,** *70* (5-6), 535.

18. Markus, M. B., The malarial hypnozoite. *Lancet* **1980,** *1* (8174), 936.

19. Haggis, A. W., Fundamental errors in the early history of cinchona. *Bull Hist Med* **1941,** *10*, 567-568.

20. Meshnick, S. R.; Sherman, I. W., From quinine to Qinghaosu: Historical perspectives. **1998**; p 341-353.

21. Honigsbaum, M., The Fever Trail: In search of the cure for malaria. *Nature Medicine* **2001**.

22. Rocco, F., Quinine: Malaria and the quest for a cure that changed the world. **2003**.

23. Vinetz, J. M.; Li, J.; McCutchan, T. F.; Kaslow, D. C., Plasmodium malariae infection in an asymptomatic 74-year-old Greek woman with splenomegaly. *The New England journal of medicine* **1998,** *338* (6), 367-71.

24. Garnham, P. C., Swellengrebel lecture. Hypnozoites and 'relapses' in Plasmodium vivax and in vivax-like malaria. *Tropical and geographical medicine* **1988,** *40* (3), 187-95.

25. R., K.; B.M., D. G., A study of monkey-malaria, and its experimental transmission to man. *Ind Med Gaz* **1932,** *67*, 301-21.

26. Kantele, A.; Jokiranta, T. S., Review of cases with the emerging fifth human malaria parasite, Plasmodium knowlesi. *Clin Infect Dis* **2011,** *52* (11), 1356-62.

27. White, N. J., Plasmodium knowlesi: the fifth human malaria parasite. *Clin Infect Dis* **2008,** *46* (2), 172-3.

28. Coatney, G. R., The simian malarias: zoonoses, anthroponoses, or both? *The American journal of tropical medicine and hygiene* **1971,** *20* (6), 795-803.

29. Ta, T. H.; Hisam, S.; Lanza, M.; Jiram, A. I.; Ismail, N.; Rubio, J. M., First case of a naturally acquired human infection with Plasmodium cynomolgi. *Malar J* **2014,** *13*, 68.

30. White, N. J., Sharing malarias. *Lancet (London, England)* **2004,** *363* (9414), 1006.

31. Abegunde, A. T., Monkey malaria in man. *Lancet (London, England)* **2004,** *364* (9441), 1217.

32. Singh, B.; Kim Sung, L.; Matusop, A.; Radhakrishnan, A.; Shamsul, S. S. G.; Cox-Singh, J.; Thomas, A.; Conway, D. J., A large focus of naturally acquired Plasmodium knowlesi infections in human beings. *Lancet (London, England)* **2004,** *363* (9414), 1017-24.

33. Meis, J. F.; Verhave, J. P., Exoerythrocytic development of malarial parasites. *Advances in parasitology* **1988,** *27*, 1-61.

34. Hollingdale, M. R., Biology and immunology of sporozoite invasion of liver cells and exoerythrocytic development of malaria parasites. *Progress in allergy* **1988,** *41*, 15-48.

35. Sherman, I. W., Malaria:Parasite Biology, Pathogenesis and Protection. ASM Press, Washington, D.C. : **1998**.

36. Cha, S. J.; Park, K.; Srinivasan, P.; Schindler, C. W.; van Rooijen, N.; Stins, M.; Jacobs-Lorena, M., CD68 acts as a major gateway for malaria sporozoite liver infection. *J Exp Med* **2015,** *212* (9), 1391-403.

37. White, N. J.; Pukrittayakamee, S.; Hien, T. T.; Faiz, M. A.; Mokuolu, O. A.; Dondorp, A. M., Malaria. *Lancet* **2014,** *383* (9918), 723-35.

38. Coatney, G. R., Relapse in malaria--an enigma. *The Journal of parasitology* **1976,** *62* (1), 3-9.

39. Schmidt, L. H., Compatibility of relapse patterns of Plasmodium cynomolgi infections in rhesus monkeys with continuous cyclical development and hypnozoite concepts of relapse. *The American*

journal of tropical medicine and hygiene **1986,** *35* (6), 1077-99.

40.   Krotoski, W. A., Discovery of the hypnozoite and a new theory of malarial relapse. *Transactions of the Royal Society of Tropical Medicine and Hygiene* **1985,** *79* (1), 1-11.

41.   Adekunle, A. I.; Pinkevych, M.; McGready, R.; Luxemburger, C.; White, L. J.; Nosten, F.; Cromer, D.; Davenport, M. P., Modeling the dynamics of Plasmodium vivax infection and hypnozoite reactivation in vivo. *PLoS Negl Trop Dis* **2015,** *9* (3), e0003595.

42.   Hulden, L.; Hulden, L., Activation of the hypnozoite: a part of Plasmodium vivax life cycle and survival. *Malar J* **2011,** *10*, 90.

43.   Krotoski, W. A., The hypnozoite and malarial relapse. *Prog Clin Parasitol* **1989,** *1*, 1-19.

44.   Galappaththy, G. N.; Tharyan, P.; Kirubakaran, R., Primaquine for preventing relapse in people with Plasmodium vivax malaria treated with chloroquine. *Cochrane Database Syst Rev* **2013,** *10*, CD004389.

45.   Dvorak, J. A.; Miller, L. H.; Whitehouse, W. C.; Shiroishi, T., Invasion of erythrocytes by malaria merozoites. *Science (New York, N.Y.)* **1975,** *187* (4178), 748-50.

46.   Egan, E. S.; Jiang, R. H.; Moechtar, M. A.; Barteneva, N. S.; Weekes, M. P.; Nobre, L. V.; Gygi, S. P.; Paulo, J. A.; Frantzreb, C.; Tani, Y.; Takahashi, J.; Watanabe, S.; Goldberg, J.; Paul, A. S.; Brugnara, C.; Root, D. E.; Wiegand, R. C.; Doench, J. G.; Duraisingh, M. T., Malaria. A forward genetic screen identifies erythrocyte CD55 as essential for Plasmodium falciparum invasion. *Science* **2015,** *348* (6235), 711-4.

47.   Aikawa, M.; Miller, L. H.; Johnson, J.; Rabbege, J., Erythrocyte entry by malarial parasites. A moving junction between erythrocyte and parasite. *The Journal of cell biology* **1978,** *77* (1), 72-82.

48.   Collins, W. E.; Jeffery, G. M., Plasmodium malariae: parasite and disease. *Clin Microbiol Rev* **2007,** *20* (4), 579-92.

49.   Garvey, G.; Neu, H. C.; Datz, M., Transfusion-induced malaria after open-heart surgery. *New York state journal of medicine* **1975,** *75* (4), 602-3.

50.   Covell, G., Congenital malaria. *Trop Dis Bull* **1950,** *47*, 1147-1167.

51.   Mwangoka, G. W.; Kimera, S. I.; Mboera, L. E., Congenital Plasmodium falciparum infection in neonates in Muheza District, Tanzania. *Malar J* **2008,** *7*, 117.

52.   Ogolla, S.; Daud, II; Asito, A. S.; Sumba, O. P.; Ouma, C.; Vulule, J.; Middeldorp, J. M.; Dent, A. E.; Mehta, S.; Rochford, R., Reduced Transplacental Transfer of a Subset of Epstein-Barr Virus-Specific Antibodies to Neonates of Mothers Infected with Plasmodium falciparum Malaria during Pregnancy. *Clin Vaccine Immunol* **2015,** *22* (11), 1197-205.

53.   Ouedraogo, A.; Tiono, A. B.; Diarra, A.; Bougouma, E. C.; Nebie, I.; Konate, A. T.; Sirima, S. B., Transplacental Transmission of Plasmodium falciparum in a Highly Malaria Endemic Area of Burkina Faso. *J Trop Med* **2012,** *2012*, 109705.

54.   Falade, C.; Mokuolu, O.; Okafor, H.; Orogade, A.; Falade, A.; Adedoyin, O.; Oguonu, T.; Aisha, M.; Hamer, D. H.; Callahan, M. V., Epidemiology of congenital malaria in Nigeria: a multi-centre study. *Trop Med Int Health* **2007,** *12* (11), 1279-87.

55.   Hanscheid, T., Diagnosis of malaria: A review of alternatives to conventional microscopy. *Clin Lab Haem* **1999,** *21*, 235-245.

56.   Gallego-Delgado, J.; Ty, M.; Orengo, J. M.; van de Hoef, D.; Rodriguez, A., A surprising role for uric acid: the inflammatory malaria response. *Curr Rheumatol Rep* **2014,** *16* (2), 401.

57.   Prakash, D.; Fesel, C.; Jain, R.; Cazenave, P. A.; Mishra, G. C.; Pied, S., Clusters of cytokines determine malaria severity in Plasmodium falciparum-infected patients from endemic areas of Central India. *J Infect Dis* **2006,** *194* (2), 198-207.

58.   WHO, Severe and complicated malaria. *Trans R Soc Trop Med Hyg* **1986,** 1-50.

59.   Wahlgren, M.; Treutiger, C. J.; Gysin, J.; Perlmann, P., Malaria: Chapter 10. Cytoadherence and rosetting in the pathogenesis of severe malaria. CRC Press: **1999;** p 289-327.

60.   Frevert, U.; Nacer, A., Fatal cerebral malaria: a venous efflux problem. *Front Cell Infect Microbiol* **2014,** *4*, 155.

61.   Cooke, B.; Coppel, R.; Wahlgren, M., Falciparum malaria: sticking up, standing out and out-standing. *Parasitol Today* **2000,** *16* (10), 416-20.

62.   Kilejian, A., Characterization of a protein correlated with the production of knob-like protrusions

on membranes of erythrocytes infected with Plasmodium falciparum. *Proc Natl Acad Sci U S A* **1979,** *76* (9), 4650-3.

63. Ruangjirachuporn, W.; Afzelius, B. A.; Paulie, S.; Wahlgren, M.; Berzins, K.; Perlmann, P., Cytoadherence of knobby and knobless Plasmodium falciparum-infected erythrocytes. *Parasitology* **1991,** *102 Pt 3*, 325-34.

64. Udeinya, I. J.; Schmidt, J. A.; Aikawa, M.; Miller, L. H.; Green, I., Falciparum malaria-infected erythrocytes specifically bind to cultured human endothelial cells. *Science (New York, N.Y.)* **1981,** *213* (4507), 555-7.

65. Chisti, A. H.; Andrabi, K. I.; Derick, L. M., Isolation of skeleton-associated knobs from human blood cells infected with the malaria parasite Plasmodium falciparum. *Mol Biochem Parasit* **1992,** *52*, 293-297.

66. Miller, L. H.; Good, M. F.; Milon, G., Malaria pathogenesis. *Science (New York, N.Y.)* **1994,** *264* (5167), 1878-83.

67. Duffy, P. E.; Fried, M., Antibodies that inhibit Plasmodium falciparum adhesion to chondroitin sulfate A are associated with increased birth weight and the gestational age of newborns. *Infection and immunity* **2003,** *71* (11), 6620-3.

68. Miller, L. H.; Smith, J. D., Motherhood and malaria. *Nature medicine* **1998,** *4* (11), 1244-5.

69. Duffy, P. E.; Fried, M., Plasmodium falciparum adhesion in the placenta. *Current opinion in microbiology* **2003,** *6* (4), 371-6.

70. Looareesuwan, S.; Ho, M.; Wattanagoon, Y.; White, N. J.; Warrell, D. A.; Bunnag, D.; Harinasuta, T.; Wyler, D. J., Dynamic alteration in splenic function during acute falciparum malaria. *The New England journal of medicine* **1987,** *317* (11), 675-9.

71. Douglas, N. M.; Anstey, N. M.; Buffet, P. A.; Poespoprodjo, J. R.; Yeo, T. W.; White, N. J.; Price, R. N., The anaemia of Plasmodium vivax malaria. *Malar J* **2012,** *11*, 135.

72. Bruneel, F.; Gachot, B.; Wolff, M.; Bedos, J. P.; Regnier, B.; Danis, M.; Vachon, F., [Blackwater fever]. *Presse medicale (Paris, France : 1983)* **2002,** *31* (28), 1329-34.

73. Ernberg, I.; Wahlgren, M.; Perlmann, P., Malaria: Molecular and Clinical Aspects: Burkitt's lymphoma and malaria. Harwood Academic Publishers, Amsterdam: **1999**; p 370-399.

74. O'Byrne, K. J.; Dalgleish, A. G., Chronic immune activation and inflammation as the cause of malignancy. *Br J Cancer* **2001,** *85* (4), 473-83.

75. Moormann, A. M.; Snider, C. J.; Chelimo, K., The company malaria keeps: how co-infection with Epstein-Barr virus leads to endemic Burkitt lymphoma. *Curr Opin Infect Dis* **2011,** *24* (5), 435-41.

76. Murray, C. J.; Ortblad, K. F.; Guinovart, C.; Lim, S. S.; Wolock, T. M.; Roberts, D. A.; Dansereau, E. A.; Graetz, N.; Barber, R. M.; Brown, J. C.; Wang, H.; Duber, H. C.; Naghavi, M.; Dicker, D.; Dandona, L.; Salomon, J. A.; Heuton, K. R.; Foreman, K.; Phillips, D. E.; Fleming, T. D.; Flaxman, A. D.; Phillips, B. K.; Johnson, E. K.; Coggeshall, M. S.; Abd-Allah, F.; Abera, S. F.; Abraham, J. P.; Abubakar, I.; Abu-Raddad, L. J.; Abu-Rmeileh, N. M.; Achoki, T.; Adeyemo, A. O.; Adou, A. K.; Adsuar, J. C.; Agardh, E. E.; Akena, D.; Al Kahbouri, M. J.; Alasfoor, D.; Albittar, M. I.; Alcala-Cerra, G.; Alegretti, M. A.; Alemu, Z. A.; Alfonso-Cristancho, R.; Alhabib, S.; Ali, R.; Alla, F.; Allen, P. J.; Alsharif, U.; Alvarez, E.; Alvis-Guzman, N.; Amankwaa, A. A.; Amare, A. T.; Amini, H.; Ammar, W.; Anderson, B. O.; Antonio, C. A.; Anwari, P.; Arnlov, J.; Arsenijevic, V. S.; Artaman, A.; Asghar, R. J.; Assadi, R.; Atkins, L. S.; Badawi, A.; Balakrishnan, K.; Banerjee, A.; Basu, S.; Beardsley, J.; Bekele, T.; Bell, M. L.; Bernabe, E.; Beyene, T. J.; Bhala, N.; Bhalla, A.; Bhutta, Z. A.; Abdulhak, A. B.; Binagwaho, A.; Blore, J. D.; Basara, B. B.; Bose, D.; Brainin, M.; Breitborde, N.; Castaneda-Orjuela, C. A.; Catala-Lopez, F.; Chadha, V. K.; Chang, J. C.; Chiang, P. P.; Chuang, T. W.; Colomar, M.; Cooper, L. T.; Cooper, C.; Courville, K. J.; Cowie, B. C.; Criqui, M. H.; Dandona, R.; Dayama, A.; De Leo, D.; Degenhardt, L.; Del Pozo-Cruz, B.; Deribe, K.; Des Jarlais, D. C.; Dessalegn, M.; Dharmaratne, S. D.; Dilmen, U.; Ding, E. L.; Driscoll, T. R.; Durrani, A. M.; Ellenbogen, R. G.; Ermakov, S. P.; Esteghamati, A.; Faraon, E. J.; Farzadfar, F.; Fereshtehnejad, S. M.; Fijabi, D. O.; Forouzanfar, M. H.; Fra Paleo, U.; Gaffikin, L.; Gamkrelidze, A.; Gankpe, F. G.; Geleijnse, J. M.; Gessner, B. D.; Gibney, K. B.; Ginawi, I. A.; Glaser, E. L.; Gona, P.; Goto, A.; Gouda, H. N.; Gugnani, H. C.; Gupta, R.; Gupta, R.; Hafezi-Nejad, N.; Hamadeh, R. R.; Hammami, M.; Hankey, G. J.; Harb, H. L.; Haro, J. M.; Havmoeller,

R.; Hay, S. I.; Hedayati, M. T.; Pi, I. B.; Hoek, H. W.; Hornberger, J. C.; Hosgood, H. D.; Hotez, P. J.; Hoy, D. G.; Huang, J. J.; Iburg, K. M.; Idrisov, B. T.; Innos, K.; Jacobsen, K. H.; Jeemon, P.; Jensen, P. N.; Jha, V.; Jiang, G.; Jonas, J. B.; Juel, K.; Kan, H.; Kankindi, I.; Karam, N. E.; Karch, A.; Karema, C. K.; Kaul, A.; Kawakami, N.; Kazi, D. S.; Kemp, A. H.; Kengne, A. P.; Keren, A.; Kereselidze, M.; Khader, Y. S.; Khalifa, S. E.; Khan, E. A.; Khang, Y. H.; Khonelidze, I.; Kinfu, Y.; Kinge, J. M.; Knibbs, L.; Kokubo, Y.; Kosen, S.; Defo, B. K.; Kulkarni, V. S.; Kulkarni, C.; Kumar, K.; Kumar, R. B.; Kumar, G. A.; Kwan, G. F.; Lai, T.; Balaji, A. L.; Lam, H.; Lan, Q.; Lansingh, V. C.; Larson, H. J.; Larsson, A.; Lee, J. T.; Leigh, J.; Leinsalu, M.; Leung, R.; Li, Y.; Li, Y.; De Lima, G. M.; Lin, H. H.; Lipshultz, S. E.; Liu, S.; Liu, Y.; Lloyd, B. K.; Lotufo, P. A.; Machado, V. M.; Maclachlan, J. H.; Magis-Rodriguez, C.; Majdan, M.; Mapoma, C. C.; Marcenes, W.; Marzan, M. B.; Masci, J. R.; Mashal, M. T.; Mason-Jones, A. J.; Mayosi, B. M.; Mazorodze, T. T.; McKay, A. C.; Meaney, P. A.; Mehndiratta, M. M.; Mejia-Rodriguez, F.; Melaku, Y. A.; Memish, Z. A.; Mendoza, W.; Miller, T. R.; Mills, E. J.; Mohammad, K. A.; Mokdad, A. H.; Mola, G. L.; Monasta, L.; Montico, M.; Moore, A. R.; Mori, R.; Moturi, W. N.; Mukaigawara, M.; Murthy, K. S.; Naheed, A.; Naidoo, K. S.; Naldi, L.; Nangia, V.; Narayan, K. M.; Nash, D.; Nejjari, C.; Nelson, R. G.; Neupane, S. P.; Newton, C. R.; Ng, M.; Nisar, M. I.; Nolte, S.; Norheim, O. F.; Nowaseb, V.; Nyakarahuka, L.; Oh, I. H.; Ohkubo, T.; Olusanya, B. O.; Omer, S. B.; Opio, J. N.; Orisakwe, O. E.; Pandian, J. D.; Papachristou, C.; Caicedo, A. J.; Patten, S. B.; Paul, V. K.; Pavlin, B. I.; Pearce, N.; Pereira, D. M.; Pervaiz, A.; Pesudovs, K.; Petzold, M.; Pourmalek, F.; Qato, D.; Quezada, A. D.; Quistberg, D. A.; Rafay, A.; Rahimi, K.; Rahimi-Movaghar, V.; Ur Rahman, S.; Raju, M.; Rana, S. M.; Razavi, H.; Reilly, R. Q.; Remuzzi, G.; Richardus, J. H.; Ronfani, L.; Roy, N.; Sabin, N.; Saeedi, M. Y.; Sahraian, M. A.; Samonte, G. M.; Sawhney, M.; Schneider, I. J.; Schwebel, D. C.; Seedat, S.; Sepanlou, S. G.; Servan-Mori, E. E.; Sheikhbahaei, S.; Shibuya, K.; Shin, H. H.; Shiue, I.; Shivakoti, R.; Sigfusdottir, I. D.; Silberberg, D. H.; Silva, A. P.; Simard, E. P.; Singh, J. A.; Skirbekk, V.; Sliwa, K.; Soneji, S.; Soshnikov, S. S.; Sreeramareddy, C. T.; Stathopoulou, V. K.; Stroumpoulis, K.; Swaminathan, S.; Sykes, B. L.; Tabb, K. M.; Talongwa, R. T.; Tenkorang, E. Y.; Terkawi, A. S.; Thomson, A. J.; Thorne-Lyman, A. L.; Towbin, J. A.; Traebert, J.; Tran, B. X.; Dimbuene, Z. T.; Tsilimbaris, M.; Uchendu, U. S.; Ukwaja, K. N.; Uzun, S. B.; Vallely, A. J.; Vasankari, T. J.; Venketasubramanian, N.; Violante, F. S.; Vlassov, V. V.; Vollset, S. E.; Waller, S.; Wallin, M. T.; Wang, L.; Wang, X.; Wang, Y.; Weichenthal, S.; Weiderpass, E.; Weintraub, R. G.; Westerman, R.; White, R. A.; Wilkinson, J. D.; Williams, T. N.; Woldeyohannes, S. M.; Wong, J. Q.; Xu, G.; Yang, Y. C.; Yano, Y.; Yentur, G. K.; Yip, P.; Yonemoto, N.; Yoon, S. J.; Younis, M.; Yu, C.; Jin, K. Y.; El Sayed Zaki, M.; Zhao, Y.; Zheng, Y.; Zhou, M.; Zhu, J.; Zou, X. N.; Lopez, A. D.; Vos, T., Global, regional, and national incidence and mortality for HIV, tuberculosis, and malaria during 1990-2013: a systematic analysis for the Global Burden of Disease Study 2013. *Lancet* **2014**, *384* (9947), 1005-70.

77.   Froebel, K.; Howard, W.; Schafer, J. R.; Howie, F.; Whitworth, J.; Kaleebu, P.; Brown, A. L.; Riley, E., Activation by malaria antigens renders mononuclear cells susceptible to HIV infection and re-activates replication of endogenous HIV in cells from HIV-infected adults. *Parasite Immunol* **2004**, *26* (5), 213-7.

78.   Mermin, J.; Lule, J. R.; Ekwaru, J. P., Association between malaria and CD4 cell count decline among persons with HIV. *J Acquir Immune Defic Syndr* **2006**, *41* (1), 129-30.

79.   Kublin, J. G.; Patnaik, P.; Jere, C. S.; Miller, W. C.; Hoffman, I. F.; Chimbiya, N.; Pendame, R.; Taylor, T. E.; Molyneux, M. E., Effect of Plasmodium falciparum malaria on concentration of HIV-1-RNA in the blood of adults in rural Malawi: a prospective cohort study. *Lancet (London, England)* **2005**, *365* (9455), 233-40.

80.   Grimwadw k; French, N., HIV infection as a cofactor for severe falciparum malaria in adults living in a region of unstable malaria transmission in South Africa. *AIDS* **2004**, *18*, 547-554.

81.   Mount, A. M.; Mwapasa, V.; Elliott, S. R.; Beeson, J. G.; Tadesse, E.; Lema, V. M.; Molyneux, M. E.; Meshnick, S. R.; Rogerson, S. J., Impairment of humoral immunity to Plasmodium falciparum malaria in pregnancy by HIV infection. *Lancet* **2004**, *363* (9424), 1860-7.

82.   Whitworth, J. A. G.; Hewitt, K. A., Effect of malaria on HIV-1 progression and transmission. *Lancet (London, England)* **2005**, *365* (9455), 196-7.

83. Chirenda, J.; Murugasampillay, S., Malaria and HIV co-infection: available evidence, gaps and possible interventions. *The Central African journal of medicine* **2003,** *49* (5-6), 66-71.
84. Patnaik, P.; Jere, C. S.; Miller, W. C.; Hoffman, I. F.; Wirima, J.; Pendame, R.; Meshnick, S. R.; Taylor, T. E.; Molyneux, M. E.; Kublin, J. G., Effects of HIV-1 serostatus, HIV-1 RNA concentration, and CD4 cell count on the incidence of malaria infection in a cohort of adults in rural Malawi. *J Infect Dis* **2005,** *192* (6), 984-91.
85. Whitworth, J.; Morgan, D.; Quigley, M.; Smith, A.; Mayanja, B.; Eotu, H.; Omoding, N.; Okongo, M.; Malamba, S.; Ojwiya, A., Effect of HIV-1 and increasing immunosuppression on malaria parasitaemia and clinical episodes in adults in rural Uganda: a cohort study. *Lancet* **2000,** *356* (9235), 1051-6.
86. Hendriksen, I. C.; Ferro, J.; Montoya, P.; Chhaganlal, K. D.; Seni, A.; Gomes, E.; Silamut, K.; Lee, S. J.; Lucas, M.; Chotivanich, K.; Fanello, C. I.; Day, N. P.; White, N. J.; von Seidlein, L.; Dondorp, A. M., Diagnosis, clinical presentation, and in-hospital mortality of severe malaria in HIV-coinfected children and adults in Mozambique. *Clin Infect Dis* **2012,** *55* (8), 1144-53.
87. Cohen, C.; Karstaedt, A.; Frean, J.; Thomas, J.; Govender, N.; Prentice, E.; Dini, L.; Galpin, J.; Crewe-Brown, H., Increased prevalence of severe malaria in HIV-infected adults in South Africa. *Clin Infect Dis* **2005,** *41* (11), 1631-7.
88. Taylor, W. R.; Hanson, J.; Turner, G. D.; White, N. J.; Dondorp, A. M., Respiratory manifestations of malaria. *Chest* **2012,** *142* (2), 492-505.
89. Allison, A. C., Protection afforded by sickle-cell trait against subtertian malarial infection. *BMJ* **1954,** *1*, 290-294.
90. Roberts, D. J.; Williams, T. N., Haemoglobinopathies and resistance to malaria. *Redox report : communications in free radical research* **2003,** *8* (5), 304-10.
91. Hill, A. V. S.; Weatherall, D. J.; Sherman, I. W., Host genetic factors in resistance to malaria. 1998; p 445-455.
92. Miller, L. H.; Mason, S. J.; Clyde, D. F.; McGinniss, M. H., The resistance factor to Plasmodium vivax in blacks. The Duffy-blood-group genotype, FyFy. *The New England journal of medicine* **1976,** *295* (6), 302-4.
93. Ferreira, A.; Marguti, I.; Bechmann, I.; Jeney, V.; Chora, A.; Palha, N. R.; Rebelo, S.; Henri, A.; Beuzard, Y.; Soares, M. P., Sickle hemoglobin confers tolerance to Plasmodium infection. *Cell* **2011,** *145* (3), 398-409.
94. Hebbel, R. P., Sickle hemoglobin instability: a mechanism for malarial protection. *Redox report : communications in free radical research* **2003,** *8* (5), 238-40.
95. Cabrera, G.; Cot, M.; Migot-Nabias, F.; Kremsner, P. G.; Deloron, P.; Luty, A. J. F., The sickle cell trait is associated with enhanced immunoglobulin G antibody responses to Plasmodium falciparum variant surface antigens. *The Journal of infectious diseases* **2005,** *191* (10), 1631-8.
96. Diallo, D. A.; Doumbo, O. K.; Dicko, A.; Guindo, A.; Coulibaly, D.; Kayentao, K.; Djimdé, A. A.; Théra, M. A.; Fairhurst, R. M.; Plowe, C. V.; Wellems, T. E., A comparison of anemia in hemoglobin C and normal hemoglobin A children with Plasmodium falciparum malaria. *Acta tropica* **2004,** *90* (3), 295-9.
97. Arie, T.; Fairhurst, R. M.; Brittain, N. J.; Wellems, T. E.; Dvorak, J. A., Hemoglobin C modulates the surface topography of Plasmodium falciparum-infected erythrocytes. *Journal of structural biology* **2005,** *150* (2), 163-9.
98. Jarolim, P.; Palek, J.; Amato, D.; Hassan, K.; Sapak, P.; Nurse, G. T.; Rubin, H. L.; Zhai, S.; Sahr, K. E.; Liu, S. C., Deletion in erythrocyte band 3 gene in malaria-resistant Southeast Asian ovalocytosis. *Proceedings of the National Academy of Sciences of the United States of America* **1991,** *88* (24), 11022-6.
99. Luzzi, G. A.; Merry, A. H.; Newbold, C. I.; Marsh, K.; Pasvol, G.; Weatherall, D. J., Surface antigen expression on Plasmodium falciparum-infected erythrocytes is modified in alpha- and beta-thalassemia. *The Journal of experimental medicine* **1991,** *173* (4), 785-91.
100. Glushakova, S.; Balaban, A.; McQueen, P. G.; Coutinho, R.; Miller, J. L.; Nossal, R.; Fairhurst, R. M.; Zimmerberg, J., Hemoglobinopathic erythrocytes affect the intraerythrocytic multiplication of Plasmodium falciparum in vitro. *J Infect Dis* **2014,** *210* (7), 1100-9.

101. Howes, R. E.; Reiner, R. C., Jr.; Battle, K. E.; Longbottom, J.; Mappin, B.; Ordanovich, D.; Tatem, A. J.; Drakeley, C.; Gething, P. W.; Zimmerman, P. A.; Smith, D. L.; Hay, S. I., Plasmodium vivax Transmission in Africa. *PLoS Negl Trop Dis* **2015,** *9* (11), e0004222.
102. Lysenko, A. J.; Beljaev, A. E., An analysis of the geographical distribution of Plasmodium ovale. *Bull World Health Organ* **1969,** *40* (3), 383-94.
103. Soe, S.; Khin Saw, A.; Htay, A.; Nay, W.; Tin, A.; Than, S.; Roussilhon, C.; Perignon, J. L.; Druilhe, P., Premunition against Plasmodium falciparum in a malaria hyperendemic village in Myanmar. *Trans R Soc Trop Med Hyg* **2001,** *95* (1), 81-4.
104. Perignon, J. L.; Druilhe, P., Immune mechanisms underlying the premunition against Plasmodium falciparum malaria. *Mem Inst Oswaldo Cruz* **1994,** *89 Suppl 2*, 51-3.
105. Biot, J.; Martin, M., [Contribution to the study of the premunition of malaria in the African adult. Apropos of 25 cases]. *Med Trop (Mars)* **1963,** *23*, 106-11.
106. Makkapati, V. V.; Rao, R. M., Ontology-based malaria parasite stage and species identification from peripheral blood smear images. *Conf Proc IEEE Eng Med Biol Soc* **2011,** *2011*, 6138-41.
107. Milne, L. M.; Kyi, M. S.; Chiodini, P. L.; Warhurst, D. C., Accuracy of routine laboratory diagnosis of malaria in the United Kingdom. *Journal of clinical pathology* **1994,** *47* (8), 740-2.
108. Wilson, M. L., Malaria rapid diagnostic tests. *Clin Infect Dis* **2012,** *54* (11), 1637-41.
109. Visser, T.; Daily, J.; Hotte, N.; Dolkart, C.; Cunningham, J.; Yadav, P., Rapid diagnostic tests for malaria. *Bull World Health Organ* **2015,** *93* (12), 862-6.
110. Mbabazi, P.; Hopkins, H.; Osilo, E.; Kalungu, M.; Byakika-Kibwika, P.; Kamya, M. R., Accuracy of two malaria rapid diagnostic tests (RDTS) for initial diagnosis and treatment monitoring in a high transmission setting in Uganda. *Am J Trop Med Hyg* **2015,** *92* (3), 530-6.
111. Gatton, M. L.; Rees-Channer, R. R.; Glenn, J.; Barnwell, J. W.; Cheng, Q.; Chiodini, P. L.; Incardona, S.; Gonzalez, I. J.; Cunningham, J., Pan-Plasmodium band sensitivity for Plasmodium falciparum detection in combination malaria rapid diagnostic tests and implications for clinical management. *Malar J* **2015,** *14*, 115.
112. Proux, S.; Suwanarusk, R.; Barends, M.; Zwang, J.; Price, R. N.; Leimanis, M.; Kiricharoen, L.; Laochan, N.; Russell, B.; Nosten, F.; Snounou, G., Considerations on the use of nucleic acid-based amplification for malaria parasite detection. *Malar J* **2011,** *10*, 323.
113. Hopkins, H.; Gonzalez, I. J.; Polley, S. D.; Angutoko, P.; Ategeka, J.; Asiimwe, C.; Agaba, B.; Kyabayinze, D. J.; Sutherland, C. J.; Perkins, M. D.; Bell, D., Highly sensitive detection of malaria parasitemia in a malaria-endemic setting: performance of a new loop-mediated isothermal amplification kit in a remote clinic in Uganda. *J Infect Dis* **2013,** *208* (4), 645-52.
114. Cook, J.; Aydin-Schmidt, B.; Gonzalez, I. J.; Bell, D.; Edlund, E.; Nassor, M. H.; Msellem, M.; Ali, A.; Abass, A. K.; Martensson, A.; Bjorkman, A., Loop-mediated isothermal amplification (LAMP) for point-of-care detection of asymptomatic low-density malaria parasite carriers in Zanzibar. *Malar J* **2015,** *14*, 43.
115. Patel, J. C.; Lucchi, N. W.; Srivastava, P.; Lin, J. T.; Sug-Aram, R.; Aruncharus, S.; Bharti, P. K.; Shukla, M. M.; Congpuong, K.; Satimai, W.; Singh, N.; Udhayakumar, V.; Meshnick, S. R., Field evaluation of a real-time fluorescence loop-mediated isothermal amplification assay, RealAmp, for the diagnosis of malaria in Thailand and India. *J Infect Dis* **2014,** *210* (8), 1180-7.
116. Plowe, C. V.; Cortese, J. F.; Djimde, A.; Nwanyanwu, O. C.; Watkins, W. M.; Winstanley, P. A.; Estrada-Franco, J. G.; Mollinedo, R. E.; Avila, J. C.; Cespedes, J. L.; Carter, D.; Doumbo, O. K., Mutations in Plasmodium falciparum dihydrofolate reductase and dihydropteroate synthase and epidemiologic patterns of pyrimethamine-sulfadoxine use and resistance. *The Journal of infectious diseases* **1997,** *176* (6), 1590-6.
117. Plowe, C. V.; Kublin, J. G.; Doumbo, O. K., P. falciparum dihydrofolate reductase and dihydropteroate synthase mutations: epidemiology and role in clinical resistance to antifolates. *Drug resistance updates : reviews and commentaries in antimicrobial and anticancer chemotherapy* **1998,** *1* (6), 389-96.
118. Sidhu, A. B. S.; Verdier-Pinard, D.; Fidock, D. A., Chloroquine resistance in Plasmodium falciparum malaria parasites conferred by pfcrt mutations. *Science (New York, N.Y.)* **2002,** *298* (5591), 210-3.

119. Mita, T.; Tachibana, S.; Hashimoto, M.; Hirai, M., Plasmodium falciparum kelch 13: a potential molecular marker for tackling artemisinin-resistant malaria parasites. *Expert Rev Anti Infect Ther* **2016,** *14* (1), 125-35.
120. Ariey, F.; Witkowski, B.; Amaratunga, C.; Beghain, J.; Langlois, A. C.; Khim, N.; Kim, S.; Duru, V.; Bouchier, C.; Ma, L.; Lim, P.; Leang, R.; Duong, S.; Sreng, S.; Suon, S.; Chuor, C. M.; Bout, D. M.; Menard, S.; Rogers, W. O.; Genton, B.; Fandeur, T.; Miotto, O.; Ringwald, P.; Le Bras, J.; Berry, A.; Barale, J. C.; Fairhurst, R. M.; Benoit-Vical, F.; Mercereau-Puijalon, O.; Menard, D., A molecular marker of artemisinin-resistant Plasmodium falciparum malaria. *Nature* **2014,** *505* (7481), 50-5.
121. Beier, J. C.; Perkins, P. V.; Wirtz, R. A.; Whitmire, R. E.; Mugambi, M.; Hockmeyer, W. T., Field evaluation of an enzyme-linked immunosorbent assay (ELISA) for Plasmodium falciparum sporozoite detection in anopheline mosquitoes from Kenya. *The American journal of tropical medicine and hygiene* **1987,** *36* (3), 459-68.
122. Baird, J. K., Effectiveness of antimalarial drugs. *The New England journal of medicine* **2005,** *352* (15), 1565-77.
123. Dondorp, A. M.; Fanello, C. I.; Hendriksen, I. C.; Gomes, E.; Seni, A.; Chhaganlal, K. D.; Bojang, K.; Olaosebikan, R.; Anunobi, N.; Maitland, K.; Kivaya, E.; Agbenyega, T.; Nguah, S. B.; Evans, J.; Gesase, S.; Kahabuka, C.; Mtove, G.; Nadjm, B.; Deen, J.; Mwanga-Amumpaire, J.; Nansumba, M.; Karema, C.; Umulisa, N.; Uwimana, A.; Mokuolu, O. A.; Adedoyin, O. T.; Johnson, W. B.; Tshefu, A. K.; Onyamboko, M. A.; Sakulthaew, T.; Ngum, W. P.; Silamut, K.; Stepniewska, K.; Woodrow, C. J.; Bethell, D.; Wills, B.; Oneko, M.; Peto, T. E.; von Seidlein, L.; Day, N. P.; White, N. J.; group, A., Artesunate versus quinine in the treatment of severe falciparum malaria in African children (AQUAMAT): an open-label, randomised trial. *Lancet* **2010,** *376* (9753), 1647-57.
124. Dondorp, A.; Nosten, F.; Stepniewska, K.; Day, N.; White, N.; South East Asian Quinine Artesunate Malaria Trial, g., Artesunate versus quinine for treatment of severe falciparum malaria: a randomised trial. *Lancet* **2005,** *366* (9487), 717-25.
125. Smithuis, F.; Shahmanesh, M.; Kyaw, M. K.; Savran, O.; Lwin, S.; White, N. J., Comparison of chloroquine, sulfadoxine/pyrimethamine, mefloquine and mefloquine-artesunate for the treatment of falciparum malaria in Kachin State, North Myanmar. *Tropical medicine & international health : TM & IH* **2004,** *9* (11), 1184-90.
126. Staedke, S. G.; Mpimbaza, A.; Kamya, M. R.; Nzarubara, B. K.; Dorsey, G.; Rosenthal, P. J., Combination treatments for uncomplicated falciparum malaria in Kampala, Uganda: randomised clinical trial. *Lancet (London, England)* **2004,** *364* (9449), 1950-7.
127. CDC, Treatment with quinidine gluconate of persons with severe Plasmodium falciparum infection: discontinuation of parenteral quinine from CDC Drug Service. *MMWR Recomm Rep* **1991,** *40* (RR-4), 21.
128. Twomey, P. S.; Smith, B. L.; McDermott, C.; Novitt-Moreno, A.; McCarthy, W.; Kachur, S. P.; Arguin, P. M., Intravenous Artesunate for the Treatment of Severe and Complicated Malaria in the United States: Clinical Use Under an Investigational New Drug Protocol. *Ann Intern Med* **2015,** *163* (7), 498-506.
129. Berkley, J. A.; Lowe, B. S.; Mwangi, I.; Williams, T.; Bauni, E.; Mwarumba, S.; Ngetsa, C.; Slack, M. P.; Njenga, S.; Hart, C. A.; Maitland, K.; English, M.; Marsh, K.; Scott, J. A., Bacteremia among children admitted to a rural hospital in Kenya. *N Engl J Med* **2005,** *352* (1), 39-47.
130. Tan, K. R.; Wiegand, R. E.; Arguin, P. M., Exchange transfusion for severe malaria: evidence base and literature review. *Clin Infect Dis* **2013,** *57* (7), 923-8.
131. Bojang, K. A.; Palmer, A.; Boele van Hensbroek, M.; Banya, W. A.; Greenwood, B. M., Management of severe malarial anaemia in Gambian children. *Trans R Soc Trop Med Hyg* **1997,** *91* (5), 557-61.
132. English, M.; Ahmed, M.; Ngando, C.; Berkley, J.; Ross, A., Blood transfusion for severe anaemia in children in a Kenyan hospital. *Lancet* **2002,** *359* (9305), 494-5.
133. Awasthi, G.; Das, A., Genetics of chloroquine-resistant malaria: a haplotypic view. *Mem Inst Oswaldo Cruz* **2013,** *108* (8), 947-61.
134. WHO, Guidelines for the treatment of malaria, 3rd ed, WHO, Geneva. http://www.who.int/malaria/publications/atoz/9789241549127/en/ *(Accessed on March 18, 2016)* **2015**.

135. Medical Letter on Drugs and Therapeutics. *Handbook of Antimicrobial Therapies* **2005**.
136. Miller, K. D.; Lobel, H. O.; Satriale, R. F.; Kuritsky, J. N.; Stern, R.; Campbell, C. C., Severe cutaneous reactions among American travelers using pyrimethamine-sulfadoxine (Fansidar) for malaria prophylaxis. *The American journal of tropical medicine and hygiene* **1986,** *35* (3), 451-8.
137. Deloron, P.; Bertin, G.; Briand, V.; Massougbodji, A.; Cot, M., Sulfadoxine/pyrimethamine intermittent preventive treatment for malaria during pregnancy. *Emerg Infect Dis* **2010,** *16* (11), 1666-70.
138. Peters, P. J.; Thigpen, M. C.; Parise, M. E.; Newman, R. D., Safety and toxicity of sulfadoxine/pyrimethamine: implications for malaria prevention in pregnancy using intermittent preventive treatment. *Drug Saf* **2007,** *30* (6), 481-501.
139. Maguire, J. D.; Krisin; Marwoto, H.; Richie, T. L.; Fryauff, D. J.; Baird, J. K., Mefloquine is highly efficacious against chloroquine-resistant Plasmodium vivax malaria and Plasmodium falciparum malaria in Papua, Indonesia. *Clin Infect Dis* **2006,** *42* (8), 1067-72.
140. Looareesuwan, S.; Wilairatana, P.; Chalermarut, K.; Rattanapong, Y.; Canfield, C. J.; Hutchinson, D. B., Efficacy and safety of atovaquone/proguanil compared with mefloquine for treatment of acute Plasmodium falciparum malaria in Thailand. *Am J Trop Med Hyg* **1999,** *60* (4), 526-32.
141. Bustos, D. G.; Canfield, C. J.; Canete-Miguel, E.; Hutchinson, D. B., Atovaquone-proguanil compared with chloroquine and chloroquine-sulfadoxine-pyrimethamine for treatment of acute Plasmodium falciparum malaria in the Philippines. *J Infect Dis* **1999,** *179* (6), 1587-90.
142. Cui, L.; Mharakurwa, S.; Ndiaye, D.; Rathod, P. K.; Rosenthal, P. J., Antimalarial Drug Resistance: Literature Review and Activities and Findings of the ICEMR Network. *Am J Trop Med Hyg* **2015,** *93* (3 Suppl), 57-68.
143. Ritchie, E. C.; Block, J.; Nevin, R. L., Psychiatric side effects of mefloquine: applications to forensic psychiatry. *J Am Acad Psychiatry Law* **2013,** *41* (2), 224-35.
144. Hill, D. R.; Baird, J. K.; Parise, M. E.; Lewis, L. S.; Ryan, E. T.; Magill, A. J., Primaquine: report from CDC expert meeting on malaria chemoprophylaxis I. *Am J Trop Med Hyg* **2006,** *75* (3), 402-15.
145. Porter, C. H.; Collins, F. H., Susceptibility of Anopheles hermsi to Plasmodium vivax. *The American journal of tropical medicine and hygiene* **1990,** *42* (5), 414-6.
146. Dhiman, S.; Veer, V., Culminating anti-malaria efforts at long lasting insecticidal net? *J Infect Public Health* **2014,** *7* (6), 457-64.
147. Lin, L. B.; Target, G. A. L., Bednets treated with pyrethroids for malaria control. 1991; p 67-82.
148. J., The western Kenya insecticide-treated bed net trial. *Am Med Hyg* **2003,** *68*, 1-173.
149. James, A. A., Mosquito molecular genetics: the hands that feed bite back. *Science (New York, N.Y.)* **1992,** *257* (5066), 37-8.
150. Gwadz, R. W., Genetic approaches to malaria control: how long the road? *The American journal of tropical medicine and hygiene* **1994,** *50* (6 Suppl), 116-25.
151. Gantz, V. M.; Jasinskiene, N.; Tatarenkova, O.; Fazekas, A.; Macias, V. M.; Bier, E.; James, A. A., Highly efficient Cas9-mediated gene drive for population modification of the malaria vector mosquito Anopheles stephensi. *Proc Natl Acad Sci U S A* **2015,** *112* (49), E6736-43.
152. Trager, W.; Jensen, J. B., Human malaria parasites in continuous culture. 1976. *J Parasitol* **2005,** *91* (3), 484-6.
153. Gardner, M. J.; Hall, N.; Fung, E.; White, O.; Berriman, M.; Hyman, R. W.; Carlton, J. M.; Pain, A.; Nelson, K. E.; Bowman, S.; Paulsen, I. T.; James, K.; Eisen, J. A.; Rutherford, K.; Salzberg, S. L.; Craig, A.; Kyes, S.; Chan, M. S.; Nene, V.; Shallom, S. J.; Suh, B.; Peterson, J.; Angiuoli, S.; Pertea, M.; Allen, J.; Selengut, J.; Haft, D.; Mather, M. W.; Vaidya, A. B.; Martin, D. M.; Fairlamb, A. H.; Fraunholz, M. J.; Roos, D. S.; Ralph, S. A.; McFadden, G. I.; Cummings, L. M.; Subramanian, G. M.; Mungall, C.; Venter, J. C.; Carucci, D. J.; Hoffman, S. L.; Newbold, C.; Davis, R. W.; Fraser, C. M.; Barrell, B., Genome sequence of the human malaria parasite Plasmodium falciparum. *Nature* **2002,** *419* (6906), 498-511.
154. Hoffmann, S. L., Malaria Vaccine Development: A Multi-Immune Response Approach. ASM Press, Washington, D.C: **1996**.
155. Miller, L. H.; Hoffman, S. L., Research toward vaccines against malaria. *Nature medicine* **1998,** *4*

(5 Suppl), 520-4.

156. Narden, E.; Wahlgren, M.; Perlmann, P., Synthetic peptides as malaria vaccines. Harwood
      Academic Publishers, Amsterdam.: **1999**; p 495-540.

157. MVI, http://www.malariavaccine.org/projects/vaccine-projects (accessed May 2016). **2016**.

158. Rts, S. C. T. P., Efficacy and safety of RTS,S/AS01 malaria vaccine with or without a booster dose
      in infants and children in Africa: final results of a phase 3, individually randomised, controlled
      trial. *Lancet* **2015,** *386* (9988), 31-45.

10. *Cryptosporidium parvum and C. hominis*

(Tyzzer 1929)

Introduction

The genus *Cryptosporidium* comprises a very large group of closely related obligate intracellular parasites that cause transient diarrheal disease in most mammal species throughout the world, including humans. All are transmitted through fecally contaminated food and water.[1-3] Most species have broad host ranges. Eight species have been shown to infect humans on a regular basis; *C. parvum*, *C. hominis*, *C. meleagridis*, *C. felis*, *C. canis*, *C. muris*, and *Cryptosporidium* pig and deer species.[4-10] The majority of human infections are caused by *C. parvum and C. hominis*, which also infects sheep, cattle, birds, rodents, and non-human primates.[11] This chapter will concentrate on *C. parvum,* with the assumption that disease in humans caused by other related species results in a similar clinical picture. In 1993, the city of Milwaukee, Wisconsin experienced the largest waterborne outbreak of diarrheal disease ever documented in the United States. Over 400,000 people suffered from infection with *C. parvum*.[12] In immunocompetent infected individuals, the most serious manifestation of infection is diarrhea of short duration, although sometimes severe. In contrast, infants, non-AIDS immunocompromised adults, and people suffering from HIV/AIDS often experience severe, protracted diarrhea, sometimes resulting in death.[13] *C. parvum* can be grown axenically *in vitro*, using monolayers of epithelial cells.[14, 15] The genome of *Cryptosporidum hominis and C. parvum* have been sequenced.[11, 16, 17]

Historical Information

In 1907, Ernest Tyzzer provided a description of cryptosporidium based on histologic sections of mouse intestine, in which the parasites were observed attached to the epithelial cells.[18] The pathogenic characteristics of cryptosporidium were not recognized until much later, when D. Slavin, in 1955, established that this protozoan caused diarrhea in turkeys.[19] F. A. Nime and coworkers, in 1976, described human diarrheal disease due to cryptosporidium, and J. L. Meisel and colleagues, in 1976, were the first to report it in immunocompromised human hosts.[20, 21] Currently various species of *Cryptosporidium* are recognized as important causes of diarrhea in cows, calves, lambs, poultry, game birds and humans.[22, 23] In 2013, the Global Enteric Multicenter Study (GEMS) evaluated the etiology of diarrheal diseases in infants and young children using nucleic acid amplification testing and identified cryptosporidium was one of the four top causes of diarrhea in children younger than 5 years of age.[24]

Life Cycle

Infection begins when the host ingests thick-walled sporulated oocysts (Fig. 10.1), each of which contains four banana-shaped sporozoites.[25] A minimum of 30 oocysts is necessary to initiate infection, while the calculated ID_{50} for healthy volunteers was 132

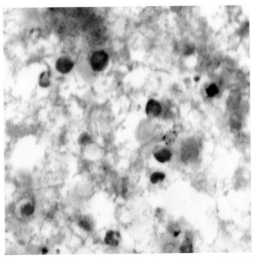

Figure 10.1. Oocysts of *Cryptosporidium parvum*. Cold acid fast stain. 5 μm.

oocysts.[26, 27] An infected individual may release as many as a billion cysts during one infection.[28]

The sporozoites excyst when the oocyst enters the small intestine. Little is known regarding excystment *in vivo*. A protein-plug in the cyst wall blocks the escape route for sporozoites.[29] *In vitro*, excystment occurs after exposure to 37° C or by pretreatment of purified oocysts with either sodium taurocholate and trypsin, or with sodium hypochlorite (bleach) alone, followed by introduction into culture medium.[30] Oocysts treated with bleach can be inhibited from excysting by exposure to human α-1-anti-trypsin inhibitor or inhibitors of arginine aminopeptidase.[31, 32] Like other enteric parasites with resistant outer structures (e.g., eggs of helminths and cysts of giardia and entamoeba), alteration of the outer surface may be a prerequisite for the organism to receive environmental cues, triggering the synthesis of enzymes of parasite origin required for emergence.

Sporozoites attach to the surface of epithelial cells (Fig. 10.2), most likely aided by numerous proteins secreted from their rhoptries and micronemes. A monoclonal antibody, designated 3E2, binds solely to the apical complex of the organism (the region where microneme- and rhoptre-specific proteins exit from the parasite), and inhibits invasion *in vitro*.[33] On Western Blot analysis, this antibody recognizes numerous epitopes, ranging from 46 kDa to 1300 kDa. Furthermore, a purified microneme-specific mucin-like 900 kDa glycoprotein can prevent invading parasites from attaching to their target cells when employed in competitive inhibition studies.[34]

After the sporozoite attaches to the cell surface, most likely mediated by thrombospondins and related adhesive proteins, microvilli in the area immediately adjacent to the parasite fuse and elongate, enveloping the parasite to create a unique intracellular environment (Fig. 10.3).[35] Apical end-associated secreted proteins may also trigger this event. A specialized membrane structure develops at the interface between the parasite and the host cell. Nutrients are thought to pass through this region, since parasite-specific ABC trans-

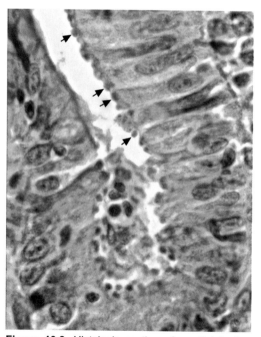

Figure 10.2. Histologic section of small intestine of patient suffering from HIV/AIDS, infected with *C. parvum* (arrows). Courtesy J. Lefkowitch.

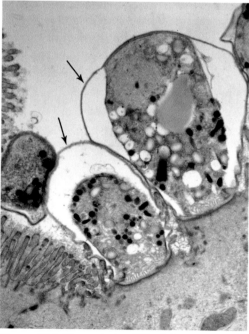

Figure 10.3. Transmission EM of *C. parvum*. Note microvillus-derived membranes encasing parasites (arrows). Courtesy J. Lefkowitch.

Cryptosporidium parvum

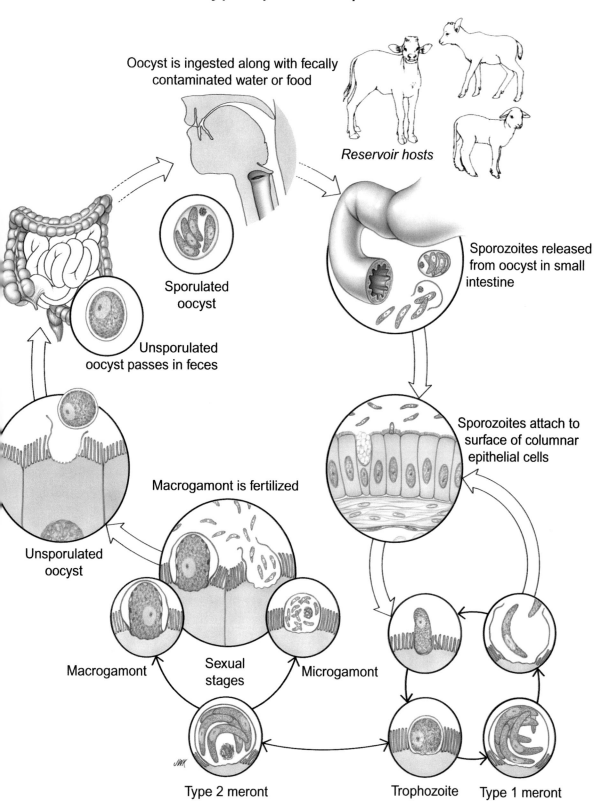

Oocyst is ingested along with fecally contaminated water or food

Reservoir hosts

Sporozoites released from oocyst in small intestine

Sporulated oocyst

Unsporulated oocyst passes in feces

Sporozoites attach to surface of columnar epithelial cells

Macrogamont is fertilized

Unsporulated oocyst

Macrogamont

Sexual stages

Microgamont

Type 2 meront

Trophozoite

Type 1 meront

porters have been identified there by means of immunofluorescent monoclonal antibodies.[36] The parasite then induces alterations in the gene expression of the invaded host cell, eliciting the upregulation of osteoprotegerin, a TNF family member known to inhibit apoptosis.[37] Such a strategy would favor the long-term survival of the parasite until it was able to complete its development to the next stage in its life cycle.[38] The sporozoite differentiates into the type I meront (Fig. 10.4) and division ensues, producing four haploid merozoites. The merozoites are released and attach to new epithelial cells, now differentiating into Type II meronts. Macrogamonts and microgamonts (pre-sex cells analogous to the gametocytes of plasmodia) are produced inside these new meronts. Following their release, microgamonts fuse with macrogamonts, forming thick-walled zygotes termed oocysts. This stage sporulates within the large intestine, and four haploid infectious sporozoites are produced. Oocysts can also be thin-walled. In this case, they sporulate and excyst within the same host, producing an autoinfection that may endure for months to years. Even in these cases, thick-walled oocysts are produced, as well.

Thick-walled oocysts pass out in feces, and can infect another host. This type of oocyst is environmentally resistant, and can remain viable for months to years in soil,

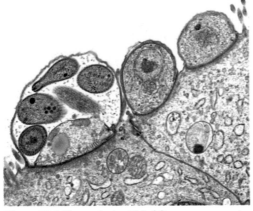

Figure 10.4. Transmission EM of *C. parvum* meronts. Courtesy M. Belosevic.

given optimum moisture conditions.[39]

Cellular and Molecular Pathogenesis

One of the most perplexing and frustrating aspects of the biology of *C. parvum* was its lack of response to a wide variety of drugs.[40-42] The altered microvillus-derived membrane complex that surrounds the parasites while they are attached to epithelial cells has proven highly impermeable to many chemotherapeutic agents. That is why speculation favors the entry of nutrients through the attachment zone between the parasite and the surface of the host cell. The fact that ABC transporters have been identified in this region is further indirect evidence in support of this hypothesis. Cellular or molecular events that result in the alteration of microvilli at the site of attachment have attracted the attention of some research groups.[43] Apparently, Cdc42 (a GTPase) and actin are recruited to the site of attachment early on in the process.[44] Actin then aggregates, forming a kind of platform on top of which the organism then elaborates its complex of membranes. Much more needs to be learned about the mechanism(s) of nutrient acquisition by *C. parvum* before rational drug design aimed at interference with this process can evolve.

Although not fully understood, the secretory diarrhea and pathogenesis of this organism are being deciphered now that the genome is fully sequenced.[16, 17] More than 25 possible factors responsible for virulence have now been isolated, and their specific roles in causing damage and diarrhea are being examined.[23] Certain virulence factors appear to be involved in excystation, adhesion and locomotion, invasion, intracellular multiplication and survival, and host cell damage.[23] Several factors such as phospholipases, proteases, and hemolysins appear to play a part in causing direct damage of host cells.[45] In addition to microbial virulence factors, pro-inflammatory cytokines such as IL-8 are possibly involved.[46]

Protection against the primary infection develops in individuals whose immune systems are not compromised. At least two classes of antibodies, IgA and IgG, and several cellular-based immune mechanisms are thought to play important roles in the elimination of the parasite from the gut tract, although the precise mechanisms responsible for this have yet to be determined.[27, 47, 48] Healthy human volunteers whose anti-*C. parvum* IgG levels were already present (exposed, immune), required a higher dose of oocysts to become infected, and developed fewer symptoms than their non-exposed (non-immune) counterparts.[27] It has also been observed that repeated infections in patients living in areas endemic for *C. parvum* have milder symptoms with repeated infections.[49] Studies carried out in experimental infections employing various strains of inbred mice have shown that IL-12, IFN-γ, and perhaps β-defensins, peptides chemically related to magainins, act in conjunction to protect against a challenge infection.[48, 50-54] Calves fed irradiated oocysts of *C. parvum* were protected from a challenge infection, implying that protection-inducing antigens are present in this stage of the infection.[55] Patients suffering from AIDS may develop an antibody response that is measureable in both serum and intestinal secretions, but this does not allow them to clear their infection.[56-58] In underserved regions of the tropics, many children born with the HIV virus who went on to develop AIDS are dying from this opportunistic infection.[59]

Clinical Disease

Infection is usually initiated through ingestion of contaminated water, directly from an infected person or animal, in tainted food, or rarely through aerosol. In immunocompetent individuals disease can vary from symptomatic infection to mild or profuse watery diarrhea. Upper abdominal cramps,

anorexia, nausea, weight loss, and vomiting are common features of the acute stage of the infection.[60] Severity of disease does not appear to correlate with the intensity of exposure.[26] In those who have already experienced clinical disease and recovered, a second infecting dose of oocysts may be asymptomatic, or they may have only a mild, transient diarrhea. Cryptosporidiosis in an immunocompetent host is self-limited, lasting for 2 weeks but may persist for longer periods of times in some individuals. In others diarrhea may be severe with several liters per day of diarrhea, and even persistent diarrhea with impacts on nutrition and growth.[61]

Children are the most severely affected group, as the diarrhea lasts longer, and there is usually some weight loss.[62] Unfortunately it is now recognized with the introduction of molecular testing that cryptosporidiosis is one of the four leading causes of diarrhea in children less than 5 years of age.[24] Those undergoing cancer chemotherapies suffer worse yet, with protracted, life-threatening diarrhea accompanied by significant weight loss.[63]

Cryptosporidiosis in patients suffering from AIDS is chronic, lasting months and even years, during which patients can lose more than three liters of fluid each day, and are in significant danger of dying; the case fatality rate can be as high as 50%. However, death is usually a result of associated conditions, such as malnutrition or superinfection with other pathogens. Extraintestinal infection in the bile duct can cause acalculous biliary disease.

Diagnosis

Diagnosis can be made by; identification of acid fast-stained oocysts seen on microscopic exam of stool (Fig. 10.1), stool antigen testing, directed polymerase chain reaction (PCR) testing or multiplex nucleic acid amplification testing (NAAT).[64, 65] Stool microscopy is perhaps the least sensitive test with sensitivities as low as 30% with single stool examinations.[66] Oocysts can be isolated from stool by flotation in sugar solution, then stained by acid-fast methods.[67] PCR testing is highly sensitive and can identify specific genotypes, which is important in outbreaks and epidemiological investigations.[68, 69] Antigen testing using monoclonal antibodies have high sensitivity, are easy to perform and can be used in both feces and tissue specimens.[70] The introduction of multiplex NAAT testing has helped to increase the number of cases of infectious diarrhea now recognized to be due to *Cryptosporidium spp.*.[24] This approach to the diagnosis of infectious diarrhea is now a highly sensitive and commercially available diagnostic option for the diagnosis of cryptosporidiosis.[71]

Treatment

Treatment of cryptosporidiosis is based on features of the infected host. In immunologically healthy children nitazoxanide is the drug of choice based on studies demonstrating early clinical improvement, earlier resolution of diarrhea and improved elimination of oocyst shedding.[40, 72-74] HIV-1-infected patients are best approached with initiation of highly active antiretroviral therapy (HAART) to reconstitute their immune systems. All patients should receive supportive care with oral rehydration when possible and intravenous therapy if required. Several clinical trials with rifamycins, azalides and paromo-mycin have demonstrated no clear benefit illustrating the difficulty of treating acute or established disease.[75]

Prevention and Control

Good hygiene is always an important approach to decreasing one's risk of exposure. Without knowledge as to the source of a given outbreak, control and prevention of infection due to *C. parvum* is not possible. In the case of waterborne epidemics, management of watersheds is the long-term solution in situations where the water supply is not filtered.[12, 76] Filtering drinking water is usually effective, but deterioration of filtration equipment and/or lack of proper maintenance can erode any progress made in controlling waterborne infections. Boiling is another option for purification of contaminated drinking water. Chlorination of water supplies is ineffective against the oocyst, but ozonation kills this stage.[77, 78] In agricultural settings, creation of vegetative barriers to curtail the spread of oocycts is effective.[79] Surveillance is key to keeping public water supplies free of pathogens with environmentally resistant stages (e.g., *Giardia lamblia, Entamoeba histolytica, Cryptosporidium parvum*). In this regard, PCR-based testing now allows for the possibility of continuous monitoring of water supplies for *C. parvum*.[80] Urban and suburban pet stores and petting zoos for children are other sources of infection that until very recently have received little attention.[81]

References

1. Laberge, I.; Griffiths, M. W., Prevalence, detection and control of Cryptosporidium parvum in food. *International journal of food microbiology* **1996,** *32* (1-2), 1-26.
2. Keusch, G. T.; Hamer, D.; Joe, A.; Kelley, M.; Griffiths, J.; Ward, H., Cryptosporidia--who is at risk? *Schweizerische medizinische Wochenschrift* **1995,** *125* (18), 899-908.
3. Guerrant, R. L., Cryptosporidiosis: an emerging, highly infectious threat. *Emerging infectious diseases* **1997,** *3* (1), 51-7.
4. Katsumata, T.; Hosea, D.; Ranuh, I. G.; Uga, S.; Yanagi, T.; Kohno, S., Short report: possible Cryptosporidium muris infection in humans. *The American journal of tropical medicine and hygiene* **2000,** *62* (1), 70-2.

5.   Ong, C. S. L.; Eisler, D. L.; Alikhani, A.; Fung, V. W. K.; Tomblin, J.; Bowie, W. R.; Isaac-Renton, J. L., Novel cryptosporidium genotypes in sporadic cryptosporidiosis cases: first report of human infections with a cervine genotype. *Emerging infectious diseases* **2002**, *8* (3), 263-8.

6.   Pedraza-Diaz, S.; Amar, C.; Fems, J.; McLauchlin, J., The identification and characterisation of an unusual genotype of Cryptosporidium from human faeces as Cryptosporidium meleagridis. *FEMS Microbiol Letters* **2000**, *189*, 189-194.

7.   Pedraza-Diaz, S.; Amar, C., Unusual Cryptosporidium species recovered from human faeces: first description of Cryptosporidium felis and Cryptosporidium 'dog type' from patients in England. *J Med Microbiol* **2001**, *50*, 293-296.

8.   Pieniazek, N. J.; Bornay-Llinares, F. J.; Slemenda, S. B.; da Silva, A. J.; Moura, I. N.; Arrowood, M. J.; Ditrich, O.; Addiss, D. G., New cryptosporidium genotypes in HIV-infected persons. *Emerging infectious diseases* **1999**, *5* (3), 444-9.

9.   Xiao, L.; Bern, C.; Arrowood, M.; Sulaiman, I.; Zhou, L.; Kawai, V.; Vivar, A.; Lal, A. A.; Gilman, R. H., Identification of the cryptosporidium pig genotype in a human patient. *The Journal of infectious diseases* **2002**, *185* (12), 1846-8.

10.   Xiao, L.; Bern, C.; Limor, J.; Sulaiman, I.; Roberts, J.; Checkley, W.; Cabrera, L.; Gilman, R. H.; Lal, A. A., Identification of 5 types of Cryptosporidium parasites in children in Lima, Peru. *The Journal of infectious diseases* **2001**, *183* (3), 492-7.

11.   Hadfield, S. J.; Pachebat, J. A.; Swain, M. T.; Robinson, G.; Cameron, S. J.; Alexander, J.; Hegarty, M. J.; Elwin, K.; Chalmers, R. M., Generation of whole genome sequences of new Cryptosporidium hominis and Cryptosporidium parvum isolates directly from stool samples. *BMC Genomics* **2015**, *16*, 650.

12.   Kramer, M. H.; Herwaldt, B. L.; Craun, G. F.; Calderon, R. L.; Juranek, D. D., Surveillance for waterborne-disease outbreaks--United States, 1993-1994. *MMWR. CDC surveillance summaries : Morbidity and mortality weekly report. CDC surveillance summaries / Centers for Disease Control* **1996**, *45* (1), 1-33.

13.   Farthing, M. J.; Kelly, M. P.; Veitch, A. M., Recently recognised microbial enteropathies and HIV infection. *The Journal of antimicrobial chemotherapy* **1996**, *37 Suppl B*, 61-70.

14.   Current, W. L.; Reese, N. C., A comparison of endogenous development of three isolates of Cryptosporidium in suckling mice. *The Journal of protozoology* **1986**, *33* (1), 98-108.

15.   Meloni, B. P.; Thompson, R. C., Simplified methods for obtaining purified oocysts from mice and for growing Cryptosporidium parvum in vitro. *The Journal of parasitology* **1996**, *82* (5), 757-62.

16.   Xu, P.; Widmer, G.; Wang, Y.; Ozaki, L. S.; Alves, J. M.; Serrano, M. G.; Puiu, D.; Manque, P.; Akiyoshi, D.; Mackey, A. J.; Pearson, W. R.; Dear, P. H.; Bankier, A. T.; Peterson, D. L.; Abrahamsen, M. S.; Kapur, V.; Tzipori, S.; Buck, G. A., The genome of Cryptosporidium hominis. *Nature* **2004**, *431* (7012), 1107-12.

17.   Abrahamsen, M. S.; Templeton, T. J.; Enomoto, S.; Abrahante, J. E.; Zhu, G.; Lancto, C. A.; Deng, M.; Liu, C.; Widmer, G.; Tzipori, S.; Buck, G. A.; Xu, P.; Bankier, A. T.; Dear, P. H.; Konfortov, B. A.; Spriggs, H. F.; Iyer, L.; Anantharaman, V.; Aravind, L.; Kapur, V., Complete genome sequence of the apicomplexan, Cryptosporidium parvum. *Science (New York, N.Y.)* **2004**, *304* (5669), 441-5.

18.   Tyzzer, E. E., A Study of Heredity in Relation to the Development of tumors in Mice. *The Journal of medical research* **1907**, *17* (2), 199-211.

19.   Slavin, D.; J., Cryptosporidium meleagridis (sp. nov.) *Pathol 346* **1955**, *65*, 262-266.

20.   Nime, F. A.; Burek, J. D.; Page, D. L.; Holscher, M. A.; Yardley, J. H., Acute enterocolitis in a human being infected with the protozoan Cryptosporidium. *Gastroenterology* **1976**, *70* (4), 592-8.

21.   Meisel, J. L.; Perera, D. R.; Meligro, C.; Rubin, C. E., Overwhelming watery diarrhea associated with a cryptosporidium in an immunosuppressed patient. *Gastroenterology* **1976**, *70* (6), 1156-60.

22.   de Graaf, D. C.; Vanopdenbosch, E.; Ortega-Mora, L. M.; Abbassi, H.; Peeters, J. E., A review of the importance of cryptosporidiosis in farm animals. *Int J Parasitol* **1999**, *29* (8), 1269-87.

23.   Bouzid, M.; Hunter, P. R.; Chalmers, R. M.; Tyler, K. M., Cryptosporidium pathogenicity and virulence. *Clin Microbiol Rev* **2013**, *26* (1), 115-34.

24.   Kotloff, K. L.; Nataro, J. P.; Blackwelder, W. C.; Nasrin, D.; Farag, T. H.; Panchalingam, S.; Wu, Y.; Sow, S. O.; Sur, D.; Breiman, R. F.; Faruque, A. S.; Zaidi, A. K.; Saha, D.; Alonso, P.

L.; Tamboura, B.; Sanogo, D.; Onwuchekwa, U.; Manna, B.; Ramamurthy, T.; Kanungo, S.; Ochieng, J. B.; Omore, R.; Oundo, J. O.; Hossain, A.; Das, S. K.; Ahmed, S.; Qureshi, S.; Quadri, F.; Adegbola, R. A.; Antonio, M.; Hossain, M. J.; Akinsola, A.; Mandomando, I.; Nhampossa, T.; Acacio, S.; Biswas, K.; O'Reilly, C. E.; Mintz, E. D.; Berkeley, L. Y.; Muhsen, K.; Sommerfelt, H.; Robins-Browne, R. M.; Levine, M. M., Burden and aetiology of diarrhoeal disease in infants and young children in developing countries (the Global Enteric Multicenter Study, GEMS): a prospective, case-control study. *Lancet* **2013,** *382* (9888), 209-22.

25.   Fayer, R., Cryptosporidium: a water-borne zoonotic parasite. *Veterinary parasitology* **2004,** *126* (1-2), 37-56.

26.   DuPont, H. L.; Chappell, C. L.; Sterling, C. R.; Okhuysen, P. C.; Rose, J. B.; Jakubowski, W., The infectivity of Cryptosporidium parvum in healthy volunteers. *The New England journal of medicine* **1995,** *332* (13), 855-9.

27.   Chappell, C. L.; Okhuysen, P. C.; Sterling, C. R.; Wang, C.; Jakubowski, W.; Dupont, H. L., Infectivity of Cryptosporidium parvum in healthy adults with pre-existing anti-C. parvum serum immunoglobulin G. *The American journal of tropical medicine and hygiene* **1999,** *60* (1), 157-64.

28.   Chappell, C. L.; Okhuysen, P. C.; Sterling, C. R.; DuPont, H. L., Cryptosporidium parvum: intensity of infection and oocyst excretion patterns in healthy volunteers. *J Infect Dis* **1996,** *173* (1), 232-6.

29.   Neuman, D.; Paraskevopoulou, P.; Psaroudakis, N.; Mertis, K.; Staples, R. J.; Stavropoulos, P., Structural and functional characteristics of rhenium clusters derived from redox chemistry of the triangular [ReIII3(mu-Cl)3] core unit. *Inorganic chemistry* **2000,** *39* (24), 5530-7.

30.   Forney, J. R.; Yang, S.; Healey, M. C., Antagonistic effect of human alpha-1-antitrypsin on excystation of Cryptosporidium parvum oocysts. *The Journal of parasitology* **1997,** *83* (4), 771-4.

31.   Okhuysen, P. C.; Chappell, C. L.; Kettner, C.; Sterling, C. R., Cryptosporidium parvum metalloaminopeptidase inhibitors prevent in vitro excystation. *Antimicrobial agents and chemotherapy* **1996,** *40* (12), 2781-4.

32.   Langer, R. C.; Riggs, M. W., Cryptosporidium parvum apical complex glycoprotein CSL contains a sporozoite ligand for intestinal epithelial cells. *Infection and immunity* **1999,** *67* (10), 5282-91.

33.   Riggs, M. W.; Stone, A. L.; Yount, P. A.; Langer, R. C.; Arrowood, M. J.; Bentley, D. L., Protective monoclonal antibody defines a circumsporozoite-like glycoprotein exoantigen of Cryptosporidium parvum sporozoites and merozoites. *Journal of immunology (Baltimore, Md. : 1950)* **1997,** *158* (4), 1787-95.

34.   Barnes, D. A.; Huang, J. X.; Bonnin, A., A novel multi-domain mucin-like glycoprotein of Cryptosporidium parvum mediates invasion. *Mol Biochem Parasitol 9693* **1998,** *110*, 1-2.

35.   Wanyiri, J.; Ward, H., Molecular basis of Cryptosporidium-host cell interactions: recent advances and future prospects. *Future Microbiol* **2006,** *1* (2), 201-8.

36.   Zapata, F.; Perkins, M. E.; Riojas, Y. A.; Wu, T. W.; Le Blancq, S. M., The Cryptosporidium parvum ABC protein family. *Molecular and biochemical parasitology* **2002,** *120* (1), 157-61.

37.   Di Genova, B. M.; Tonelli, R. R., Infection Strategies of Intestinal Parasite Pathogens and Host Cell Responses. *Front Microbiol* **2016,** *7*, 256.

38.   Castellanos-Gonzalez, A.; Yancey, L. S.; Wang, H. C.; Pantenburg, B.; Liscum, K. R.; Lewis, D. E.; White, A. C., Jr., Cryptosporidium infection of human intestinal epithelial cells increases expression of osteoprotegerin: a novel mechanism for evasion of host defenses. *J Infect Dis* **2008,** *197* (6), 916-23.

39.   Brasseur, P.; Uguen, C.; Moreno-Sabater, A.; Favennec, L.; Ballet, J. J., Viability of Cryptosporidium parvum oocysts in natural waters. *Folia parasitologica* **1998,** *45* (2), 113-6.

40.   Smith, H. V.; Corcoran, G. D., New drugs and treatment for cryptosporidiosis. *Current opinion in infectious diseases* **2004,** *17* (6), 557-64.

41.   Blagburn, B. L.; Soave, R.; C., C. R., Prophylaxis and chemotherapy: Human and animal. 1997; p 113-130.

42.   Clark, D. P., New insights into human cryptosporidiosis. *Clinical microbiology reviews* **1999,** *12* (4), 554-63.

43.   Huang, B. Q.; Chen, X.-M.; LaRusso, N. F., Cryptosporidium parvum attachment to and

internalization by human biliary epithelia in vitro: a morphologic study. *The Journal of parasitology* **2004,** *90* (2), 212-21.

44.   Chen, X.-M.; Huang, B. Q.; Splinter, P. L.; Orth, J. D.; Billadeau, D. D.; McNiven, M. A.; LaRusso, N. F., Cdc42 and the actin-related protein/neural Wiskott-Aldrich syndrome protein network mediate cellular invasion by Cryptosporidium parvum. *Infection and immunity* **2004,** *72* (5), 3011-21.

45.   Okhuysen, P. C.; Chappell, C. L., Cryptosporidium virulence determinants--are we there yet? *Int J Parasitol* **2002,** *32* (5), 517-25.

46.   Kirkpatrick, B. D.; Noel, F.; Rouzier, P. D.; Powell, J. L.; Pape, J. W.; Bois, G.; Alston, W. K.; Larsson, C. J.; Tenney, K.; Ventrone, C.; Powden, C.; Sreenivasan, M.; Sears, C. L., Childhood cryptosporidiosis is associated with a persistent systemic inflammatory response. *Clin Infect Dis* **2006,** *43* (5), 604-8.

47.   Jenkins, M. C.; O'Brien, C.; Trout, J.; Guidry, A.; Fayer, R., Hyperimmune bovine colostrum specific for recombinant Cryptosporidium parvum antigen confers partial protection against cryptosporidiosis in immunosuppressed adult mice. *Vaccine* **1999,** *17* (19), 2453-60.

48.   McDonald, V., Host cell-mediated responses to infection with Cryptosporidium. *Parasite immunology* **2000,** *22* (12), 597-604.

49.   Okhuysen, P. C.; Chappell, C. L.; Sterling, C. R.; Jakubowski, W.; DuPont, H. L., Susceptibility and serologic response of healthy adults to reinfection with Cryptosporidium parvum. *Infect Immun* **1998,** *66* (2), 441-3.

50.   Urban, J. F.; Fayer, R.; Chen, S. J.; Gause, W. C.; Gately, M. K.; Finkelman, F. D., IL-12 protects immunocompetent and immunodeficient neonatal mice against infection with Cryptosporidium parvum. *J Immunol* **1998,** *156* (1), 263-268.

51.   Tarver, A. P.; Clark, D. P.; Diamond, G.; Russell, J. P.; Erdjument-Bromage, H.; Tempst, P.; Cohen, K. S.; Jones, D. E.; Sweeney, R. W.; Wines, M.; Hwang, S.; Bevins, C. L., Enteric beta-defensin: molecular cloning and characterization of a gene with inducible intestinal epithelial cell expression associated with Cryptosporidium parvum infection. *Infection and immunity* **1998,** *66* (3), 1045-56.

52.   Giacometti, A.; Cirioni, O.; Barchiesi, F.; Caselli, F.; Scalise, G., In-vitro activity of polycationic peptides against Cryptosporidium parvum, Pneumocystis carinii and yeast clinical isolates. *The Journal of antimicrobial chemotherapy* **1999,** *44* (3), 403-6.

53.   Ludtke, S. J.; He, K.; Heller, W. T.; Harroun, T. A.; Yang, L.; Huang, H. W., Membrane pores induced by magainin. *Biochemistry* **1996,** *35* (43), 13723-8.

54.   Huang, H. W., Peptide-lipid interactions and mechanisms of antimicrobial peptides. *Novartis Foundation symposium* **1999,** *225,* 188-200; discussion 200.

55.   Jenkins, M.; Higgins, J.; Kniel, K.; Trout, J.; Fayer, R., Protection of calves against cryptosporiosis by oral inoculation with gamma-irradiated Cryptosporidium parvum oocysts. *The Journal of parasitology* **2004,** *90* (5), 1178-80.

56.   Benhamou, Y.; Kapel, N.; Hoang, C.; Matta, H.; Meillet, D.; Magne, D.; Raphael, M.; Gentilini, M.; Opolon, P.; Gobert, J. G., Inefficacy of intestinal secretory immune response to Cryptosporidium in acquired immunodeficiency syndrome. *Gastroenterology* **1995,** *108* (3), 627-35.

57.   Cozon, G.; Biron, F.; Jeannin, M.; Cannella, D.; Revillard, J. P., Secretory IgA antibodies to Cryptosporidium parvum in AIDS patients with chronic cryptosporidiosis. *J Infect Dis* **1994,** *169* (3), 696-9.

58.   Ravera, M.; Reggiori, A.; Cocozza, E., Prevalence of Cryptosporidium parvum in AIDS and immunocompetent patients in Uganda. *Int J STD AIDS* **1994,** *5* (4), 302-3.

59.   Guarino, A.; Bruzzese, E.; De Marco, G.; Buccigrossi, V., Management of gastrointestinal disorders in children with HIV infection. *Paediatric drugs* **2004,** *6* (6), 347-62.

60.   Farthing, M. J., Clinical aspects of human cryptosporidiosis. *Contributions to microbiology* **2000,** *6,* 50-74.

61.   Checkley, W.; Epstein, L. D.; Gilman, R. H.; Black, R. E.; Cabrera, L.; Sterling, C. R., Effects of Cryptosporidium parvum infection in Peruvian children: growth faltering and subsequent catch-up growth. *Am J Epidemiol* **1998,** *148* (5), 497-506.

62. Cicirello, H. G.; Kehl, K. S.; Addiss, D. G.; Chusid, M. J.; Glass, R. I.; Davis, J. P.; Havens, P. L., Cryptosporidiosis in children during a massive waterborne outbreak in Milwaukee, Wisconsin: clinical, laboratory and epidemiologic findings. *Epidemiology and infection* **1997**, *119* (1), 53-60.

63. Burgner, D.; Pikos, N.; Eagles, G.; McCarthy, A.; Stevens, M., Epidemiology of Cryptosporidium parvum in symptomatic paediatric oncology patients. *Journal of paediatrics and child health* **1999**, *35* (3), 300-2.

64. Blackman, E.; Binder, S.; Gaultier, C.; Benveniste, R.; Cecilio, M., Cryptosporidiosis in HIV-infected patients: diagnostic sensitivity of stool examination, based on number of specimens submitted. *The American journal of gastroenterology* **1997**, *92* (3), 451-3.

65. Coupe, S.; Sarfati, C.; Hamane, S.; Derouin, F., Detection of cryptosporidium and identification to the species level by nested PCR and restriction fragment length polymorphism. *Journal of clinical microbiology* **2005**, *43* (3), 1017-23.

66. Blanshard, C.; Jackson, A. M.; Shanson, D. C.; Francis, N.; Gazzard, B. G., Cryptosporidiosis in HIV-seropositive patients. *Q J Med* **1992**, *85* (307-308), 813-23.

67. Ignatius, R.; Eisenblatter, M.; Regnath, T., Efficacy of different methods for detection of low Cryptosporidium parvum oocyst numbers or antigen concentrations in stool specimens. *Eur J* **1997**.

68. Morgan, U. M.; Pallant, L.; Dwyer, B. W.; Forbes, D. A.; Rich, G.; Thompson, R. C., Comparison of PCR and microscopy for detection of Cryptosporidium parvum in human fecal specimens: clinical trial. *J Clin Microbiol* **1998**, *36* (4), 995-8.

69. Morgan, U. M.; Thompson, R. C., PCR detection of cryptosporidium: the way forward? *Parasitol Today* **1998**, *14* (6), 241-5.

70. Garcia, L. S.; Shimizu, R. Y., Evaluation of nine immunoassay kits (enzyme immunoassay and direct fluorescence) for detection of Giardia lamblia and Cryptosporidium parvum in human fecal specimens. *J Clin Microbiol* **1997**, *35* (6), 1526-9.

71. Buss, S. N.; Leber, A.; Chapin, K.; Fey, P. D.; Bankowski, M. J.; Jones, M. K.; Rogatcheva, M.; Kanack, K. J.; Bourzac, K. M., Multicenter evaluation of the BioFire FilmArray gastrointestinal panel for etiologic diagnosis of infectious gastroenteritis. *J Clin Microbiol* **2015**, *53* (3), 915-25.

72. Fox, L. M.; Saravolatz, L. D., Nitazoxanide: a new thiazolide antiparasitic agent. *Clinical infectious diseases : an official publication of the Infectious Diseases Society of America* **2005**, *40* (8), 1173-80.

73. Rossignol, J. F.; Ayoub, A.; Ayers, M. S., Treatment of diarrhea caused by Cryptosporidium parvum: a prospective randomized, double-blind, placebo-controlled study of Nitazoxanide. *J Infect Dis* **2001**, *184* (1), 103-6.

74. Rossignol, J. F.; Kabil, S. M.; el-Gohary, Y.; Younis, A. M., Effect of nitazoxanide in diarrhea and enteritis caused by Cryptosporidium species. *Clin Gastroenterol Hepatol* **2006**, *4* (3), 320-4.

75. Checkley, W.; White, A. C., Jr.; Jaganath, D.; Arrowood, M. J.; Chalmers, R. M.; Chen, X. M.; Fayer, R.; Griffiths, J. K.; Guerrant, R. L.; Hedstrom, L.; Huston, C. D.; Kotloff, K. L.; Kang, G.; Mead, J. R.; Miller, M.; Petri, W. A., Jr.; Priest, J. W.; Roos, D. S.; Striepen, B.; Thompson, R. C.; Ward, H. D.; Van Voorhis, W. A.; Xiao, L.; Zhu, G.; Houpt, E. R., A review of the global burden, novel diagnostics, therapeutics, and vaccine targets for cryptosporidium. *Lancet Infect Dis* **2015**, *15* (1), 85-94.

76. Steiner, T. S.; Thielman, N. M.; Guerrant, R. L., Protozoal agents: what are the dangers for the public water supply? *Annual review of medicine* **1997**, *48*, 329-40.

77. Clancy, J. L.; Hargy, T. M.; Marshall, M. M.; Dykesen, J. E.; J., UV light inactivation of Cryptosporidium oocysts. *Water Works Assoc* **1998**, *90* 92-102.

78. Gyurek, L. L.; Finch, G. R.; Li, H.; Belosevic, M.; J., Ozone inactivation kinetics of Cryptosporidium parvum in phosphate buffer. *Engine* **2000**, *125*, 913-924.

79. Tate, K. W.; Pereira, M. D. G. C.; Atwill, E. R., Efficacy of vegetated buffer strips for retaining Cryptosporidium parvum. *Journal of environmental quality* **2004**, *33* (6), 2243-51.

80. Hallier-Soulier, S.; Guillot, E., An immunomagnetic separation polymerase chain reaction assay for rapid and ultra-sensitive detection of Cryptosporidium parvum in drinking water. *FEMS microbiology letters* **1999**, *176* (2), 285-9.

81. Itoh, N.; Oohashi, Y.; Ichikawa-Seki, M.; Itagaki, T.; Ito, Y.; Saeki, H.; Kanai, K.; Chikazawa,

S.; Hori, Y.; Hoshi, F.; Higuchi, S., Molecular detection and characterization of Cryptosporidium species in household dogs, pet shop puppies, and dogs kept in a school of veterinary nursing in Japan. *Vet Parasitol* **2014,** *200* (3-4), 284-8.

11. *Toxoplasma gondii*
(Nicolle and Manceaux 1908)

Introduction

Toxoplasma gondii is an obligate intracellular parasite that has a worldwide distribution. Its biology is similar to members of the Phylum Apicomplexa, which includes the *Plasmodium* spp., *Cytoisospora* spp., *Babesia* spp., *Cyclospora* spp., and *Cryptosporidium* spp.. *T. gondii* infects most species of warm-blooded animals including domesticated and wild birds.[1] Although reliable information is not available in many parts of the world, it is estimated based on sero-prevalence studies that in some areas of the world such as Brazil and parts of Indonesia, the majority of individuals living in these countries are infected.[2] *Toxoplasma gondii* is one of the most successful parasites on earth, even when one takes into account all the viruses and bacteria that infect this large group of vertebrates. It has even emerged as a serious pathogen of some marine mammals such as sea otters.[3] It can remain alive as a dormant infection for the life of the host. When immunity breaks down, it can reactivate, often with clinical consequences. In this regard, *Toxoplasma* behaves similarly to other infectious agents whose reproduction is held in check by host-acquired protective immune responses (e.g., herpes simplex virus, *Mycobacterium tuberculosis*).

Toxoplasma gondii is easily cultured and can be experimentally transfected, facilitating studies on its genetics, cell, and molecular biology.[4-6] Its genome is now sequenced and available.[7, 8] Toxoplasma is usually acquired through the ingestion of infected, raw, or undercooked meats, but several recent outbreaks were traced back to drinking water supplies contaminated with the oocysts.[9, 10] The domestic cat and other feline species serve as the definitive host, harboring the sexual stages of the parasite.

In immunocompetent humans, infection rarely leads to serious illness. In contrast, when *T. gondii* infects immunocompromised individuals, or when a previously acquired infection is reactivated, the clinical disease that follows can often be life-threatening.[11] Congenital infection also occurs and can occasionally lead to devastating pathological consequences for the developing fetus.

Historical Information

In 1908, Charles Nicolle and Louis Manceaux described the organism which they isolated from the gondi (*Ctenodactylus gondii*), a gerbil-like desert inhabiting mammal.[12] In the same year, Alfonso Splendore, working in Brazil, described the identical parasite, which he identified in the tissues of rabbits.[13] They published their results at the same time, but in different publications, so neither was aware of the other's findings. In 1923, Josef Janku, described the congenital manifestations of the infection, which he accurately characterized as causing hydrocephalus and chorioretinitis.[14] Janku was unable to isolate the organism from the brains of its victims. In 1939, Abner Wolf and colleagues confirmed Janku's clinical description, and went on to experimentally transfer the infection from infected brain tissue to mice and rabbits.[15] H. Pinkerton and W. R. Henderson, and Alfred Sabin independently described cases of adult-acquired toxoplasmosis in 1941.[16, 17] In 1970, John Frenkel and colleagues identified the sexual stages of the life cycle working in cats, as did William M. Hutchinson and co-workers in that same year.[18, 19]

Life Cycle

Definitive Host Cycle
Felidae are the definitive host for *T. gondii*.[4] Domestic cats acquire the infection in one of three ways; 1. ingesting oocysts in

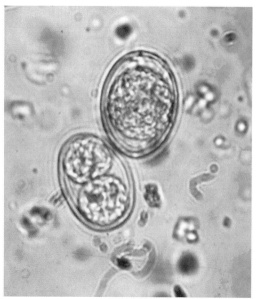

Figure 11.1. Sporulated oocysts of *Toxoplasma gondii*. 12 µm.

contaminated cat feces (Fig. 11.1), 2. ingesting the tissue cysts (Fig. 11.2) harbored by infected prey (e.g., mice, rats, rabbits, squirrels), 3. ingesting tissue cysts fed to them by their unwitting owners in the form of left over bits of ground meats (particularly pork and lamb). The cycle usually involves cats and rodents or birds. Rodents acquire the asexual tissue cyst stage of the parasite by ingesting food or water tainted with cat feces containing oocysts. Although feces is likely the main source of infectious oocysts, this stage may be present in other body fluids such as saliva, milk, sputum, tears, semen and urine.[20, 21]

T. gondii can follow two paths of development, the enteric and the extraintestinal. It is only in felidae that the enteric pathway with the sexual stage can occur. Infection in cats is usually initiated when they consume tissue cysts. The tissue cyst contains hundreds of infectious units, termed bradyzoites. When the cat eats this stage, the cyst wall becomes partially digested in the stomach and fully ruptures in the small intestine, releasing its complement of bradyzoites. This stage invades epithelial cells, developing into merozoites. The intracellular merozoite undergoes multiple cycles of division by a process termed endodyogeny. Finally, sheer numbers of parasites overwhelms the cell and they are released into the lumen of the small intestine. Each merozoite can infect other epithelial cells, continuing the infection. Alternatively, merozoites can develop into gametocytes (male and female). The two sexual forms fuse, forming an oocyst that passes out with the fecal mass. This completes the portion of the enteric cycle that occurs inside the felidae. Oocysts sporulate outside the host, producing haploid sporozoites, the infectious stage for the intermediate host, or for another cat. Cats do not develop a high enough level of protective immunity after exposure to a primary infection to prevent reinfection with the oocyst stage. Long-term, full protection can be induced in experimental situations, giving hope for the eventual development of an effective vaccine.[22] There currently is a live vaccine using a mutant strain of *T. gondii* that reduces cyst development in sheep and inhibits sexual development of *T. gondii* in the feline intestinal tract. [23]

Domestic and feral cats are implicated as the host most commonly responsible for transmission of the infection to farm animals (e.g., cattle, pigs, sheep, dogs, etc.). In addition, as will be described in full under clinical aspects, house cats may be considered a health hazard to pregnant women.

Intermediate Host Cycle

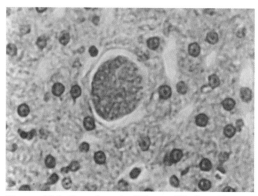

Figure 11.2. Pseudocyst of *T. gondii* in liver biopsy.

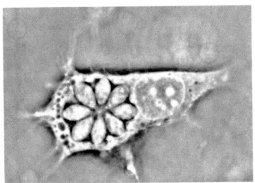

Figure 11.3. Tachyzoites of *T. gondii* in parasitophorous vacuoles of infected fibroblast.

The oocyst stage contains the infectious sporozoites. Ingestion of this stage leads to infection in mammals and birds. Sporozoites are released by exposure of the oocyst to digestive enzymes in the small intestine. The freed parasites then penetrate the intestinal wall, and are taken up by macrophages. *T. gondii* now can follow the extraintestinal pathway. Once inside a cell (Fig. 11.3), the organisms are referred to as tachyzoites. This stage resides in its own membrane-bound parasitophorous vacuole.[24] Infected cells are not able to destroy tachyzoites, due to the fact that *T. gondii* inhibits the process of fusion between the lysosomal vessels and this specialized intracellular niche (Figs. 11.4, 11.5).[25] Replication occurs inside the macrophages and parasites are passively carried to all parts of the body. Approximately 8 to 20 tachyzoites are produced inside each infected cell. Macrophages eventually succumb to the infection, releasing tachyzoites into the surrounding tissues. Cells take up freed parasites adjacent to the site of release (e.g., glial cells, astrocytes, hepatocytes, neutrophils, cardiac muscle). *T. gondii* undergoes another round of replication until protective immune responses are elicited. As the result, extensive tissue damage can be incurred, often accompanied by a constellation of clinical signs and symptoms. An effective immune response, mediated by IL-12 and IFN-γ, and involving monocytes, dendritic cells, neutrophils, T cells and NK cells limits the rate of parasite division.[26] Antibodies are thought not to play a role in controlling this phase of the infection. Apparently, protective immunity does not result in the death of the parasite. Rather, in response to host defense mechanisms, tachyzoites are forced to differentiate into a second asexual stage known as the bradyzoite. This form divides both by endodyogeny and endopolygeny, then organizes into a tissue cyst.[27] IFN-γ-dependent, nitric oxide-mediated effector mechanisms maintain this state of latency by eliminating any parasites emerging from the cysts.[28] Bradyzoites lie dormant in the tissues for as long as host defenses remain active. Although all tissues can harbor tissue cysts, the brain, kidney, heart, and liver are a favored sites for the long-term survival of the tissue cyst.[29]

In addition to ingesting oocysts, intermediate as well as paratenic hosts can be infected by ingesting tissue cysts contained in the flesh of another intermediate host species. This route of transmission is most common among

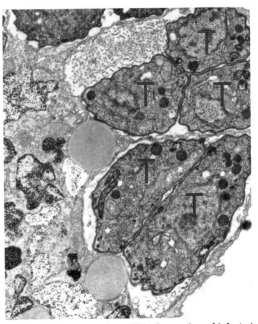

Figure 11.4. Transmission EM of a portion of infected macrophage. Note numerous tachyzoites (T). All parasites are alive; thus, the fusion of lysosomes with the parasitophorous vacuole is inhibited. Courtesy T. Jones.

Table 11.1. Congenital toxoplasmosis following maternal infection during first and second trimester*

Not Infected	73%
Subclinical Infection	13%
Mild Infection	7%
Severe Infection	6%

*From Desmonts and Couvier, NEJM 290:1110, 1974

carnivores and scavengers. This is often a means of acquisition for humans who tend to ingest insufficiently cooked meat. Lamb, beef and pork are the most common meats implicated in transmission worldwide.[30-32] The suggested internal temperature of 145 °F for cooking of beef to kill *T. gondii* is the final cooked temperature of a medium rare steak.

Congenital transmission occurs during infection of the mother, when tachyzoites cross the placenta. The role of specific antibodies in limiting infection to the mother and not the fetus has yet to be defined, while INF-γ and CD8+ T cells appear to be necessary in preventing congenital infection in mouse models.[33]

Cellular and Molecular Pathogenesis

Since toxoplasma infection is not restricted by cell type, entry does not depend upon tissue-specific receptor molecules. The pro-

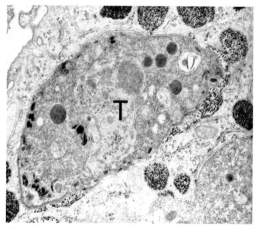

Figure 11.5. Transmission EM of a portion of macrophage that ingested a heat-killed tachyzoite. Note fusion of lysosomes with the parasitophorous vacuole (see top right fusion event. T = tachyzoite, Courtesy T. Jones.

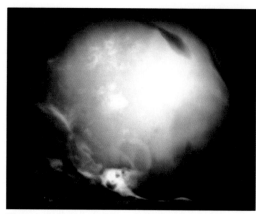

Figure 11.6. X-ray of the skull of an infant born with congenital toxoplasmosis. Infection was acquired most likely during the first or second trimester. Note calcifications.

cess is nevertheless complex, and involves the coordinated, sequential deployment of a set of specialized subcellular organelles; micronemes, rhoptries (lysosome-like granules), dense granules and the glideosome.[34, 35] As the result of the biological activities unleashed upon the host cell by these organelles, the tachyzoite is able to assume its intracellular life without hindrance from host defense mechanisms related to phagocytosis. *T. gondii* employs an entry scheme referred to as a 'kiss and spit' approach, whereby it injects virulence factors onto potential host cells, as well as into already infected host cells.[36] Rhoptries, located at the apical end of the tachyzoite, and micronemes both secrete adhesin-like molecules.[35, 37-40] Parasite-specific secreted serine and cysteine proteases are required for the engineering of the parasitophorous vacuole in which the tachyzoite lives and reproduces.[37, 41, 42] These secreted serine and cysteine proteases are released and enable the parasite to deform the cell membrane of the target cell and re-model the inner membrane of the vacuole. Inhibition of these two proteases prevents *T. gondii* from entering the cell.[37, 41] The cDNA-encoding proteins from these organelles have been cloned and sequenced, and their amino acid sequences deduced.[43-45] The Myr1 protein appears to be a key factor enabling transit of molecules

Toxoplasma gondii

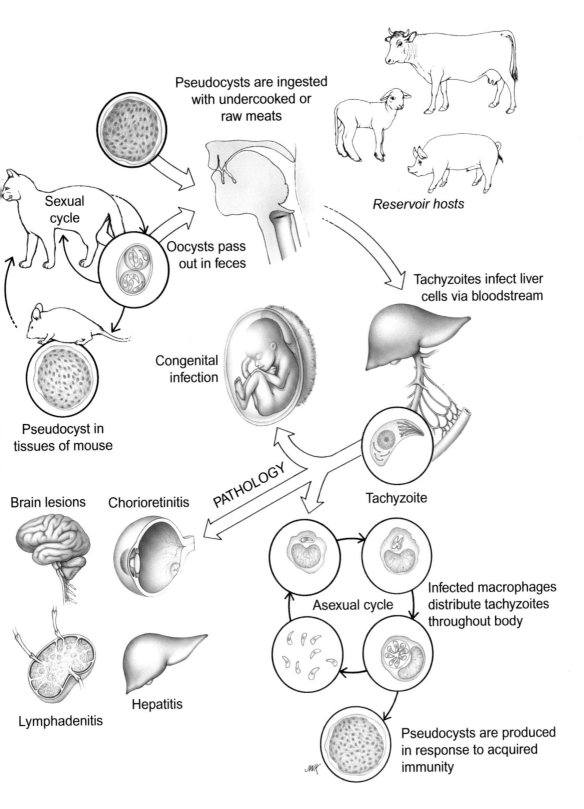

Pseudocysts are ingested with undercooked or raw meats

Reservoir hosts

Sexual cycle

Oocysts pass out in feces

Tachyzoites infect liver cells via bloodstream

Congenital infection

Pseudocyst in tissues of mouse

Brain lesions

Chorioretinitis

PATHOLOGY

Tachyzoite

Infected macrophages distribute tachyzoites throughout body

Asexual cycle

Lymphadenitis

Hepatitis

Pseudocysts are produced in response to acquired immunity

Table 11.2. Differential diagnosis of lymphadenopathy

	Toxoplasmosis	Inf. Mono	Lymphoma
Lymphadenopathy without other symptoms	+++	+	+++
Pharyngitis	+	+++	+
Monocytosis, eosinophilia	+++	+	+++
Atypical lymphocytes	+	++++	+++
Anemia	0	+	+++
Positive heterophil	0	++++	0
Altered liver function	0	++++	++
Hilar lymphadenopathy	+	+	+++
Lymph node pathology	Reticulum cells	Germinal cells	Bizarre cells

from the parasitophorous vacuole and is responsible for the organisms' virulence.[46]

The parasite affects the arrangement of host cell organelles, including the mitochondria, which aggregate around the parasitophorous vacuole.[47] Division depends upon the ability of the parasite to inhibit lysosomal fusion and inhibition of acidification of the parasitophorous vacuole.[48] Congenital toxoplasmosis is characterized by lesions of the central nervous system, which lead to various states of clinical disease.[49] Inflammatory lesions become necrotic and eventually calcify. Chorioretinitis is frequently associated with congenital toxoplasmosis.[50] The retina is inflamed and becomes necrotic, and the pigmented layer becomes disrupted by infiltration of inflammatory cells. Eventually, granulation tissue forms, and invades the vitreous humor. Calcification of brain tissue (Fig. 11.6) is common when the fetus acquires infection during the first trimester. Hydrocepha-

lus may result. Learning deficits in children who became infected in the second or third trimesters have been documented, but are less common for those whose infection occurred in the third trimester. In adult-acquired toxoplasmosis, lesions are less intense, giving rise to foci of inflammation around tachyzoites in muscle and other tissues, such as spleen, liver, and lymph nodes. Interstitial pneumonitis may also accompany infection.[51, 52] Adult patients with AIDS who harbor latent infection with *T. gondii* suffer the most from reactivation of the infection.[53] This is due largely to the fact that the HIV virus down regulates IL-12 production and reduces the number of parasite-specific CD4[+] and CD8[+] T cells.[54-56] This reduces dramatically the INF-γ dependent inhibition of parasite multiplication. Bradyzoites resume replication within tissue cysts, and eventually rupture into the tissues, initiating infection in neighboring cells. Toxoplasma encephalitis results when reactivation

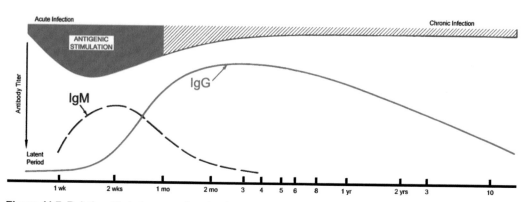

Figure 11.7. Relationship between antigenic stimulation, antibody production, and stages of infection (latent period, acute, and chronic infection). Redrawn after Remington.

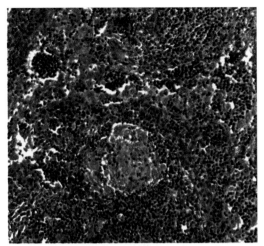

Figure 11.8. Histologic section of lymph node positive for macrophages infected with *T. gondii*. These cells are referred to as Piringa-Kuchenka cells.

occurs in the brain.[57] Reactivation can also occur in the lung, gastrointestinal tract, heart, eye, and liver. However, with the introduction of effective chemoprophylaxis for toxoplasmosis and HAART for HIV, the incidence of clinical toxoplasmosis has been markedly reduced in recent years, even in resource-limited parts of the world.[58]

Clinical Disease

There are three main manifestations of toxoplasmosis; congenital toxoplasmosis, acquired acute toxoplasmosis in the immunocompetent individual, and toxoplasmosis in the immunocompromised patient.[59, 60]

Congenital Toxoplasmosis

Congenital infection varies from asymptomatic to severe damage to the central nervous system (CNS) and stillbirth.[61] (Table 11.1) Transmission typically occurs when a pregnant woman acquires a primary infection while pregnant. Transmission to the fetus is lowest when acute infection occurs during the first trimester, with only ~6% of fetuses acquiring infection. The percentage rises with gestational age of the fetus to over 70% if infection is acquired late in the third trimester.[62] Fetal damage is most severe and

likely when infection occurs early in the pregnancy.[62] Infection later in pregnancy constitutes the majority of congenital toxoplasmosis with most affected children asymptomatic, however they may show the less severe pathological consequences of infection several months to years later. The classic triad of chorioretinitis, hydrocephalus, and intracranial calcifications is present in less than 10% of cases.[63] Congenital toxoplasmosis can present as a subclinical infection, severe neonatal disease, disease in the first few months of life, or later as a relapse. Relapses often occur as ocular (e.g., chorioretinitis) manifestations when congenital infection has gone unnoted and untreated.[64] Of the infants that do acquire infection in utero, about 15% have severe clinical manifestations.[49] Chorioretinitis leading to blindness, cerebral calcifications, and learning disabilities are the most frequent consequences.[65] Severely affected infants may have hepatosplenomegaly, liver failure, thrombocytopenia, convulsions, and hydrocephalus.[66] Without treatment new lesions may continue to develop, increasing the likelihood that severe impairment to the CNS will occur.[67]

Acute Acquired Toxoplasmosis in the Immunocompetent Patient

It is estimated that 80-90% of acquired infections are asymptomatic. Those that are clinically apparent usually present as mild self-limited disease. Symptomatic acute toxoplasmosis in the immunocompetent individual is often characterized by generalized lymphadenopathy, with predominant enlargement of the cervical nodes, sometimes associated with a low-grade fever (Table 11.2). The disease mimics infectious mononucleosis and, to a lesser extent, Hodgkin's-type lymphoma. Rarely, adult-acquired toxoplasmosis is severe, involving major vital organs and systems. These patients may suffer myocarditis and encephalitis.[68, 69] Chorioretinitis in acquired toxoplasmosis is rare, but *T. gondii* is one of the most common pathogens to cause this posterior uveitis in immunocompetent hosts.

Toxoplasmosis in the Immunocompromised Patient

Encephalitis due to *T. gondii* is one of the causes of CNS disease in patients with AIDS.[57, 70, 71] Toxoplasmosis in this setting is almost uniformly due to reactivation of latent *T. gondii* acquired previously. HIV-infected patients at significant risk are those with CD4+ T cell counts <100 cells μl who have serological evidence of prior infection.[72] Brain imaging usually reveals multiple ring enhancing lesions. There can be extracerebral manifestation of toxoplasmosis in the immunocompromised patient. The lung is the next most common organ involved in reactivated toxoplasmosis, often manifesting as an interstitial pneumonitis.[51, 52] The gastrointestinal tract, liver, and heart may also be involved. Cutaneous toxoplasmosis presents as a prominent macular and papular rash on the palms and soles.[73] An unusual form of acquired toxoplasmosis has been described in seronegative recipients of organ transplants from *T. gondii*-infected donors. Heart transplant recipients are particularly at risk, and can develop a myocarditis or disseminated infection.[74] Severe recrudescent toxoplasmosis has also been described in patients undergoing immune suppression during bone marrow transplantation.[75]

Diagnosis

Definitive diagnosis is made by demonstrating the organism in histological sections, or by using polymerase chain reaction.[76-79] PCR tests are especially useful in identifying organisms in ocular, amniotic, or CSF fluids.[80] Identification of tachyzoites in tissue sections without the aid of antibody-based staining methods is very challenging, even for a seasoned histopathologist. Indirect evidence of infection includes the application of a wide variety of commercially available serological tests of several modalities (Fig. 11.7).[81] These tests depend on the identification of specific immunoglobulins - IgG and IgM. A wide variety of laboratory-based methods take advantage of these host responses to insure an accurate diagnosis of both active and inactive infection.

In most infections among otherwise healthy adults, IgM antibodies appear within five days to two weeks after infection, and usually reach titers of 1:80 or more during the first 2-3 months after infection. They return to normal shortly thereafter. IgG antibody titers rise 2-3 weeks after infection, and usually achieve levels above 1:1024. Specific IgG antibodies are detectable for life. Significant rises in titers of IgG antibodies between acute and convalescent serum specimens are highly correlated with acute infection. A single elevated IgM titer early in the infection is also diagnostic.

In certain regions of the world, women at increased risk are recommended to undergo screening during pregnancy.[82] Sero-conversion during pregnancy can then be documented early on in infection and closely monitored. Congenital infection can be confirmed when specific IgM antibodies are detected in the infant's serum. About 25% of newborns with congenital toxoplasmosis have IgM antibodies. In contrast, infants with IgG antibodies pose a problem to the clinician in deciding whether or not the fetus was ever infected or whether the IgG represents passive transfer of maternal antibody. Careful clinical and serological follow-up of the child is indicated to determine whether intrauterine infection has occurred.

Diagnosing toxoplasmosis in patients with AIDS often involves making a presumptive diagnosis and then administration of a therapeutic trial.[83] The triad of a compatible clinical syndrome, a positive toxoplasma IgG, and typical brain imaging demonstrating multiple ring enhancing lesions is associated with greater than a 90% positive predictive value for the diagnosis of CNS toxoplasmosis in an HIV infected patient with a CD4 T cell count <100 cells/μl.[72] Histologic examination of lymph node tissue (Fig. 11.8) obtained at biopsy may show abnormal histiocytes, but this evidence is not pathognomonic for toxoplasmosis.

Treatment

Mild infection in the immunocompetent patient does not require therapy. Unless the patient is pregnant and being treated to prevent infection of the fetus, pyrimethamine and sulfadiazine are the drugs of choice.[84] Unfortunately for a number of reasons, alternative less studied regimens are often necessary. If pyrimethamine is not available due to supply issues or cost, patients can be treated with trimethoprim-sulfamethoxazole or atovaquone.[85] In patients unable to tolerate sulfadiazine, alternative regimens containing atovaquone or azithromycin may be utilized. Unfortunately the combination of pyrimethamine and sulfadiazine is teratogenic in animals and there is concern regarding its use in pregnancy, particularly early trimesters. As a consequence, women who become acutely infected during pregnancy are usually treated with the macrolide antibiotic spiramycin. The ability of this agent to concentrate in the placenta is thought to help prevent transmission to the fetus.[86, 87] Some physicians will treat women who acquire acute infection during later trimesters with pyrimethamine and sulfadiazine, but in some settings women will choose to terminate their pregnancies, as it is not clear that initiation of treatment after the development of intracranial calcifications has any benefit.[88]

Prevention and Control

Most infections can be prevented by eating only well-cooked meats and avoiding the inadvertent ingestion of cat feces contaminated with toxoplasma oocysts. These preventive measures often fail because of cultural or individual cuisine preferences. In France, where the rate of infection is over 85% among those over the age of 50, the most common source of infection is raw meat served as "steak" tartar, most of which is actually lamb or horse meat. Many other cultures also have numerous recipes calling for undercooked or raw meat as a main ingredient. A number of Alaskan native peoples still eat some of their meat raw, and are therefore at the mercy of the pathogens lurking inside each carcass.[89] In Ethiopia, the practice of eating raw meat with melted butter, *kitfo*, is a popular but risky dietary choice.[90] Prevention of infection from oocysts requires care when handling cat feces, especially when cleaning litter boxes.[91] Pregnant women diminish their risk of infection by avoiding these activities. Rarely, toxoplasmosis is acquired as the result of inhaling dust, or drinking water contaminated with oocysts.[92] Vaccines potentially offer another set of strategies for controlling this infection, but carefully defined susceptible at risk populations, such as sero-negative women of child-bearing age, would need to be clearly articulated prior to committing the necessary resources to vaccine development.[93]

References

1. Dubey, J. P., A review of toxoplasmosis in wild birds. *Vet Parasitol* **2002**, *106* (2), 121-53.
2. Pappas, G.; Roussos, N.; Falagas, M. E., Toxoplasmosis snapshots: global status of Toxoplasma gondii seroprevalence and implications for pregnancy and congenital toxoplasmosis. *Int J Parasitol* **2009**, *39* (12), 1385-94.

3.   Miller, M. A.; Grigg, M. E.; Kreuder, C.; James, E. R.; Melli, A. C.; Crosbie, P. R.; Jessup, D. A.; Boothroyd, J. C.; Brownstein, D.; Conrad, P. A., An unusual genotype of Toxoplasma gondii is common in California sea otters (Enhydra lutris nereis) and is a cause of mortality. *International journal for parasitology* **2004,** *34* (3), 275-84.

4.   Kim, K.; Weiss, L. M., Toxoplasma gondii: the model apicomplexan. *International journal for parasitology* **2004,** *34* (3), 423-32.

5.   Gubbels, M.-J.; Striepen, B., Studying the cell biology of apicomplexan parasites using fluorescent proteins. *Microscopy and microanalysis : the official journal of Microscopy Society of America, Microbeam Analysis Society, Microscopical Society of Canada* **2004,** *10* (5), 568-79.

6.   Boothroyd, J. C., Toxoplasma gondii: 25 years and 25 major advances for the field. *Int J Parasitol* **2009,** *39* (8), 935-46.

7.   Kissinger, J. C.; Gajria, B.; Li, L.; Paulsen, I. T.; Roos, D. S., ToxoDB: accessing the Toxoplasma gondii genome. *Nucleic acids research* **2003,** *31* (1), 234-6.

8.   Khan, A.; Bohme, U.; Kelly, K. A.; Adlem, E.; Brooks, K.; Simmonds, M.; Mungall, K.; Quail, M. A.; Arrowsmith, C.; Chillingworth, T.; Churcher, C.; Harris, D.; Collins, M.; Fosker, N.; Fraser, A.; Hance, Z.; Jagels, K.; Moule, S.; Murphy, L.; O'Neil, S.; Rajandream, M. A.; Saunders, D.; Seeger, K.; Whitehead, S.; Mayr, T.; Xuan, X.; Watanabe, J.; Suzuki, Y.; Wakaguri, H.; Sugano, S.; Sugimoto, C.; Paulsen, I.; Mackey, A. J.; Roos, D. S.; Hall, N.; Berriman, M.; Barrell, B.; Sibley, L. D.; Ajioka, J. W., Common inheritance of chromosome Ia associated with clonal expansion of Toxoplasma gondii. *Genome Res* **2006,** *16* (9), 1119-25.

9.   Pozio, E., Foodborne and waterborne parasites. *Acta microbiologica Polonica* **2003,** *52 Suppl,* 83-96.

10.   Dubey, J. P., Toxoplasmosis - a waterborne zoonosis. *Vet Parasitol* **2004,** *126* (1-2), 57-72.

11.   Halonen, S. K.; Weiss, L. M., Toxoplasmosis. *Handb Clin Neurol* **2013,** *114,* 125-45.

12.   Nicolle, C.; Manceaux, L. H.; R., C., Sur une infection a coyes de Leishman (ou organismes voisins) du gondi. *Seance Acad Sci* **1908,** *147,* 763-766.

13.   Splendore, A., Un nuovo protozoa parassita dei conigli: incontrato nelle lesioni anatomiche d'ua maittia che ricorda in molti punti ii Kala-azar dell'uomo. . *Rev Soc Sci Sao Paulo* **1908,** *3* 109-112.

14.   Janku, J.; J., Pathogenesis and pathologic anatomy of the "congenital coloboma" of the maculalutea in an eye of normal size, with microscopic detection of parasites in the retina. *Phys* **1923,** *62,* 1021-1027.

15.   Wolf, A.; Cowen, D.; Paige, B., HUMAN TOXOPLASMOSIS: OCCURRENCE IN INFANTS AS AN ENCEPHALOMYELITIS VERIFICATION BY TRANSMISSION TO ANIMALS. *Science (New York, N.Y.)* **1939,** *89* (2306), 226-7.

16.   Pinkerton, H.; Henderson, R. G., Adult toxoplasmosis: a previously unrecognized disease entity simulating the typhus-spotted fever group. *JAMA* **1941,** *116* 807-814.

17.   Sabin, A. B., Toxoplasmic encephalitis in children. *JAMA* **1941,** *116* 801-807.

18.   Frenkel, J. K.; Dubey, J. P.; Miller, N. L., Toxoplasma gondii in cats: fecal stages identified as coccidian oocysts. *Science (New York, N.Y.)* **1970,** *167* (3919), 893-6.

19.   Hutchison, W. M.; Dunachie, J. F.; Siim, J. C.; Work, K., Coccidian-like nature of Toxoplasma gondii. *Br Med J* **1970,** *1* (5689), 142-4.

20.   Bresciani, K. D.; Costa, A. J.; Toniollo, G. H.; Sabatini, G. A.; Moraes, F. R.; Paulillo, A. C.; Ferraudo, A. S., Experimental toxoplasmosis in pregnant bitches. *Vet Parasitol* **1999,** *86* (2), 143-5.

21.   Tenter, A. M.; Heckeroth, A. R.; Weiss, L. M., Toxoplasma gondii: from animals to humans. *Int J Parasitol* **2000,** *30* (12-13), 1217-58.

22.   Bhopale, G. M., Development of a vaccine for toxoplasmosis: current status, Microbes Infect. **2003,** *5,* 457-462.

23.   Verma, R.; Khanna, P., Development of Toxoplasma gondii vaccine: A global challenge. *Hum Vaccin Immunother* **2013,** *9* (2), 291-3.

24.   Jones, T. C.; Hirsch, J. G., The interaction between Toxoplasma gondii and mammalian cells. II. The absence of lysosomal fusion with phagocytic vacuoles containing living parasites. *The Journal of experimental medicine* **1972,** *136* (5), 1173-94.

25.   Dlugonska, H.; J., Molecular modifications of host cells by Toxoplasma gondii. *Pol* **2004,** *53* 45-54.

26.   Hunter, C. A.; Sibley, L. D., Modulation of innate immunity by Toxoplasma gondii virulence effectors. *Nat Rev Microbiol* **2012,** *10* (11), 766-78.

27.   Dzierszinski, F.; Nishi, M.; Ouko, L.; Roos, D. S., Dynamics of Toxoplasma gondii differentiation. *Eukaryotic cell* **2004,** *3* (4), 992-1003.

28.   Scharton-Kersten, T. M.; Yap, G.; Magram, J.; Sher, A., Inducible nitric oxide is essential for host control of persistent but not acute infection with the intracellular pathogen Toxoplasma gondii. *The Journal of experimental medicine* **1997,** *185* (7), 1261-73.

29.   Dadimoghaddam, Y.; Daryani, A.; Sharif, M.; Ahmadpour, E.; Hossienikhah, Z., Tissue tropism and parasite burden of Toxoplasma gondii RH strain in experimentally infected mice. *Asian Pac J Trop Med* **2014,** *7* (7), 521-4.

30.   Williams, R. H.; Morley, E. K.; Hughes, J. M.; Duncanson, P.; Terry, R. S.; Smith, J. E.; Hide, G., High levels of congenital transmission of Toxoplasma gondii in longitudinal and cross-sectional studies on sheep farms provides evidence of vertical transmission in ovine hosts. *Parasitology* **2005,** *130* (Pt 3), 301-7.

31.   Dubey, J. P.; Gamble, H. R.; Hill, D.; Sreekumar, C.; Romand, S.; Thuilliez, P., High prevalence of viable Toxoplasma gondii infection in market weight pigs from a farm in Massachusetts. *J Parasitol* **2002,** *88* (6), 1234-8.

32.   Dubey, J. P.; Ott-Joslin, J.; Torgerson, R. W.; Topper, M. J.; Sundberg, J. P., Toxoplasmosis in black-faced kangaroos (Macropus fuliginosus melanops). *Vet Parasitol* **1988,** *30* (2), 97-105.

33.   Abou-Bacar, A.; Pfaff, A. W.; Letscher-Bru, V.; Filisetti, D.; Rajapakse, R.; Antoni, E.; Villard, O.; Klein, J. P.; Candolfi, E., Role of gamma interferon and T cells in congenital Toxoplasma transmission. *Parasite immunology* **2004,** *26* (8-9), 315-8.

34.   Carruthers, V. B.; Blackman, M. J., A new release on life: emerging concepts in proteolysis and parasite invasion. *Molecular microbiology* **2005,** *55* (6), 1617-30.

35.   Keeley, A.; Soldati, D., The glideosome: a molecular machine powering motility and host-cell invasion by Apicomplexa. *Trends in cell biology* **2004,** *14* (10), 528-32.

36.   Boothroyd, J. C.; Dubremetz, J. F., Kiss and spit: the dual roles of Toxoplasma rhoptries. *Nat Rev Microbiol* **2008,** *6* (1), 79-88.

37.   Que, X.; Ngo, H.; Lawton, J.; Gray, M.; Liu, Q.; Engel, J.; Brinen, L.; Ghosh, P.; Joiner, K. A.; Reed, S. L., The cathepsin B of Toxoplasma gondii, toxopain-1, is critical for parasite invasion and rhoptry protein processing. *The Journal of biological chemistry* **2002,** *277* (28), 25791-7.

38.   Ngo, H. M.; Yang, M.; Joiner, K. A., Are rhoptries in Apicomplexan parasites secretory granules or secretory lysosomal granules?Mol Microbiol. **2004,** *52* 1531-41.

39.   Carruthers, V. B.; Giddings, O. K.; Sibley, L. D., Secretion of micronemal proteins is associated with toxoplasma invasion of host cells. *Cellular microbiology* **1999,** *1* (3), 225-35.

40.   Huynh, M.-H.; Rabenau, K. E.; Harper, J. M.; Beatty, W. L.; Sibley, L. D.; Carruthers, V. B., Rapid invasion of host cells by Toxoplasma requires secretion of the MIC2-M2AP adhesive protein complex. *The EMBO journal* **2003,** *22* (9), 2082-90.

41.   Conseil, V.; Soête, M.; Dubremetz, J. F., Serine protease inhibitors block invasion of host cells by Toxoplasma gondii. *Antimicrobial agents and chemotherapy* **1999,** *43* (6), 1358-61.

42.   Kim, K., Role of proteases in host cell invasion by Toxoplasma gondii and other Apicomplexa. *Acta tropica* **2004,** *91* (1), 69-81.

43.   Ajioka, J. W.; Boothroyd, J. C.; Brunk, B. P.; Hehl, A.; Hillier, L.; Manger, I. D.; Marra, M.; Overton, G. C.; Roos, D. S.; Wan, K. L.; Waterston, R.; Sibley, L. D., Gene discovery by EST sequencing in Toxoplasma gondii reveals sequences restricted to the Apicomplexa. *Genome research* **1998,** *8* (1), 18-28.

44.   Yahiaoui, B.; Dzierszinski, F.; Bernigaud, A.; Slomianny, C.; Camus, D.; Tomavo, S., Isolation and characterization of a subtractive library enriched for developmentally regulated transcripts expressed during encystation of Toxoplasma gondii. *Molecular and biochemical parasitology* **1999,** *99* (2), 223-35.

45.   Bradley, P. J.; Li, N.; Boothroyd, J. C., A GFP-based motif-trap reveals a novel mechanism of

targeting for the Toxoplasma ROP4 protein. *Molecular and biochemical parasitology* **2004,** *137* (1), 111-20.

46. Franco, M.; Panas, M. W.; Marino, N. D.; Lee, M. C.; Buchholz, K. R.; Kelly, F. D.; Bednarski, J. J.; Sleckman, B. P.; Pourmand, N.; Boothroyd, J. C., A Novel Secreted Protein, MYR1, Is Central to Toxoplasma's Manipulation of Host Cells. *MBio* **2016,** *7* (1), e02231-15.

47. Lindsay, D. S.; Mitschler, R. R.; Toivio-Kinnucan, M. A.; Upton, S. J.; Dubey, J. P.; Blagburn, B. L., Association of host cell mitochondria with developing Toxoplasma gondii tissue cysts. *American journal of veterinary research* **1993,** *54* (10), 1663-7.

48. Shaw, M. K.; Roos, D. S.; Tilney, L. G., Acidic compartments and rhoptry formation in Toxoplasma gondii. *Parasitology* **1998,** *117 (Pt 5)*, 435-43.

49. Remington, J. S.; McLeod, R.; Desmonts, G.; Remington, J. O.; S., J., Toxoplasmosis. In: Infectious Diseases of the Fetus and Newborn Infant. 1995.

50. Mets, M. B.; Holfels, E.; Boyer, K. M.; Swisher, C. N.; Roizen, N.; Stein, L.; Stein, M.; Hopkins, J.; Withers, S.; Mack, D.; Luciano, R.; Patel, D.; Remington, J. S.; Meier, P.; McLeod, R., Eye manifestations of congenital toxoplasmosis. *American journal of ophthalmology* **1997,** *123* (1), 1-16.

51. Campagna, A. C., Pulmonary toxoplasmosis. *Seminars in respiratory infections* **1997,** *12* (2), 98-105.

52. Mariuz, P.; Bosler, E. M.; Luft, B. J., Toxoplasma pneumonia. *Seminars in respiratory infections* **1997,** *12* (1), 40-3.

53. Kaplan, J. E.; V., H. I., Diagnosis, treatment, and prevention of selected common HIV-related opportunistic infections in the Caribbean region. *Top* **2005,** *12*, 136-41.

54. Vanham, G.; Penne, L.; Devalck, J.; Kestens, L.; Colebunders, R.; Bosmans, E.; Thielemans, K.; Ceuppens, J. L., Decreased CD40 ligand induction in CD4 T cells and dysregulated IL-12 production during HIV infection. *Clinical and experimental immunology* **1999,** *117* (2), 335-42.

55. Sartori, A.; Ma, X.; Gri, G.; Showe, L.; Benjamin, D.; Trinchieri, G., Interleukin-12: an immunoregulatory cytokine produced by B cells and antigen-presenting cells. *Methods (San Diego, Calif.)* **1997,** *11* (1), 116-27.

56. Alonso, K.; Pontiggia, P.; Medenica, R.; Rizzo, S., Cytokine patterns in adults with AIDS. *Immunological investigations* **1997,** *26* (3), 341-50.

57. Luft, B. J.; Remington, J. S., Toxoplasmic encephalitis in AIDS. *Clinical infectious diseases : an official publication of the Infectious Diseases Society of America* **1992,** *15* (2), 211-22.

58. Hari, K. R.; Modi, M. R.; Mochan, A. H.; Modi, G., Reduced risk of toxoplasma encephalitis in HIV-infected patients--a prospective study from Gauteng, South Africa. *Int J STD AIDS* **2007,** *18* (8), 555-8.

59. Hill, D.; Dubey, J. P., Toxoplasma gondii: transmission, diagnosis and prevention. *Clinical microbiology and infection : the official publication of the European Society of Clinical Microbiology and Infectious Diseases* **2002,** *8* (10), 634-40.

60. Montoya, J. G.; Liesenfeld, O., Toxoplasmosis. *Lancet (London, England)* **2004,** *363* (9425), 1965-76.

61. Desmont, G.; Couvrer, J.; N.; J., Congenital toxoplasmosis: a prospecstudy of 378 pregnancies. **1974,** *290 S*, 1110-1116.

62. Montoya, J. G.; Remington, J. S., Management of Toxoplasma gondii infection during pregnancy. *Clin Infect Dis* **2008,** *47* (4), 554-66.

63. Tamma, P., Toxoplasmosis. *Pediatr Rev* **2007,** *28* (12), 470-1.

64. Wilson, C. B.; Remington, J. S.; Stagno, S.; Reynolds, D. W., Development of adverse sequelae in children born with subclinical congenital Toxoplasma infection. *Pediatrics* **1980,** *66* (5), 767-74.

65. Kravetz, J. D.; Federman, D. G., Toxoplasmosis in pregnancy. *The American journal of medicine* **2005,** *118* (3), 212-6.

66. Koppe, J. G.; Loewer-Sieger, D. H.; de Roever-Bonnet, H., Results of 20-year follow-up of congenital toxoplasmosis. *Lancet (London, England)* **1986,** *1* (8475), 254-6.

67. Bhopale, G. M., Pathogenesis of toxoplasmosis. *Comparative immunology, microbiology and*

infectious diseases **2003,** *26* (4), 213-22.

68.   Kirchhoff, L. V.; Weiss, L. M.; Wittner, M.; Tanowitz, H. B., Parasitic diseases of the heart. *Frontiers in bioscience : a journal and virtual library* **2004,** *9*, 706-23.

69.   Wilson, E. H.; Hunter, C. A., The role of astrocytes in the immunopathogenesis of toxoplasmic encephalitis. *International journal for parasitology* **2004,** *34* (5), 543-8.

70.   Nath, A.; Sinai, A. P., Cerebral Toxoplasmosis. *Current treatment options in neurology* **2003,** *5* (1), 3-12.

71.   Leyva, W. H.; Santa Cruz, D. J., Cutaneous toxoplasmosis. *Journal of the American Academy of Dermatology* **1986,** *14* (4), 600-5.

72.   Belanger, F.; Derouin, F.; Grangeot-Keros, L.; Meyer, L., Incidence and risk factors of toxoplasmosis in a cohort of human immunodeficiency virus-infected patients: 1988-1995. HEMOCO and SEROCO Study Groups. *Clin Infect Dis* **1999,** *28* (3), 575-81.

73.   Janitschke, K.; Held, T.; Krüiger, D.; Schwerdtfeger, R.; Schlier, G.; Liesenfeld, O., Diagnostic value of tests for Toxoplasma gondii-specific antibodies in patients undergoing bone marrow transplantation. *Clinical laboratory* **2003,** *49* (5-6), 239-42.

74.   Wreghitt, T. G.; Hakim, M.; Gray, J. J.; Balfour, A. H.; Stovin, P. G.; Stewart, S.; Scott, J.; English, T. A.; Wallwork, J., Toxoplasmosis in heart and heart and lung transplant recipients. *J Clin Pathol* **1989,** *42* (2), 194-9.

75.   Mele, A.; Paterson, P. J.; Prentice, H. G.; Leoni, P.; Kibbler, C. C., Toxoplasmosis in bone marrow transplantation: a report of two cases and systematic review of the literature. *Bone Marrow Transplant* **2002,** *29* (8), 691-8.

76.   Bergstrom, T.; Ricksten, A.; Nenonen, N.; J., Congenital Toxoplasma gondii infection diagnosed by PCR amplification of peripheral mononuclear blood cells from a child and mother. *Scand Dis* **1998,** *30* (2), 202-4.

77.   Danise, A.; Cinque, P.; Vergani, S.; Candino, M.; Racca, S.; De Bona, A.; Novati, R.; Castagna, A.; Lazzarin, A., Use of polymerase chain reaction assays of aqueous humor in the differential diagnosis of retinitis in patients infected with human immunodeficiency virus. *Clinical infectious diseases : an official publication of the Infectious Diseases Society of America* **1997,** *24* (6), 1100-6.

78.   Nimri, L.; Pelloux, H.; Elkhatib, L., Detection of Toxoplasma gondii DNA and specific antibodies in high-risk pregnant women. *Am J Trop Med Hyg* **2004,** *71* (6), 831-5.

79.   Wilson, M.; Remington, J. S.; Clavet, C.; Varney, G.; Press, C.; Ware, D., Evaluation of six commercial kits for detection of human immunoglobulin M antibodies to Toxoplasma gondii. The FDA Toxoplasmosis Ad Hoc Working Group. *Journal of clinical microbiology* **1997,** *35* (12), 3112-5.

80.   Costa, J. G.; Carneiro, A. C.; Tavares, A. T.; Andrade, G. M.; Vasconcelos-Santos, D. V.; Januario, J. N.; Menezes-Souza, D.; Fujiwara, R. T.; Vitor, R. W., Real-time PCR as a prognostic tool for human congenital toxoplasmosis. *J Clin Microbiol* **2013,** *51* (8), 2766-8.

81.   Petersen, E.; Borobio, M. V.; Guy, E.; Liesenfeld, O.; Meroni, V.; Naessens, A.; Spranzi, E.; Thulliez, P., European multicenter study of the LIAISON automated diagnostic system for determination of Toxoplasma gondii-specific immunoglobulin G (IgG) and IgM and the IgG avidity index. *Journal of clinical microbiology* **2005,** *43* (4), 1570-4.

82.   Paquet, C.; Yudin, M. H.; Society of, O.; Gynaecologists of, C., Toxoplasmosis in pregnancy: prevention, screening, and treatment. *J Obstet Gynaecol Can* **2013,** *35* (1), 78-81.

83.   Malla, N.; Sengupta, C.; Dubey, M. L.; Sud, A.; Dutta, U., Antigenaemia and antibody response to Toxoplasma gondii in human immunodeficiency virus-infected patients. *British journal of biomedical science* **2005,** *62* (1), 19-23.

84.   Petersen, E.; Schmidt, D. R., Sulfadiazine and pyrimethamine in the postnatal treatment of congenital toxoplasmosis: what are the options? *Expert review of anti-infective therapy* **2003,** *1* (1), 175-82.

85.   Torre, D.; Casari, S.; Speranza, F.; Donisi, A.; Gregis, G.; Poggio, A.; Ranieri, S.; Orani, A.; Angarano, G.; Chiodo, F.; Fiori, G.; Carosi, G., Randomized trial of trimethoprim-sulfamethoxazole versus pyrimethamine-sulfadiazine for therapy of toxoplasmic encephalitis in

patients with AIDS. Italian Collaborative Study Group. *Antimicrob Agents Chemother* **1998,** *42* (6), 1346-9.

86.   Chang, H. R.; Pechere, J. C., In vitro effects of four macrolides (roxithromycin, spiramycin, azithromycin [CP-62,993], and A-56268) on Toxoplasma gondii. *Antimicrob Agents Chemother* **1988,** *32* (4), 524-9.

87.   Couvreur, J.; Desmonts, G.; Thulliez, P., Prophylaxis of congenital toxoplasmosis. Effects of spiramycin on placental infection. *J Antimicrob Chemother* **1988,** *22 Suppl B*, 193-200.

88.   Cortina-Borja, M.; Tan, H. K.; Wallon, M.; Paul, M.; Prusa, A.; Buffolano, W.; Malm, G.; Salt, A.; Freeman, K.; Petersen, E.; Gilbert, R. E.; European Multicentre Study on Congenital, T., Prenatal treatment for serious neurological sequelae of congenital toxoplasmosis: an observational prospective cohort study. *PLoS Med* **2010,** *7* (10).

89.   Boyer, K. M.; Holfels, E.; Roizen, N.; Swisher, C.; Mack, D.; Remington, J.; Withers, S.; Meier, P.; McLeod, R.; Toxoplasmosis Study, G., Risk factors for Toxoplasma gondii infection in mothers of infants with congenital toxoplasmosis: Implications for prenatal management and screening. *American journal of obstetrics and gynecology* **2005,** *192* (2), 564-71.

90.   Muleta, D.; Ashenafi, M., Salmonella, Shigella and growth potential of other food-borne pathogens in Ethiopian street vended foods. *East Afr Med J* **2001,** *78* (11), 576-80.

91.   Teutsch, S. M.; Juranek, D. D.; Sulzer, A.; Dubey, J. P.; Sikes, R. K., Epidemic toxoplasmosis associated with infected cats. *N Engl J Med* **1979,** *300* (13), 695-9.

92.   Isaac-Renton, J.; Bowie, W. R.; King, A.; Irwin, G. S.; Ong, C. S.; Fung, C. P.; Shokeir, M. O.; Dubey, J. P., Detection of Toxoplasma gondii oocysts in drinking water. *Applied and environmental microbiology* **1998,** *64* (6), 2278-80.

93.   Beghetto, E.; Nielsen, H. V.; Del Porto, P.; Buffolano, W.; Guglietta, S.; Felici, F.; Petersen, E.; Gargano, N., A combination of antigenic regions of Toxoplasma gondii microneme proteins induces protective immunity against oral infection with parasite cysts. *J Infect Dis* **2005,** *191* (4), 637-45.

12. *Entamoeba histolytica*
(Schaudinn 1903)

Introduction

Entamoeba histolytica is the causative agent of amoebic dysentery in humans.[1, 2] While most species of amoebae are free-living, many other members of this genus (e.g., *Entamoeba dispar* and *Entamoeba moshkovskii),* can inhabit the human large intestine, but none other than *E. histolytica* are clearly pathogenic. (There is some controversy regarding the role of *E. moshkovskii* in childhood diarrhea in Bangledesh.) *Entamoeba histolytica* is transmitted from person to person via the fecal-oral route, taking up residence in the wall of the large intestine.[3, 4] Protracted infection can progress from watery diarrhea to dysentery (bloody diarrhea) that may prove fatal if left untreated. In addition, *E. histolytica* can spread to extra-intestinal sites causing serious disease.[5] *E. histolytica* lives as a trophozoite in the tissues of the host and as a resistant cyst in the outside environment. Sanitation programs designed to limit exposure to food and water-borne diarrheal disease agents are effective in limiting infection with *E. histolytica*. Some animals (non-human primates and domestic dogs) can become infected with *E. histolytica*, but none serve as important reservoirs for human infection.

Entamoeba dispar and *E. moshkovskii* are morphologically identical amoebae that can be misidentified as *E. histolytica* during microscopic examination of fecal samples.[6] Commercially available stool antigen detection tests and nucleic acid amplification tests are now widely available that are sensitive and specific, allowing for discrimination between *E. histolytica* and nonpathogenic amoeba.[7, 8] Fortunately, much is now known about the basic biology and clinical aspects of infection with *Entamoeba histolytica,* and the genome has also been sequenced.[9-11]

Historical Information

Although reports of what appears to be amoebiasis can be found in the writings of Hippocrates (460-377 BCE), and the Old Testament, appreciation for its significance as a pathogen began when Fedor Losch, in 1875, described clinical features of infection with *E. histolytica,* and reproduced some aspects of the disease in experimentally infected dogs.[12, 13] In 1893, Heinrich Quincke and Ernst Roos distinguished *E. histolytica* from *Entamoeba coli,* a non-pathogenic amoeba acquired by the fecal-oral route and often found in the stool of asymptomatic individuals.[14] In 1903, Fritz Schaudinn described the trophozoites and cysts of *E. histolytica.*[15] He died at the age of 35 of overwhelming amoebiasis, a tragic outcome of self-experimentation. In 1891, William Councilman and Henri Lafleur described the main features of the intestinal pathogenesis caused by *E. histolytica.* William Boeck, in 1925, was the first to culture *E. histolytica*, while Clifford Dobell, in 1928, fully elucidated its life cycle.[16-18]

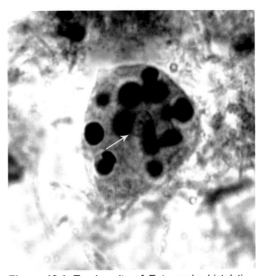

Figure 12.1. Trophozoite of *Entamoeba histolytica.* Note nucleus (arrow) and numerous ingested red cells. 35 μm.

Life Cycle

The trophozoite (Fig. 12.1) is a facultative anaerobe metabolizing glucose as its main source of energy.[19] The trophozoite measures 20-30 μm in diameter, and the cytoplasm contains a single nucleus with a centrally located nucleolus, often termed the karyosome. In addition, surface soluble lysosomes, and a remnant mitochondrion organelle called a "crypton," or mitosome, are present.[20-22] *Entamoeba* spp. evolved after the introduction of the mitochondrial containing eukaryotes arose, and the mitosome is thought to be a remnant organelle resulting from organelle decay of the mitochondria.[23, 24] Evidence suggests that the mitosome no longer contains any DNA and likely lost its prior genome through reductive evolution.[23] Discovery of a calreticulin-like molecule of 51 kDa suggested the presence of an endoplasmic reticulum and further work has now verified the presence of a continuous ER in *Entamoeba histolytica*.[25, 26]

The cyst (Fig. 12.2) is smaller than the trophozoite (10-15 μm in diameter), and at full maturity contains four typically round *E. histolytica* nuclei. Each nucleus ultimately will give rise to an individual trophozoite. Immature cysts may contain a single, smooth-ended chromatoidal bar, a crystalline-like condensation of ribosomes, and any number of nuclei up to four.

Ingestion of a single cyst is all that is necessary to initiate infection, making this organism one of the most efficient pathogenic protozoa known to infect humans.[27] Each cyst undergoes excystation in the small intestine. Excystation is complex, involving actin cytoskeletal reorganization.[28, 29] The cyst must receive certain specific environmental cues from the host, including sequential exposure to an acidic and a basic pH environment, in order for the four trophozoites contained within cyst to exit through the cyst wall and enter the small intestine. The four newly emerged trophozoites then divide, and the resulting eight parasites are carried by peristalsis to the large intestine. There is no sexual phase, and consequently replication is clonal.[5]

In the large intestine the trophozoite penetrates the perimucosal space and attaches to epithelial cells using lectin-galactose interactions.[30] This event is cytotoxic.[31] The amoeba engulfs and kills only living cells (Fig. 12.3).[30] Trophozoites divide by binary fission, occupying increasingly larger areas of tissue as they do so.[18] This activity eventually causes

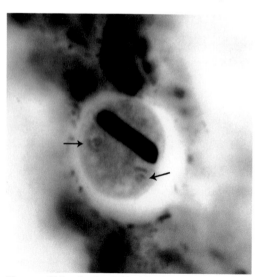

Figure 12.2. Cyst of *E. histolytica*. Two nuclei (arrows) and a smooth-ended chromatoidal bar can be seen. 15 μm.

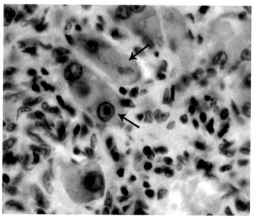

Figure 12.3. Trophozoites of *E. histolytica* in liver abscess (arrows). Note ingested host cells inside parasites.

Entamoeba histolytica

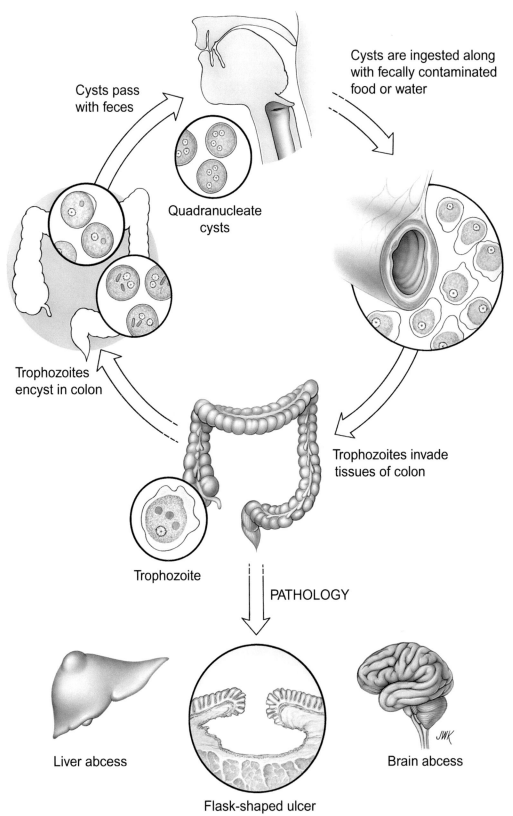

Cysts pass with feces

Cysts are ingested along with fecally contaminated food or water

Quadranucleate cysts

Trophozoites encyst in colon

Trophozoites invade tissues of colon

Trophozoite

PATHOLOGY

Liver abcess

Flask-shaped ulcer

Brain abcess

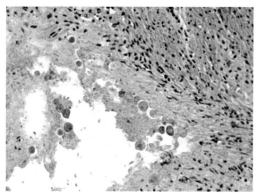

Figure 12.4. Low-magnification histologic section of amoebic ulcer in small intestine. Organisms can be seen at living margin of ulcer.

flask-shaped ulcers to develop (Fig. 12.4). Hematogenous or lymphatic spread is then possible, but this aspect does not play a role in the life cycle.

Some trophozoites, instead of dividing, encyst in the lumen of the ulcer. Encystation also involves actin cytoskeletal reorganization that is likely triggered by means of the Gal/Gal-NAc-specific lectin.[28, 29] Amoebic proteasome activity may also be necessary for the process, since treating cultures with lactacystin caused marked inhibition of cyst formation.[32, 33] Although early work required feeder cells to culture *E. histolytica*, it can now be cultured in cell-free media, with

excellent results, particularly when a layer of mineral oil is overlaid to enhance the anaerobic conditions.[34] During infection in the GI tract, cysts may be continuously produced and exit the host in feces. Cysts can survive in warm, moist conditions for weeks without losing infectivity.

Cellular and Molecular Pathogenesis

There is a complex process underlying the pathogenesis of intra-intestinal and extra-intestinal amoebiasis.[10, 11, 35-39] Amoebae must attach to host tissues as a necessary prerequisite for parasite-mediated cytotoxicity. Attachment is dependent upon interactions between epithelial cell membrane-bound N-acetyl-glucosamine and N-acetyl-galactosamine and at least two surface lectin proteins. The genes for both of the parasite lectins have been cloned and their cDNAs sequenced. One lectin is a 260 kDa protein, while the other is 220 kDa.[40] The heavy subunit of the 260 kDa lectin has a single transmembrane–spanning domain and a cytoplasmic domain related to β-2-integrins, which may also participate in the attachment process.[41, 42] These surface lectins apparently also facilitate the parasite's evasion of the complement mem-

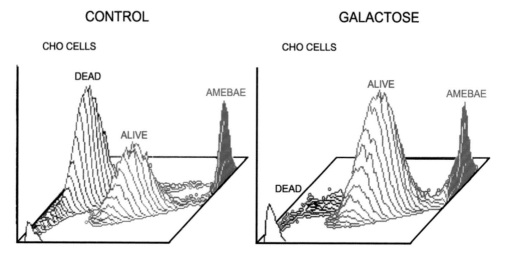

Figure 12.5. *In vitro* experiment showing that galactose-containing surface proteins are important for parasite cytotoxicy. Free galactose prevents attachment of amoebae to their target cells. CHO cells=Chinese hamster ovary cells. Redrawn after J. I. Ravdin.

brane attack complex.[43] *In vitro, E. histolytica* can be inhibited from attaching to its target cells simply by adding free galactose to the medium (Fig. 12.5).[44] In this situation, cells and trophozoites coexist. Attachment leads to cell death, which, at least *in vitro*, is calcium-dependent.[45] Several possible mechanisms for the actual killing of host cells have been proposed, all of which involve enzymes such as serine proteases.[46] A recent finding has shown that trophozoites can "nibble" off a portion of their target cells just before actually killing them; a process termed trogocytosis.[47] Apparently, *E. histolytica* needs to sample its meal before fully committing to ingesting it. So this pathogen may turn out to be a fussier eater that previously thought. Although inflammation and the release of cytokines may play a role in the tissue destruction associated with acute infection, there is a significant amount of tissue destruction present in chronic ulcerations that is out of proportion to the degree of inflammation seen at this stage of infection.[48]

The trophozoite's surface membrane contains phospholipase A, neuraminidase, and a metallocollagenase.[49] In addition, it secretes a minimum of four cysteine proteases.[50] These enzymes may also aid the parasite in moving through the extracellular matrix. Attachment elicits the secretion of a pore-forming peptide that is biochemically related both in structure and function to saposins.[51, 52] The pore-forming protein presumably plays a central role in lysing the host cell membrane. During attachment, the intracellular calcium levels of the target cell increase by 20-fold.[53] One intriguing finding is that the trophozoite may actually "lure in" new target cells, in this case lymphocytes, to the site of infection by upregulating the lymphotactic IL-8 in the surrounding colonic epithelial cells, while simultaneously inhibiting the upregulation of other cytokines known to play a role in inflammation.[54, 55]

Protective immune mechanisms are short-lived and depend on the development of sIgA antibodies directed against parasite surface proteins involved in adherence to target cells, such as the carbohydrate-recognition domain of Gal/GalNAc lectin.[56-60] In addition, cell-mediated killing of parasites can occur by induction of nitric oxide by the 220 kDa lectin, which up-regulates IFN-γ.[61, 62] The importance of CD4+ T cells may be minimal as patients with HIV-1-infection and impaired T cell function do not seem to suffer dramatically increased rates of invasive disease.[63] In experimental infections, polyclonal and monoclonal antibodies have been shown to be effective in protecting the host when they are directed against carbohydrate-binding lectins of the parasite, emphasizing the central role these parasite proteins play in the pathogenesis of disease.[64, 65]

Clinical Disease

Intestinal amoebiasis

Most exposed individuals are asymptomatic, but a number will go on to experience clinical disease or become chronic carriers. Host factors such as genetic background, age, immune status, nutritional status, pregnancy and co-morbidities may determine whether a host becomes symptomatic, as well as the severity and type of manifestation. Those who are symptomatic may experience a wide range of clinical disease.[37, 66] The most common manifestation is diarrhea, lasting more than a few days, and in some cases for weeks, months or years if not treated appropriately.[37, 66] Although a large number of patients do not report blood or excess mucous in their stools, almost all stools are heme-positive if tested.[67] Involvement of the entire bowel can be associated with colicky pain, flatulence, alteration in the pattern of bowel movements, bloody stools, and eventually dysentery, which must be distinguished clinically from ulcerative colitis. Although patients may be afebrile, a large percentage of patients will report fever at clinical presentation.[67]

Generalized abdominal tenderness, with particular accentuation in the iliac fossae is frequently encountered on physical examination. Dysentery can either worsen, possibly resulting in a life-threatening situation, or resolve into a chronic state of ill-health characterized by bouts of diarrhea, abdominal cramping, and abdominal discomfort. In the chronic condition, amoeboma (large granuloma consisting of eosinophils, amoebae, and necrotic colonic tissue) are possible, presenting as palpable masses. Amoeboma are often misdiagnosed on barium enema as malignancies. If disease progresses, the colon may become atonic and may perforate at one or several points of ulceration (Fig. 12.6). If perforation occurs, symptoms and signs of peritonitis may develop. Acute colitis occurs more frequently in children.[37]

The perforated, inflamed bowel may adhere to the abdominal wall, and the perforation may extend to the skin, causing cutaneous amoebiasis, which can progress rapidly.[68] This situation may also occur in the perianal area as the result of invasion of the skin by the trophozoites emerging from the rectum.

Extraintestinal amoebiasis

Amoebae can erode the wall of the large intestine until the circulation of the submucosa is breached. In that case, parasites are thought to enter mainly via the portal circulation and disseminate throughout the body.

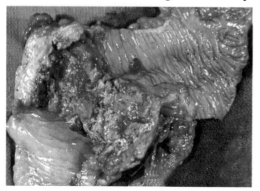

Figure 12.6. Portion of transverse colon showing extensive ulceration due to intestinal infection with *E. histolytica*.

The most common extraintestinal site is the liver, occasionally presenting as a medical emergency.[66, 69] Invasion of liver tissue may occur after symptomatic intestinal amoebiasis, or in cases where the colonic infection is asymptomatic. Nearly half of all patients with amoebic liver abscess do not have a history suggestive of amoebic colitis.

Hepatic amoebiasis is a slowly progressive, insidious disease that typically begins as a nonspecific febrile illness, with pain and tenderness in the right upper quadrant of the abdomen. Frequently this presents as referred pain to the shoulder region. Examination at that time may reveal only a slightly enlarged, tender liver, or it may reveal a mass. In some cases pressure exerted between the ribs, the so called 'intercostal sign', will detect tenderness.[5] Most patients with hepatic amoebiasis have involvement of the right hepatic lobe, but the left lobe of the liver can also be infected; the enlargement and tenderness can be central or even left-sided.

The lungs are the next most common extraintestinal sites of infection.[70, 71] Direct extension to the right pleural space and the lung is the most common form of intrathoracic amoebiasis, but hematogenous spread may cause metastatic amoebiasis in other portions of the lung and the pleura, as well as in other organs, notably the brain. Amoebic pericarditis can occur in the same manner. The major pleuropulmonary manifestations include effusion, pleurisy, empyema, and lung abscess. Occasionally, a hepatobronchial fistula forms, resulting in a productive cough, with large amounts of amoebae-containing necrotic material. Embolism is rare. Rupture into the pericardium is usually fatal.

Cerebral amoebiasis rarely occurs. The onset is usually abrupt and is associated with a high mortality rate unless diagnosed early on in the infection.[72]

It is now recognized that many populations infected with HIV-1 have higher exposures and asymptomatic colonization rates for *E.*

histolytica. There may be some increase in the incidence of invasive disease in these patients compared to those without HIV-infection.[73-76]

Diagnosis

The site, as well as duration of infection, dictates the most appropriate diagnostic test. Stool testing for heme is positive in almost all cases of intestinal amoebiasis if performed properly, while stool test for leukocytes tend to be negative due to the ability of the amoeba to destroy leukocytes despite the invasive nature of this disease. Definitive diagnosis depends upon; detection of antigens in stool, nucleic acid amplification testing (NAAT) on stool or tissue samples, or microscopy coupled with species identification by one of the first two testing modalities.[7, 77] Antigen detection and NAAT testing are replacing microscopy, based on their sensitivity, specificity, rapidity, ease of execution, and cost. An ELISA-based test is now in common use that is both rapid and specific for distinguishing *Entamoeba histolytica* from its non-pathogenic *doppelgängers.*[7] Molecular testing with NAAT is reported to have a sensitivity 100x that of stool antigen testing, and is now available and in routine use in many centers as part of a gastrointestinal diagnostic panel.[73, 78]

Microscopy is still the only diagnostic modality in many facilities. Stool culture is not clinically available and does not play a role in the routine diagnosis of this disease. The trophozoites of *E. histolytica* are more often described as showing evidence of erythophagocytosis, and this has been suggested to allow for definitive diagnosis using microscopy. There are both *in vitro* and *in vivo* reports that nonpathogenic amoebae phagocytize red cells, and in one study over 15% of cases of *E. dispar* showed erythrophagocytosis on stool microscopy.[79-82] If red blood cells are seen in the cytoplasm, particularly more than 2 rbcs per trophozoite, then *Entamoeba histolytica* is more likely.[82] (Fig.

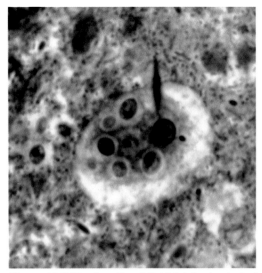

Figure 12.7. Trophozoite of *E. histolytica* in stool of patient suffering from amoebic dysentery. Note Charcot-Leyden crystal "pointing" to nucleus. Also note numerous red cells in parasite cytoplasm. 30 µm.

12.7)

The Charcot-Leyden crystals (Fig. 12.8) in stool are frequently present when patients are suffering from disease caused by *E. histolytica*, but they are also seen with heavy infection caused by *Trichuris trichiura* and *Strongyloides stercoralis*, and therefore are not pathognomonic for amoebiasis. PCR can also be useful for diagnosis of liver disease when used on aspirates derived from the abscess.[83]

Since infection with *E. histolytica* invariably leads to long-lasting antibody production, antibody-based tests are sometimes

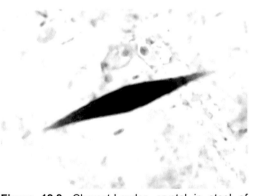

Figure 12.8. Charcot-Leyden crystal in stool of patient suffering from amoebic dysentery. These crystals can also be found in patients infected with *Trichuris trichiura* and *Strongyloides stercoralis*.

difficult to interpret, especially when done during chronic infection.[84] Serological testing will become positive, even in intestinal amoebiaisis infection, 5-7 days after onset of symptoms and usually remain positive for years, consequently limiting their utility in endemic areas where up to 35% of the population may have seropositivity due to prior exposure.[85] The IHA and IFA tests are used together to rule in the possibility of extraintestinal disease, but are not definitive proof of infection. Intestinal amoebiasis must always be considered in any patient with protracted diarrhea and in all patients with dysentery. The diagnosis must also be considered in patients presenting with intraluminal colonic masses, because of the development of amoebomas that resemble carcinoma of the colon. In extraintestinal amoebiasis, identification of the lesion by the various modalities and the presence of a travel history compatible with amoebiasis, in parallel with identification of amoebae in the colon, points to the diagnosis.

Extraintestinal amoebiasis is often a more challenging diagnosis. Intestinal and extraintestinal amoebiasis do not usually occur simultaneously, and stool testing is usually negative in the setting of extraintestinal amoebiasis. Serology is usually positive in cases of extraintestinal amoebiasis, but may be negative during the first 7 days. Imaging tests play a critical role in the diagnosis of extraintestinal amoebiasis. Radiography of the abdomen may show enlargement of the liver and a fixed, raised diaphragm. In cases of perforation of the diaphragm, there may be evidence of consolidation one of the lower lobes of the lung or its lower segment, and a pleural effusion. A radionuclide or a CT scan often reveals the abscess; it may also show additional abscesses, which are rare. On ultrasonography, an amoebic liver abscess usually appears as a round hypodense area that is contiguous to the liver capsule, usually without significant wall echoes.[86] Direct extension to the right pleural space and the lung is the most common form of intrathoracic amoebiasis, but hematogenous spread may cause metastatic amoebiasis in other portions of the lung and the pleura, as well as in other organs, notably the brain. Amoebic pericarditis can occur in the same manner.[87]

If the diagnosis is still in doubt after serological testing and imaging, the cyst can be aspirated. The obtained fluid from an hepatic amoebic abscess is often a brown fluid containing necrotic hepatocytes, and has been likened to anchovy paste. In some cases, the fluid may be clear or yellow in color. Amoebic forms are rarely present and antigen testing or NAAT is helpful in confirming the diagnosis. Abscesses may be secondarily infected with bacteria, so sending the fluid for bacterial culture is recommended. Although eosinophils may play some role in local tissue control early in the course of hepatic amoebiasis, very few patients have elevated eosinophils in the peripheral circulation, and patients may even become eosinopenic in severe infections.[88-90]

Treatment

All forms of symptomatic amoebiasis are considered invasive and consequently should be treated with an agent that is active against the tissue invasive forms that reaches adequate levels at the sites of infection. Metronidazole is the drug of choice for the intestinal and extraintestinal infection.[91] It can be given in equivalent doses orally or intravenously. This drug also has a few limitations and some adverse side effects. Use of alcohol is prohibited during treatment, as it induces a side-effect similar to that caused by disulfiram (antabuse) therapy. Alternative agents include tinidazole and second-line agents that may be inferior in efficacy, such as nitazoxinide or ornidazole. Since these drugs do not target the cyst stage, a second intraluminal agent to target the intraluminal cysts is also recommended for all symptomatic patients. Treatment of asymptomatic carriers of E hys-

tolytica to prevent disease or transmission is controversial.[92] A cysticidal intraluminal agent alone may be adequate for asymptomatic cyst passers and those with nondysenteric amoebic colitis. The intraluminal agent paromomycin is widely used in the United States for this indication, while other agents, such as diloxanide furoate and iodoquinol (diidohydroxyquin), are both effective at killing cysts and should be considered.[93] Additional antibiotics are appropriate in patients in whom a secondary bacterial infection is suspected.

No naturally occurring metronidazole-resistant strains of *E. histolytica* have been reported to date, but they can be easily induced under laboratory conditions.[94, 95] It is probably only a matter of time before they appear in human populations. Liver abscesses resolve slowly, despite treatment with the recommended high doses of metronidazole. Aspiration of an amoebic liver abscess may serve not only to confirm the diagnosis, but also as a therapeutic intervention. There are established indications for therapeutic drainage of an amoebic liver abscess and for surgery, in cases of severe colitis. A surgeon or interventional radiologist should be involved if; 1. if there is no clinical improvement within 48-72 hours despite appropriate medical therapy, 2. for abscesses greater than 10 cm in diameter, 3. when there is marked elevation of the diaphragm, 4. for abscesses in the left lobe, and 5. when there is negative serology, which might raise suspicion of a pyogenic abscess.[66, 96, 97]

There are few reports of patients surviving amoebic abscess of the brain, since, unfortunately, they are typically diagnosed too late.[72] In the case of infection involving the pleural cavity, quick aspiration of an expanding pericardial effusion, combined with aggressive anti-amoebic therapy, has saved the lives of most of those suffering from this rare manifestation of the infection.[98]

Prevention and Control

Good public health practice, starting with ensuring the safety of drinking water supplies, and in some cases, watershed management, are the best long-term approaches to controlling most waterborne diarrheal disease agents. Screening of food handlers with periodic stool examinations can identify carriers whose occupations would place the general public at risk. Recurrent outbreaks of amoebiasis in mental institutions can be prevented by strictly adhering to appropriate sanitary practices, coupled with routine stool examinations of the patients. All infected individuals should receive treatment.

Vaccine targets against both the intestinal and extraintestinal infection have been identified. Successful development of vaccines based on these findings will require extensive non-clinical and clinical studies before a vaccine is considered for the highest risk groups including children in endemic areas and other high-risk groups such as travelers.[99]

References

1. Bercu, T. E.; Petri, W. A.; Behm, J. W., Amebic colitis: new insights into pathogenesis and treatment. *Curr Gastroenterol Rep* **2007,** *9* (5), 429-33.
2. Heredia, R. D.; Fonseca, J. A.; Lopez, M. C., Entamoeba moshkovskii perspectives of a new agent to be considered in the diagnosis of amebiasis. *Acta Trop* **2012,** *123* (3), 139-45.
3. Marciano-Cabral, F., Free-living amoebae as agents of human infection. *J Infect Dis* **2009,** *199* (8), 1104-6.
4. Kotloff, K. L.; Nataro, J. P.; Blackwelder, W. C.; Nasrin, D.; Farag, T. H.; Panchalingam, S.; Wu, Y.; Sow, S. O.; Sur, D.; Breiman, R. F.; Faruque, A. S.; Zaidi, A. K.; Saha, D.; Alonso, P. L.; Tamboura, B.; Sanogo, D.; Onwuchekwa, U.; Manna, B.; Ramamurthy, T.; Kanungo, S.;

Ochieng, J. B.; Omore, R.; Oundo, J. O.; Hossain, A.; Das, S. K.; Ahmed, S.; Qureshi, S.; Quadri, F.; Adegbola, R. A.; Antonio, M.; Hossain, M. J.; Akinsola, A.; Mandomando, I.; Nhampossa, T.; Acacio, S.; Biswas, K.; O'Reilly, C. E.; Mintz, E. D.; Berkeley, L. Y.; Muhsen, K.; Sommerfelt, H.; Robins-Browne, R. M.; Levine, M. M., Burden and aetiology of diarrhoeal disease in infants and young children in developing countries (the Global Enteric Multicenter Study, GEMS): a prospective, case-control study. *Lancet* **2013**, *382* (9888), 209-22.

5. Haque, R.; Huston, C. D.; Hughes, M.; Houpt, E.; Petri, W. A., Jr., Amebiasis. *N Engl J Med* **2003**, *348* (16), 1565-73.

6. Tannich, E., Royal Society of Tropical Medicine and Hygiene Meeting at Manson House, London, 19 February 1998. Amoebic disease. Entamoeba histolytica and E. dispar: comparison of molecules considered important for host tissue destruction. *Transactions of the Royal Society of Tropical Medicine and Hygiene* **1998**, *92* (6), 593-6.

7. Anane, S.; Khaled, S., [Entamoeba histolytica and Entamoeba dispar: differentiation methods and implications]. *Annales de biologie clinique* **2005**, *63* (1), 7-13.

8. Blessmann, J.; Buss, H.; Nu, P. A.; Dinh, B. T.; Ngo, Q. T.; Van, A. L.; Alla, M. D.; Jackson, T. F.; Ravdin, J. I.; Tannich, E., Real-time PCR for detection and differentiation of Entamoeba histolytica and Entamoeba dispar in fecal samples. *J Clin Microbiol* **2002**, *40* (12), 4413-7.

9. Reed, S.; Ravdin, J. I.; Blazer, M. J.; Smith, P. D.; Greenberg, H. B.; Guerrant, R. L., Amoebiasis In: Infections of the Gastrointestinal Tract 2nd ed. 2002; p 961-978.

10. Martinez-Paloma, A.; Cantellano, M.; Collier, L.; Balows, A.; Sussman, M.; Cox, F. E. G.; Kreier, J. P.; Wakelin, D., Topley and Wilson's Microbiology and Microbial Infections 9th ed. 1998; p 157-177.

11. Loftus, B.; Anderson, I.; Davies, R.; Alsmark, U. C. M.; Samuelson, J.; Amedeo, P.; Roncaglia, P.; Berriman, M.; Hirt, R. P.; Mann, B. J.; Nozaki, T.; Suh, B.; Pop, M.; Duchene, M.; Ackers, J.; Tannich, E.; Leippe, M.; Hofer, M.; Bruchhaus, I.; Willhoeft, U.; Bhattacharya, A.; Chillingworth, T.; Churcher, C.; Hance, Z.; Harris, B.; Harris, D.; Jagels, K.; Moule, S.; Mungall, K.; Ormond, D.; Squares, R.; Whitehead, S.; Quail, M. A.; Rabbinowitsch, E.; Norbertczak, H.; Price, C.; Wang, Z.; Guillén, N.; Gilchrist, C.; Stroup, S. E.; Bhattacharya, S.; Lohia, A.; Foster, P. G.; Sicheritz-Ponten, T.; Weber, C.; Singh, U.; Mukherjee, C.; El-Sayed, N. M.; Petri, W. A.; Clark, C. G.; Embley, T. M.; Barrell, B.; Fraser, C. M.; Hall, N., The genome of the protist parasite Entamoeba histolytica. *Nature* **2005**, *433* (7028), 865-8.

12. Losch, F. A., Massenhafte Entwicklung von Amoben in Dickdarm. *Arch Pathol Anat Phys Klm Med Virchow* **1875**, *65*, 196-211.

13. Tanyuksel, M.; Petri, W. A., Jr., Laboratory diagnosis of amebiasis. *Clin Microbiol Rev* **2003**, *16* (4), 713-29.

14. Quincke, H. I.; Roos, E., Uber Amoben-enteritis. *Berl Klm Wochenschr* **1893**, *30* 1089-1094.

15. Schaudinn, F., Untersuchungen uber Fortpflanzung einiger Rhizopoden (vorlaufige Mitteilung). Arb Kaiserlichen Ges. **1903**, *19* 547-576.

16. Councilman, W. T.; Lafleur, H. A., Amoebic dysentery. *Johns Hopkins Hosp Rep* **1891**, *2*, 395-548.

17. Boeck, W. C.; J., Cultivation of Entamoeba histolytica. *Am* **1925**, *5* 371-407.

18. Dobell, C., Researches on the intestinal protozoa of monkeys and man. *Parasitology* **1928**, *20* 357-412.

19. Saavedra, E.; Encalada, R.; Pineda, E.; Jasso-Chávez, R.; Moreno-Sánchez, R., Glycolysis in Entamoeba histolytica. Biochemical characterization of recombinant glycolytic enzymes and flux control analysis. *The FEBS journal* **2005**, *272* (7), 1767-83.

20. Mai, Z.; Ghosh, S.; Frisardi, M.; Rosenthal, B.; Rogers, R.; Samuelson, J., Hsp60 is targeted to a cryptic mitochondrion-derived organelle ("crypton") in the microaerophilic protozoan parasite Entamoeba histolytica. *Molecular and cellular biology* **1999**, *19* (3), 2198-205.

21. Tovar, J.; Fischer, A.; Clark, C. G., The mitosome, a novel organelle related to mitochondria in the amitochondrial parasite Entamoeba histolytica. *Molecular microbiology* **1999**, *32* (5), 1013-21.

22. Nakada-Tsukuii, K.; Nozaki, T., Molecular Basis of the Trafficking of Cysteine Proteases and Other Soluble Lysosomal Proteins in Entamoeba histolytica. *Amebiasis Springer Japan* **2015**.

23. Aguilera, P.; Barry, T.; Tovar, J., Entamoeba histolytica mitosomes: organelles in search of a

function. *Exp Parasitol* **2008,** *118* (1), 10-6.

24. Bakatselou, C.; Beste, D.; Kadri, A. O.; Somanath, S.; Clark, C. G., Analysis of genes of mitochondrial origin in the genus Entamoeba. *The Journal of eukaryotic microbiology* **2003,** *50* (3), 210-4.

25. Gozalez, E.; Rico, G.; J., Calreticulin-like molecule in trophozoites of Entamoeba histolytica. *Am Med Hyg* **2002,** *67*, 636-639.

26. Teixeira, J. E.; Huston, C. D., Evidence of a continuous endoplasmic reticulum in the protozoan parasite Entamoeba histolytica. *Eukaryot Cell* **2008,** *7* (7), 1222-6.

27. Walker, E. L.; Sellards, A. W.; J.; B., Experimental entamoebic dysentery. *Phillipine Med* **1913,** *8* 253-330.

28. Makioka, A.; Kumagai, M.; Hiranuka, K.; Kobayashi, S.; Takeuchi, T., Expression analysis of Entamoeba invadens profilins in encystation and excystation. *Parasitol Res* **2012,** *110* (6), 2095-104.

29. Eichinger, D., A role for a galactose lectin and its ligands during encystment of Entamoeba. *J Eukaryot Microbiol* **2001,** *48* (1), 17-21.

30. Ravdin, J. I.; Guerrant, R. L., Role of adherence in cytopathogenic mechanisms of Entamoeba histolytica. Study with mammalian tissue culture cells and human erythrocytes. *J Clin Invest* **1981,** *68* (5), 1305-13.

31. Saffer, L. D.; Petri, W. A., Jr., Role of the galactose lectin of Entamoeba histolytica in adherence-dependent killing of mammalian cells. *Infect Immun* **1991,** *59* (12), 4681-3.

32. Makioka, A.; Kumagai, M.; Ohtomo, H.; Kobayashi, S.; Takeuchi, T., Effect of proteasome inhibitors on the growth, encystation, and excystation of Entamoeba histolytica and Entamoeba invadens. *Parasitology research* **2002,** *88* (5), 454-9.

33. Eichinger, D., Encystation of entamoeba parasites. *BioEssays : news and reviews in molecular, cellular and developmental biology* **1997,** *19* (7), 633-9.

34. Pires-Santos, G. M.; Santana-Anjos, K. G.; Vannier-Santos, M. A., Optimization of Entamoeba histolytica culturing in vitro. *Exp Parasitol* **2012,** *132* (4), 561-5.

35. Carrero, J. C.; Laclette, J. P., Molecular biology of Entamoeba histolytica: a review. *Archives of medical research* **1996,** *27* (3), 403-12.

36. Lohia, A., The cell cycle of Entamoeba histolytica. *Molecular and cellular biochemistry* **2003,** *253* (1-2), 217-22.

37. Petrin, D.; Delgaty, K.; Bhatt, R.; Garber, G., Clinical and microbiological aspects of Trichomonas vaginalis. *Clinical microbiology reviews* **1998,** *11* (2), 300-17.

38. Stauffer, W.; Ravdin, J. I., Entamoeba histolytica: an update. *Current opinion in infectious diseases* **2003,** *16* (5), 479-85.

39. Begum, S.; Quach, J.; Chadee, K., Immune Evasion Mechanisms of Entamoeba histolytica: Progression to Disease. *Front Microbiol* **2015,** *6*, 1394.

40. Dodson, J. M.; Lenkowski, P. W.; Eubanks, A. C.; Jackson, T. F.; Napodano, J.; Lyerly, D. M.; Lockhart, L. A.; Mann, B. J.; Petri, W. A., Infection and immunity mediated by the carbohydrate recognition domain of the Entamoeba histolytica Gal/GalNAc lectin. *The Journal of infectious diseases* **1999,** *179* (2), 460-6.

41. Rosales-Encina, J. L.; Meza, I.; López-De-León, A.; Talamás-Rohana, P.; Rojkind, M., Isolation of a 220-kilodalton protein with lectin properties from a virulent strain of Entamoeba histolytica. *The Journal of infectious diseases* **1987,** *156* (5), 790-7.

42. Vines, R. R.; Ramakrishnan, G.; Rogers, J. B.; Lockhart, L. A.; Mann, B. J.; Petri, W. A., Regulation of adherence and virulence by the Entamoeba histolytica lectin cytoplasmic domain, which contains a beta2 integrin motif. *Molecular biology of the cell* **1998,** *9* (8), 2069-79.

43. Braga, L. L.; Ninomiya, H.; McCoy, J. J.; Eacker, S.; Wiedmer, T.; Pham, C.; Wood, S.; Sims, P. J.; Petri, W. A., Inhibition of the complement membrane attack complex by the galactose-specific adhesion of Entamoeba histolytica. *The Journal of clinical investigation* **1992,** *90* (3), 1131-7.

44. Kain, K. C.; Ravdin, J. I., Galactose-specific adhesion mechanisms of Entamoeba histolytica: model for study of enteric pathogens. *Methods in enzymology* **1995,** *253*, 424-39.

45. Arias-Negrete, S.; Muñoz, M. d. L.; Murillo-Jasso, F., Expression of in vitro virulence by

Entamoeba histolytica: effect of calmodulin inhibitors. *APMIS : acta pathologica, microbiologica, et immunologica Scandinavica* **1999,** *107* (9), 875-81.

46.   McKerrow, J. H.; Sun, E.; Rosenthal, P. J.; Bouvier, J., The proteases and pathogenicity of parasitic protozoa. *Annual review of microbiology* **1993,** *47,* 821-53.

47.   Ralston, K. S.; Solga, M. D.; Mackey-Lawrence, N. M.; Somlata; Bhattacharya, A.; Petri, W. A., Jr., Trogocytosis by Entamoeba histolytica contributes to cell killing and tissue invasion. *Nature* **2014,** *508* (7497), 526-30.

48.   Brandt, H.; Tamayo, R. P., Pathology of human amebiasis. *Hum Pathol* **1970,** *1* (3), 351-85.

49.   Reed, S. L.; Ember, J. A.; Herdman, D. S.; DiScipio, R. G.; Hugli, T. E.; Gigli, I., The extracellular neutral cysteine proteinase of Entamoeba histolytica degrades anaphylatoxins C3a and C5a. *Journal of immunology (Baltimore, Md. : 1950)* **1995,** *155* (1), 266-74.

50.   Franco, E.; de Araujo Soares, R. M.; Meza, I., Specific and reversible inhibition of Entamoeba histolytica cysteine-proteinase activities by Zn2+: implications for adhesion and cell damage. *Archives of medical research* **1999,** *30* (2), 82-8.

51.   Leippe, M.; Muller-Eberhard, H. J., The pore-forming peptide of Entamoeba histolytica, the protozoan parasite causing human amoebiasis. *Toxicology* **1994,** *18,* 1-3.

52.   Vaccaro, A. M.; Salvioli, R.; Tatti, M.; Ciaffoni, F., Saposins and their interaction with lipids. *Neurochemical research* **1999,** *24* (2), 307-14.

53.   Ravdin, J. I.; Moreau, F.; Sullivan, J. A.; Petri, W. A.; Mandell, G. L., Relationship of free intracellular calcium to the cytolytic activity of Entamoeba histolytica. *Infection and immunity* **1988,** *56* (6), 1505-12.

54.   Yu, Y.; Chadee, K., Secreted Entamoeba histolytica proteins stimulate interleukin-8 mRNA expression and protein production in human colonic epithelial cells. *Archives of medical research* **1997,** *28 Spec No,* 223-4.

55.   Utrera-Barillas, D.; Velazquez, J. R.; Enciso, A.; Cruz, S. M.; Rico, G.; Curiel-Quesada, E.; Teran, L. M.; Kretschmer, R. R., An anti-inflammatory oligopeptide produced by Entamoeba histolytica down-regulates the expression of pro-inflammatory chemokines. *Parasite immunology* **2003,** *25* (10), 475-82.

56.   Choudhuri, G.; Prakash, V.; Kumar, A.; Shahi, S. K.; Sharma, M., Protective immunity to entamoeba histolytica infection in subjects with antiamoebic antibodies residing in a hyperendemic zone. *Scandinavian journal of infectious diseases* **1991,** *23* (6), 771-6.

57.   Lotter, H.; Zhang, T.; Seydel, K. B.; Stanley, S. L.; Tannich, E., Identification of an epitope on the Entamoeba histolytica 170-kD lectin conferring antibody-mediated protection against invasive amebiasis. *The Journal of experimental medicine* **1997,** *185* (10), 1793-801.

58.   Ravdin, J. I.; Kelsall, B. L., Role of mucosal secretory immunity in the development of an amebiasis vaccine. *The American journal of tropical medicine and hygiene* **1994,** *50* (5 Suppl), 36-41.

59.   Abou-el-Magd, I.; Soong, C. J.; el-Hawey, A. M.; Ravdin, J. I., Humoral and mucosal IgA antibody response to a recombinant 52-kDa cysteine-rich portion of the Entamoeba histolytica galactose-inhibitable lectin correlates with detection of native 170-kDa lectin antigen in serum of patients with amebic colitis. *The Journal of infectious diseases* **1996,** *174* (1), 157-62.

60.   Stanley, S. L. J., Protective immunity to amoebiasis: new insights and new challenges. *Dis* **2001,** *184,* 504-6.

61.   Ghadirian, E.; Denis, M., In vivo activation of macrophages by IFN-gamma to kill Entamoeba histolytica trophozoites in vitro. *Parasite immunology* **1992,** *14* (4), 397-404.

62.   Seguin, R.; Mann, B. J.; Keller, K.; Chadee, K., The tumor necrosis factor alpha-stimulating region of galactose-inhibitable lectin of Entamoeba histolytica activates gamma interferon-primed macrophages for amebicidal activity mediated by nitric oxide. *Infect Immun* **1997,** *65* (7), 2522-7.

63.   Nagata, N.; Shimbo, T.; Akiyama, J.; Nakashima, R.; Nishimura, S.; Yada, T.; Watanabe, K.; Oka, S.; Uemura, N., Risk factors for intestinal invasive amebiasis in Japan, 2003-2009. *Emerg Infect Dis* **2012,** *18* (5), 717-24.

64.   Ravdin, J. I.; Shain, D. C.; Kelsall, B. L., Antigenicity, immunogenicity and vaccine efficacy of the galactose-specific adherence protein of Entamoeba histolytica. *Vaccine* **1993,** *11* (2), 241-6.

65. Marinets, A.; Zhang, T.; Guillén, N.; Gounon, P.; Bohle, B.; Vollmann, U.; Scheiner, O.; Wiedermann, G.; Stanley, S. L.; Duchêne, M., Protection against invasive amebiasis by a single monoclonal antibody directed against a lipophosphoglycan antigen localized on the surface of Entamoeba histolytica. *The Journal of experimental medicine* **1997**, *186* (9), 1557-65.

66. Wells, C. D.; Arguedas, M., Amebic liver abscess. *Southern medical journal* **2004**, *97* (7), 673-82.

67. Das, S. K.; Chisti, M. J.; Malek, M. A.; Salam, M. A.; Ahmed, T.; Faruque, A. S.; Mondal, D., Comparison of clinical and laboratory characteristics of intestinal amebiasis with shigellosis among patients visiting a large urban diarrheal disease hospital in Bangladesh. *Am J Trop Med Hyg* **2013**, *89* (2), 339-44.

68. Parshad, S.; Grover, P. S.; Sharma, A.; Verma, D. K.; Sharma, A., Primary cutaneous amoebiasis: case report with review of the literature. *International journal of dermatology* **2002**, *41* (10), 676-80.

69. Hoffner, R. J.; Kilaghbian, T.; Esekogwu, V. I.; Henderson, S. O., Common presentations of amebic liver abscess. *Annals of emergency medicine* **1999**, *34* (3), 351-5.

70. Lyche, K. D.; Jensen, W. A., Pleuropulmonary amebiasis. *Seminars in respiratory infections* **1997**, *12* (2), 106-12.

71. Mbaye, P. S.; Koffi, N.; Camara, P.; Burgel, P. R.; Hovette, P.; Klotz, F., [Pleuropulmonary manifestations of amebiasis]. *Revue de pneumologie clinique* **1998**, *54* (6), 346-52.

72. Sundaram, C.; Prasad, B. C. M.; Bhaskar, G.; Lakshmi, V.; Murthy, J. M. K., Brain abscess due to Entamoeba histolytica. *The Journal of the Association of Physicians of India* **2004**, *52*, 251-2.

73. Hung, C.-C.; Deng, H.-Y.; Hsiao, W.-H.; Hsieh, S.-M.; Hsiao, C.-F.; Chen, M.-Y.; Chang, S.-C.; Su, K.-E., Invasive amebiasis as an emerging parasitic disease in patients with human immunodeficiency virus type 1 infection in Taiwan. *Archives of internal medicine* **2005**, *165* (4), 409-15.

74. Hung, C. C.; Ji, D. D.; Sun, H. Y.; Lee, Y. T.; Hsu, S. Y.; Chang, S. Y.; Wu, C. H.; Chan, Y. H.; Hsiao, C. F.; Liu, W. C.; Colebunders, R., Increased risk for Entamoeba histolytica infection and invasive amebiasis in HIV seropositive men who have sex with men in Taiwan. *PLoS Negl Trop Dis* **2008**, *2* (2), e175.

75. Park, W. B.; Choe, P. G.; Jo, J. H.; Kim, S. H.; Bang, J. H.; Kim, H. B.; Kim, N. J.; Oh, M. D.; Choe, K. W., Amebic liver abscess in HIV-infected patients, Republic of Korea. *Emerg Infect Dis* **2007**, *13* (3), 516-7.

76. Wu, K. S.; Tsai, H. C.; Lee, S. S.; Liu, Y. C.; Wann, S. R.; Wang, Y. H.; Mai, M. H.; Chen, J. K.; Sy, C. L.; Chen, K. M.; Chen, Y. J.; Chen, Y. S., Comparison of clinical characteristics of amebic liver abscess in human immunodeficiency virus (HIV)-infected and non-HIV-infected patients. *J Microbiol Immunol Infect* **2008**, *41* (6), 456-61.

77. Mirelman, D.; Nuchamowitz, Y.; Stolarsky, T., Comparison of use of enzyme-linked immunosorbent assay-based kits and PCR amplification of rRNA genes for simultaneous detection of Entamoeba histolytica and E. dispar. *Journal of clinical microbiology* **1997**, *35* (9), 2405-7.

78. Buss, S. N.; Leber, A.; Chapin, K.; Fey, P. D.; Bankowski, M. J.; Jones, M. K.; Rogatcheva, M.; Kanack, K. J.; Bourzac, K. M., Multicenter evaluation of the BioFire FilmArray gastrointestinal panel for etiologic diagnosis of infectious gastroenteritis. *J Clin Microbiol* **2015**, *53* (3), 915-25.

79. Talamas-Lara, D.; Chavez-Munguia, B.; Gonzalez-Robles, A.; Talamas-Rohana, P.; Salazar-Villatoro, L.; Duran-Diaz, A.; Martinez-Palomo, A., Erythrophagocytosis in Entamoeba histolytica and Entamoeba dispar: a comparative study. *Biomed Res Int* **2014**, *2014*, 626259.

80. Boettner, D. R.; Huston, C. D.; Sullivan, J. A.; Petri, W. A., Jr., Entamoeba histolytica and Entamoeba dispar utilize externalized phosphatidylserine for recognition and phagocytosis of erythrocytes. *Infect Immun* **2005**, *73* (6), 3422-30.

81. Gonzalez-Ruiz, A.; Haque, R.; Aguirre, A.; Castanon, G.; Hall, A.; Guhl, F.; Ruiz-Palacios, G.; Miles, M. A.; Warhurst, D. C., Value of microscopy in the diagnosis of dysentery associated with invasive Entamoeba histolytica. *J Clin Pathol* **1994**, *47* (3), 236-9.

82. Haque, R.; Neville, L. M.; Hahn, P.; Petri, W. A., Jr., Rapid diagnosis of Entamoeba infection by using Entamoeba and Entamoeba histolytica stool antigen detection kits. *J Clin Microbiol* **1995**, *33* (10), 2558-61.

83.   Zengzhu, G.; Bracha, R.; Nuchamowitz, Y.; Cheng-I, W.; Mirelman, D., Analysis by enzyme-linked immunosorbent assay and PCR of human liver abscess aspirates from patients in China for Entamoeba histolytica. *Journal of clinical microbiology* **1999**, *37* (9), 3034-6.

84.   Lotter, H.; Jackson, T. F.; Tannich, E., Evaluation of three serological tests for the detection of antiamebic antibodies applied to sera of patients from an area endemic for amebiasis. *Tropical medicine and parasitology : official organ of Deutsche Tropenmedizinische Gesellschaft and of Deutsche Gesellschaft fur Technische Zusammenarbeit (GTZ)* **1995**, *46* (3), 180-2.

85.   Samie, A.; Obi, L. C.; Bessong, P. O.; Stroup, S.; Houpt, E.; Guerrant, R. L., Prevalence and species distribution of E. Histolytica and E. Dispar in the Venda region, Limpopo, South Africa. *Am J Trop Med Hyg* **2006**, *75* (3), 565-71.

86.   Petri, W. A., Jr., Pathogenesis of amebiasis. *Curr Opin Microbiol* **2002**, *5* (4), 443-7.

87.   Shamsuzzaman, S. M.; Hashiguchi, Y., Thoracic amebiasis. *Clinics in chest medicine* **2002**, *23* (2), 479-92.

88.   Lopez-Osuna, M.; Perez-Tamayo, R.; Frenk, P.; Kretschmer, R., [The eosinophil and Entamoeba histolytica. II. Testicular amebic lesions produced in eosinophilic rats]. *Arch Invest Med (Mex)* **1990**, *21 Suppl 1*, 263-5.

89.   Lopez-Osuna, M.; Velazquez, J. R.; Kretschmer, R. R., Does the eosinophil have a protective role in amebiasis? *Mem Inst Oswaldo Cruz* **1997**, *92 Suppl 2*, 237-40.

90.   Schulte, C.; Krebs, B.; Jelinek, T.; Nothdurft, H. D.; von Sonnenburg, F.; Loscher, T., Diagnostic significance of blood eosinophilia in returning travelers. *Clin Infect Dis* **2002**, *34* (3), 407-11.

91.   Rosenblatt, J. E., Antiparasitic agents. *Mayo Clinic proceedings* **1992**, *67* (3), 276-87.

92.   Blessmann, J.; Ali, I. K.; Nu, P. A.; Dinh, B. T.; Viet, T. Q.; Van, A. L.; Clark, C. G.; Tannich, E., Longitudinal study of intestinal Entamoeba histolytica infections in asymptomatic adult carriers. *J Clin Microbiol* **2003**, *41* (10), 4745-50.

93.   McAuley, J. B.; Herwaldt, B. L., Diloxanide furoate for treating asymptomatic Entamoeba histolytica cyst passers: 14 years' experience in the United States. *Clin Infect Dis* **1992**, *15* 464-468.

94.   Bansal, D.; Sehgal, R.; Chawla, Y.; Mahajan, R. C.; Malla, N., In vitro activity of antiamoebic drugs against clinical isolates of Entamoeba histolytica and Entamoeba dispar. *Annals of clinical microbiology and antimicrobials* **2004**, *3*, 27.

95.   Upcroft, P.; Upcroft, J. A., Drug targets and mechanisms of resistance in the anaerobic protozoa. *Clinical microbiology reviews* **2001**, *14* (1), 150-64.

96.   Gibney, E. J., Amoebic liver abscess. *The British journal of surgery* **1990**, *77* (8), 843-4.

97.   de la Rey Nel, J.; Simjee, A. E.; Patel, A., Indications for aspiration of amoebic liver abscess. *S Afr Med J* **1989**, *75* (8), 373-6.

98.   Kirchhoff, L. V.; Weiss, L. M.; Wittner, M.; Tanowitz, H. B., Parasitic diseases of the heart. *Frontiers in bioscience : a journal and virtual library* **2004**, *9*, 706-23.

99.   Quach, J.; St-Pierre, J.; Chadee, K., The future for vaccine development against Entamoeba histolytica. *Hum Vaccin Immunother* **2014**, *10* (6), 1514-21.

13. *Balantidium coli*

(Malmsten 1857)

Introduction

Balantidium coli is the only ciliated pro-tozoan that routinely infects humans. Balan-tidiasis occurs throughout the world, but the prevalence of human infection is not known. It is endemic in Japan, New Guinea, Micro-nesia, Seychelles Islands, Thailand, South Africa, Central and South America, and Europe.[1-6] Sporadic epidemics have occurred in institutionalized populations. *B. coli* locates to the large intestine, where it causes dysen-tery, occasionally leading to fatalities. It has many reservoir hosts, including both domes-tic and wild mammals (non-human primates, guinea pigs, horses, cattle, pigs, wild boars, and rats).[1] When patients suffering from HIV encounter *B. coli*, the infection can locate to sites other than the GI tract.[7]

Historical Information

In 1857, Pehr Malmsten described in detail *B. coli* organisms in two patients from Stock-holm, Sweden, suffering from acute diarrheal disease.[8] One patient went on to recover, while the other succumbed to the infection. In 1861, Rudolph Leuckart described this same

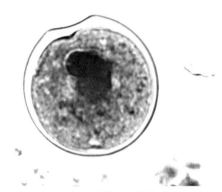

Figure 13.2. Cyst of *Balantidium coli*. Note macronu-cleus. 65 µm.

organism that he isolated from the intestine of a pig.[9] These two isolates were equated by F. Stein, and they were both named *Bal-antidium coli*.[9, 10] Currently there is still some controversy about whether the pig-associated organism, *Balantidium suis*, and the human-associated organism, *Balantidium coli*, are the same species.[9]

Life Cycle

There are two stages produced by *Balan-tidium coli*; the trophozoite (Fig. 13.1), and the cyst (Fig. 13.2). The invasive stage is the trophozoite. *B. coli* resides in the tissues of the large intestine (Fig. 13.3) in a similar habitat to that of *Entamoeba histolytica* (Figs. 12.4, 12.6), from which it must be clinically distinguished. The trophozoite of *B. coli* ingests living cells and causes ulcerations to develop at the site of infection. While the cyst of *Entamoeba histolytica* is only 10-20 µm in diameter and is often present in loose stools, the cyst stage of *Balantidium coli* measures 65 µm in diameter is usually only seen in formed stools.[9]

Infection begins by ingestion of the cyst, usually by means of consumption of contami-nated food or water. The trophozoite excysts in the small intestine then relocates to the large intestine. The preferred site of infection is the epithelium of the transverse and descending

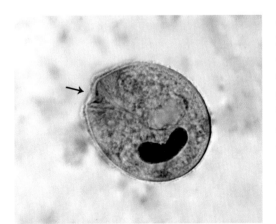

Figure 13.1. Trophozoite of *Balantidium coli*. Note large macronucleus and cytostome (arrow). 150 µm.

Balantidium coli

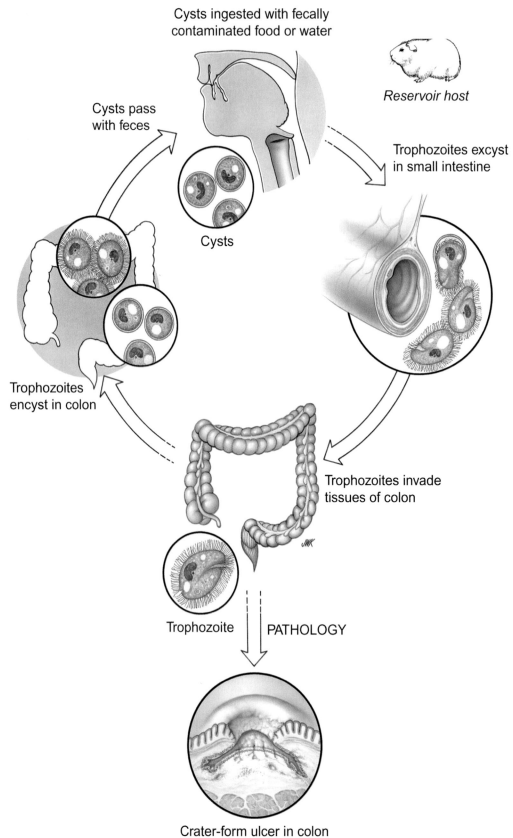

Cysts ingested with fecally contaminated food or water

Reservoir host

Cysts pass with feces

Cysts

Trophozoites excyst in small intestine

Trophozoites encyst in colon

Trophozoites invade tissues of colon

Trophozoite

PATHOLOGY

Crater-form ulcer in colon

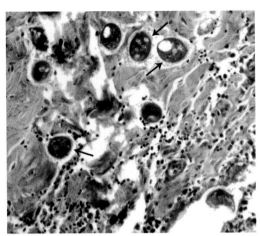

Figure 13.3. Histologic section of small intestine infected with *B. coli* (arrows).

colon. *B. coli* is usually limited to the bowel, although a case involving liver abscess has been reported, as well as infection in the lungs and heart.[6, 11, 12] The trophozoite divides by simple binary fission within the host, but in culture, it behaves like all other free-living ciliates, undergoing syngamy, a specialized type of sexual reproduction similar to conjugation.[13]

The trophozoites cause extensive destruction to the surrounding tissue (Fig. 13.3). During prolonged infection, some trophozoites enter the lumen of the colon, where they secrete an impervious, hyaline, acellular layer resulting in the formation of the cyst stage. The cyst exits from the host in the fecal mass and is immediately infectious without the requirement for an intermediate host, allowing for direct human-to-human transmission. In many ecological settings, pigs are the presumed reservoirs, since infection is more common where pigs live in close association with human habitats. Guinea pigs are thought to harbor *B. coli* as a commensal, and have been the source of some human infections.[6]

Pathogenesis

Balantidium coli survives in anaeroebic as well as aerobic conditions and uses carbohydrates as its main source of energy.[9] The trophozoite possesses a hyaluronidase which is presumed to facilitate lysis of cells and disruption of the mucosal epithelial cells.[14] Proteases, most likely lysosomal in origin, released within food vacuoles (phagolysosomes), participate in the process of digestion of cell debris that enters through the peristome (mouth-like opening) that is located at the narrowed end of the trophozoite.

Clinical Disease

The four main presentations that can result after human exposure to *B. coli* are; a lack of symptoms with carriage or clearance, acute colitis, chronic infection, and invasive disease.[4, 12, 15-17] Although it appears that most exposed individuals will remain asymptomatic, a minority will go on to develop acute balantidiasis with watery diarrhea or dysentery.[12] Fever, nausea, vomiting, and asthenia (physical weakness or lack of energy) have been described, and there have been some deaths associated with intestinal perforation and consequent sepsis.[16] Chronic infection has been studied in endemic areas and may be responsible for negative impacts on growth in infected children.[18] Rarely, *B. coli* causes ulcerative and granulomatous disease in the colon and appendix leading to typhlitis (inflammation of the cecum) and appendicitis.[19] Individuals who are immune compromised due to malnutrition, HIV infection or from other causes may develop invasive disease with organisms invading, the lungs, urinary tract, liver and heart.[6, 7, 11, 12, 20]

Diagnosis

Definitive diagnosis is by identifying the organism (trophozoite or cyst; see Figs 13.1, 13.2) by microscopy in a sample of stool, or on a stained section of tissue from a biopsy of an ulcer identified by colonoscopy.[21] One might find trophozoites in freshly obtained watery stool, while only the cyst stage is present in formed stools. There are no established diagnostic serological or molecular tests available.[22] Culture is also not routinely used for diagnosis, so microscopy on stool specimens is the only diagnostic test.[22]

Treatment

Although there is limited data to guide therapy, tetracycline, metronidazole, iodoquinol, paromomycin, nitazoxanide and chloroquine have been used to treat balantidiasis.[9, 21, 23] Surgery (bowel resection) is sometimes necessary in severe cases of dysentery.

Prevention and Control

Good sanitation and a clean source of drinking water are prerequisites for controlling the spread of *B. coli*. The usual concentration of chlorine used to purify water is not adequate to destroy the cyst stage of *Balantidium coli*.[9] Domestic pigs would need to be restricted from releasing infective cysts into waters that would end up in the municipal water supplies to interrupt transmission. Considering that a high percentage of swine in many parts of the world are infected with *Balantidium coli*, when pigs share the same space with humans, as is the case in many parts of the less-developed world, the risk of infection is high.[24, 25]

References

1. Nakauchi, K., The prevalence of Balantidium coli infection in fifty-six mammalian species. *The Journal of veterinary medical science / the Japanese Society of Veterinary Science* **1999,** *61* (1), 63-5.
2. Nuti, M.; Comarmond, C.; Dac, C., An endemic focus of balantidiasis in the Seychelles Islands. *In Abstracts of the 10th Internat Congr Trop Med Malaria p* **1980,** *13*
3. Chavalittamrong, B.; Jirapinyo, P., Intestinal parasites in pediatric patients with diarrhoeal diseases in Bangkok. *The Southeast Asian journal of tropical medicine and public health* **1984,** *15* (3), 385-8.
4. Currie, A. R., Human balantidiasis. A case report. *South African journal of surgery. Suid-Afrikaanse tydskrif vir chirurgie* **1990,** *28* (1), 23-5.
5. Clyti, E.; Aznar, C.; Couppie, P.; el Guedj, M.; Carme, B.; Pradinaud, R., [A case of coinfection by Balantidium coli and HIV in French Guiana]. *Bulletin de la Societe de pathologie exotique (1990)* **1998,** *91* (4), 309-11.
6. Hindsbo, O.; Nielsen, C. V.; Andreassen, J.; Willingham, A. L.; Bendixen, M.; Nielsen, M. A.; Nielsen, N. O., Age-dependent occurrence of the intestinal ciliate Balantidium coli in pigs at a Danish research farm. *Acta veterinaria Scandinavica* **2000,** *41* (1), 79-83.
7. Vasilakopoulos, A.; Dimarongona, K.; J., Balantidium coli pneumonia in an immunocompromised patient. *Scand Dis* **2003,** *35* 144-146.
8. Malmsten, P. H., Infusorien als intestinal-Tiere beim Menschen. *Arch Pathol Anat Physiol Klin Med Virchow* **1857,** *12* 302-309.
9. Schuster, F. L.; Ramirez-Avila, L., Current world status of Balantidium coli. *Clin Microbiol Rev* **2008,** *21* (4), 626-38.
10. Chistyakova, L. V.; Kostygov, A. Y.; Kornilova, O. A.; Yurchenko, V., Reisolation and redescription of Balantidium duodeni Stein, 1867 (Litostomatea, Trichostomatia). *Parasitol Res* **2014,** *113* (11), 4207-15.
11. Wenger, R., [On differential electro-vectorcardiographic diagnosis of hypertrophy of the right ventricle]. *Atti della Societa italiana di cardiologia* **1967,** *2*, 91-2.
12. Arean, V. M.; Koppisch, E.; J., Balantidiasis: a review and report of cases. *Am* **1956,** *32*, 1089-1117.

13.	Martinez-Paloma, A.; Cantellano, M.; Collier, L.; Balows, A.; Sussman, M.; Cox, F. E. G.; Kreier, J. P.; Wakelin, D., Topley and Wilson's Microbiology and Microbial Infections 9th ed. 1998; p 157-177.

14.	Tempelis, C. H.; Lysenko, M. G., The production of hyaluronidase by B coli. *Exp Parasitol* **1957,** *6*, 31-36.

15.	Young, M. D., Attempts to transmit human Balantidium coli. *Am J Trop Med Hyg* **1950,** *30* (1), 71.

16.	Ladas, S. D.; Savva, S.; Frydas, A.; Kaloviduris, A.; Hatzioannou, J.; Raptis, S., Invasive balantidiasis presented as chronic colitis and lung involvement. *Dig Dis Sci* **1989,** *34* (10), 1621-3.

17.	Dorfman, S.; Rangel, O.; Bravo, L. G., Balantidiasis: report of a fatal case with appendicular and pulmonary involvement. *Trans R Soc Trop Med Hyg* **1984,** *78* (6), 833-4.

18.	Esteban, J. G.; Aguirre, C.; Angles, R.; Ash, L. R.; Mas-Coma, S., Balantidiasis in Aymara children from the northern Bolivian Altiplano. *Am J Trop Med Hyg* **1998,** *59* (6), 922-7.

19.	Dodd, L. G., Balantidium coli infestation as a cause of acute appendicitis. *The Journal of infectious diseases* **1991,** *163* (6), 1392.

20.	Karuna, T.; Khadanga, S., A rare case of urinary balantidiasis in an elderly renal failure patient. *Trop Parasitol* **2014,** *4* (1), 47-9.

21.	Castro, J.; Vazquez-Iglesias, J. L.; Arnal-Monreal, F., Dysentery caused by Balantidium coli--report of two cases. *Endoscopy* **1983,** *15* (4), 272-4.

22.	McHardy, I. H.; Wu, M.; Shimizu-Cohen, R.; Couturier, M. R.; Humphries, R. M., Detection of intestinal protozoa in the clinical laboratory. *J Clin Microbiol* **2014,** *52* (3), 712-20.

23.	Ochoa, T. J.; White, A. C., Jr., Nitazoxanide for treatment of intestinal parasites in children. *Pediatr Infect Dis J* **2005,** *24* (7), 641-2.

24.	Morris, R. G.; Jordan, H. E.; Luce, W. G.; Coburn, T. C.; Maxwell, C. V., Prevalence of gastrointestinal parasitism in Oklahoma swine. *Am J Vet Res* **1984,** *45* (11), 2421-3.

25.	Solaymani-Mohammadi, S.; Rezaian, M.; Hooshyar, H.; Mowlavi, G. R.; Babaei, Z.; Anwar, M. A., Intestinal protozoa in wild boars (Sus scrofa) in western Iran. *J Wildl Dis* **2004,** *40* (4), 801-3.

14. Protozoans of Minor Medical Importance

Babesia spp.

Babesia spp. comprises a group of genetically-related intracellular protozoa that infect red blood cells.[1] They are closely related to the malarias, belonging to the phylum Apicomplexa. *Babesia* spp. are all vector-borne infections transmitted by the bite of ticks. Babesiosis in humans can manifest as a mild fever or progress to a severe, life threatening illness. There are over 100 species that infect numerous hosts, but very few are responsible for the majority of human infections. This is a disease that not only impacts on human health, but also on domestic cattle. As an example, *Babesia bigemina* occasionally infects humans, but primarily infects cows, causing extensive economic loss wherever it is endemic. *B. microti* is the most common species infecting rodents and humans in the United States.[2] A number of species infect dogs as well as cats that in some instances may be responsible for human infection, and some human cases have been reported.[3,4] The occurrence of babesiosis in humans was considered a rarity, yet 139 cases were reported from New York State between 1982 and 1993.[5] Currently babesiosis is as prevalent in some areas as Lyme disease, and consequently is now classified as an emerging infection by the Centers for Disease Control and Prevention.[6]

B. divergens is the most frequently occurring species in Europe, and is also considered an emerging infection in that region of the world.[7] Many species overlap in their geographic distribution, but most have discrete ecological niches largely determined by their restriction to only certain species of ticks.

Historical Information

In 1888, the Romanian pathologist Victor Babes, after whom the genus is named, identified these intraerythrocytic microorganisms as causing febrile hemoglobulinuria in cattle.[8] Theobald Smith and Frederick L. Kilbourne, in 1893, demonstrated that ticks were the vectors of *Babesia bigemina*, the cause of Texas Cattle Fever in the Southwestern United States, making this infectious agent the first one shown to be transmitted by the bite of an arthropod.[9] Their finding inspired others to look for additional vector-borne diseases. Shortly thereafter, the mosquito vectors for the yellow fever virus and *Plasmodium* spp. were described. *Babesia* spp. were not recognized as human pathogens until 1957, when a case report was published on *Babesia divergens* as an infectious agent in a splenectomized herdsman.[10] In 1969, a case of babesiosis was identified in an immunocompetent individual living on Nantucket Island, a small island off the cost of Massachusettes in the United States.[11] After additional cases were reported this became known in some areas as "Nantucket fever".[6]

Life Cycle

The sexual part of the life cycle takes place in the tick. Infection begins by the introduction of sporozoites contained within salivary secretions of the larval tick. *Ixodes scapularis* is the vector for *B. microti* in the many parts of the United States (the same one that transmits Lyme Disease), and *Ixodes ricinus* is the main vector for *B. divergens* in Europe. Because *Babesia* spp. infects red cells, infections can also be acquired by blood transfusion.[12] The sporozoites bind to glycosaminoglycans and sialoglycoproteins on erythrocytes and enter these cells (Fig. 14.1) by inducing a deformation in the membrane, creating a parasitophorous vacuole.[13-16] There it grows and develops, maturing into mero-

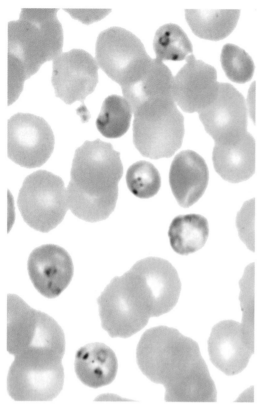

Figure 14.1. Red cells infected with various stages of *Babesia microti*.

zoites that then divide. Simultaneously, the parasitophorous vacuole breaks down, leaving the organism bathed in the naked red cell cyosol. It is inferred by its ecological niche that babesia ingests and utilizes hemoglobin as a nutritional source. In contrast with plasmodium, babesia does not discard haemazoin within the red blood cells. Reproduction is by schizogony. Egress from the red cells results in rupture of host erythrocytes. Levels of parasitized red blood cells are usually in the range of 1-10%, but can be as high as 80%, sometimes without pathological consequences.[17-19]

The sexual cycle takes place in the tick gut where gametocytes differentiate into gametes. Gametes migrate into the hemolymph where, two weeks after ingesting organisms, ookinetes develop. Ookinetes migrate to the tick salivary glands ultimately leading to infectious haploid sporozoites.[6] Larval

ticks remain infected throughout the winter months. After developing to the nymph stage, they can transmit the infection to another host (mouse, bovine, dog, or human).[20]

Clinical Disease

Usually after a gradual onset of nonspecific symptoms patients experience high fever. In the United States, infected individuals typically present in one of two ways. Immunocompetent individuals develop a self-limiting disease of mild duration, lasting two to four weeks.[21-23] The self-limiting disease in immunocompetent patients is typically mild and likely often goes unnoticed without a visit to a physician. The second presentation is in the immunocompromised person. Those who are asplenic, HIV-infected, have cancer, or on immunosuppressive medication may have a more fulminant course. Patients with generalized myalgias often experience fever, malaise, headache, and occasionally bradycardia with lymphopenia.[24] The severity appears to be dictated by the immune status of the patient, with fatality rates over 20% in some immunosuppressed populations.[19] Patients without spleens are at greatest risk of dying from babesiosis.[25-28] Patients may also be coinfected with other tick-borne pathogens, such as *Borrelia burgdorferi* (Lyme disease) and *Ehrlichia* species (ehrlichiosis), complicating the clinical picture.[29-34] In Europe, infection due to *B. divergens* is usually more severe.[22,23] Intravascular hemolysis and hemaglobinuria is common, and may necessitate whole body transfusion as an emergency procedure.

In human infection with *B. microti*, the ratio of CD4+ T cells to CD8+ T cells decreases during infection, while natural killer (NK) cells, IFN-γ, TNF, IL-2 and IL-6 increase. These results indicate that NK cells may be important in modulation of infection.[35] B cells may also be important, as severe infections have developed in patients on B cell depleting therapies such as the monoclonal antibody rituximab.[36] Patients with HIV/AIDS may develop a long-term chronic infection despite specific therapy for babesiosis.[37]

Diagnosis

Diagnosis is typically made by examination of Wright or Giemsa-stained thin blood smears. [38, 39] Intraerythrocytic as well as extracellular rings can be seen and rarely the pathognomonic finding of tetrads of merozoites appearing as a "Maltese Cross" can be visualized on thin blood smear.[40] PCR is sensitive and specific for the diagnosis of babesiosis.[41] An ELISA-based test has been developed for both IgM as well as IgG for *B. microti,* but this test will not detect antibodies to other *Babesia* spp.[6, 42]

Treatment

Combination therapy with atovaquone/azithromycin is the treatment of choice for most mild to moderate cases in immunocompetent patients, while the combination of clindamycin/quinine is recommended for severe cases, or in patients who are immunocompromised.[6, 43] In some individuals, the infection may persist, even after receiving combination therapy with clindamycin and quinine.[44] Exchange transfusion is sometimes employed when patients have levels of parasitemia >10%, are multisystem compromised, or are infected with *B. divergens*.[23]

Prevention and control

Since *Babesia* spp. infects a number of reservoir host species, some domestic and some wild, avoiding environments in which infection occurs is often difficult or undesirable. Prevention at an individual level includes checking for nymphal stage ticks (note: this stage of ixodes is quite difficult to see) at the end of each trip into a wooded area, and taking precautions to cover up the lower portion of

pants with socks. This advice is particularly relevant for those living in the Northeastern regions of United States, where the prevalence of *Borrelia burgdorferi* in some populations of *Ixodes* ticks have been shown to be as high as 50%. DEET sprayed at the bottom of pants may also help. There are no vaccines against babesia for humans, but ones for use in cattle are under development.[45] Burning understory in wooded, tick-infested regions may prove useful in ecologically controlling infection in ticks.[46]

Cytoisospora belli (Formerly known as Isospora belli)
(Wenyon 1923)

Cytoisospora belli is an Apicomplexan intracellular parasite of humans that lives within enterocytes of the small intestine.[47] *C. belli* is a rare infection in immunocompetent individuals, but in recent years it has emerged as a serious diarrheal disease in patients suffering from HIV/AIDS, and in other immunosuppressed individuals.[48, 49]

Life Cycle

Infection is initiated by ingestion of the infective sporulated oocyst in fecally contaminated food or beverages. Oocysts require a period of 1-2 days outside the host in order to undergo sporulation and become infectious to a new host. Direct person-to-person transmis-

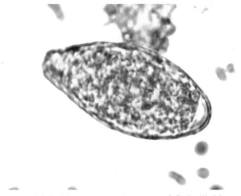

Figure 14.2. Unsporulated oocyst of *C. belli*. 20 μm.

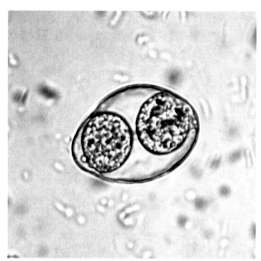

Figure 14.3. Sporulated oocyst of *C. belli*. 20 μm.

sion is thought not to occur.[50, 51] The oocyst (Figs. 14.2, 14.3) measures approximately 25 μm by 15 μm. Four sporozoites reside within each of the two sporocysts contained by the oocyst. Digestion of the cyst wall causes the release of the sporozoites into the lumen of the small intestine, and there they enter columnar epithelial cells. Asexual reproduction follows, leading to increased numbers of meronts and zoites. *C. belli* infection in humans is similar to the sexual phase of *Toxoplasma gondii* in the cat. Occasionally, gametocytes may develop, resulting in the production of an oocyst. The molecular events controlling oocyst formation have yet to be elucidated. Oocysts are passed in the fecal mass unsporulated and are non-infectious. The oocysts require 1-2 days to sporulate after reaching the external environment. In HIV/AIDS patients, *C. belli* can invade and reproduce in other organs, such as the gall bladder, liver, spleen, and lymph nodes.[52-54]

Pathogenesis

C. belli causes a protracted, secretory diarrhea in AIDS patients with depressed CD4+ T cell counts. In patients suffering from other varieties of immunosuppression, disease resembles that induced by *Cryptosporid-*

ium.[55-58] In most immunocompetent patient populations, infection is either subclinical or the diarrhea is transitory. Malabsorption of fats in immunocompromised patients has been reported.[59]

Clinical Disease

Patients infected with *Cytoisospora belli* may experience fever, abdominal cramping, diarrhea, malaise, and weight loss. HIV/AIDS patients may present with severe disease, including watery non-bloody diarrhea, malabsorption syndrome with steatorrhea, foul smelling stools, vomiting, and dehydration.[60] Patients may die from wasting associated with protracted weight loss and electrolyte imbalance.[61] Usually symptoms resolve with specific treatment of the infection or reconstitution of the immune system with highly active antiretroviral therapy (HAART).

Diagnosis

C. belli, along with *Dientamoeba fragilis* and *Sarcocystis* spp., is one of the few protozoan pathogens that causes peripheral blood eosinophilia.[62-64] This can be a clue to considering this pathogen in the differential diagnosis of a patient with diarrhea. Identifying the unsporulated oocysts by microscopy is the definitive diagnostic test of choice. The oocysts can be visualized with modified acid-fast staining and show autofluorescence when illuminated with an ultraviolet light in the 330-380 nm wavelength range.[49] At times, duodenal aspirates are required to make the diagnosis and biopsy of small intestinal tissue in heavy infections often reveals the intracellular parasites.

Treatment

Trimethoprim-sulfamethoxazole is the therapy of choice. Its use for prophylaxis in the HIV-infected population along with

HAART has effectively decreased the incidence of this pathogen in many parts of the world.[65] Pyrimethamine is an alternative therapy for infection in adults and ciprofloxacin is a second line agent that is a less effective option.[66] Although associated with some failures, nitazoxanide is another option with some degree of efficacy in the treatment of *C. belli*.[67, 68]

Prevention and control

Avoiding fecal contamination of food, and proper disposal of human feces is the best way to prevent infection. In many areas of the world, these recommendations are difficult or impossible to follow.

Cyclospora cayetanensis

Cyclospora cayetanensis causes watery diarrhea in humans and is acquired from contaminated food and water.[69-71] Although at one time this infection was virtually unknown, it has been recognized as a significant cause of diarrhea throughout the world including the United States where approximately 15,000 cases occur per year, with some requiring hospitalization.[72, 73] In some populations, particularly in tropical regions of Peru, Brazil, and Haiti, it is endemic, causing more mild disease in children and adults, but more severe disease in immunocompromised individuals, such as those with HIV/AIDS.[74, 75]

In regions of the world where this disease is endemic, epidemics tend to be seasonal, and in studies conducted in Guatemala coincided with the spring raspberry harvest.[76-78] In the United States most cases are seen in returning travelers or after ingestion of imported contaminated foods such as raspberries, basil, snow peas, and mesculin lettuce.[79-81] Several outbreaks in the United States have been caused by ingestion of fecally contaminated imported raspberries that may have come from Guatemala.[82-84]

The life cycle can be completed in a single host species, but little is known about the details of the life cycle, or the role of reservoir hosts in maintaining infection in the environment.[85-87] Studies surveying feces from multiple animals have reported the presence of *Cyclospora* oocysts in numerous animal species suggesting a role in maintaining this organism in the environment while others report not detecting oocysts and multiple unsuccessful attempts to infect multiple types of animals.[88]

Historical Information

In 1979, Bailey Ashford described several cases of diarrhea in Papua New Guinea with a coccidian detected in the stool.[89] In 1986, Rosemary Soave reported several cases of diarrhea in returning travelers that may have been due to a coccidial pathogen.[90] In 1991, Ynes R. Ortega characterized this organism as a new coccidian species and named this organism, *C. cayetanensis,* after her alma mater the Peruvian University Cayetano Heredia in Lima Peru.[91]

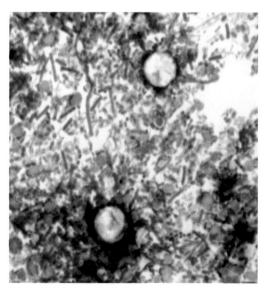

Figure 14.4. Oocyst of *C. cayetanensis*. 10 µm.

Life Cycle

Unsporulated oocysts are released into the environment by an infected host. A period of 1-2 weeks is required before oocysts sporulate, and become infectious. Ingestion of a sporulated oocyst begins the next round of infection (Fig. 14.4). Excystation of sporozoites occurs in the small intestine where they attach to epithelial cells. An initial asexual stage divides, then develops into the sexual stage, resulting in the production of unsporulated oocysts that are then shed into the environment.[88]

Clinical Disease

The clinical presentation and frequency of asymptomatic infected individuals varies in different parts of the world where *C. cayetanensis* is endemic. In general, infections tend to decrease in severity and duration after repeated exposures.[92] Following initial infection, watery diarrhea with 5-15 bowel movements per day ensues within a week or two, depending upon the initial number of oocysts ingested. In some cases, the onset of symptoms may be as long as 2 months after exposure.[93] In immunocompetent individuals, symptoms can last up to 2-3 weeks.[94] In those with HIV/AIDS, diarrhea can be protracted.[95] Nausea, vomiting, anorexia, and abdominal cramping are frequent symptoms during the acute phase of the infection.[86] Less common presentations, such as biliary disease, have been recorded. Post-infectious immune-mediated complications such as Guillian-Barre syndrome and reactive arthritis have been reported.[96, 97]

Diagnosis

Diagnosis can be made by nucleic acid amplification testing (NAAT), or by microscopic identification of oocysts in stool samples (Fig. 14.4). *C. cayetanensis* oocysts can be seen without staining, but the use of modified acid fast staining techniques can improve the sensitivity up to about 30%.[95] PCR was initially introduced to monitor foods. Currently, molecular testing is in use clinically and is now included in fecal NAAT panels, such as the BioFire Film Array GI panel.[98, 99]

Treatment, Control, and Prevention

The drug of choice for treatment of infection with *C. cayetanensis* is trimethoprim-sulfamethoxazole.[100, 101] Ciprofloxacin is an alternative for patients with sulfa allergies but this option may result in lower cure rates.[102] Nitazoxanide may also be an option for treatment.[103]

The source of infection is typically fecally contaminated food, so prevention and control at the community level is possible by employing good public health practices, especially in agricultural settings.

Naegleria fowleri and *Acanthamoeba* spp.
(Culbertson 1970)

Several groups of free-living amoebae cause serious disease in humans; *Naegleria fowleri*, various species of Acanthamoeba (*A. astronyxis, A. culbertsoni, A. castellanii, A. polyphaga, A. rhysodes,* and *A. hatchetti*), and *Balamuthia mandrillaris*.[104] All of these species are worldwide in distribution and have been isolated from all types of freshwater habitats and soils. *N. fowleri* is thermophylic, thriving in standing freshwater environments such as hot springs, heated swimming pools, and hot tubs.

Naegleria fowleri

N. fowleri, commonly known as the brain-eating amoeba, is a robust thermophilic free-living amoeba found around the world in warm freshwater.[105] The trophozoite (Fig.

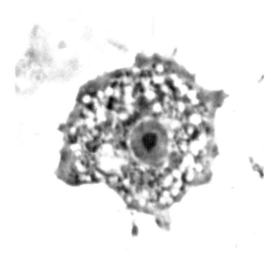

Figure 14.5. Trophozoite of *Naeglaria fowleri*. Phase contrast. 25 µm.

14.5) measures 20-30 µm in diameter, while its cyst is smaller, measuring 8-10 µm in diameter. *N. fowleri* was found in abundance in the thermal spas built by a Roman legion in what is now Bath, England.[106] Its discovery there caused the spa to be temporarily closed, and the resulting archeological dig through the sediments that had built up over the centuries led to fascinating glimpses into the lives of this ancient army during its occupation of that region.

Clinical Disease

N. fowleri causes a serious, often fatal, fulminating infection in the central nervous system, referred to as primary amoebic meningoencephalitis (PAM).[107, 108] Cases of PAM have occurred in the United States, Europe, Australia, South and Central America, and Southeast Asia.

The infection is typically acquired by swimming or bathing in water above 37°C. It is presumed that this unusual environment results in the selection of an abundance of thermally-tolerant organisms, including *N. fowleri*.[109] Diving or playful splashing activity can force heated water containing the trophozoites up into the nose and through the cribiform plate. *N. fowleri* invades and migrates along the base of the brain, and then penetrates deeply into the cortex producing an acute inflammatory reaction with extensive areas of lysis. Amoebae lyse their way through tissue, probably aided by a pore-forming protein similar to that of *Entamoeba histolytica*.[110] Symptoms include severe frontal headache, vomiting, confusion, fever and coma, followed by death.[111]

Diagnosis

Motile *N. fowleri* trophozoites can sometimes be isolated from cerebrospinal fluid and visualized with microscopy. In this case, the fluid should be concentrated, a smear made, stained with Giemsa or Wright's stain, and examined microscopically. An immunofluorescent assay, culture techniques and multiplex PCR have been introduced to improve the sensitivity of detection.[112, 113] Biopsy is another option that may reveal organisms. However, diagnosis can be delayed by the fact that PAM resembles symptoms of meningitis, a more commonly occurring clinical entity. Since death often ensues within five days after the acquisition of PAM, rapid diagnosis is essential. *N. fowleri* may be suspected in any otherwise healthy young adult with a recent history of contact with heated water. DNA probes specific for *N. fowleri* have been developed for its detection in water samples.[114]

Treatment and Prevention

Amphotericin B was the initial therapeutic agent used to treat patients, but mortality remained greater than 95% despite administration.[115] In 2013, two young children in the United States were treated with miltefosine added to their treatment regimen and both children survived.[116, 117]

N. fowleri is ubiquitous in distribution. One study conducted in Oklahoma showed that the number of pathogenic free-living amoeba species varied throughout the seasons, and were most prevalent in natural water sources (i.e., lakes and impoundments) in the spring and fall. This suggests that the organisms are normally found in benthic situations, and only gain access to the water column during periods of lake "turn over."[118] There are certain behaviors such as the use of netty pots and religious ablutions where warm water potentially containing these amoebae are forced up the nose. Modifications of these behaviors or only using water that does not contain these amoebae could reduce certain risks.

Due to the rarity of this disease, most situations leading to infection must be classified as incidents of unlucky circumstance, especially when one considers the number of visits to hot tubs, spas and natural hot springs, and the number of user hours spent relaxing in them.

Acanthamoeba spp.

Clinical Disease

Acanthamoeba is a free-living amoeba that is associated with both keratitis and granulomatous amoebic encephalitis (GAE). *Acanthamoeba* spp. infections most commonly occur in immunocompromised patients, especially those with HIV/AIDS, but in the case of keratitis due to contaminated contact lens solutions immunocompetent individuals can be infected.[119, 120] Both the growing number of immunocompromised individuals and the increase in contact lens wearers are contributing to the rise in human cases.[121]

Acanthamoeba has both a trophozoite and a cyst stage. The trophozoite as well as the cyst are both approximately 13-23 µm in diameter.[122] The route of infection of *Acanthamoeba* spp. is most likely via the lungs or skin, resulting in multiple foci of infection.[123] It is likely that with the ubiquitous nature of this organism almost all human beings encounter this organism at some point during their lives,

and disease is then due to either a particular type of exposure or due to a particular host susceptibility feature.[124] *Acanthamoeba* spp. have the ability to invade the central nervous system.[125] In the brain, a slowly developing, ulcerative granulomatous disease develops, characterized by diplopia, frontal headache, seizures, and occasionally death. Patients with HIV/AIDS may experience overwhelming disseminated infection.[119, 126]

Ulcerative keratitis of the eye caused by *Acanthamoeba* spp. occurs primarily in those who use contact lenses that are routinely washed in unfiltered tap water.[127] This is now considered a rare situation, primarily due to targeted public health education programs, and the availability of sterile lens cleaning solutions. Infection begins with the excystation of the trophozoite under the contact lens after it is applied to the eye. Amoebae invade the cornea and begin to erode the surface, creating the sensation of burning and a perceived "gritty" consistency under the lid when the eye is closed. A ring-enhancing lesion develops, impairing vision. Partial or total blindness may ensue if left untreated.

Diagnosis

Definitive diagnosis depends upon microscopically identifying the amoebae in biopsy tissue, CSF, or lachrymal secretions, or through the use of PCR.[128] A reliable staining method is available, employing Field's staining reagent.[129] This test is rapid, taking only 20 minutes to carry out, and is also a valuable adjunct for field surveys.

Treatment and Prevention

Although different treatments have been used for both keratitis and GAE, choosing the best treatment is problematic, owing to both a lack of clinical experience and absence of controlled trials evaluating therapies.[122, 130] Few patients with GAE survive, regardless of treatment, particularly those suffering from HIV/AIDS. Keratitis is also difficult to treat, but some drugs show promise, particularly topical miconazole, propamidine and neosporin.[130] Prevention of keratitis is straightforward and simple: use only sterile contact lens cleaning solutions. These products are easily obtained at any drug store as over-the-counter preparations. In contrast, HIV/AIDS predisposes individuals to topical or inhalational entry routes, and since acanthamoebae are found in countless ecological settings, it is nearly impossible to advise a method of avoiding contact with this ubiquitous group of organisms.

Balamuthia mandrillaris

Clinical Disease

Balamuthia mandrillaris is another free-living amoeba that can cause granulomatous amoebic encephalitis (GAE). It was discovered in 1986 in the brain of a mandrill, an Old World monkey that died of encephalitis in the San Diego Wildlife Park.[131] Its name was derived from the late parasitologist William Balamuth and the mandrill from which it was first identified.[132] *B. mandrillaris* is found in soil, and the route of initial infection is likely via the skin, but inhalation can also occur, resulting in an initial localized infection with the potential for spread to the brain.[133] *B. mandrillaris* encephalitis can occur in immunocompetent individuals. Like acanthamoeba, *B. mandrillaris* has both a trophozoite (15-60 μm in diameter) and a dormant cyst stage (13-30 μm in diameter).[132] Current investigations support a role for hematogenous spread from an initial locus of infection to distal sites such as the kidneys, lungs, adrenal glands, pancreas, thyroid, and brain. *B. mandrillaris* appears to enter the brain through the choroid plexus.[134] GAE can then develop. Most patients initially present with painless nodules and skin changes at the site

of entry, followed by meningeal symptoms, such as fever, stiff neck, and headache that may progress to severe encephalitic manifestations with incomprehensible speech.[135] *B. mandrillaris* is not an infection limited to the tropics, as a large number of cases have been recognized in the United States.

Diagnosis

Although *B. mandrillaris* may be seen on biopsy specimens from the skin lesions or from distal sites such as the brain, expert knowledge is required to recognize the morphological characteristics of this pathogen. Identification of an amoeba seen on microscopic evaluation can be confirmed with both nucleic acid amplification testing (NAAT) and through the use of immunofluorescent antibodies specific for *B. mandrillaris*.[136] The DNA sequence of this organism is now known.[137] The Centers for Disease Control and Prevention (CDC) offers diagnostic assistance.

Treatment and Prevention

This disease has been associated with a very high mortality once there is brain involvement and GAE manifests. Initial attempts at treating patients with amphotericin were associated with patient deterioration, but the use of multi-drug regimens containing 4-5 agents such as amphotericin, fluconazole, albendazole and miltefosine has resulted in some patients surviving and doing well, despite treatment initiation after the onset of GAE. Other medications such as voriconazole, flucytosine, pentamidine, azithromycin, clarithromycin, trimethoprim-sulfamethoxazole and sulfadiazine may have a role in the treatment of this pathogen.[136]

With the limited number of cases seen and no readily identifiable host susceptibility factors in most cases, advice for prevention is currently limited.

Blastocystis hominis

Blastocystis hominis is an anaerobic protozoan of uncertain taxonomic status.[138] *B. hominis* has been described in detail at the electron microscope level, and this study recognized only two stages; the vacuolar stage (Fig. 14.6) and the cyst.[139] Other investigators have described four major forms, while in reality the extensive variation in forms is just one more aspect of this organism that makes the study of its biology challenging.[140] Division is by binary fission. No sexual aspect to its life cycle has been documented. The fecal-oral route is presumed to be the way *B. hominis* infects, and the cyst stage may be important in transmission. The cyst is small, measuring 2 to 5 μm in diameter, and is protected by a multilayer cyst wall.[141] It can be grown in axenic culture, permitting studies on its biochemical, genetic and biological properties.[142, 143]

B. hominis is a very common finding on routine stool examination worldwide, even in asymptomatic individuals.[144] This organism is also frequently encountered with other more clinically defined pathogens, and this fact alone has made deciding on its status as pathogen, based upon its epidemiology, nearly impossible. Nonetheless, it is frequently associated with gastrointestinal (GI) symptoms. Several cases have been described that defy any interpretation other

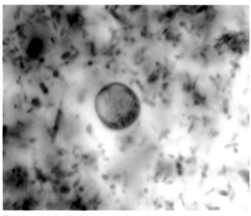

Figure 14.6. *Blastocystis hominis.* 6 μm.

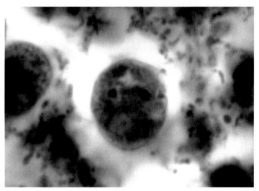

Figure 14.7. *Dientamoeba fragilis.* Note the two nuclei. 10 μm

than illness caused by *B. hominis*, based upon an extensive negative laboratory finding regarding all other known pathogens of the GI tract. In one case, gastroenteritis accompanied by diarrhea and hypoalbuminemia in the complete absence of all other pathogens was reported.[145]

Many genetically distinct strains of *B. hominis* have been characterized, so it is possible that some variants are pathogenic, while others are not.[146, 147] This could explain the high degree of variability in its clinical presentation.[148, 149] Most patients with HIV/AIDS do not have an increased prevalence of *B. hominis* infection, nor do they appear to be any more affected by its presence than those harboring it in the general immunocompetent population. Exceptions have been reported, in which the patient was symptomatic with diarrhea and was treated successfully after diagnosis of *B. hominis* infection, only.[150] The very elderly may represent an exception, under certain as-yet-undefined conditions.[151]

Diagnosis is generally made by detection of organisms on stained smears or wet mounts of stool specimens, and PCR has being developed.[152] Treatment of heavily-infected individuals with metronidazole, a proven antimicrobial agent against most anaerobes, was effective in eradicating *B. hominis* and improving symptoms in a high percentage of treated patients.[153] Paromomycin is another therapy suggested by some investigators to be an alternative first line therapy.[153] Trimethoprim-sulfamethoxazole has shown efficacy in the treatment of symptomatic patients and achieved high rates of *B. hominis* eradication from stool.[154] Nitazoxanide shows promise as an effective alternative therapeutic approach but studies have been confounded by its impact on other intestinal pathogens.[150]

Dientamoeba fragilis
(Jepps and Dobell 1918)

Dientamoeba fragilis is taxonomically related to *Histomonas* spp., a flagellated protozoan, but it has the morphology of an amoeba.[155, 156] Each trophozoite (Fig. 14.7) has two nuclei. For many years investigators had been unable to identify a cyst form, but cysts were finally identified both in a mouse model and in human feces.[157] Despite many years of controversy regarding whether or not this organism was pathogenic, it is now generally agreed that *D. fragilis* is responsible for causing a related series of gastroenteritis-like symptoms, including diarrhea and nausea with a duration often of more than 2 weeks.[158] *D. fragilis* is similar to *Cystoisospora belli* in that a peripheral eosinophilia can accompany infection, and patients may develop a form of eosinophilic colitis.[62, 159]

Diagnosis is either by direct examination of stool by microscopy, or by PCR, but since trophozoites are fragile and not easily detectable on wet mounts, fixed, stained stool samples are more sensitive.[160]

Many drugs have been shown to have some efficacy in treating infections.[156] Although large randomized clinical trials have yet to be carried out, metronidazole or paromomycin are recommended.[161, 162] Nitazoxanide, tetracycline, and iodoquinol are potential options for treatment of *D. fragilis* based on *in vitro* susceptibility testing.[163]

References

1. Beugnet, F.; Moreau, Y., Babesiosis. *Rev Sci Tech* **2015,** *34* (2), 627-39.
2. Eskow, E. S.; Krause, P. J.; Spielman, A.; Freeman, K.; Aslanzadeh, J., Southern extension of the range of human babesiosis in the eastern United States. *Journal of clinical microbiology* **1999,** *37* (6), 2051-2.
3. Herwaldt, B. L.; Kjemtrup, A. M.; Conrad, P. A.; Barnes, R. C.; Wilson, M.; McCarthy, M. G.; Sayers, M. H.; Eberhard, M. L., Transfusion-transmitted babesiosis in Washington State: first reported case caused by a WA1-type parasite. *J Infect Dis* **1997,** *175* (5), 1259-62.
4. Telford, S. R.; Speilman, A.; Collier, L.; Balows, A.; Sussman, M.; Cox, F. E. G.; Kreier, J.; Wakelin, D., Topley and Wilson's Microbiology and Microbial Infections. 1998; p 349-359.
5. White, D. J.; Talarico, J.; Chang, H. G.; Birkhead, G. S.; Heimberger, T.; Morse, D. L., Human babesiosis in New York State: Review of 139 hospitalized cases and analysis of prognostic factors. *Archives of internal medicine* **1998,** *158* (19), 2149-54.
6. Vannier, E.; Krause, P. J., Human babesiosis. *N Engl J Med* **2012,** *366* (25), 2397-407.
7. Gray, J. S., Babesia sp.: emerging intracellular parasites in Europe. *Polish journal of microbiology / Polskie Towarzystwo Mikrobiologow = The Polish Society of Microbiologists* **2004,** *53 Suppl,* 55-60.
8. Babes, V., Sur l'hemoglobinurie bacterienne de boeuf. *C R Acad Sci* **1888,** *107,* 692-4.
9. Smith, T.; Kilobourne, F. L., Investigations into the Nature, Causation, and Prevention of Texas or Southern Cattle Fever. **1893.**
10. Skrabalo, Z.; Deanovic, Z., Piroplasmosis in man; report of a case. *Doc Med Geogr Trop* **1957,** *9* (1), 11-6.
11. Western, K. A.; Benson, G. D.; Gleason, N. N.; Healy, G. R.; Schultz, M. G., Babesiosis in a Massachusetts resident. *N Engl J Med* **1970,** *283* (16), 854-6.
12. Leiby, D. A.; Gill, J. E., Transfusion-transmitted tick-borne infections: a cornucopia of threats.

Transfusion medicine reviews **2004,** *18* (4), 293-306.

13. Rudzinska, M. A.; Kreier, J. P.; Ristic, M., Morphological aspects of host-cell-parasite relationships in babesiosis. 1981; p 87-141.

14. Okubo, K.; Wilawan, P.; Bork, S.; Okamura, M.; Yokoyama, N.; Igarashi, I., Calcium-ions are involved in erythrocyte invasion by equine Babesia parasites. *Parasitology* **2006,** *133* (Pt 3), 289-94.

15. Yokoyama, N.; Okamura, M.; Igarashi, I., Erythrocyte invasion by Babesia parasites: current advances in the elucidation of the molecular interactions between the protozoan ligands and host receptors in the invasion stage. *Vet Parasitol* **2006,** *138* (1-2), 22-32.

16. Lobo, C. A.; Rodriguez, M.; Cursino-Santos, J. R., Babesia and red cell invasion. *Curr Opin Hematol* **2012,** *19* (3), 170-5.

17. Christianson, D.; Pollack, R. J., Persistent parasitemia after acute babesiosis. *N E J M* **1998,** *339* 160-5.

18. Shih, C. M.; Liu, L. P.; Chung, W. C.; Ong, S. J.; Wang, C. C., Human babesiosis in Taiwan: asymptomatic infection with a Babesia microti-like organism in a Taiwanese woman. *Journal of clinical microbiology* **1997,** *35* (2), 450-4.

19. Hatcher, J. C.; Greenberg, P. D.; Antique, J.; Jimenez-Lucho, V. E., Severe babesiosis in Long Island: review of 34 cases and their complications. *Clin Infect Dis* **2001,** *32* (8), 1117-25.

20. Piesman, J.; Mather, T. N.; Dammin, G. J.; Telford, S. R.; Lastavica, C. C.; Spielman, A., Seasonal variation of transmission risk of Lyme disease and human babesiosis. *American journal of epidemiology* **1987,** *126* (6), 1187-9.

21. Boustani, M. R.; Gelfand, J. A., Babesiosis. *Clinical infectious diseases : an official publication of the Infectious Diseases Society of America* **1996,** *22* (4), 611-5.

22. Gorenflot, A.; Moubri, K.; Precigout, E.; Carcy, B.; Schetters, T. P., Human babesiosis. *Annals of tropical medicine and parasitology* **1998,** *92* (4), 489-501.

23. Uguen, C.; Girard, L.; Brasseur, P.; Leblay, R., [Human babesiosis in 1997]. *La Revue de medecine interne / fondee ... par la Societe nationale francaise de medecine interne* **1997,** *18* (12), 945-51.

24. Kim, N.; Rosenbaum, G. S.; Cunha, B. A., Relative bradycardia and lymphopenia in patients with babesiosis. *Clinical infectious diseases : an official publication of the Infectious Diseases Society of America* **1998,** *26* (5), 1218-9.

25. Herwaldt, B.; Persing, D. H.; Précigout, E. A.; Goff, W. L.; Mathiesen, D. A.; Taylor, P. W.; Eberhard, M. L.; Gorenflot, A. F., A fatal case of babesiosis in Missouri: identification of another piroplasm that infects humans. *Annals of internal medicine* **1996,** *124* (7), 643-50.

26. Slovut, D. P.; Benedetti, E.; Matas, A. J., Babesiosis and hemophagocytic syndrome in an asplenic renal transplant recipient. *Transplantation* **1996,** *62* (4), 537-9.

27. Bonoan, J. T.; Johnson, D. H.; Cunha, B. A., Life-threatening babesiosis in an asplenic patient treated with exchange transfusion, azithromycin, and atovaquone. *Heart & lung : the journal of critical care* **1998,** *27* (6), 424-8.

28. Hohenschild, S., [Babesiosis--a dangerous infection for splenectomized children and adults]. *Klinische Padiatrie* **1999,** *211* (3), 137-40.

29. Persing, D. H., The cold zone: a curious convergence of tick-transmitted diseases. *Clin Infect Dis 25 Suppl* **1997,** *1*, S35-42.

30. Hilton, E.; DeVoti, J.; Benach, J. L.; Halluska, M. L.; White, D. J.; Paxton, H.; Dumler, J. S., Seroprevalence and seroconversion for tick-borne diseases in a high-risk population in the northeast United States. *The American journal of medicine* **1999,** *106* (4), 404-9.

31. Krause, P. J.; Telford, S. R.; Spielman, A.; Sikand, V.; Ryan, R.; Christianson, D.; Burke, G.; Brassard, P.; Pollack, R.; Peck, J.; Persing, D. H., Concurrent Lyme disease and babesiosis. Evidence for increased severity and duration of illness. *JAMA* **1996,** *275* (21), 1657-60.

32. Mitchell, P. D.; Reed, K. D.; Hofkes, J. M., Immunoserologic evidence of coinfection with Borrelia burgdorferi, Babesia microti, and human granulocytic Ehrlichia species in residents of Wisconsin and Minnesota. *Journal of clinical microbiology* **1996,** *34* (3), 724-7.

33. Magnarelli, L. A.; Ijdo, J. W.; Anderson, J. F.; Padula, S. J.; Flavell, R. A.; Fikrig, E., Human

exposure to a granulocytic Ehrlichia and other tick-borne agents in Connecticut. *Journal of clinical microbiology* **1998,** *36* (10), 2823-7.

34.   dos Santos, C. C.; Kain, K. C., Two tick-borne diseases in one: a case report of concurrent babesiosis and Lyme disease in Ontario. *CMAJ : Canadian Medical Association journal = journal de l'Association medicale canadienne* **1999,** *160* (13), 1851-3.

35.   Shaio, M. F.; Lin, P. R., A case study of cytokine profiles in acute human babesiosis. *Am J Trop Med Hyg* **1998,** *58* (3), 335-7.

36.   Kelesidis, T.; Daikos, G.; Boumpas, D.; Tsiodras, S., Does rituximab increase the incidence of infectious complications? A narrative review. *Int J Infect Dis* **2011,** *15* (1), e2-16.

37.   Falagas, M. E.; Klempner, M. S., Babesiosis in patients with AIDS: a chronic infection presenting as fever of unknown origin. *Clinical infectious diseases : an official publication of the Infectious Diseases Society of America* **1996,** *22* (5), 809-12.

38.   Krause, P. J., Babesiosis diagnosis and treatment. *Vector borne and zoonotic diseases (Larchmont, N.Y.)* **2003,** *3* (1), 45-51.

39.   Homer, M. J.; Aguilar-Delfin, I.; Telford, S. R.; Krause, P. J.; Persing, D. H., Babesiosis. *Clinical microbiology reviews* **2000,** *13* (3), 451-69.

40.   Conrad, P. A.; Kjemtrup, A. M.; Carreno, R. A.; Thomford, J.; Wainwright, K.; Eberhard, M.; Quick, R.; Telford, S. R., 3rd; Herwaldt, B. L., Description of Babesia duncani n.sp. (Apicomplexa: Babesiidae) from humans and its differentiation from other piroplasms. *Int J Parasitol* **2006,** *36* (7), 779-89.

41.   Teal, A. E.; Habura, A.; Ennis, J.; Keithly, J. S.; Madison-Antenucci, S., A new real-time PCR assay for improved detection of the parasite Babesia microti. *J Clin Microbiol* **2012,** *50* (3), 903-8.

42.   Loa, C. C.; Adelson, M. E.; Mordechai, E.; Raphaelli, I.; Tilton, R. C., Serological diagnosis of human babesiosis by IgG enzyme-linked immunosorbent assay. *Current microbiology* **2004,** *49* (6), 385-9.

43.   Shaio, M. F.; Yang, K. D., Response of babesiosis to a combined regimen of quinine and azithromycin. *Transactions of the Royal Society of Tropical Medicine and Hygiene* **1997,** *91* (2), 214-5.

44.   Krause, P. J.; Spielman, A.; Telford, S. R.; Sikand, V. K.; McKay, K.; Christianson, D.; Pollack, R. J.; Brassard, P.; Magera, J.; Ryan, R.; Persing, D. H., Persistent parasitemia after acute babesiosis. *N Engl J Med* **1998,** *339* (3), 160-5.

45.   Beniwal, R. P.; Nichani, A. K.; Rakha, N. K.; Sharma, R. D.; Sarup, S., An immunisation trial with in vitro produced Babesia bigemina exoantigens. *Tropical animal health and production* **1997,** *29* (4 Suppl), 124S-126S.

46.   Stafford, K. C.; Ward, J. S.; Magnarelli, L. A., Impact of controlled burns on the abundance of Ixodes scapularis (Acari: Ixodidae). *Journal of medical entomology* **1998,** *35* (4), 510-3.

47.   Wenyon, C. M., Coccidiosis of cats and dogs and the status of the Isospora of man. *Ann Trop Med Parasitol* **1923,** *17* 231-39.

48.   Joshi, M.; Chowdhary, A. S.; Dalal, P. J.; Maniar, J. K., Parasitic diarrhoea in patients with AIDS. *The National medical journal of India* **2002,** *15* (2), 72-4.

49.   Curry, A.; Smith, H. V., Emerging pathogens: Isospora, Cyclospora and microsporidia. *Parasitology* **1998,** *117 Suppl*, S143-59.

50.   Jongwutiwes, S.; Putaporntip, C.; Charoenkorn, M.; Iwasaki, T.; Endo, T., Morphologic and molecular characterization of Isospora belli oocysts from patients in Thailand. *Am J Trop Med Hyg* **2007,** *77* (1), 107-12.

51.   Ryan, E. T.; Cronin, C. G.; Branda, J. A., Case records of the Massachusetts General Hospital. Case 38-2011. A 34-year-old man with diarrhea and weakness. *N Engl J Med* **2011,** *365* (24), 2306-16.

52.   Benator, D. A.; French, A. L.; Beaudet, L. M.; Levy, C. S.; Orenstein, J. M., Isospora belli infection associated with acalculous cholecystitis in a patient with AIDS. *Annals of internal medicine* **1994,** *121* (9), 663-4.

53.   Michiels, J. F.; Hofman, P.; Bernard, E.; Saint Paul, M. C.; Boissy, C.; Mondain, V.; LeFichoux,

Y.; Loubiere, R., Intestinal and extraintestinal Isospora belli infection in an AIDS patient. A second case report. *Pathology, research and practice* **1994,** *190* (11), 1089-93; discussion 1094.

54.   Restrepo, C.; Macher, A. M.; Radany, E. H., Disseminated extraintestinal isosporiasis in a patient with acquired immune deficiency syndrome. *American journal of clinical pathology* **1987,** *87* (4), 536-42.

55.   Heyworth, M. F., Parasitic diseases in immunocompromised hosts. Cryptosporidiosis, isosporiasis, and strongyloidiasis. *Gastroenterology clinics of North America* **1996,** *25* (3), 691-707.

56.   Sahu, A. R.; Koticha, A. H.; Kuyare, S. S.; Khopkar, U. S., Isospora induced diarrhea in a pemphigus vulgaris patient. *Indian J Dermatol Venereol Leprol* **2014,** *80* (4), 342-3.

57.   Kim, M. J.; Kim, W. H.; Jung, H. C.; Chai, J. W.; Chai, J. Y., Isospora belli Infection with Chronic Diarrhea in an Alcoholic Patient. *Korean J Parasitol* **2013,** *51* (2), 207-12.

58.   Stein, J.; Tannich, E.; Hartmann, F., An unusual complication in ulcerative colitis during treatment with azathioprine and infliximab: Isospora belli as 'Casus belli'. *BMJ Case Rep* **2013,** *2013*.

59.   Kitsukawa, K.; Kamihira, S.; Kinoshita, K.; Amagasaki, T.; Ichimaru, M., [An autopsy case of T-cell lymphoma associated with disseminated varicella and malabsorption syndrome due to Isospora belli infection (author's transl)]. *[Rinsho ketsueki] The Japanese journal of clinical hematology* **1981,** *22* (2), 258-65.

60.   DeHovitz, J. A.; Pape, J. W.; Boncy, M.; Johnson, W. D., Jr., Clinical manifestations and therapy of Isospora belli infection in patients with the acquired immunodeficiency syndrome. *N Engl J Med* **1986,** *315* (2), 87-90.

61.   Pape, J. W.; Johnson, W. D., Isospora belli infections. *Progress in clinical parasitology* **1991,** *2,* 119-27.

62.   Gray, T. J.; Kwan, Y. L.; Phan, T.; Robertson, G.; Cheong, E. Y.; Gottlieb, T., Dientamoeba fragilis: a family cluster of disease associated with marked peripheral eosinophilia. *Clin Infect Dis* **2013,** *57* (6), 845-8.

63.   Navaneethan, U.; Venkatesh, P. G.; Downs-Kelly, E.; Shen, B., Isospora belli superinfection in a patient with eosinophilic gastroenteritis--a diagnostic challenge. *J Crohns Colitis* **2012,** *6* (2), 236-9.

64.   Fayer, R.; Esposito, D. H.; Dubey, J. P., Human infections with Sarcocystis species. *Clin Microbiol Rev* **2015,** *28* (2), 295-311.

65.   Mohanty, I.; Panda, P.; Sahu, S.; Dash, M.; Narasimham, M. V.; Padhi, S.; Parida, B., Prevalence of isosporiasis in relation to CD4 cell counts among HIV-infected patients with diarrhea in Odisha, India. *Adv Biomed Res* **2013,** *2,* 61.

66.   St. Georgiev, V., Opportunistic infections: treatment and developmental therapeutics of cryptosporidiosis and isosporiasis. *Drug Develop Res* **1993,** *28,* 445-59.

67.   Bialek, R.; Overkamp, D.; Rettig, I.; Knobloch, J., Case report: Nitazoxanide treatment failure in chronic isosporiasis. *Am J Trop Med Hyg* **2001,** *65* (2), 94-5.

68.   Doumbo, O.; Rossignol, J. F.; Pichard, E.; Traore, H. A.; Dembele, T. M.; Diakite, M.; Traore, F.; Diallo, D. A., Nitazoxanide in the treatment of cryptosporidial diarrhea and other intestinal parasitic infections associated with acquired immunodeficiency syndrome in tropical Africa. *Am J Trop Med Hyg* **1997,** *56* (6), 637-9.

69.   Ortega, Y. R.; Sterling, C. R.; Gilman, R. H., Cyclospora cayetanensis. *Advances in parasitology* **1998,** *40,* 399-418.

70.   Rose, J. B.; Slifko, T. R., Giardia, Cryptosporidium, and Cyclospora and their impact on foods: a review. *Journal of food protection* **1999,** *62* (9), 1059-70.

71.   Mansfield, L. S.; Gajadhar, A. A., Cyclospora cayetanensis, a food- and waterborne coccidian parasite. *Vet Parasitol* **2004,** *126* (1-2), 73-90.

72.   Sterling, C. R.; Ortega, Y. R., Cyclospora: an enigma worth unraveling. *Emerging infectious diseases* **1999,** *5* (1), 48-53.

73.   Mead, P. S.; Slutsker, L.; Dietz, V.; McCaig, L. F.; Bresee, J. S.; Shapiro, C.; Griffin, P. M.; Tauxe, R. V., Food-related illness and death in the United States. *Emerg Infect Dis* **1999,** *5* (5),

607-25.

74.   Eberhard, M. L.; Nace, E. K.; Freeman, A. R.; Streit, T. G.; da Silva, A. J.; Lammie, P. J., Cyclospora cayetanensis infections in Haiti: a common occurrence in the absence of watery diarrhea. *Am J Trop Med Hyg* **1999,** *60* (4), 584-6.

75.   Pape, J. W.; Verdier, R. I.; Boncy, M.; Boncy, J.; Johnson, W. D., Cyclospora infection in adults infected with HIV. Clinical manifestations, treatment, and prophylaxis. *Annals of internal medicine* **1994,** *121* (9), 654-7.

76.   Bern, C.; Hernandez, B.; Lopez, M. B.; Arrowood, M. J.; De Merida, A. M.; Klein, R. E., The contrasting epidemiology of Cyclospora and Cryptosporidium among outpatients in Guatemala. *Am J Trop Med Hyg* **2000,** *63* (5-6), 231-5.

77.   Bern, C.; Arrowood, M. J.; Eberhard, M.; Maguire, J. H., Cyclospora in Guatemala: further considerations. *J Clin Microbiol* **2002,** *40* (2), 731-2.

78.   Bern, C.; Hernandez, B.; Lopez, M. B.; Arrowood, M. J.; de Mejia, M. A.; de Merida, A. M.; Hightower, A. W.; Venczel, L.; Herwaldt, B. L.; Klein, R. E., Epidemiologic studies of Cyclospora cayetanensis in Guatemala. *Emerg Infect Dis* **1999,** *5* (6), 766-74.

79.   Chalmers, R. M.; Nichols, G.; Rooney, R., Foodborne outbreaks of cyclosporiasis have arisen in North America. Is the United Kingdom at risk? *Commun Dis Public Health* **2000,** *3* (1), 50-5.

80.   Manuel, D.; Neamatullah, S.; Shahin, R.; Reymond, D.; Keystone, J.; Carlson, J.; Le Ber, C.; Herwaldt, B.; Werker, D., An outbreak of cyclosporiasis in 1996 associated with consumption of fresh berries- Ontario. *Can J Infect Dis* **2000,** *11* (2), 86-92.

81.   Centers for Disease, C.; Prevention, Outbreak of cyclosporiasis associated with snow peas--Pennsylvania, 2004. *MMWR Morb Mortal Wkly Rep* **2004,** *53* (37), 876-8.

82.   Caceres, V. M.; Ball, R. T.; J., A foodborne outbreak of cyclosporiasis caused by imported raspberries. *Pract* **1998,** *47* 231-4.

83.   Koumans, E. H.; Katz, D. J.; Malecki, J. M.; Kumar, S.; Wahlquist, S. P.; Arrowood, M. J.; Hightower, A. W.; Herwaldt, B. L., An outbreak of cyclosporiasis in Florida in 1995: a harbinger of multistate outbreaks in 1996 and 1997. *Am J Trop Med Hyg* **1998,** *59* (2), 235-42.

84.   Herwaldt, B. L.; Beach, M. J., The return of Cyclospora in 1997: another outbreak of cyclosporiasis in North America associated with imported raspberries. Cyclospora Working Group. *Annals of internal medicine* **1999,** *130* (3), 210-20.

85.   Shields, J. M.; Olson, B. H., Cyclospora cayetanensis: a review of an emerging parasitic coccidian. *International journal for parasitology* **2003,** *33* (4), 371-91.

86.   Ortega, Y. R.; Nagle, R.; Gilman, R. H.; Watanabe, J.; Miyagui, J.; Quispe, H.; Kanagusuku, P.; Roxas, C.; Sterling, C. R., Pathologic and clinical findings in patients with cyclosporiasis and a description of intracellular parasite life-cycle stages. *J Infect Dis* **1997,** *176* (6), 1584-9.

87.   Smith, H. V.; Paton, C. A.; Girdwood, R. W.; Mtambo, M. M., Cyclospora in non-human primates in Gombe, Tanzania. *The Veterinary record* **1996,** *138* (21), 528.

88.   Ortega, Y. R.; Sanchez, R., Update on Cyclospora cayetanensis, a food-borne and waterborne parasite. *Clin Microbiol Rev* **2010,** *23* (1), 218-34.

89.   Ashford, R. W., Occurrence of an undescribed coccidian in man in Papua New Guinea. *Ann Trop Med Parasitol* **1979,** *73* (5), 497-500.

90.   Soave, R.; Armstrong, D., Cryptosporidium and cryptosporidiosis. *Rev Infect Dis* **1986,** *8* (6), 1012-23.

91.   Ortega, Y. R.; Sterling, C. R.; Gilman, R. H.; Cama, V. A.; Diaz, F., Cyclospora species--a new protozoan pathogen of humans. *N Engl J Med* **1993,** *328* (18), 1308-12.

92.   Connor, B. A.; Reidy, J.; Soave, R., Cyclosporiasis: clinical and histopathologic correlates. *Clin Infect Dis* **1999,** *28* (6), 1216-22.

93.   Shlim, D. R.; Cohen, M. T.; Eaton, M.; Rajah, R.; Long, E. G.; Ungar, B. L., An alga-like organism associated with an outbreak of prolonged diarrhea among foreigners in Nepal. *Am J Trop Med Hyg* **1991,** *45* (3), 383-9.

94.   Fleming, C. A.; Caron, D.; Gunn, J. E.; Barry, M. A., A foodborne outbreak of Cyclospora cayetanensis at a wedding: clinical features and risk factors for illness. *Arch Intern Med* **1998,** *158* (10), 1121-5.

95.   Blanshard, C.; Jackson, A. M.; Shanson, D. C.; Francis, N.; Gazzard, B. G., Cryptosporidiosis in

HIV-seropositive patients. *Q J Med* **1992**, *85* (307-308), 813-23.

96.   Richardson, R. F.; Remler, B. F.; Murad, M. H.; Katirji, B., Guillain-Barre syndrome after Cyclospora infection. *Muscle Nerve* **1998**, *21* (5), 669-71.

97.   Connor, B. A.; Johnson, E. J.; Soave, R., Reiter syndrome following protracted symptoms of Cyclospora infection. *Emerg Infect Dis* **2001**, *7* (3), 453-4.

98.   Jinneman, K. C.; Wetherington, J. H.; J., An oligonucleotide-ligation assay for the differentiation between Cyclospora and Eimeria spp polymerase chain reaction amplification products *Prot 62*, 682-5.

99.   Buss, S. N.; Leber, A.; Chapin, K.; Fey, P. D.; Bankowski, M. J.; Jones, M. K.; Rogatcheva, M.; Kanack, K. J.; Bourzac, K. M., Multicenter evaluation of the BioFire FilmArray gastrointestinal panel for etiologic diagnosis of infectious gastroenteritis. *J Clin Microbiol* **2015**, *53* (3), 915-25.

100.   Madico, G.; Gilman, R. H.; Miranda, E.; Cabrera, L.; Sterling, C. R., Treatment of Cyclospora infections with co-trimoxazole. *Lancet* **1993**, *342* (8863), 122-3.

101.   Hoge, C. W.; Shlim, D. R.; Ghimire, M.; Rabold, J. G.; Pandey, P.; Walch, A.; Rajah, R.; Gaudio, P.; Echeverria, P., Placebo-controlled trial of co-trimoxazole for Cyclospora infections among travellers and foreign residents in Nepal. *Lancet* **1995**, *345* (8951), 691-3.

102.   Verdier, R. I.; Fitzgerald, D. W.; Johnson, W. D., Jr.; Pape, J. W., Trimethoprim-sulfamethoxazole compared with ciprofloxacin for treatment and prophylaxis of Isospora belli and Cyclospora cayetanensis infection in HIV-infected patients. A randomized, controlled trial. *Ann Intern Med* **2000**, *132* (11), 885-8.

103.   Zimmer, S. M.; Schuetz, A. N.; Franco-Paredes, C., Efficacy of nitazoxanide for cyclosporiasis in patients with sulfa allergy. *Clin Infect Dis* **2007**, *44* (3), 466-7.

104.   Schuster, F. L.; Visvesvara, G. S., Amebae and ciliated protozoa as causal agents of waterborne zoonotic disease. *Vet Parasitol* **2004**, *126* (1-2), 91-120.

105.   Baig, A. M.; Khan, N. A., Tackling infection owing to brain-eating amoeba. *Acta Trop* **2015**, *142*, 86-8.

106.   Kilvington, S.; Beeching, J., Identification and epidemiological typing of Naegleria fowleri with DNA probes. *Applied and environmental microbiology* **1995**, *61* (6), 2071-8.

107.   Rodriguez, R.; Mendez, O.; Molina, O., Infection del sistema nervioso central por amoebas de vida libre: comunicacion de tres nuevos casos venezolanos. *Rev Neurologia* **1998**, *26*, 1005-8.

108.   Okuda, D. T.; Hanna, H. J.; Coons, S. W.; Bodensteiner, J. B., Naegleria fowleri hemorrhagic meningoencephalitis: report of two fatalities in children. *Journal of child neurology* **2004**, *19* (3), 231-3.

109.   Visvesvara, G. S.; Stehr-Green, J. K., Epidemiology of free-living ameba infections. *The Journal of protozoology* **1990**, *37* (4), 25S-33S.

110.   Herbst, R.; Marciano-Cabral, F.; Leippe, M., Antimicrobial and pore-forming peptides of free-living and potentially highly pathogenic Naegleria fowleri are released from the same precursor molecule. *The Journal of biological chemistry* **2004**, *279* (25), 25955-8.

111.   Martinez, A. J., Free-living amoebic meningoencephalitides: comparative study. *NeurologiaNeurocirugiaPsiquiatria 18 Suppl 391* **1977**, *401*, 2-3.

112.   Visvesvara, G. S.; Peralta, M. J.; Brandt, F. H.; Wilson, M.; Aloisio, C.; Franko, E., Production of monoclonal antibodies to Naegleria fowleri, agent of primary amebic meningoencephalitis. *J Clin Microbiol* **1987**, *25* (9), 1629-34.

113.   Qvarnstrom, Y.; Visvesvara, G. S.; Sriram, R.; da Silva, A. J., Multiplex real-time PCR assay for simultaneous detection of Acanthamoeba spp., Balamuthia mandrillaris, and Naegleria fowleri. *J Clin Microbiol* **2006**, *44* (10), 3589-95.

114.   Behets, J.; Seghi, F.; Declerck, P.; Verelst, L.; Duvivier, L.; Van Damme, A.; Ollevier, F., Detection of Naegleria spp. and Naegleria fowleri: a comparison of flagellation tests, ELISA and PCR. *Water science and technology : a journal of the International Association on Water Pollution Research* **2003**, *47* (3), 117-22.

115.   Schuster, F. L.; Visvesvara, G. S., Opportunistic amoebae: challenges in prophylaxis and treatment. *Drug resistance updates : reviews and commentaries in antimicrobial and anticancer chemotherapy* **2004**, *7* (1), 41-51.

116.   Linam, W. M.; Ahmed, M.; Cope, J. R.; Chu, C.; Visvesvara, G. S.; da Silva, A. J.; Qvarnstrom, Y.; Green, J., Successful treatment of an adolescent with Naegleria fowleri primary amebic meningoencephalitis. *Pediatrics* **2015,** *135* (3), e744-8.

117.   Capewell, L. G.; Harris, A. M.; Yoder, J. S.; Cope, J. R.; Eddy, B. A.; Roy, S. L.; Visvesvara, G. S.; Fox, L. M.; Beach, M. J., Diagnosis, Clinical Course, and Treatment of Primary Amoebic Meningoencephalitis in the United States, 1937-2013. *J Pediatric Infect Dis Soc* **2015,** *4* (4), e68-75.

118.   John, D. T.; Howard, M. J., Seasonal distribution of pathogenic free-living amebae in Oklahoma waters. *Parasitology research* **1995,** *81* (3), 193-201.

119.   Paltiel, M.; Powell, E.; Lynch, J.; Baranowski, B.; Martins, C., Disseminated cutaneous acanthamebiasis: a case report and review of the literature. *Cutis* **2004,** *73* (4), 241-8.

120.   Marciano-Cabral, F.; Cabral, G., Acanthamoeba spp. as agents of disease in humans. *Clinical microbiology reviews* **2003,** *16* (2), 273-307.

121.   Khan, N. A., Acanthamoeba: biology and increasing importance in human health. *FEMS Microbiol Rev* **2006,** *30* (4), 564-95.

122.   Siddiqui, R.; Khan, N. A., Biology and pathogenesis of Acanthamoeba. *Parasit Vectors* **2012,** *5,* 6.

123.   Martinez, A. J., Infection of the central nervous system due to Acanthamoeba. *Rev of Infect Dis 13 Suppl* **1991,** *5* S399-402.

124.   Brindley, N.; Matin, A.; Khan, N. A., Acanthamoeba castellanii: high antibody prevalence in racially and ethnically diverse populations. *Exp Parasitol* **2009,** *121* (3), 254-6.

125.   Koide, J.; Okusawa, E.; Ito, T.; Mori, S.; Takeuchi, T.; Itoyama, S.; Abe, T., Granulomatous amoebic encephalitis caused by Acanthamoeba in a patient with systemic lupus erythematosus. *Clinical rheumatology* **1998,** *17* (4), 329-32.

126.   Sison, J. P.; Kemper, C. A.; Loveless, M.; McShane, D.; Visvesvara, G. S.; Deresinski, S. C., Disseminated acanthamoeba infection in patients with AIDS: case reports and review. *Clinical infectious diseases : an official publication of the Infectious Diseases Society of America* **1995,** *20* (5), 1207-16.

127.   Auran, J. D.; Starr, M. B.; Jakobiec, F. A., Acanthamoeba keratitis. A review of the literature. *Cornea* **1987,** *6* (1), 2-26.

128.   Goldschmidt, P.; Degorge, S.; Benallaoua, D.; Saint-Jean, C.; Batellier, L.; Alouch, C.; Laroche, L.; Chaumeil, C., New tool for the simultaneous detection of 10 different genotypes of Acanthamoeba available from the American Type Culture Collection. *Br J Ophthalmol* **2009,** *93* (8), 1096-100.

129.   Pirehma, M.; Suresh, K.; Sivanandam, S.; Anuar, A. K.; Ramakrishnan, K.; Kumar, G. S., Field's stain--a rapid staining method for Acanthamoeba spp. *Parasitology research* **1999,** *85* (10), 791-3.

130.   Seal, D., Treatment of Acanthamoeba keratitis. *Expert review of anti-infective therapy* **2003,** *1* (2), 205-8.

131.   Schuster, F. L.; Dunnebacke, T. H.; Booton, G. C.; Yagi, S.; Kohlmeier, C. K.; Glaser, C.; Vugia, D.; Bakardjiev, A.; Azimi, P.; Maddux-Gonzalez, M.; Martinez, A. J.; Visvesvara, G. S., Environmental isolation of Balamuthia mandrillaris associated with a case of amebic encephalitis. *J Clin Microbiol* **2003,** *41* (7), 3175-80.

132.   Matin, A.; Siddiqui, R.; Jayasekera, S.; Khan, N. A., Increasing importance of Balamuthia mandrillaris. *Clin Microbiol Rev* **2008,** *21* (3), 435-48.

133.   Siddiqui, R.; Khan, N. A., Balamuthia amoebic encephalitis: an emerging disease with fatal consequences. *Microb Pathog* **2008,** *44* (2), 89-97.

134.   Jayasekera, S.; Sissons, J.; Tucker, J.; Rogers, C.; Nolder, D.; Warhurst, D.; Alsam, S.; White, J. M.; Higgins, E. M.; Khan, N. A., Post-mortem culture of Balamuthia mandrillaris from the brain and cerebrospinal fluid of a case of granulomatous amoebic meningoencephalitis, using human brain microvascular endothelial cells. *J Med Microbiol* **2004,** *53* (Pt 10), 1007-12.

135.   Martinez, A. J.; Visvesvara, G. S., Balamuthia mandrillaris infection. *J Med Microbiol* **2001,** *50* (3), 205-7.

136. Parija, S. C.; Dinoop, K.; Venugopal, H., Management of granulomatous amebic encephalitis: Laboratory diagnosis and treatment. *Trop Parasitol* **2015,** *5* (1), 23-8.
137. Detering, H.; Aebischer, T.; Dabrowski, P. W.; Radonic, A.; Nitsche, A.; Renard, B. Y.; Kiderlen, A. F., First Draft Genome Sequence of Balamuthia mandrillaris, the Causative Agent of Amoebic Encephalitis. *Genome Announc* **2015,** *3* (5).
138. Nasirudeen, A. M. A.; Tan, K. S. W., Isolation and characterization of the mitochondrion-like organelle from Blastocystis hominis. *Journal of microbiological methods* **2004,** *58* (1), 101-9.
139. Windsor, J. J.; Stenzel, D. J.; Macfarlane, L., Multiple reproductive processes in Blastocystis hominis. *Trends in parasitology* **2003,** *19* (7), 289-90; author reply 291.
140. Tan, K. S., New insights on classification, identification, and clinical relevance of Blastocystis spp. *Clin Microbiol Rev* **2008,** *21* (4), 639-65.
141. Chen, X. Q.; Singh, M.; Howe, J.; Ho, L. C.; Tan, S. W.; Yap, E. H., In vitro encystation and excystation of Blastocystis ratti. *Parasitology* **1999,** *118 (Pt 2)*, 151-60.
142. Zaman, V.; Zaki, M.; Manzoor, M.; Howe, J.; Ng, M., Postcystic development of Blastocystis. *Parasitol Res* **1999,** *27* (8), 941-5.
143. Carbajal, J. A.; Castillo, L., del Karyotypic diversity among Blastocystis hominis isolates. *Parasitol Res* **1999,** *85*, 437-40.
144. Aguiar, J. I.; Goncalves, A. Q.; Sodre, F. C.; Pereira Sdos, R.; Boia, M. N.; de Lemos, E. R.; Daher, R. R., Intestinal protozoa and helminths among Terena Indians in the State of Mato Grosso do Sul: high prevalence of Blastocystis hominis. *Rev Soc Bras Med Trop* **2007,** *40* (6), 631-4.
145. Nassir, E.; Awad, J.; Abel, A. B.; Khoury, J.; Shay, M.; Lejbkowicz, F., Blastocystis hominis as a cause of hypoalbuminemia and anasarca. *European journal of clinical microbiology & infectious diseases : official publication of the European Society of Clinical Microbiology* **2004,** *23* (5), 399-402.
146. Clark, C. G., Extensive genetic diversity in Blastocystis hominis. *Molecular and biochemical parasitology* **1997,** *87* (1), 79-83.
147. Bohm-Gloning, B.; Knobloch, J.; Walderich, B., Five subgroups of Blastocystis hominis from symptomatic and asymptomatic patients revealed by restriction site analysis of PCR-amplified 16S-like rDNA. *Trop Med Internat Health* **1997,** *2* 771-8.
148. Horiki, N.; Maruyama, M.; Fujita, Y.; Yonekura, T.; Minato, S.; Kaneda, Y., Epidemiologic survey of Blastocystis hominis infection in Japan. *Am J Trop Med Hyg* **1997,** *56* (4), 370-4.
149. Jelinek, T.; Peyerl, G.; Löscher, T.; von Sonnenburg, F.; Nothdurft, H. D., The role of Blastocystis hominis as a possible intestinal pathogen in travellers. *The Journal of infection* **1997,** *35* (1), 63-6.
150. Cimerman, S.; Ladeira, M. C. T.; Iuliano, W. A., Blastocystosis: nitazoxanide as a new therapeutic option. *Revista da Sociedade Brasileira de Medicina Tropical* **2003,** *36* (3), 415-7.
151. Levy, Y.; George, J.; Shoenfeld, Y., Severe Blastocystis hominis in an elderly man. *The Journal of infection* **1996,** *33* (1), 57-9.
152. Jones, M. S., 2nd; Ganac, R. D.; Hiser, G.; Hudson, N. R.; Le, A.; Whipps, C. M., Detection of Blastocystis from stool samples using real-time PCR. *Parasitol Res* **2008,** *103* (3), 551-7.
153. Sekar, U.; Shanthi, M., Blastocystis: Consensus of treatment and controversies. *Trop Parasitol* **2013,** *3* (1), 35-9.
154. Ertug, S.; Dost, T.; Ertabaklar, H.; Gultekin, B., The effect of trimethoprim-sulfamethoxazole in Blastocystis hominis infection. *Turkiye Parazitol Derg* **2009,** *33* (4), 270-2.
155. Silberman, J. D.; Clark, C. G.; Sogin, M. L., Dientamoeba fragilis shares a recent common evolutionary history with the trichomonads. *Molecular and biochemical parasitology* **1996,** *76* (1-2), 311-4.
156. Johnson, E. H.; Windsor, J. J.; Clark, C. G., Emerging from obscurity: biological, clinical, and diagnostic aspects of Dientamoeba fragilis. *Clin Microbiol Rev Jul* **2004,** *17*, 553-70.
157. Stark, D.; Garcia, L. S.; Barratt, J. L.; Phillips, O.; Roberts, T.; Marriott, D.; Harkness, J.; Ellis, J. T., Description of Dientamoeba fragilis cyst and precystic forms from human samples. *J Clin Microbiol* **2014,** *52* (7), 2680-3.

158.   Stark, D.; Barratt, J.; Roberts, T.; Marriott, D.; Harkness, J.; Ellis, J., A review of the clinical presentation of dientamoebiasis. *Am J Trop Med Hyg* **2010,** *82* (4), 614-9.

159.   Cuffari, C.; Oligny, L.; Seidman, E. G., Dientamoeba fragilis masquerading as allergic colitis. *J Pediatr Gastroenterol Nutr* **1998,** *26* (1), 16-20.

160.   Peek, R.; Reedeker, F. R.; van Gool, T., Direct amplification and genotyping of Dientamoeba fragilis from human stool specimens. *Journal of clinical microbiology* **2004,** *42* (2), 631-5.

161.   Roser, D.; Simonsen, J.; Stensvold, C. R.; Olsen, K. E.; Bytzer, P.; Nielsen, H. V.; Molbak, K., Metronidazole therapy for treating dientamoebiasis in children is not associated with better clinical outcomes: a randomized, double-blinded and placebo-controlled clinical trial. *Clin Infect Dis* **2014,** *58* (12), 1692-9.

162.   van Hellemond, J. J.; Molhoek, N.; Koelewijn, R.; Wismans, P. J.; van Genderen, P. J., Is paromomycin the drug of choice for eradication of Blastocystis in adults? *J Infect Chemother* **2013,** *19* (3), 545-8.

163.   Nagata, N.; Marriott, D.; Harkness, J.; Ellis, J. T.; Stark, D., In vitro susceptibility testing of Dientamoeba fragilis. *Antimicrob Agents Chemother* **2012,** *56* (1), 487-94.

15. Non-Pathogenic Protozoa

Introduction

We are constantly confronted with a plethora of microbes whose sole purpose is to colonize us and take advantage of our biochemical systems. The human body can be viewed as a series of ecological niches that select for numerous entities, including viruses, bacteria, fungi, protozoa, helminths, and arthropods. They enter through the gastrointestinal, urogenital, and respiratory tracts, through abrasions, and other portalsw of entry. Most of the world's microbes are incapable of remaining on or within these environments and are repelled. This is mainly due to the inadequacy of their fundamental biological makeup, preventing them from thriving on or in us, and the resiliency of our microbiome.[1] The majority of those that have succeeded do us little or no harm. In fact, the great majority of cells on and in us are foreigners! We refer to them collectively as our microbiome (see: http://hmpdacc.org/). Commensals do us no harm, and are just along for the ride, so to speak. Symbionts actively help maintain our homeostatic mechanisms. For example, the oral cavity harbors some 700 different species of bacteria (see: http://www.homd.org/), serving to exclude those that would lead to various states of ill health. Our intestinal tract is another good example of "peaceful" coexistence between our symbiotic microbes and us, harboring some 500 species of "friendly" bacteria.[2]

A few that have managed to run the gauntlet of our immune system and overcome the physiological barriers established by our complex metabolic regimes can and often do cause pathology leading to clinical conditions. This chapter is devoted to a brief mention of a few of those eukaryotic organisms that we routinely harbor, and which do us no harm. The clinician will undoubtedly receive a diagnostic slip from the laboratory with the

name of one or more of them on it. How these "hitchhiker" species should be approached in the context of the clinical setting is the subject of this brief chapter.

A number of commensal protozoans have been selected for life within us. Under unusual conditions, a few have been shown to be associated with disease, but have never been implicated as the primary cause of illness. When a person is placed at risk from infection (e.g., surgery, immunosuppression, or infection with another pathogenic organism), some commensal organisms become opportunistic pathogens, growing and extending their territory at the expense of our now compromised microbiome. At those times, the clinician has a difficult time determining who did what to whom. The diagnostic microbiology laboratory now assumes a role of major importance, helping to catalogue microbes into the good, the bad, and the ugly. Resolving the primary cause of the disease often reverses the growth pattern of the opportunist. None of the organisms listed in the tables, except for rare cases of *Entamoeba dispar* and *E. gingivalis* have ever been associated with actual infection, and in these exceptions, no serious disease due to the protozoan occurred. [3-5]

It is critical for the clinician to recognize the fact that even though the organism reported is not a pathogen, it is potentially a marker of the patient's exposure to a situation that may have led to the acquisition of another organism that may be pathogenic. The search should focus on all other agents transmitted by the same route. A representative of each organism mentioned in the following summaries can be found in Appendix C.

Commensal flagellated protozoa

Trichomonas tenax, T. hominis, Enteromonas hominis, Retortamonas intestinalis, and *Chilomastix mesnili* all only colonize the human host, and are considered nonpathogenic by all standard criteria.[6] *T. tenax* lives in the oral cavity in plaque, and the rest of them are intestinal dwellers. Only *C. mesnili* has a cyst stage. All are considered amitochondriate, aerotolerant anaerobic protists.[7] Heavy growth of *T. tenax* was found concurrently with abscesses and tumors of the oral cavity.[8, 9] In addition, *T. tenax* has been isolated from cases of inhalation pneumonia, and from pleural effusions from a patient in which ulceration of the esophagus resulted in communication with the pleural cavity. A PCR test for detecting *T. tenax* in dental plaque has been reported.[10, 11] Due to the overwhelming number of people harboring this flagellate who do not experience any discomfort, *T. tenax* remains on the list of commensals.

A single case of *Enteromonas hominis* has been reported in which the patient experienced diarrhea and was treated successfully with metronidazole.[12] Neither *R. intestinalis* nor *C. mesnili* have ever been linked to any abnormal health condition.

Commensal amoebae

Entamoeba dispar, E. hartmanni, E. coli, Endolimax nana, and *Iodamoeba bütschlii* are organisms often identified in routine stool examination, and whose reporting often elic-

its confusion among clinicians seeking the causes for diarrheal disease in their patients. Some bear a resemblance to *Entamoeba histolytica*, especially to the inexperienced laboratory technician, and they sometimes err on the side of this pathogen, rather than the commensal. Hence, the patient receives treatment for an entity that is not causing the problem. After treatment, the illness often "recurs," and drug failure is blamed. Commensal amoebae do not respond to the standard drugs used to eradicate *Entamoeba histolytica*, the pathogen most often confused with *E. dispar* or *E. hartmanni*. The use of PCR allows for definitive diagnosis of the pathogenic amoebae.[13] Another approach uses monoclonal antibodies to distinguish *E. histolytica* cysts from those of *E. dispar* and other commensal amoebae, facilitating their use in an antigen capture mode for routine diagnosis.[14]

Entamoeba polecki is an inhabitant of the gut tract of pigs that sometimes finds its way into humans, while *E. gingivalis* lives in the gingival flaps of a small subset of humans not yet defined, and is associated with, but does not cause pyorrhea. *E. gingivalis* was diagnosed by fine needle aspiration of an abscess of the neck, following radiation therapy.[15]

References

1. Bull, M. J.; Plummer, N. T., Part 1: The Human Gut Microbiome in Health and Disease. *Integr Med (Encinitas)* **2014**, *13* (6), 17-22.
2. Qin, J.; Li, R.; Raes, J.; Arumugam, M.; Burgdorf, K. S.; Manichanh, C.; Nielsen, T.; Pons, N.; Levenez, F.; Yamada, T.; Mende, D. R.; Li, J.; Xu, J.; Li, S.; Li, D.; Cao, J.; Wang, B.; Liang, H.; Zheng, H.; Xie, Y.; Tap, J.; Lepage, P.; Bertalan, M.; Batto, J. M.; Hansen, T.; Le Paslier, D.; Linneberg, A.; Nielsen, H. B.; Pelletier, E.; Renault, P.; Sicheritz-Ponten, T.; Turner, K.; Zhu, H.; Yu, C.; Li, S.; Jian, M.; Zhou, Y.; Li, Y.; Zhang, X.; Li, S.; Qin, N.; Yang, H.; Wang, J.; Brunak, S.; Dore, J.; Guarner, F.; Kristiansen, K.; Pedersen, O.; Parkhill, J.; Weissenbach, J.; Meta, H. I. T. C.; Bork, P.; Ehrlich, S. D.; Wang, J., A human gut microbial gene catalogue established by metagenomic sequencing. *Nature* **2010**, *464* (7285), 59-65.
3. Allison-Jones, E.; Mindel, A.; N.; J., Entamoeba histolytica as a commensal intestinal parasite in homosexual men. **1986**, *315*, 353-6.
4. Haque, R.; Neville, L. M.; Wood, S.; Petri, W. A., Jr., Short report: detection of Entamoeba histolytica and E. dispar directly in stool. *Am J Trop Med Hyg* **1994**, *50* (5), 595-6.
5. Lucht, E.; Evengård, B.; Skott, J.; Pehrson, P.; Nord, C. E., Entamoeba gingivalis in human immunodeficiency virus type 1-infected patients with periodontal disease. *Clinical infectious diseases : an official publication of the Infectious Diseases Society of America* **1998**, *27* (3), 471-3.

6.   Aucott, J. N.; Ravdin, J. I., Amebiasis and "nonpathogenic" intestinal protozoa. *Infectious disease clinics of North America* **1993**, *7* (3), 467-85.

7.   Coombs, G. H.; Sleigh, M. A.; Vickerman, K.; Warren, A., Evolutionary Relationships Among Protozoa 1998; p 110-132.

8.   Duboucher, C.; Mogenet, M.; Périé, G., Salivary trichomoniasis. A case report of infestation of a submaxillary gland by Trichomonas tenax. *Archives of pathology & laboratory medicine* **1995**, *119* (3), 277-9.

9.   Shiota, T.; Arizono, N.; Morimoto, T.; Shimatsu, A.; Nakao, K., Trichomonas tenax empyema in an immunocompromised patient with advanced cancer. *Parasite (Paris, France)* **1998**, *5* (4), 375-7.

10.   El Kamel, A.; Rouetbi, N.; Chakroun, M.; Battikh, M., Pulmonary eosinophilia due to Trichomonas tenax. *Thorax* **1996**, *51* (5), 554-5.

11.   Kikuta, N.; Yamamoto, A.; Fukura, K.; Goto, N., Specific and sensitive detection of Trichomonas tenax by the polymerase chain reaction. *Lett Appl Microbiol* **1999**, *24* (3), 193-7.

12.   Spriegel, J. R.; Saag, K. G.; Tsang, T. K., Infectious diarrhea secondary to Enteromonas hominis. *The American journal of gastroenterology* **1989**, *84* (10), 1313-4.

13.   Acuna-Soto, R.; Samuelson, J.; De Girolami, P.; Zarate, L.; Millan-Velasco, F.; Schoolnick, G.; Wirth, D., Application of the polymerase chain reaction to the epidemiology of pathogenic and nonpathogenic Entamoeba histolytica. *The American journal of tropical medicine and hygiene* **1993**, *48* (1), 58-70.

14.   Walderich, B.; Burchard, G. D.; Knobloch, J.; Müller, L., Development of monoclonal antibodies specifically recognizing the cyst stage of Entamoeba histolytica. *The American journal of tropical medicine and hygiene* **1998**, *59* (3), 347-51.

15.   Perez-Jaffe, L.; Katz, R.; Gupta, P. K., Entamoeba gingivalis identified in a left upper neck nodule by fine-needle aspiration: a case report. *Diagnostic cytopathology* **1998**, *18* (6), 458-61.

V. The Nematodes

Nematodes are non-segmented round-worms belonging to the phylum Nematoda, and are among the most abundant life forms on earth. The great majority of nematodes are free-living, inhabiting most essential niches in soil and freshwater and saltwater, as well as other, more specialized ones. Only a small fraction of the total number of species is parasitic, and only some of these infect the human host. Most parasitic nematodes have developed a highly specific biologic dependence on a particular species of host, and are incapable of survival in any other. Only a few have succeeded in adapting to a variety of hosts. Best known by far among the free-living nematodes is *Caenorhabditis elegans*, whose entire genome has been sequenced (20,512 genes). In contrast, the genome of *Trichinella spiralis*, a parasitic nematode, has more total DNA than *C. elegans*, and only 60% of it is homologous with its free-living relative. However, there have only been 15,808 coding regions identified, implying that this parasite needs fewer, not more genes than its free-living relatives. Virulence factors, and other specialized compounds needed to resist digestion or immune attack are likely to be encoded by genes that permit the invader to live comfortably in the face of an exquisitely developed immune system.

Infections caused by nematodes are among the most prevalent, affecting nearly all of us at one time in our lives. The most common nematodes are three types of soil-transmitted helminths (STHs), the common roundworm *Ascaris lumbricoides*, the whipworm *Trichuris trichiura*, and the hookworms *Necator americanus* and *Ancylostoma duodenale*. Children are particularly susceptible to acquiring large numbers of these parasites, and consequently suffer greater morbidity. In many developing countries, children frequently harbor all three types of STHs (hence the moniker "the unholy trinity") and suffer from childhood malnutrition, physical growth retardation, and deficits in cognitive and intellectual development as a result.

The typical nematode, both larva and adult, is surrounded by a flexible, durable outer coating, the acellular cuticle, that is resistant to chemicals. It is a complex structure composed of a variety of layers, each of which has many components, including structural proteins, enzymes, and lipids. The cuticle of each species has a unique structure and composition; it not only protects the worm but may also be involved in active transport of small molecules, including water, electrolytes, and organic compounds. A further layer, the epicuticle, surrounds the cuticle of a few parasitic species, making them even more resistant to attack from enzymes, antibodies, and other host resistance factors.

All nematodes have a well-developed muscular system. The muscle cells form an outer ring of tissue lying just underneath the cuticle, and their origins and insertions are in cuticular processes. In addition, there is some muscle tissue surrounding the buccal cavity and esophageal and sub-esophageal regions of the gut tract. These muscles are particularly important elements of the feeding apparatus in both parasitic and free-living nematodes. Each muscle cell consists of filaments, mitochondria, and cytoplasmic processes that connect it with a single nerve fiber. The nervous system consists of a dorsal nerve ring or a series of ganglia that give rise to the peripheral nerves - two lateral, one dorsal, and one ventral branch. Commissures connect the branches and allow for integration of signaling, which results in fluid, serpiginous movements. Several classes of drugs interfere only with nematode nerve signaling, and are thus effective treatments for nematode infections in humans.

Nematodes have a complete, functional gut tract; the oral (i.e., buccal) cavity and esophagus, the midgut, and the hindgut with anus. The oral cavity and hindgut are usually lined by cuticle; the midgut consists of columnar cells, complete with microvilli. The function of the midgut is to absorb ingested nutrients, whereas the usually muscular esophagus serves to deliver food to the midgut.

In addition, a number of specialized exocrine glands open into the lumen of the digestive tract, usually in the region of the esophagus. These glands are thought to be largely concerned with digestion, but may be related to other functions as well. For example, in hookworms, the cephalic glands secrete an anticoagulant. In other instances, there is a single row of cells called stichocytes that empty their products directly into the esophagus via a cuticular-lined duct. These cells occupy a large portion of the body mass of trichinella, trichuris, and capillaria, for example. The function of these cells is not fully understood, and may vary from species to species.

Nematodes excrete solid and fluid wastes. Excretion of solids takes place through the digestive tract. Fluids are eliminated by means of the excretory system, consisting of two or more collecting tubes connected at one end to the ventral gland (a primitive kidney-like organ) and at the other end to the excretory pore.

The adult female nematode has a large portion of her body devoted to reproduction. One or two ovaries lead to the vagina by way of a tubular oviduct and uterus. A seminal receptacle for storage of sperm is connected to the uterus. The male has a single testis connected to the vas deferens, seminal vesicle, ejaculatory duct, and cloaca. In addition, males of many species have specialized structures to aid in transfer of sperm to the female during mating. Their identification is often based on morphology of these structures. Most nematodes lay eggs, but some are viviparous. More about the biology of nematodes will be given within the text for each infectious agent as they are discussed, whenever it relates to the pathogenesis of the disease.

16. *Enterobius vermicularis*
   (Linnaeus 1758)

Introduction

Enterobius vermicularis (pinworm) is the most prevalent nematode infection of humans, its only host. In the United States, pinworm still occurs with one estimate indicating that it may affect up to 40 million individuals or more.[1] It is likely that the prevalence of enterobiasis has diminished considerably over the last decade. In some communities in Europe, the prevalence rates may be as high as 50% in children, especially in the poorer countries of Eastern Europe and the Balkans.[1,2] *Enterobius vermicularis* is mainly an infection of school-aged children, but infections have been diagnosed in the elderly and in certain other populations, such as institutionalized and immunosuppressed individuals.[3-6] Transmission of enterobius is especially frequent in elementary schools and daycare centers.[6] A syndrome of eosinophilic colitis associated with *E. vermicularis* larvae has recently been described, but is notable for not causing a peripheral eosinophilia.[7]

Historical Information

In 1758, Carl Linnaeus named this organism *Enterobius vermicularis*.[8] Later, in 1824, Johann Bremser distinguished this roundworm from the other oxyurid and ascarid nematodes, and provided an accurate description of it that forms the basis for today's modern classification scheme.[9] Pinworm ova have been recovered from human coprolites found in numerous archeological sites, some as old as 10,000 years, and enterobius DNA has been detected in ancient DNA from North and South American human coprolites.[10, 11]

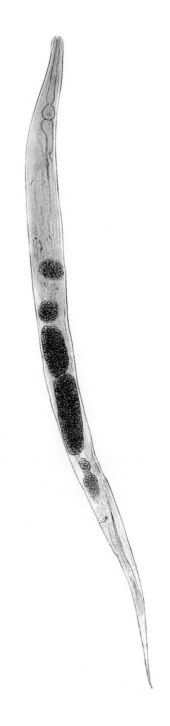

Figure 16.1. Adult female *Enterobius vermicularis*. 10mm.

Enterobius vermicularis

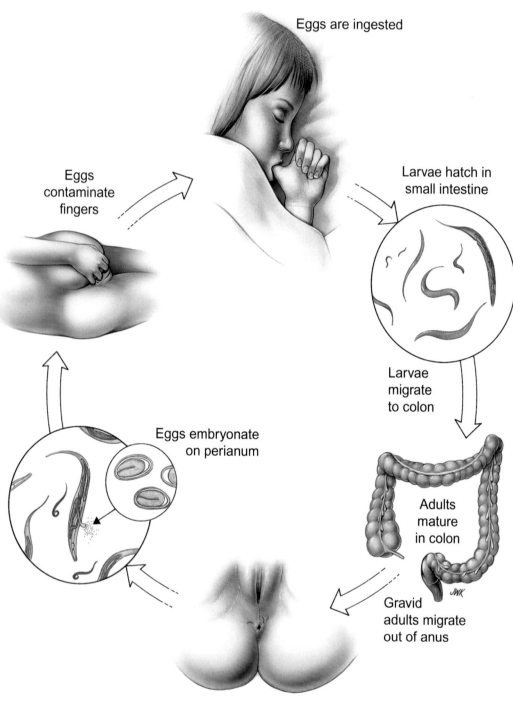

Eggs are ingested

Larvae hatch in
small intestine

Eggs
contaminate
fingers

Larvae
migrate
to colon

Eggs embryonate
on perianum

Adults
mature
in colon

JWK

Gravid
adults migrate
out of anus

Adults lay eggs on perianum

Parasitic Diseases 6th Ed. Parasites Without Borders www.parasiteswithoutborders.com

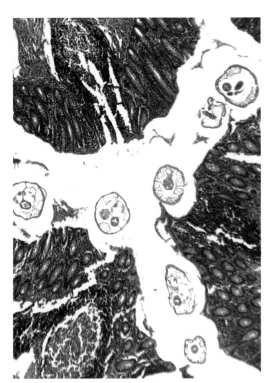

Figure 16.2. Cross sections of adult *E. vermicularis* in appendix.

Life Cycle

The lifecycle of pinworm is one of the simplest among parasites, and has a typical nematode pattern of development; four larval stages (L1-L4), and the adult stage. Adult worms live freely in the lumen of the transverse and descending colon, and in the rectum. The female (Fig. 16.1) measures 8-13 mm in length and 0.3-0.6 mm in width. The male is typically smaller, measuring 2-5 mm by 0.2 mm. The tail of the male contains a single curved copulatory spicule. Adult pinworms feed on our microbiome.

The adult worms mate, and within 6 weeks, each female contains approximately 10,000 fertilized, non-embryonated eggs. Males die shortly after copulation. The gravid female migrates out the anus onto the perianal skin at night, most likely stimulated to do so by the drop in body temperature of the host. There, she experiences a prolapse of the uterus, expels all her eggs, and then dies.

Expulsion can be so intense that the eggs become airborne. The eggs rapidly embryonate and become infective within 6 hours of being laid, exhibiting one of most rapid embryological developmental cycles among all nematode species.

An uncomfortable perianal pruritis develops, called *pruritis ani,* that may be severe enough to cause sleeping disturbance.[12] Scratching of the perianal area can often lead to eggs lodging under the fingernails. Ingestion of these eggs can occur when a child places infective hands into their mouth. The embryonated eggs (Fig. 16.2) are swallowed and hatch as L1 larvae. Once they reach the small intestine, they shed their cuticle (molt) becoming L2 larvae. Development to the third and fourth stages also occurs in the small intestine. L4 larvae feed and then molt, transforming into adults that travel to the large intestine, where they take up residence. (Figure 16.3.) The entire cycle is completed within 4-6 weeks after ingestion of the infectious egg. Alternatively, eggs can hatch on the skin at the site of deposition, and the L2 larvae can crawl back through the anus into the rectum, and eventually the colon, where they develop into reproducing adults. This is referred to as retro-infection.

In female patients, the larvae that hatch on the skin near the anus occasionally crawl into the vagina instead of the rectum, establishing an aberrant infection. Less frequently, gravid parasites infect the fallopian tubes. Aberrant infections also include pelvic peritonitis, ovarian infection, granuloma of the liver, and the appendix.[13-18]

Cellular and Molecular Pathogenesis

All stages of *E. vermicularis* develop in the gut tract, so the host does not experience any systemic reactions unless the worm burden is particularly high, or there is ectopic infection. The parasite elicits a mild, local inflammatory response, and while eosinophilic colitis has

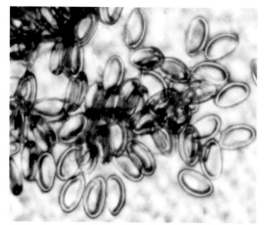

Figure 16.3. Embryonated eggs of *E. vermicularis*.

been described, circulating eosinophilia does not develop[7, 19].

A few patients develop pruritus resulting from allergic responses to worm proteins. Whether pinworm infection causes secondary problems, such as appendicitis or pelvic inflammatory disease, is unclear.[17] Pinworms have been found in these organs at autopsy with no evidence of an inflammatory reaction. In other circumstances, pinworms have been implicated as an appendicolith that might have led to the chain of events leading to clinical appendicitis.[20]

Although there are no comparable studies in humans, experimental evidence has shown that the immune status of the host affects the outcome of the infection. *Syphacia oblevata* is a pinworm species that infects mice only, and reaches much larger numbers in nude (athymic) mice than it does in the same mice into which a subcutaneous implant of thymic tissue from syngeneic donors was introduced.[21] In one unusual case, intense infiltration of the colon with eosinophils and neutrophils led to clinical eosinophilic enteritis in an 18-year old homosexual male who passed numerous *E. vermicularis* larvae. The larvae were definitively identified on the basis of characteristic 28S ribosomal RNA and 5S rRNA spacer genes by PCR.[9] Susceptibility to pinworm infection decreases with age in humans, but the reasons for this are not clear.

It remains to be determined whether this difference in susceptibility has an immunological or physiological basis.

Clinical Disease

The great majority of infected individuals are free of symptoms. Those few who are symptomatic experience intense itching of the perianal area, which in rare instances leads to cellulitis.[22] Aberrant vaginal infection leads to vaginal itching and sometimes serous discharge. Enuresis has been attributed to infection with pinworm, but no causal relation has been established.[23] Gnashing of teeth and sleep disturbances have not been definitely related to the pinworm either. Patients who experience abdominal pain during infection may do so because of co-infection with *Dientamoeba fragilis*. Eosinophilic enteritis caused by *E. vermicularis* can be hemorrhagic and presents with abdominal pain and melena. Rarely, enterobiasis has been linked to clinical appendicitis.[16]

Diagnosis

The infection is usually diagnosed by visualization of pinworm eggs or adult worms. Since eggs are deposited on the perianal skin and not released into feces, stool examination for ova and parasites is of little utility in diagnosing this infection. Eggs are best obtained by harvesting of these from the perianal area using clear (not frosted) adhesive tape or the commercially available adhesive pinworm paddle. The adhesive tape or paddle should be applied to the perianal region in the early hours of the morning as the patient sleeps or as soon as the patient awakens (i.e., before a bath or bowel movement). The tape or paddle is then examined using light microscopy. The characteristic eggs (Figs. 16.2, C.37) can be readily detected in this manner. On occasion, thread like female worms may be directly visible on the perianal skin. These female worms are 8-13mm long and very thin having the appearance of small white pieces of thread. Serologic tests specific for *E. vermicularis* are not used clinically for the diagnosis of this infection.

Adult pinworms can be readily identified when they are seen on histologic sections because of bilateral cuticular projections known as alae. In patients with abdominal pain or other gastrointestinal symptoms, a fecal examination may be necessary to rule out co-infection with other infectious agents. Colonoscopy of a patient with eosinophilic enteritis from *E. vermicularis* showed a purulent discharge from the rectum to the terminal ileum and ulcerations. One patient described with this syndrome was noted to pass larvae instead of eggs or adult worms, which required PCR for identification.[7]

Treatment

Pyrantel pamoate in a single dose [11 mg/kg (max. 1 gram)], or either albendazole (400 mg) or mebendazole (100 mg) in a single dose is the recommended therapy, with improved efficacy approaching 100 percent if a second dose is given two weeks after the first.[24-27] In the United States pyrantel palmoate is an inexpensive and effective over the counter option while treatment with alternative medications, if prescribed by a physician unaware of drug prices, can cost hundreds of dollars. None of these drugs kills the eggs or developing larvae, therefore, "blind" re-treatment is the reason for a second treatment 2 weeks after the original therapy. This second round of therapy destroys worms that have hatched from eggs ingested after the first treatment.[24-27] Since eggs can survive 2 to 3 weeks on clothing, inanimate objects, and bedding reinfection can continue to occur only for this limited period of time

and thus only the one retreatment is usually sufficient. Knowing that the entire cycle takes 4-6 weeks after ingestion of the infectious egg can help with identification of any contacts that might be infected as well as identification of the patient's exposure. Since eggs can survive 2 to 3 weeks before being ingested, the timing of exposure for an infected patient is 1 to 2 months prior to appearance of adult female worms capable of producing infective eggs. Treatment of exposed contacts, all household members, and source patients, if not household members, is recommended and has been successful in both households and institutions. (http://www.cdc.gov/parasites/pinworm/treatment.html)

Prevention and Control

In the young child, infection and reinfection is frequent, because of the ready transmissibility of the pinworm. The groups showing highest prevalence of infection are school children and institutionalized individuals. Compounding the problem is the fact that the eggs can survive for several days under conditions of high humidity and intermediate to low temperatures. There are no predilections on the basis of sex, race, or socioeconomic class.

Thorough washing of hands with soap and water after; using the toilet, changing diapers, or caring for school age children should help to reduce transmission.[3] Trimming of fingernails has been suggested to decrease the possibility of eggs collecting and to reduce the risk of skin breaks in the perianal area from scratching. In institutions, daycare centers, schools, or other areas with pinworm infections, mass treatment during outbreaks can be successful.[28]

References

1.   Burkhart, C. N.; Burkhart, C. G., Assessment of frequency, transmission, and genitourinary complications of enterobiasis (pinworms). *Int J Dermatol* **2005,** *44* (10), 837-40.
2.   Hotez, P. J.; Gurwith, M., Europe's neglected infections of poverty. *Int J Infect Dis* **2011,** *15* (9), e611-9.
3.   Snow, M., Pinning down pinworms. *Nursing* **2006,** *36* (5), 17.
4.   Agholi, M.; Hatam, G. R.; Motazedian, M. H., HIV/AIDS-associated opportunistic protozoal diarrhea. *AIDS Res Hum Retroviruses* **2013,** *29* (1), 35-41.
5.   Schupf, N.; Ortiz, M.; Kapell, D.; Kiely, M.; Rudelli, R. D., Prevalence of intestinal parasite infections among individuals with mental retardation in New York State. *Ment Retard* **1995,** *33* (2), 84-9.
6.   Crawford, F. G.; Vermund, S. H., Parasitic infections in day care centers. *The Pediatric infectious disease journal* **1987,** *6* (8), 744-9.
7.   Liu, L. X.; Chi, J.; Upton, M. P.; Ash, L. R., Eosinophilic colitis associated with larvae of the pinworm Enterobius vermicularis. *Lancet (London, England)* **1995,** *346* (8972), 410-2.
8.   Cox, F. E., History of human parasitology. *Clin Microbiol Rev* **2002,** *15* (4), 595-612.
9.   Bremser, J. G., Oxyure vermiculaire. *In Traite zoologique et physiologique sur les vers intestinaux de lhomme CLF Panchouke Paris pp* **1824,** 149-157.
10.   Horne, P. D., First evidence of enterobiasis in ancient Egypt. *J Parasitol* **2002,** *88* (5), 1019-21.
11.   Iniguez, A. M.; Reinhard, K. J.; Araujo, A.; Ferreira, L. F.; Vicente, A. C., Enterobius vermicularis: ancient DNA from North and South American human coprolites. *Mem Inst Oswaldo Cruz 98 Suppl* **2003,** *1*, 67-9.
12.   Jones, J. E., Pinworms. *Am Fam Physician* **1988,** *38* (3), 159-64.
13.   Pearson, R. D.; Irons, R. P., Chronic pelvic peritonitis due to the pinworm Enterobius vermicularis. *JAMA* **1981,** *245* (13), 1340-1.
14.   Beckman, E. N.; Holland, J. B., Ovarian enterobiasis--a proposed pathogenesis. *The American journal of tropical medicine and hygiene* **1981,** *30* (1), 74-6.
15.   Daly, J. J.; Baker, G. F., Pinworm granuloma of the liver. *The American journal of tropical medicine and hygiene* **1984,** *33* (1), 62-4.
16.   Arca, M. J.; Gates, R. L.; Groner, J. I.; Hammond, S.; Caniano, D. A., Clinical manifestations of appendiceal pinworms in children: an institutional experience and a review of the literature. *Pediatric surgery international* **2004,** *20* (5), 372-5.
17.   Lala, S.; Upadhyay, V., Enterobius vermicularis and its role in paediatric appendicitis: protection or predisposition? *ANZ J Surg* **2016.**
18.   Powell, G.; Sarmah, P.; Sethi, B.; Ganesan, R., Enterobius vermicularis infection of the ovary. *BMJ Case Rep* **2013,** *2013.*
19.   Cacopardo, B.; Onorante, A.; Nigro, L.; Patamia, I.; Tosto, S.; Romano, F.; Zappala, C.; Bruno, S.; Nunnari, A., Eosinophilic ileocolitis by Enterobius vermicularis: a description of two rare cases. *Ital J Gastroenterol Hepatol* **1997,** *29* (1), 51-3.
20.   Ahmed, M. U.; Bilal, M.; Anis, K.; Khan, A. M.; Fatima, K.; Ahmed, I.; Khatri, A. M.; Shafiq ur, R., The Frequency of Enterobius Vermicularis Infections in Patients Diagnosed With Acute Appendicitis in Pakistan. *Glob J Health Sci* **2015,** *7* (5), 196-201.
21.   Jacobson, R. H.; Reed, N. D., The thymus dependency of resistance to pinworm infection in mice. *The Journal of parasitology* **1974,** *60* (6), 976-9.
22.   Ockert, G., [Epidemiology of Dientamoeba fragilis Jepps and Dobell 1918. 1. Spread of the species in child collectives]. *Journal of hygiene, epidemiology, microbiology, and immunology* **1972,** *16* (2), 213-21.
23.   Hotez, P. J., The other intestinal protozoa: enteric infections caused by Blastocystis hominis, Entamoeba coli, and Dientamoeba fragilis. *Sem Pedi Infect Dis* **2000.**
24.   St. Georgiev, V., Opportunistic infections: treatment and developmental therapeutics of cryptosporidiosis and isosporiasis. *Drug Develop Res* **1993,** *28*, 445-59.
25.   Wang, B. R.; Wang, H. C.; Li, L. W.; Zhang, X. L.; Yue, J. Q.; Wang, G. X.; Shi, X. Q.; Xiao, F. R.,

Comparative efficacy of thienpydin, pyrantel pamoate, mebendazole and albendazole in treating ascariasis and enterobiasis. *Chin Med J (Engl)* **1987,** *100* (11), 928-30.

26.   Lormans, J. A.; Wesel, A. J.; Vanparus, O. F., Mebendazole (R 17635) in enterobiasis. A clinical trial in mental retardates. *Chemotherapy* **1975,** *21* (3-4), 255-60.

27.   St Georgiev, V., Chemotherapy of enterobiasis (oxyuriasis). *Expert Opin Pharmacother* **2001,** *2* (2), 267-75.

28.   Ashford, R. W.; Hart, C. A.; Williams, R. G., Enterobius vermicularis infection in a children's ward. *J Hosp Infect* **1988,** *12* (3), 221-4.

17. *Trichuris trichiura*
(Linnaeus 1771)

Introduction

Trichuris trichiura, commonly known as "whipworm" because of its characteristic shape, is one of the three major soil-transmitted helminths (STHs) that cause serious morbidity in developing countries.[1-4] Trichuris infection is frequently coincident with infections caused by the other STHs, *Ascaris lumbricoides* and the hookworms. The prevalence of trichuriasis is approximately 477 million worldwide, with the largest numbers of infections in Asia, Sub-Saharan Africa, and the tropical regions of the Americas.[5] Whether or not trichuriasis still occurs in the southeastern region of the United States is unknown.[1-3, 6]

T. trichiura has no reservoir hosts. Other species of trichuris infect a wide range of mammals (e.g., *T. vulpis* in caenidae, *T. muris* in the mouse, *T. suis* in the pig). Worm burdens due to trichuris are usually higher in children than in adults, and disease is consequently more severe in that age group.[6] School-aged children are particularly affected. Heavily infected children often go on to develop colitis and stunted growth, and those with chronic infections can even develop intellectual and cognitive deficits.[6, 7]

Historical Information

In 1740, Giovanni Morgagni accurately described the location of *T. trichiura* in the cecum and transverse colon.[8] In 1761, a report by Johannes Roederer, depicted the external morphology of *T. trichiura*.[9] Roederer's report was accompanied by scientific renderings that are still deemed highly accurate. Carl Linnaeus classified this parasite, then called "teretes," as a nematode in 1771.[10] Finding the petrified, characteristic eggs in coprolites of prehistoric humans has identified human

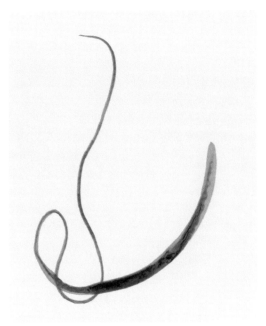

Figure 17.1. Adult female *Trichuris trichiura*.

infection with trichuris as a pathogen infecting humans for over 5,000 years.[10]

Life Cycle

The adult female (Fig. 17.1) measures 30-50 mm, while the male (Fig. 17.2) is 30-45 mm in length. Infection begins when the embryonated egg (Fig. 17.3) is swallowed. The L1 larva hatches in the small intestine, penetrates the columnar epithelium, and comes to lie just above the lamina propria.

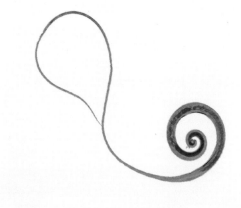

Figure 17.2. Adult male *Trichuris trichiura*.

Trichuris trichiura

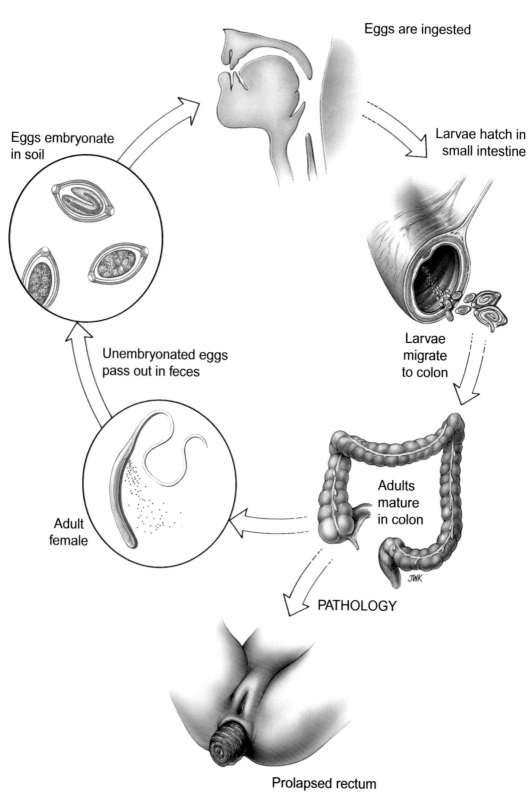

Eggs are ingested

Larvae hatch in small intestine

Larvae migrate to colon

Eggs embryonate in soil

Unembryonated eggs pass out in feces

Adults mature in colon

Adult female

PATHOLOGY

Prolapsed rectum

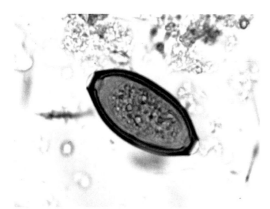

Figure 17.3. Fertilized, non-embryonated egg of *T. trichiura*. 50 μm x 20 μm.

Four molts later, the immature adult emerges, is passively carried to the large intestine, where it re-embeds itself in the columnar cells, and then induces its essential niche. Adult *Trichuris trichiura* live in the transverse and descending colon (Fig 17.4). The anterior, narrow, elongate esophagus is embedded within a syncytium of host cells created by the worm. This syncytium probably results from exposure of the host to worm secretions emanating from its stichosome. The posterior abdomen protrudes into the lumen, allowing eggs to escape. Nothing is known about the nutritional requirements of this parasite, but experimental evidence on related species suggests that they do not ingest blood.[11] The parasites grow and mature in the large intestine, where mating also occurs.

Patency (i.e., the first time eggs are detectable in the feces) is about 90 days following the time of ingestion of embryonated eggs. Females can produce up to 3,000-5,000 eggs per day, and are live for 1.5-2.0 years.[12, 13] Fertilized eggs are deposited in soil with feces, and must embryonate in the soil before becoming infectious. Environmental factors, including high humidity, sandy or loamy soil, and a warm temperature (20-30° C), favor rapid development of the embryo.[14] Under optimal conditions, embryonic development takes place over an 18-22 day period.[15]

Cellular and Molecular Pathogenesis

In trichuris-endemic areas, pediatric populations, typically harbor the largest whipworm burdens, with highest burdens in children between age 5-15 years. It is not known why these heavy worm burdens diminish in older age groups. Some studies indicate that susceptibility to heavy trichuris infections may depend on an inability to mount a strong T helper cell type 2 response.[16] There also appears to be a genetic component to susceptibility.[17]

The presence of adult whipworms in the large intestine induces structural defects in the epithelium.[18] In order to invade the colonic mucosa, adult trichuris release a novel pore-forming and channel-forming protein.[19] *In vitro*, these secreted proteins induce ion-conducting pores in lipid bilayers. Pore formation in epithelial cell membranes may facilitate invasion and enable the parasite to maintain its syncytial environment in the cecal epithelium. Genes encoding these novel proteins are comprised of repeats.[20]

Despite the immunomodulatory capacity of adult trichuris, in some cases, a low-grade inflammatory response to the presence of the adults can occur, together with the upregulation of inflammatory biomarkers and a clinical picture resembling inflammatory bowel

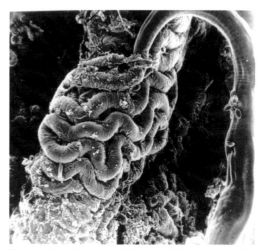

Figure 17.4. Scanning EM of adult trichuris, *in situ*. Courtesy K. Wright.

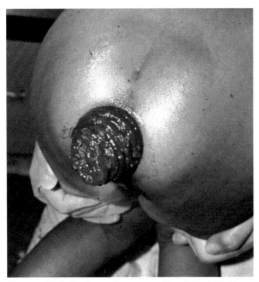

Figure 17.5. Prolapsed rectum with adult *T. trichiura*.

disease (IBD) of ulcerative colitis or Crohn's disease can occur.[21] The latter conditions are characterized by more extensive histopathologic damage to the gut. With heavy infections, the population of whipworms may extend from the proximal to the terminal end of the ileum and cause ileitis. Anemia results from a combination of capillary damage and erosion leading to blood loss and anemia of chronic inflammation.[21] Generally, the anemia resulting from heavy infection with *T. trichiura* is much less severe than hookworm-related anemia.

In contrast to situations where there is a low-grade inflammation, immunomodulatory effects of adult trichuris can predominate. Ironically these features of the whipworm have been exploited to develop a novel treatment for Crohn's disease. Ingestion of embryonated eggs of the porcine whipworm *T. suis* have been shown to reduce the symptoms of Crohn's disease for short periods of time without significant adverse effects on the patient.[22, 23] The precise mechanism of how *T. suis* reduces host inflammation is still being actively studied, but current evidence suggests that *T. suis* shifts the immune system from a Th1 to a Th2 response and changes the levels of certain cytokines, possibly in part

through changes in the gut microbiome.[24, 25] Research suggests that excreted/secreted products affect intestinal epithelium, macrophage, and dendritic cells and suppress the pro-inflammatory cytokine production by these cells.[26, 27]

Clinical Disease

Clinical disease occurs mainly in children.[28] Those with very heavy trichuris infections can either present with dysentery or with chronic colitis. Trichuris-induced dysentery results in weight loss, emaciation, and anemia. Because of the extensive mucosal swelling of the rectum, the urge to strain as if feces were present (tenesmus) can occur. Protracted tenesmus can lead to rectal prolapse (Fig. 17.5).[18]

Chronic trichuris colitis in pediatric patients can resemble characteristics of better-known forms of inflammatory bowel disease, such as Crohn's disease and ulcerative colitis. Children suffering from heavy trichuriasis develop chronic malnutrition, short stature, anemia, and finger clubbing.[18] Following specific chemotherapy, many of these conditions abate, often resulting in rapid catch-up growth.

Increasing evidence suggests that in addition to the physical symptoms of trichuriasis, chronic infection can also produce long-term deficits in child cognitive and intellectual development.[7] The mechanism by which this occurs is not yet known.

Diagnosis

Trichuris eggs have a characteristic appearance and are easily identified. In cases of light infection, the concentration of feces prior to microscopic examination may be required to identify the eggs. Charcot-Leyden crystals in the stool should lead to further examination even in the absence of identifying eggs on a first stool examination. A search for pathogenic protozoa, such as *Entamoeba histolytica* or *Giardia lamblia,* is indicated in given the high frequency of multiple infections. While identification of trichuris eggs is relatively easy, finding giardia or entamoeba is more difficult, and requires an experienced microscopist. Adult trichuris worms can also be identified by direct visualization on colonoscopy.[29] When doubt exists, it is reasonable to treat the patient for trichuris infection and request expert advice if the patient's symptoms do not abate. Failure to control diarrhea after trichuris is eradicated mandates a more thorough evaluation of other causes of diarrhea. Stool cultures should be used to determine the possible presence of enteric prokaryotic or viral pathogens. In histologic preparations, trichuris adults can be readily identified by the characteristic variability of their diameter in different sections.

Treatment

A benzimidazole — mebendazole or albendazole — is the treatment of choice for trichuriasis.[1] The primary mechanism of these drugs is to inhibit microtubule polymerization by affinity binding to the unique beta-tubulin of invertebrates. Although most global anthelminthic de-worming programs rely on using a single dose of either drug, several doses are usually required for cure of trichuriasis.[30] Alternatively, trichuris de-worming can sometimes be improved by adding either ivermectin or oxantel.[31] In Africa it is currently common to combine albendazole with ivermectin in programs that simultaneously target intestinal helminth infections including trichuriasis and lymphatic filariasis or onchocerciasis.[32]

Both albendazole and mebendazole have an excellent safety profile in children. In the doses used to treat soil-transmitted helminth (STH) infections, neither drug causes significant systemic toxicity in routine use, although transient abdominal pain, diarrhea, nausea and dizziness have been reported. Long-term use has been associated with bone marrow suppression, alopecia and hepatotoxicity. There is a single report that in children with asymptomatic trichuriasis, albendazole resulted in impaired growth, although this observation has not been confirmed in other studies.[28]

Mebendazole and albendazole are teratogenic and embryotoxic in pregnant laboratory rats at doses of 10 mg/kg. In view of these findings, the World Health Organization recommends use of these drugs in pregnancy only after the first trimester and when the benefits of de-worming to the health of the mother and unborn fetus outweigh the risks. In anticipation of using mebendazole and albendazole among large pediatric populations in developing countries, the WHO convened an informal consultation on their use in children under the age of 2.[33] From this it was concluded that the incidence of side effects are likely to be the same in this population as in older children, and that both agents could be used to treat children as young as 12 months using reduced dosages.

Prevention and Control

Trichuris trichiura infection is common in tropical areas, where prevalence as high as 80% has been documented. Most infections are light and asymptomatic. Warm, moist soils in tropical and subtropical regions favor the maintenance of eggs, which can remain alive for months under these optimum conditions. As with ascaris eggs, exposure of *T. trichiura* eggs to direct sunlight for 12 hours or exposure to temperatures in excess of 40° C for 1 hour kills the embryo inside the egg. Eggs are relatively resistant to chemical disinfectants, and can survive for protracted periods of time in raw or treated sewage. Proper disposal of feces is the primary means of prevention. In areas of the world where untreated human feces is used to fertilize crops, control of this infection is impossible.

Because school-aged children typically harbor the heaviest trichuris (and ascaris) infections, and specific anthelmintic chemotherapy with either albendazole or mebendazole can result in catch-up growth and improved cognition for heavily-infected individuals, these agents have been used in school-based programs throughout the developing world.[6, 34, 35] In 2001, the World Health Assembly passed a resolution that recommended its member states administer single dose albendazole and mebendazole on a frequent and periodic basis (1-3 times per year) in order to control STH (ascaris, trichuris, hookworm) morbidity. Because school-aged children contribute the most to trichuris and ascaris transmission in the community, there is also some optimism that widespread treatment could theoretically interrupt transmission. High rates of post-treatment soil-transmitted helminth re-infection require that children must be treated at least on an annual basis. While there are clear health and educational benefits for school-based intervention, there are concerns that single doses of albendazole or mebendazole are often not sufficient to cure trichuris infections, so that addition of ivermectin or oxantel maybe warranted.

References

1. Keiser, J.; Utzinger, J., Efficacy of current drugs against soil-transmitted helminth infections: systematic review and meta-analysis. *JAMA* **2008**, *299* (16), 1937-48.

2. Bethony, J.; Brooker, S.; Albonico, M.; Geiger, S. M.; Loukas, A.; Diemert, D.; Hotez, P. J., Soil-transmitted helminth infections: ascariasis, trichuriasis, and hookworm. *Lancet* **2006**, *367* (9521), 1521-32.

3. Lammie, P. J.; Fenwick, A.; Utzinger, J., A blueprint for success: integration of neglected tropical disease control programmes. *Trends Parasitol* **2006**, *22* (7), 313-21.

4. Webster, J. P.; Molyneux, D. H.; Hotez, P. J.; Fenwick, A., The contribution of mass drug administration to global health: past, present and future. *Philos Trans R Soc Lond B Biol Sci* **2014**, *369* (1645), 20130434.

5. Global Burden of Disease Study, C., Global, regional, and national incidence, prevalence, and years lived with disability for 301 acute and chronic diseases and injuries in 188 countries, 1990-2013: a systematic analysis for the Global Burden of Disease Study 2013. *Lancet* **2015**, *386* (9995), 743-800.

6. Piraja de Silva, M. A., Contribucao para o estudo da schistosomiasena Bahia. *Brazil Med* **1908**, *2* 281-283.

7. Cooper, E. S.; Bundy, D. A., Trichuris is not trivial. *Parasitology today (Personal ed.)* **1988**, *4* (11), 301-6.

8. Nokes, C.; Grantham-McGregor, S. M.; Sawyer, A. W.; Cooper, E. S.; Robinson, B. A.; Bundy, D. A., Moderate to heavy infections of Trichuris trichiura affect cognitive function in Jamaican school children. *Parasitology* **1992**, *104 (Pt 3)*, 539-47.

9. Morgagni, G. B.; Anatomica, X. I. V., Epistolarum anatomicarum duodeviginti ad script pertinentium celeberrimi yin Antonii Marie Valsalvae pars Altera. *Epistola Apud Franciscum Pitheri Venice* **1740**.

10. Cox, F. E., History of human parasitology. *Clin Microbiol Rev* **2002**, *15* (4), 595-612.

11. Roederer, J. G., Nachrichten von der Trichuriden, der Societat der Wissenschaften in Gottingen. *Gottingische Anzeigen von gelebrten Sachen Unter der Aufsicht der Konigliche Gesellschaft der Wissenschaften Part* **1761**, *25*, 243-245.

12. Pike, E. H., Bionomics, blood and 51Cr: investigations of Trichuris muris and studies with two related species. *Doctoral dissertation Columbia University pp* **1963**, 1-207.

13. Brown, H. W.; West, D., The Whipworm of Man (Seminar) (Vol 16). Merck Sharp & PA, pp. **1954**, 19-22.

14. Belding, D.; New, M., Textbook of Parasitology. *pp* **1965**, 397-398.

15. Brown, H. W., Studies on the rate of development and viability of the eggs of Ascaris lumbricoides and Trichuris trichiura under field conditions. *Parasitology* **1927**, *14*, 1-15.

16. Jackson, J. A.; Turner, J. D.; Rentoul, L.; Faulkner, H.; Behnke, J. M.; Hoyle, M.; Grencis, R. K.; Else, K. J.; Kamgno, J.; Boussinesq, M.; Bradley, J. E., T helper cell type 2 responsiveness predicts future susceptibility to gastrointestinal nematodes in humans. *The Journal of infectious diseases* **2004**, *190* (10), 1804-11.

17. Williams-Blangero, S.; McGarvey, S. T.; Subedi, J.; Wiest, P. M.; Upadhayay, R. P.; Rai, D. R.; Jha, B.; Olds, G. R.; Guanling, W.; Blangero, J., Genetic component to susceptibility to Trichuris trichiura: evidence from two Asian populations. *Genetic epidemiology* **2002**, *22* (3), 254-64.

18. MacDonald, T. T.; Choy, M. Y.; Spencer, J.; Richman, P. I.; Diss, T.; Hanchard, B.; Venugopal, S.; Bundy, D. A.; Cooper, E. S., Histopathology and immunohistochemistry of the caecum in children with the Trichuris dysentery syndrome. *Journal of clinical pathology* **1991**, *44* (3), 194-9.

19. Drake, L.; Korchev, Y.; Bashford, L.; Djamgoz, M.; Wakelin, D.; Ashall, F.; Bundy, D., The major secreted product of the whipworm, Trichuris, is a pore-forming protein. *Proceedings. Biological sciences / The Royal Society* **1994**, *257* (1350), 255-61.

20. Bennett, A. B.; Barker, G. C.; Bundy, D. A., A beta-tubulin gene from Trichuris trichiura. *Molecular and biochemical parasitology* **1999**, *103* (1), 111-6.

21. Bundy, D. A.; Cooper, E. S., Trichuris and trichuriasis in humans. *Advances in parasitology* **1989**, *28*, 107-73.

22. Summers, R. W.; Elliott, D. E.; Urban, J. F.; Thompson, R.; Weinstock, J. V., Trichuris suis therapy in Crohn's disease. *Gut* **2005**, *54* (1), 87-90.

23. Sandborn, W. J.; Elliott, D. E.; Weinstock, J.; Summers, R. W.; Landry-Wheeler, A.; Silver, N.; Harnett, M. D.; Hanauer, S. B., Randomised clinical trial: the safety and tolerability of Trichuris suis ova in patients with Crohn's disease. *Aliment Pharmacol Ther* **2013**, *38* (3), 255-63.

24. Reddy, A.; Fried, B., The use of Trichuris suis and other helminth therapies to treat Crohn's disease. *Parasitol Res* **2007**, *100* (5), 921-7.

25. Ramanan, D.; Bowcutt, R.; Lee, S. C.; Tang, M. S.; Kurtz, Z. D.; Ding, Y.; Honda, K.; Gause, W. C.; Blaser, M. J.; Bonneau, R. A.; Lim, Y. A.; Loke, P.; Cadwell, K., Helminth infection promotes colonization resistance via type 2 immunity. *Science* **2016**, *352* (6285), 608-12.

26. Hiemstra, I. H.; Klaver, E. J.; Vrijland, K.; Kringel, H.; Andreasen, A.; Bouma, G.; Kraal, G.; van Die, I.; den Haan, J. M., Excreted/secreted Trichuris suis products reduce barrier function and suppress inflammatory cytokine production of intestinal epithelial cells. *Mol Immunol* **2014**, *60* (1), 1-7.

27. Ottow, M. K.; Klaver, E. J.; van der Pouw Kraan, T. C.; Heijnen, P. D.; Laan, L. C.; Kringel, H.; Vogel, D. Y.; Dijkstra, C. D.; Kooij, G.; van Die, I., The helminth Trichuris suis suppresses TLR4-induced inflammatory responses in human macrophages. *Genes Immun* **2014**, *15* (7), 477-86.

28. Gilman, R. H.; Chong, Y. H.; Davis, C.; Greenberg, B.; Virik, H. K.; Dixon, H. B., The adverse consequences of heavy Trichuris infection. *Transactions of the Royal Society of Tropical Medicine and Hygiene* **1983**, *77* (4), 432-8.

29. Joo, J. H.; Ryu, K. H.; Lee, Y. H.; Park, C. W.; Cho, J. Y.; Kim, Y. S.; Lee, J. S.; Lee, M. S.; Hwang, S. G.; Shim, C. S., Colonoscopic diagnosis of whipworm infection. *Hepato-gastroenterology* **1998**, *45* (24), 2105-9.

30. Sirivichayakul, C.; Pojjaroen-Anant, C.; Wisetsing, P.; Praevanit, R.; Chanthavanich, P.; Limkittikul, K., The effectiveness of 3, 5 or 7 days of albendazole for the treatment of Trichuris trichiura infection. *Annals of tropical medicine and parasitology* **2003**, *97* (8), 847-53.

31. Speich, B.; Ame, S. M.; Ali, S. M.; Alles, R.; Huwyler, J.; Hattendorf, J.; Utzinger, J.; Albonico, M.; Keiser, J., Oxantel pamoate-albendazole for Trichuris trichiura infection. *N Engl J Med* **2014**, *370* (7), 610-20.

32. Hotez, P. J., Mass drug administration and integrated control for the world's high-prevalence neglected tropical diseases. *Clin Pharmacol Ther* **2009**, *85* (6), 659-64.

33. Montresor, A.; Awasthi, S.; Crompton, D. W. T., Use of benzimidazoles in children younger than 24 months for the treatment of soil-transmitted helminthiasis. *Acta tropica* **2003**, *86* (2-3), 223-32.

34. Nokes, C.; Grantham-McGregor, S. M.; Sawyer, A. W.; R., Moderate to high infections of Trichuris trichiura and cognitive function in Jamaican school children. *Proc* **1991,** *247*, 77-81.

35. Albonico, M.; Engels, D.; Savioli, L., Monitoring drug efficacy and early detection of drug resistance in human soil-transmitted nematodes: a pressing public health agenda for helminth control. *International journal for parasitology* **2004,** *34* (11), 1205-10.

18. *Ascaris lumbricoides*
(Linnaeus, 1758)

Introduction

Ascaris lumbricoides is one of the largest nematodes to infect humans. The adult lives in the small intestine where it can grow to a length of more than 30 cm. This worm infection is found almost wherever poverty occurs in developing countries. Current estimates indicate that over 800 million people are infected.[1-3] The most severe consequences of ascaris infection occur in children who are predisposed to suffer from heavier worm burdens than adults living under similar conditions. Ascaris eggs thrive in warm, moist soil, and are highly resistant to a variety of environmental conditions. The eggs can survive in the sub-arctic regions.[4] In some developing countries, ascaris eggs are ubiquitous, and have been recovered on a wide variety of environmental surfaces including poorly washed hands. Ascaris eggs have even been isolated from the paper currency.[5, 6] The ability of ascaris eggs to survive in these harsh

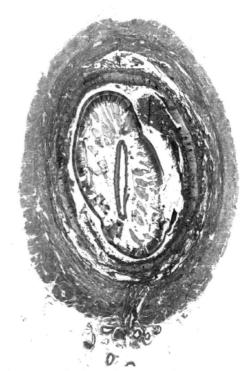

Figure 18.2. Adult ascaris in appendix.

environments accounts for the urban transmission of ascariasis in large cities.

It is controversial as to whether pigs can serve as an animal reservoir for *A. lumbricoides*, or whether the related parasite, *Ascaris suum*, is also transmissible to humans.[7] It has been suggested that human infection arose in association with pig domestication, possibly in China.[8] However, the available evidence suggests that ascaris in humans and pigs comprise reproductively isolated populations, suggesting that zoonotic transmission is not common.[8]

Historical Information

In 1683, Edward Tyson described the anatomy of *A. lumbricoides*, then known as *Lumbricus teres*.[9] Carl Linnaeus gave it its current name on the basis of its remarkable similarity to the earth-worm, *Lumbricus terrestrias*, which he also named.[10] The worm's life cycle was accurately described by Brayton Ransom.[11] In 1922, Shimesu Koino

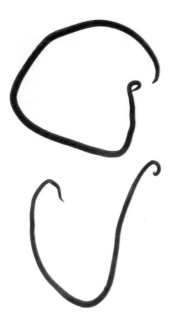

Figure 18.1. Adult female (upper) and male (lower) *Ascaris lumbricoides*. 13-18 cm in length.

Ascaris lumbricoides

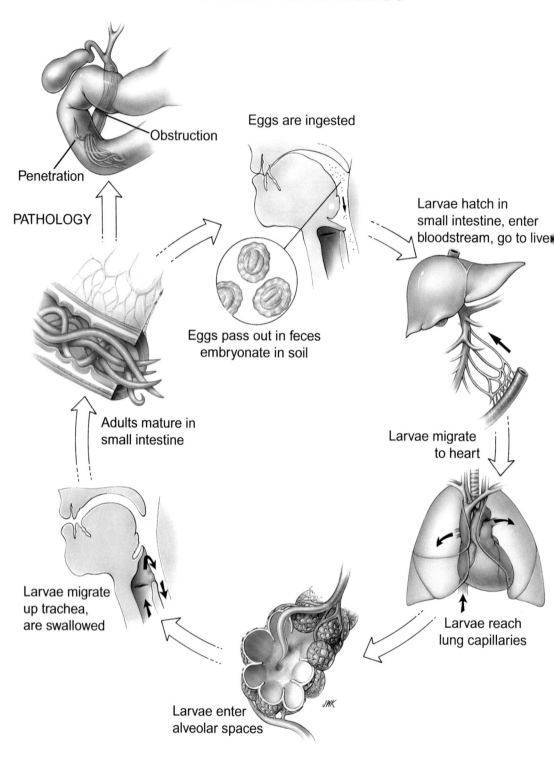

Eggs are ingested

Obstruction

Penetration

PATHOLOGY

Eggs pass out in feces
embryonate in soil

Larvae hatch in
small intestine, enter
bloodstream, go to liver

Adults mature in
small intestine

Larvae migrate
to heart

Larvae migrate
up trachea,
are swallowed

Larvae reach
lung capillaries

Larvae enter
alveolar spaces

JWK

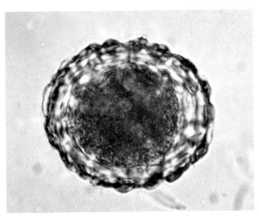

Figure 18.3. Fertilized, unembryonated egg of *A. lumbricoides*. 60 µm x 40 µm

reported on a series of experiments, in which he infected both himself and his younger brother.[12] For his brother, Koino chose to use *A. suum* eggs, instead of *A. lumbricoides* eggs. The pig ascarid usually fails to complete its life cycle in humans, thus sparing the younger Koino from an overwhelming infection. It is now known that in some cases, *A. suum* in humans can result in the development of adult worms.[12] The older Koino brother gave himself 500 *A. lumbricoides* eggs, and demonstrated that a pneumonia-like syndrome developed during the early phase of the infection, caused by L3 larvae migrating through the lungs on their way to the stomach. The older Koino became seriously ill, but did not suffer permanent disability.

Life Cycle

The adult worms (Figs. 18.1, 18.2) occupy the lumen of the upper small intestine, where they live off predigested food, or chyme, as well as host cellular debris. The worms maintain themselves in the lumen of the small intestine by assuming an S-shaped configuration, pressing their cuticular surfaces against the columnar epithelium of the intestine, and continually moving against the peristalsis. The worms are covered with a tough, thick cuticle composed of collagens and unusual lipids, enabling them to successfully resist

being digested by hydrolases. The adult worms produce a battery of protease inhibitors, some of which may also interfere with host digestion.

The egg production of the adult female worm is prolific, producing, on average, 200,000 eggs per day, each of which can survive up to 10 years in the right conditions.[13] Her uterus may contain up to 27 million eggs at any one time. To synthesize the amount of sterol necessary for massive egg production, ascaris possesses a special biochemical pathway to carry out this oxygen-dependent reaction in the low-oxygen folds of the small intestine. It assembles the components of the reaction on a special oxygen-avid hemoglobin.[14] Since ascaris is probably an obligate anaerobe, its hemoglobin might actually serve to detoxify its environment by removing oxygen through a unique chemical coupling with nitric oxide.[15, 16]

Fertilized eggs (Fig. 18.3) pass out of the adult, but they are not yet embryonated. Eggs become incorporated into the fecal mass and exit the host in feces. Embryonation takes place outside the host in soil, and is completed by week 2-4 after being deposited there. Eggs not reaching soil immediately (e.g., municipal sewage sludge) can survive in moist environments for up to 2 months.[17] A unique lipoprotein, known as ascaroside, occupies a portion of the inner layer of the egg, and may confer a number of the environmental resistance properties attributed to ascaris eggs. A second mucopolysaccharide component on the ova's surface provides adhesive properties, allowing them to accumulate on various environmental surfaces. Embryonated eggs must be swallowed for the life cycle to continue. The L1 larva develops into the L2 larva inside the egg, but the worm retains the L2 cuticle around its body.

In the host, the L2 larva is stimulated to hatch by a combination of alkaline conditions in the small intestine, and the solubilization of certain outer layers of the eggshell, facilitated by bile salts. These conditions induce a worm-specific proteolytic enzyme, facilitating hatching. The egg protease is activated by alkaline conditions, insuring that it will hatch in the right anatomic location inside the host. The infectious process is accompanied by a dramatic shift in ascaris metabolism from aerobic to anaerobic.[18]

The immature parasite, now in the intestinal lumen, penetrates the intestinal wall, enters the lamina propria, penetrates a capillary, and is carried by the portal circulation to the liver. In the liver, the worm feeds on parenchymal (*foie gras d'homme*) tissue and grows (Fig. 18.4.). It then migrates via the bloodstream to the heart, and into the pulmonary circulation. The larva molts once more and grows larger, both in length and in diameter. It becomes stuck in an alveolar capillary, since its diameter is now much greater than that of the vessel's. The worm receives a thigmotactic (touch) signal, initiating a behavior that results in its breaking out into the alveolar spaces (Fig. 18.5.). This is the phase of the infection that caused Koino to experience "*verminous*" pneumonia.

The larva migrates up the bronchi into the trachea and across the epiglottis; it is swallowed, finally reaching the lumen of the small intestine for a second time. There, after two additional molts, the worms grow prodigiously, maturing to adulthood in about 6 weeks. Adult worms then mate. Occasionally,

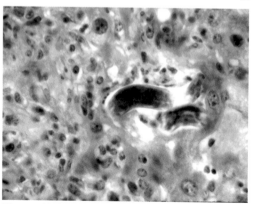

Figure 18.4. Larvae of *A. lumbricoides* in liver of experimentally infected mouse.

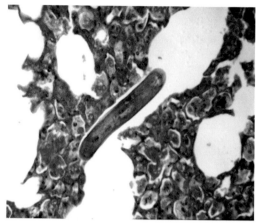

Figure 18.5. Larva of *A. lumbricoides* in lung of an experimentally infected mouse.

egg production may precede mating. When this occurs, the worm releases infertile eggs. Rarely, a single female worm is acquired, also resulting in infertile egg production.

Cellular and Molecular Pathogenesis

The most intense host reactions occur during the migratory phase of infection. Ascaris antigens released during the molting process have allergenic properties that cause inflammation associated with eosinophilic infiltration of the tissues, peripheral eosinophilia, and an antibody response leading to an increase in serum immunoglobulin E (IgE) levels. At least one of these allergens is known as ABA-1. It has been suggested that IgE responses to ABA-1 and related antigens confer resistance to ascaris infections.[19] Because of the links between IgE levels, eosinophilia and ascaris infections, a number of hypotheses have been made to examine the impact of helminth infections such as ascariasis on the atopic state of the host. Among them is the notion that atopy evolved as an adaptive mechanism to promote resistance to helminths.[20] Through the above mechanisms, ascaris larvae trigger allergic responses in the lungs that resemble the pathogenesis of asthma.[21] Both processes may be linked to polymorphisms of the β-2-adrenoreceptor gene.[22] In addition, ascaris adults secrete an anti-trypsin factor that enables it to ingest a portion of any meal before it is absorbed by the host. In-depth proteomic studies of the excretory/secretory products produced by *A. lumbricoides* and *A. suum* are not only helping to improve our understanding of how this helminth influences the host, but may also serve as targets for vaccine development.[23]

School-aged children are predisposed to heavy infections with ascaris, although the reason for this remains unclear. Many of the same children also harbor large numbers of *Trichuris trichiura*. Such children may suffer from impairments in their physical growth and cognitive and intellectual development.[24] It has been hypothesized that ascaris interferes with host nutrition, possibly through competition for nutrients, but this hypothesis is as yet unproven. Other studies indicate that ascaris-infected children can develop malabsorption of fat, protein and vitamin A, lactose intolerance from damaged intestinal mucosa, impaired intestinal permeability, and anorexia.[25] It has been further hypothesized that chronic intestinal inflammation leads to anorexia and cachexia, although there is no strong evidence for this. There have been a number of longitudinal studies in Asia and Africa comparing the growth of ascaris-infected children to that of children given anthelminthics, with most studies showing a significant improvement in weight after treatment.[26] In some of these studies, children who were treated also had a greater increase in height compared to those untreated. The effects on growth were more pronounced in children with the heaviest infections. Additional studies also suggest that ascaris may impair mental processing.[27]

Clinical Disease

Migratory Phase

The intensity of the systemic response to the larva of ascaris is directly related to the number of worms migrating at any one time. If infection is light, and only a few parasites traverse the tissues, the host response is negligible, and infected individuals remain asymptomatic. In heavy infections, such as after ingestion of hundreds to thousands of eggs, the patient can experience intense pneumonitis, enlargement of the liver, and generalized toxicity that may last up to two weeks. The pneumonitis, known as Löeffler's syndrome, presents with eosinophilic infiltrates, an elevated IgE, and bronchospasm that clinically resembles asthma. Similar phenomena have also been described among uninfected laboratory workers who develop bronchospasm after previous sensitization to ascaris allergens.[20]

Intestinal Phase

Although adult worms in the intestine usually cause few symptoms, when they are numerous their sheer bulk may cause fullness and even obstruction. Adult worms migrate when they are irritated (high fevers, drugs, etc.), which may lead them to perforate the intestine, penetrate the liver, obstruct the biliary tract, or cause peritonitis. Individuals with mild and moderate infections are rarely symptomatic. Most commonly, these individuals become aware of the infection through casual examination of the stools for another reason, because of passage of an adult worm in the stool, or by regurgitation of it during an episode of vomiting. Heavy infections may lead to the formation of a large bolus of adults that obstructs the intestinal lumen, especially the ileum (Figs. 18.6, 18.7). In developing countries throughout the tropics, acute ascaris intestinal obstruction is a leading cause of a "surgical abdomen" in children, accounting for up to 35% of all intestinal obstruction in these regions, and 10,000 deaths annually.[27,28]

Hepatobiliary Ascariasis (HPA)

Adult worms may migrate into the biliary tree, causing hepatobiliary and pancreatic ascariasis. This problem occurs more commonly in small children who harbor large numbers of worms. Migration of adult worms into the hepatobiliary tree can lead to cholecystitis, cholangitis, hepatic abscess, pancreatitis, and death may ensue.[29, 30] An ultrasound screen of the general population in Kashmir, India determined that 0.5% of the adults in this region had evidence of hepatobiliary ascariasis.[30]

Neonatal Ascariasis

Neonatal ascariasis may occur when ascaris larvae enter the placenta.[31, 32] Although transplacental transmission is common among animal ascarids, the true extent of this phenomenon among humans is not known.

Diagnosis

A. lumbricoides infection cannot be specifically diagnosed solely on the basis of

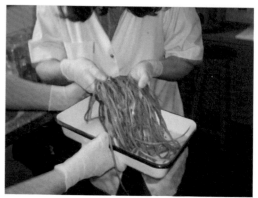

Figure 18.7. Adult ascaris recovered from child in Fig. 18.6. after treatment with mebendazole.

signs or symptoms during the migratory or intestinal phases of the infection. Hepatobiliary ascariasis is difficult to diagnose by conventional radiographic techniques, as the worms often move out of the bile or pancreatic duct after eliciting symptoms. In some endemic areas, ultrasonography and endoscopic retrograde cholangiopancreatography (ERCP) have been used diagnostically.[29, 30, 33] The clinical suspicion of infection with intestinal helminths is the usual reason to request a stool examination.

Ascaris eggs (Figs. 18.3, Fig. C.39) are easily recognized on stool examination. If only a few eggs are present, they may be missed, but can be identified if the stool specimen is concentrated by any of several standard techniques (see Appendix C). Since so many eggs are passed each day by individual female worms the likelihood of finding them, even in patients with light infections, is high. The presence of infertile ascaris eggs is diagnostically significant, as the presence of even a single female worm may have serious clinical consequences if it were to migrate. Occasionally, defective eggs missing the outer mamillations are observed. Serological tests to detect antibodies to *A. lumbricoides* are available but are generally only used in epidemiological studies rather than clinically due to concerns with cost and specificity.[34-36] While available for other helminths, antigen tests are not available for *A. lumbricoides*,

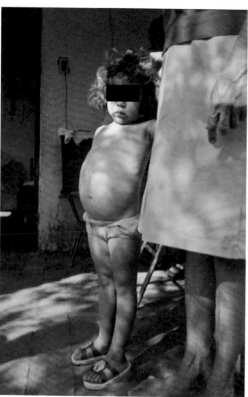

Figure 18.6. Child with distended abdomen due to large bolus of *A. lumbricoides* adult worms in small intestines.

but molecular tests have been developed with sensitivities high enough to detect a single ascaris egg.[37]

Treatment

Albendazole and mebendazole are the treatments of choice for ascariasis.[38, 39] For school-based de-worming programs, usually a single dose of albendazole (400 mg) or mebendazole (500 mg) is effective. The older drug pyrantel pamoate is also effective. Piperazine citrate can be used in cases of intestinal obstruction because it paralyzes the worm's myoneural junctions, allowing them to be expelled by peristalsis, although this drug is no longer widely available. The migratory (parenteral) phase of the infection is transitory, seldom diagnosed, and not typically treated. If infection is heavy, a pneumonia-like syndrome may alert the physician, and patients may be treated symptomatically with corticosteroids.[40]

Surgical intervention is sometimes necessary if a large number of worms result in an intestinal or biliary obstruction. These conditions often present as a medical emergency due to anaerobic necrosis of intestinal tissue. In some cases the adult worms can be removed endoscopically.

Prevention and Control

A. lumbricoides is present in temperate and sub-tropical zones, but is at its highest prevalence in tropical, rural areas where sanitation is all but absent. Because ascaris are hardy it is not uncommon to also find ascariasis cases in urban slums. In some regions of Africa, 95% of the population is infected, and in parts of Central and South America 45% are infected. In the United States, infection was at one time prevalent in southern, rural communities, but no more recent studies have been conducted.[40, 41] Sex or race is of no epidemiological consequence in the distribution of ascariasis. Although persons of all ages are susceptible, the infection predominates among school-aged children, who typically harbor the highest intensity infections. This observation, along with the health and educational benefits of de-worming, led by the 2001 World Health Assembly to recommend the use of single-dose treatments of children with albendazole or mebendazole as a cornerstone of a global de-worming program. Through such programs of mass drug administration the global prevalence of ascariasis is believed to have diminished by approximately 25% over the last two decades.[3]

Ascaris eggs are destroyed by exposure to direct sunlight for 12 hours, and die when exposed to temperatures in excess of 40°C. Exposure to cold, however, does not adversely affect the eggs. They have been known to survive the ordinary freezing temperatures of winter months in the temperate zones. The eggs are also resistant to many commonly used chemical disinfectants, and can thrive in treated sewage for many months to years.

References

1. DeSilva, N. R.; Brooker, S., Soil-transmitted helminth infections: updating the global picture. *Trends Parasitol* **2003,** *19* 547-51.
2. Hotez, P. J.; Brindley, P. J.; Bethony, J. M.; King, C. H.; Pearce, E. J.; Jacobson, J., Helminth infections: the great neglected tropical diseases. *J Clin Invest* **2008,** *118* (4), 1311-21.
3. Global Burden of Disease Study, C., Global, regional, and national incidence, prevalence, and years lived with disability for 301 acute and chronic diseases and injuries in 188 countries, 1990-2013: a systematic analysis for the Global Burden of Disease Study 2013. *Lancet* **2015,** *386*

(9995), 743-800.

4. Embil, J. A.; Pereira, L. H.; White, F. M.; Garner, J. B.; Manuel, F. R., Prevalence of Ascaris lumbricoides infection in a small Nova Scotian community. *The American journal of tropical medicine and hygiene* **1984,** *33* (4), 595-8.

5. Jeandron, A.; Ensink, J. H.; Thamsborg, S. M.; Dalsgaard, A.; Sengupta, M. E., A quantitative assessment method for Ascaris eggs on hands. *PLoS One* **2014,** *9* (5), e96731.

6. Saturnino, A. C.; Freira, A. C.; Silva, E. M.; Nunes, J. F., [Transmission of enteropasitosis through currency notes]. *Acta Cir Bras* **2005,** *20 Suppl 1*, 262-5.

7. Mruyama, H.; Nawa, Y.; Noda, S.; Mimori, T.; E., S.; J., An outbreak of ascariasis with marked eosinophilia in the southern part of Kyushu District, Japan, caused by infection with swine ascaris. *Med Public Health 28 Suppl* **1997,** *1* 194-6.

8. Peng, W.; Anderson, T. J.; Zhou, X.; Kennedy, M. W., Genetic variation in sympatric Ascaris populations from humans and pigs in China. *Parasitology* **1998,** *117 (Pt 4)*, 355-61.

9. Tyson, E., Lumbricus teres, or some anatomical observations on the roundworm bred on the human bodies. *Philos Trans* **1683,** *13* 153-161.

10. Cox, F. E., History of human parasitology. *Clin Microbiol Rev* **2002,** *15* (4), 595-612.

11. Ransom, R. H.; Foster, W. D.; J., Life history of Ascaris lumbricoides and related forms. *Res* **1917,** *11*, 395-398.

12. Koino, S., Experimental infections on human body with ascarides. *Jpn Med World* **1922,** *2*, 317-320.

13. Khuroo, M. S., Ascariasis. *Gastroenterol Clin North Am* **1996,** *25* (3), 553-77.

14. Sherman, D. R.; Guinn, B.; Perdok, M. M.; Goldberg, D. E., Components of sterol biosynthesis assembled on the oxygen-avid hemoglobin of Ascaris. *Science (New York, N.Y.)* **1992,** *258* (5090), 1930-2.

15. Minning, D. M.; Gow, A. J.; Bonaventura, J.; Braun, R.; Dewhirst, M.; Goldberg, D. E.; Stamler, J. S., Ascaris haemoglobin is a nitric oxide-activated 'deoxygenase'. *Nature* **1999,** *401* (6752), 497-502.

16. Goldberg, D. E., Oxygen-Avid Hemoglobin of Ascaris. *Chemical reviews* **1999,** *99* (12), 3371-3378.

17. Bryan, F. D.; J., Diseases transmitted by foods contaminated by waste water. *Protein* **1977,** *40* 45-56.

18. Harmych, S.; Arnette, R.; Komuniecki, R., Role of dihydrolipoyl dehydrogenase (E3) and a novel E3-binding protein in the NADH sensitivity of the pyruvate dehydrogenase complex from anaerobic mitochondria of the parasitic nematode, Ascaris suum. *Molecular and biochemical parasitology* **2002,** *125* (1-2), 135-46.

19. McSharry, C.; Xia, Y.; Holland, C. V.; Kennedy, M. W., Natural immunity to Ascaris lumbricoides associated with immunoglobulin E antibody to ABA-1 allergen and inflammation indicators in children. *Infection and immunity* **1999,** *67* (2), 484-9.

20. Lynch, N. R.; Hagel, I. A.; Palenque, M. E.; Di Prisco, M. C.; Escudero, J. E.; Corao, L. A.; Sandia, J. A.; Ferreira, L. J.; Botto, C.; Perez, M.; Le Souef, P. N., Relationship between helminthic infection and IgE response in atopic and nonatopic children in a tropical environment. *The Journal of allergy and clinical immunology* **1998,** *101* (2 Pt 1), 217-21.

21. Buendia, E.; Zakzuk, J.; Mercado, D.; Alvarez, A.; Caraballo, L., The IgE response to Ascaris molecular components is associated with clinical indicators of asthma severity. *World Allergy Organ J* **2015,** *8* (1), 8.

22. Ramsay, C. E.; Hayden, C. M.; Tiller, K. J.; Burton, P. R.; Hagel, I.; Palenque, M.; Lynch, N. R.; Goldblatt, J.; LeSouëf, P. N., Association of polymorphisms in the beta2-adrenoreceptor gene with higher levels of parasitic infection. *Human genetics* **1999,** *104* (3), 269-74.

23. Wang, T.; Van Steendam, K.; Dhaenens, M.; Vlaminck, J.; Deforce, D.; Jex, A. R.; Gasser, R. B.; Geldhof, P., Proteomic analysis of the excretory-secretory products from larval stages of Ascaris suum reveals high abundance of glycosyl hydrolases. *PLoS Negl Trop Dis* **2013,** *7* (10), e2467.

24. Hadidjaja, P.; Bonang, E.; Suyardi, M. A.; Abidin, S. A.; Ismid, I. S.; Margono, S. S., The effect of intervention methods on nutritional status and cognitive function of primary school children

infected with Ascaris lumbricoides. *The American journal of tropical medicine and hygiene* **1998**, *59* (5), 791-5.

25.   Crompton, D. W. T.; Nesheim, M. C., Nutritional impact of intestinal helminthiasis during the human life cycle. *Annual review of nutrition* **2002**, *22*, 35-59.

26.   O'Lorcain, P.; Holland, C. V., The public health importance of Ascaris lumbricoides. *Parasitology* **2000**, *121*, S51-71.

27.   Crompton, D. W., Ascaris and ascariasis. *Advances in parasitology* **2001**, *48*, 285-375.

28.   Andrade, A. M.; Perez, Y.; Lopez, C.; Collazos, S. S.; Andrade, A. M.; Ramirez, G. O.; Andrade, L. M., Intestinal Obstruction in a 3-Year-Old Girl by Ascaris lumbricoides Infestation: Case Report and Review of the Literature. *Medicine (Baltimore)* **2015**, *94* (16), e655.

29.   Khuroo, M. S.; Zargar, S. A.; Mahajan, R., Hepatobiliary and pancreatic ascariasis in India. *Lancet (London, England)* **1990**, *335* (8704), 1503-6.

30.   Khuroo, M. S., Hepatobiliary and pancreatic ascariasis. *Indian journal of gastroenterology : official journal of the Indian Society of Gastroenterology* **2001**, *20 Suppl 1*, C28-32.

31.   Costa-Macedo, L. M. D.; Rey, L., Ascaris lumbricoides in neonate: evidence of congenital transmission of intestinal nematodes. *Rev Inst Med Trop Sao Paulo* **1990**, *32* 351-354.

32.   Synovia, C. B.; Narayanan, P. R.; Vivakanandan, S., Fetal response to maternal ascariasis as evidenced by anti-Ascaris lumbricoides IgM antibodies in the cord blood. *Acta Paediatr Scand* **1991**, *80*, 1134-1138.

33.   Schulman, A., Ultrasound appearances of intra- and extrahepatic biliary ascariasis. *Abdominal imaging* **1998**, *23* (1), 60-6.

34.   Bhattacharyya, T.; Santra, A.; Majumder, D. N.; Chatterjee, B. P., Possible approach for serodiagnosis of ascariasis by evaluation of immunoglobulin G4 response using Ascaris lumbricoides somatic antigen. *J Clin Microbiol* **2001**, *39* (8), 2991-4.

35.   Santra, A.; Bhattacharya, T.; Chowdhury, A.; Ghosh, A.; Ghosh, N.; Chatterjee, B. P.; Mazumder, D. N., Serodiagnosis of ascariasis with specific IgG4 antibody and its use in an epidemiological study. *Trans R Soc Trop Med Hyg* **2001**, *95* (3), 289-92.

36.   Lamberton, P. H.; Jourdan, P. M., Human Ascariasis: Diagnostics Update. *Curr Trop Med Rep* **2015**, *2* (4), 189-200.

37.   Leles, D.; Araujo, A.; Vicente, A. C.; Iniguez, A. M., ITS1 intra-individual variability of Ascaris isolates from Brazil. *Parasitol Int* **2010**, *59* (1), 93-6.

38.   Aubry, M. L.; Cowell, P.; Davey, M. J.; Shevde, S., Aspects of the pharmacology of a new anthelmintic: pyrantel. *British journal of pharmacology* **1970**, *38* (2), 332-44.

39.   Chevarria, A. P.; Schwartzwelder, J. C.; J., Mebendazole, an effective broad spectrum anthelminthic. *Am Med Hyg* **1973**, *22* 592-595.

40.   Blumenthal, D. S.; Schultz, M. G., Incidence of intestinal obstruction in children infected with Ascaris lumbricoides. *The American journal of tropical medicine and hygiene* **1975**, *24* (5), 801-5.

41.   Starr, M. C.; Montgomery, S. P., Soil-transmitted Helminthiasis in the United States: a systematic review--1940-2010. *Am J Trop Med Hyg* **2011**, *85* (4), 680-4.

19. The Hookworms:

Necator americanus
(Stiles 1902)

Ancylostoma duodenale
(Dubini 1843)

Introduction

Two species of hookworm account for most human infections; *Necator americanus* and *Ancylostoma duodenale*.[1, 2] *N. americanus* is by far the more common human hookworm except in some focal areas of Egypt, India, and China. A third species, *Ancylostoma ceylanicum*, is also found as a human parasite in Southeast Asia.[3] Adult hookworms inhabit the small intestine and feed on intestinal villi and blood. Blood loss resulting from adult hookworms in the intestine leads to protein and iron deficiency, as well as anemia. Hookworms infect approximately 472 million people in the developing nations of the tropics, making this one of the most prevalent human infections worldwide, and one of the most common causes of iron-deficiency anemia.[4-6] According to some estimates, hookworm ranks with schistosomiasis as the leading helminth infection in terms of deaths and disability adjusted life years (DALYs)

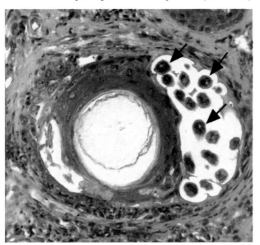

Figure 19.1. Hookworm larvae (arrows) in skin of experimentally infected dog.

lost than any other human helminth infection.[1, 7]

Children heavily infected with hookworms are likely to develop deficits in both physical and cognitive development, and are more susceptible to other intercurrent infections.[1, 7-9] Hookworm is an important health threat for women of reproductive age. An estimated 44 million pregnant women are infected with hookworms in endemic countries.[5] The resulting iron deficiency and malnutrition during pregnancy adversely affects intrauterine growth, birth weight and even maternal survival.[9] Hookworm also increases the likelihood of premature birth, and may contribute to maternal mortality.[10]

The distribution of the two species was thought at one time to be discrete and not overlapping, but both species have been shown to occupy at least some of the same regions of Africa, South America, and Asia. *N. americanus* is the predominant hookworm worldwide, with the highest rates in Sub-Saharan Africa, tropical regions of the Americas, South China, and Southeast Asia.[1] *A. duodenale* is more focally endemic in parts of China, India, North Africa, Sub-Saharan Africa, and a few regions of the Americas. A third species, *Ancylostoma ceylanicum*, is found mainly in cats, but also in humans living in Malaysia and elsewhere in Asia.[11-15] The canine hookworm, *A. caninum,* has been implicated as the cause of eosinophilic enteritis syndrome in parts of northern Queensland, Australia.[16] *A. braziliense*, whose definitive hosts are dogs and cats, causes cutaneous larva migrans.[17]

There are no known reservoirs for *A. duodenale* or *N. americanus*. The dog is the primary host for *A. caninum*, but it has not been well-established whether this hookworm causes mature human infection, save for a few reported cases in Australia.

Necator americanus

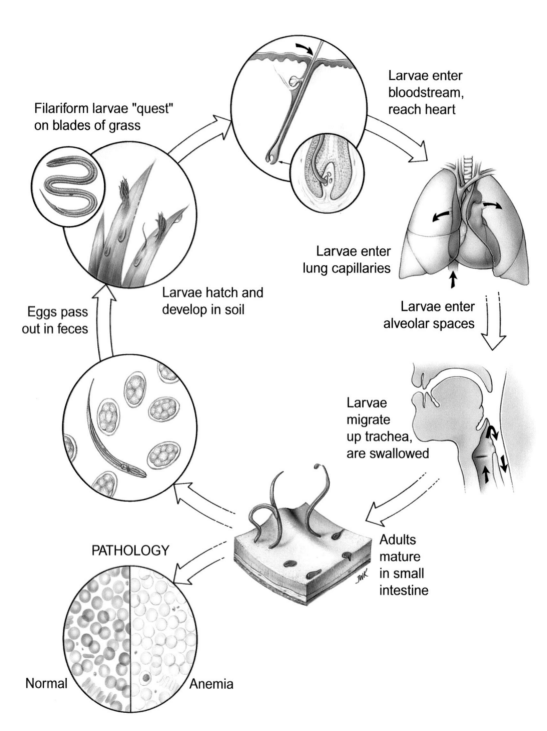

Filariform larvae "quest" on blades of grass

Larvae enter bloodstream, reach heart

Larvae enter lung capillaries

Larvae hatch and develop in soil

Eggs pass out in feces

Larvae enter alveolar spaces

Larvae migrate up trachea, are swallowed

Adults mature in small intestine

PATHOLOGY

Normal

Anemia

Historical Information

Necator americanus likely originated in Asia, while *Ancylostoma duodenale* most likely originally came from Africa.[18] Hookworms appear to have been infecting humans for thousands of years in the Old World, while controversy exists as to whether hookworm was present in the Americas prior to European exploration and colonization.[18, 19] Hookworm infection had been common in the United States in the past (primarily in the rural South), as well as in Puerto Rico.[20, 21] Because hookworm disease was thought to be a major obstacle to the economic development in the South following the Civil War, John D. Rockefeller, Sr. established the Rockefeller Sanitary Commission (which later became the Rockefeller Foundation) in 1909, for the sole purpose of eliminating hookworm from the United States and Puerto Rico.[21] In 1902, Charles W. Stiles, first described *N. americanus*, and was largely responsible for convincing Frederick Gates, a Baptist minister and Rockefeller's key advisor, to establish the Commission.[22] The prevalence of hookworm infection in the United States has been reduced almost to the point of eradication, but this resulted less from any planned intervention than from the general improvement in socioeconomic conditions. Economic development also accounts in a large part for the control of malaria and typhoid fever in the United States. However, much of our knowledge regarding the natural history and pathogenesis of hookworm infection was based on the work of investigators funded by the Rockefeller philanthropies, including William Cort, Auriel O. Foster, Asa C. Chandler, J. Allen Scott, and Norman Stoll. Stoll described hookworm as "the great infection of mankind."[23] Angelo Dubini first reported human infection with *A. duodenale* in 1843; but it was Arthur Looss, working in Egypt, who demonstrated percutaneous transmission of hookworm infection and clarified its life cycle.[24] The life cycle was further defined by Gerald Schad, who demonstrated the ability of *A. duodenale* larvae to remain in a dormant arrested state in human tissues.[25]

Life Cycle

Infection begins when the L3 (filariform) larvae actively penetrate the cutaneous tissues, usually through a hair follicle (Fig. 19.1) or an abraded area. Skin invasion may be facilitated by the release of hydrolytic enzymes. Once in the subcutaneous tissues, larvae enter capillaries and are carried passively through the bloodstream to the capillaries of the lungs. The L3 larvae break out of the alveolar capillaries and complete the migratory phase of the life cycle by crawling up the bronchi and trachea, over the epiglottis, and into the pharynx. They are swallowed, and proceed into the stomach. This portion of the life cycle (i.e., parenteral phase) closely parallels those of *Ascaris lumbricoides* and *Strongyloides stercoralis*. Two molts take place in the small intestine, resulting in the development of an adult worm (Fig. 19.2, 19.3).

Ancylostoma duodenale larvae are also infective orally.[26] In some regions, oral ingestion may be the predominant mode of

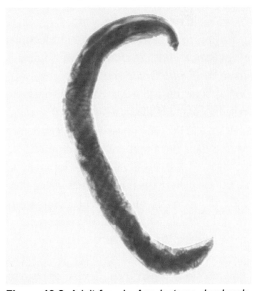

Figure 19.2. Adult female *Ancylostoma duodenale*. 10 mm.

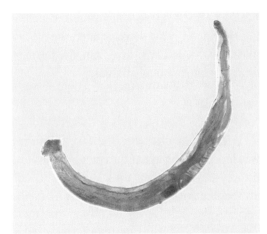

Figure 19.3. Adult male *A. duodenale*. Note hand-like bursa at tail end. 8 mm.

transmission. Larvae that infect orally may undergo two molts to adulthood without leaving the gastrointestinal tract, and a syndrome known as Wakana disease, characterized by nausea, vomiting, cough and difficulty breathing can develop.[27]

Forty days following maturation and copulation, the female worms begin laying eggs (Fig. 19.4), completing the life cycle. In some cases of infection with *A. duodenale*, larvae may stay longer in tissues before transiting to the intestine, with a resultant delay in egg production.[28] Adult worms live an average of one year in the case of *A. duodenale* and 3-5 years in the case of *N. americanus*.[29] The maximum recorded survival time is 15 years.[30]

In endemic areas, where reinfections are continual, the development of some L3 larvae of *A. duodenale* (but not *N. americanus*) is interrupted. After entering the host, these larvae penetrate into bundles of skeletal muscles and become dormant. They can later resume their development and complete the life cycle.[25] Larval arrested development in human tissues occurs during times of the year when the external environmental conditions are unfavorable to parasite development in the soil. Larval arrest also occurs during pregnancy, and development resumes at the onset of parturition. When these larvae appear in breast milk, vertical transmission of *A. duo-*

denale infection in neonates may result.[31]

The adult worms feed on intestinal villi and blood in the small intestine (Fig. 19.5). Morphologically, each species can be differentiated on the basis of the mouth-parts of the adults. *A. duodenale* possesses cutting teeth (Fig. 19.6), whereas *N. americanus* has rounded cutting plates (Fig. 19.7). Moreover, their body sizes differ. The adult male hookworms are differentiated from the females by the presence of a copulatory bursa.

Ancylostoma duodenale and *N. americanus* exhibit major differences in their life cycles and pathogenicity. *A. duodenale* is generally considered the more virulent of the two species because it is larger, causes more blood loss, produces more eggs, and has several modes of transmission other than penetrating skin.[1, 2] The female passes eggs into the lumen of the small intestine. *A. duodenale* produces about 28,000 eggs per day, and *N. americanus* about 10,000. The eggs embryonate to the four-cell and eight-cell stages immediately after they are passed. In warm, moist, sandy, or loamy soil the embryo develops to the L1, (rhabditiform) larva within 48 hours of deposition in the soil. After hatching, the larva feeds on debris in the immediate surroundings, and grows, then molts twice to develop into the infective L3 (filariform) larva. Filariform larvae do not

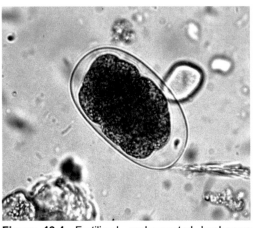

Figure 19.4. Fertilized, embryonated hookworm egg. 65 μm x 40 μm.

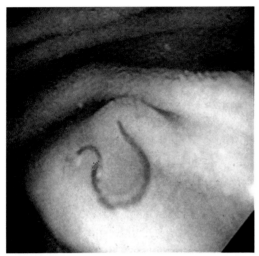

Figure 19.5. Hookworm adult, diagnosed by colonoscopy.

consume food, and are generally considered to be in a developmentally arrested state.[32] However, these larvae do not lie motionless; rather, they actively seek out the highest point in the environment (e.g., the tops of grass blades, small rocks), where they are more likely to come into direct contact with human skin. This activity is known as "questing." In endemic areas, it is common for many L3 larvae to aggregate on dewy grass, increasing the chances for multiple infections of the same host. Sandy soils, such as those found in coastal areas, are particularly favorable for

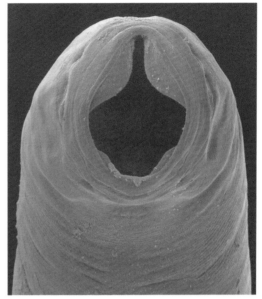

Figure 19.7. Scanning EM of head of *Necator americanus*. Note cutting plates. Photo by D. Scharf.

hookworm larval migrations and hookworm transmission.

Cellular and Molecular Pathogenesis

The L3 hookworm larvae penetrate unbroken skin with the aid of secreted enzymes that include a metalloprotease and a family of cysteine-rich secretory proteins, known as the Ancylostoma secreted proteins (ASPs).[33, 34] Repeated infection results in an immediate hypersensitivity and other inflammatory responses comprising hookworm dermatitis. Subsequent larval migration through the lungs may result in pulmonary inflammation, resulting in a pneumonitis.

Most of the pathology of hookworm infection results from the presence of adult hookworms in the small intestine. The adult worms derive their nourishment from eating villous tissue. They also suck blood directly from their site of attachment to the intestinal mucosa and submucosa. Adult worms possess a well-developed esophageal bulb, enabling them to pump blood from the capillary bed of the mucosa. Adult parasites secrete an anticoagulant that blocks the action of host factor Xa and the VIIa/ tissue factor complex.[35, 36]

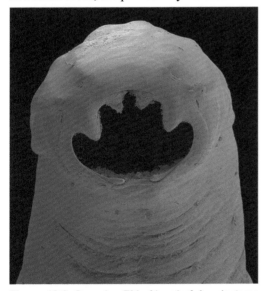

Figure 19.6. Scanning EM of head of *Ancylostoma duodenale*. Note teeth. Photo D. Scharf.

Hookworms also secrete a protein that functions as a platelet inhibitor through blockade of GPIIb/IIIa.[37-39] Blood loss continues after the worms move to a new location through the combined activity of these products. Each *A. duodenale* adult sucks 0.1-0.2 ml of blood per day, while each *N. americanus* adult worm sucks 0.01-0.02 ml of blood per day.[40] Following blood ingestion, the adult hookworms rupture the red blood cells with the aid of hemolysins,[41] and then break down host hemoglobin in an ordered manner through the activities of specific hemoglobin-specific proteases.[42]

In addition to blood loss, there can be protein loss that contributes to protein malnutrition, a problem that is already existent in the locations where hookworm infection is still endemic.[43] Production of a hookworm serine protease inhibitor that interferes with pancreatic enzyme-based digestion may also interfere with breakdown of ingested foods, leading to malabsorption and consequent retardation of growth and development.[44]

Repeated exposure to hookworm infection does not necessarily result in protective immunity.[45] Although a humoral antibody response to numerous hookworm antigens can be demonstrated in naturally-infected individuals, the presence of specific antibodies often does not correlate with resistance to infection.[46] Some immunoglobulins may even serve as a marker for hookworm infection.[47] The absence of effector immunity may explain why the intensity of hookworm infection often increases with age in endemic regions, in contrast to the other major soil-transmitted helminth infections (e.g., ascaris and trichuris) for which the intensity peaks in childhood.[7] A concerning feature of hookworm infection is it may actually induce immune suppression through its excretory/secretory products (ESPs). Hookworm ESPs appear to impair dendritic cell function, trigger secretion of immunosuppressive cytokines, induce regulatory T cells, modulate immune

cells through nitric oxide release, and induce apoptosis of effector T cells.[48-52] A persistent impact on the immune system could also explain why continued infection with hookworms and reinfection with hookworms can occur within just a few months of anthelmintic treatment.[53] It may account for the difficulties associated with the control of hookworm and increased incidence of other infections such as malaria in infected patients.[54] The absence of resistance to hookworms may reflect the parasite's ability to escape host immunity, but some success with the development of a human hookworm vaccine suggest that an effective protective human immune response may be inducible.[55-58]

Recent studies using animal models for human intestinal helminth infections (hookworm-like nematodes, and *Trichinella spiralis*), have demonstrated that tuft cells (chemosensory cells), may be responsible for initiating the development of the expulsion mechanism, in which goblet cells proliferate and, combined with specific sIgA antibodies, act together to limit infection in a primary exposure.[59] This study offers some hope for the eventual development of effective vaccines against intestinal helminths.

Clinical Disease

In general, there are four potential manifestations of hookworm disease that are determined by the stage of the infection, the route of acquisition and the degree of worm burden.[1] Initial penetration of the skin by L3 larvae may not result in symptoms in previously uninfected individuals. However, those experiencing repeated infections may develop a pruritic papular vesicular dermatitis at the site of larval entry, known as ground itch, or dew itch.

In heavily-infected individuals, there may be symptoms of pneumonia during the migratory phase of the developmental cycle of these worms. Whether this develops with any regularity is unknown, as pulmonary symptoms attributable to hookworm infection have not been observed in experimentally-infected volunteers.[28, 60] The tissue migrating larval stages do induce circulating eosinophilia one to two months after exposure.[60, 61]

The intestinal phase can be asymptomatic, although it can result in epigastric pain and abdominal discomfort. A syndrome known as Wakana disease occurs when large numbers of larvae are ingested, and is associated with nausea, vomiting, dyspnea, and eosinophilia.[27, 62]

Severe illness resulting from hookworm infection results only when large numbers of adult worms are present in the small intestine. In most endemic areas, hookworm infections "aggregated."[63] Anywhere from two-thirds to three-fourths of the infections in a given area are sufficiently light in terms of intensity (numbers of worms) that they are clinically silent. The clinical features of hookworm disease usually occur only in 10-30% of individuals who harbor large numbers of worms. In some regions, certain individuals might be predisposed to acquiring heavy infections on the basis of genetics or infectious exposures.[63, 64]

The major clinical feature of hookworm disease is iron-deficiency anemia, which occurs as the result of blood loss in the intestinal tract.[1, 7, 65-68] Intestinal blood loss is proportional to the number of hookworms present in the intestine, although whether or not true iron-deficiency anemia subsequently develops depends upon the predominant species of hookworm in the intestine (*A. duodenale* is associated with larger blood loss than *N. americanus*), the iron reserves of the host, and the daily intake of iron.[65-68] Severe anemia is associated with lassitude, palpitations, and exertional dyspnea. This can be associated with a impaired growth and development in the young, and may lead to angina pectoris and congestive heart failure in older individuals. The physical signs of hookworm anemia include the signs of iron deficiency, such as pale sclera, fingernail concavities (koilonychia), and cheilitis. In addition, children may manifest a yellow-green discoloration of the skin known as chlorosis due to the similarity in color to plant leaves deficient in chlorophyll.[69] Children with severe hookworm infection also show signs of protein malnutrition that result from hookworm-associated plasma protein loss, and they may develop abdominal distension, facial edema, and hair loss.

A syndrome of infantile ancylostomiasis has been described, associated with severe anemia, melena, abdominal distension and failure to thrive.[31, 70] There is evidence suggesting that these neonates ingested *A. duodenale* through breast milk.[31]

Chronic hookworm anemia during childhood causes physical growth retardation, as well as deficits in child cognition and intellectual development.[1, 7-9] As with other soil-transmitted helminth infections, growth retardation is often reversible by administration of anthelminthic therapy, but intellectual and cognitive defects cannot always be reversed by therapy.[71] Chronic hookworm anemia during pregnancy can result in prematurity or low birth weight.[9] Many of these chronic sequelae account for the tremendous impact of hookworms on maternal child health. In its World Development Report, the World Bank cited hookworm as a leading cause of morbidity among school-aged children.[72]

Diagnosis

Serological tests are not available and consequently diagnosis is usually established by the microscopic identification of characteristic eggs in the stool (Figs. 19.4, C.42). Quantitative methods for determining the number of eggs per gram of feces are also available. Under some circumstances these provide an estimate of the overall worm burden. No distinction can be made among eggs of any of the hookworm species based purely on microscopy. Differentiation by light microscopy depends upon the examination of either L3 larvae (Fig. 19.8), or by recovering adult worms. PCR tests have been developed that have increased sensitivity for diagnosis and allow for species differentiation, but these assays are not in routine use in most parts of the world endemic for hookworm.[73, 74]

Treatment

Adult hookworms are often susceptible to the two major benzimidazole anthelmintic drugs, albendazole and mebendazole, although albendazole is more effective in a single dose compared with single dose mebendazole.[75] Failures of a single dose of mebendazole or albendazole to remove hookworms from the gastrointestinal tract have been reported, and twice daily dosing for three days results in higher cure rates.[76-78] Pyrantel pamoate can be given for three days as an alternate therapy, but ivermectin has poor efficacy.[77, 79]

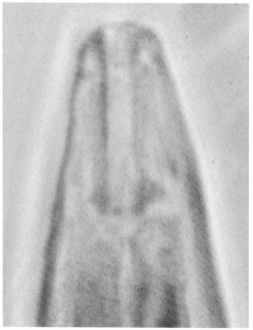

Figure 19.8. Buccal cavity of hookworm rhabditiform larva. It is longer than that of the same stage of *Strongyloides stercoralis* (see Fig. 20.7).

Very young children and pregnant women are considered especially vulnerable to the effects of hookworm anemia. In Africa, hookworm was found to make a substantial contribution to anemia in preschool children, while in Nepal hookworm was a significant cause of anemia in pregnancy.[80, 81] Pregnant women who received antenatal albendazole were shown to exhibit significant improvements in maternal anemia, birthweight, and infant mortality.[82] The concerns about the toxicities of the benzimidazoles need to be weighed against their potentially important benefits in pregnancy.[83, 84]

Albendazole and mebendazole work by binding to the microtubules of the parasite.[85] Anthelminthic resistance to the benzimidazoles has been well-described among nematodes of veterinary importance, and occurs via mutations in the parasite tubulin alleles.[86] Reports on the outright failure of mebendazole to treat human hookworm infections in Mali, and the reduced efficacy of mebendazole with frequent and periodic use, have raised possible concerns that benzimidazole drug resistance may be emerging among hookworms.[76, 82] Efficacy of these drugs will need to be monitored, as they are used in mass de-worming campaigns.[82]

Most children and adults with hookworm infection can be treated with benzimidazole anthelminthics alone and do not require iron supplementation. Pregnant women with severe hookworm anemia and their unborn children have been shown to benefit from simultaneous oral supplementation with iron such as ferrous sulfate along with anthelminthic drugs.[81]

Prevention and Control

The traditional methods of hookworm control in endemic areas have included; sanitary disposal of feces through the implementation of latrines, health education, drinking clean safe water, hand washing, cooking of food and encouraging use of shoes or other footwear.[87] Despite decades of widespread attempts to control hookworm through these traditional methods, the global prevalence and intensity of hookworm remained the same. Among the reasons why traditional methods have failed are the ability of *A. duodenale* hookworm larvae to infect humans through ingestion, the ability of *N. americanus* larvae to penetrate all aspects of the body including the hands and abdomen, the high rate of occupational exposure to hookworm that occurs during agricultural pursuits, and the continued reliance on human feces for fertilizing crops.[88]

At the World Health Assembly in 2001, member states were urged to control the global morbidity of hookworm and other soil-transmitted helminth (STH) infections through the frequent and periodic use of anthelminthic drugs (www.who.int/worm-control). In 2012, The London Declaration on Neglected Tropical Diseases was put forth as a plan to control hookworm among other diseases that involved several components including mass drug administration.[89] There are concerns that this approach might have less of an impact on hookworm than the other STH infections such as Trichuris and Ascaris. The highest hookworm intensities in a community are often not in children, so that targeting children is not expected to reduce hookworm transmission.[90] High rates of post-treatment hookworm reinfection occur in many communities, especially those with high levels of transmission, which sometimes requires thrice-yearly anthelminthic treatment.[53] As noted above, outright drug failure with both mebendazole and albendazole has been described, while the diminishing efficacy of mebendazole with frequent and periodic use has raised concerns about emerging drug resistance and the impact this will have on mass drug treatment programs. A recent analysis through the Global Burden of Disease Study found that the prevalence rate of hookworm has decreased only 5% over the last two decades, despite comparatively greater reductions of 25% for ascariasis.[6]

As a complementing control strategy, the Human Hookworm Vaccine Initiative of the Sabin Vaccine Institute product development partnership has developed a recombinant vaccine that targets adult hookworm blood feeding by eliciting anti-enzyme antibodies that block parasite hemoglobin digestion.[56] This vaccine is in phase 1 clinical trials for safety and immunogenicity in Brazil and Gabon. Mathematical modeling of the vaccine indicates that it could reduce hookworm transmission, which would not be possible using pediatric anthelmintic drug de-worming approaches, while economic modeling indicates that a hookworm vaccine could be highly cost-effective.[91, 92]

References

1. Hotez, P. J.; Brooker, S.; Bethony, J. M.; Bottazzi, M. E.; Loukas, A.; Xiao, S., Hookworm infection. *The New England journal of medicine* **2004**, *351* (8), 799-807.
2. Bethony, J.; Brooker, S.; Albonico, M.; Geiger, S. M.; Loukas, A.; Diemert, D.; Hotez, P. J., Soil-transmitted helminth infections: ascariasis, trichuriasis, and hookworm. *Lancet* **2006**, *367* (9521), 1521-32.
3. Ngui, R.; Lim, Y. A.; Traub, R.; Mahmud, R.; Mistam, M. S., Epidemiological and genetic data supporting the transmission of Ancylostoma ceylanicum among human and domestic animals. *PLoS Negl Trop Dis* **2012**, *6* (2), e1522.
4. DeSilva, N. R.; Brooker, S., Soil-transmitted helminth infections: updating the global picture. *Trends Parasitol* **2003**, *19* 547-51.
5. Pullan, R. L.; Smith, J. L.; Jasrasaria, R.; Brooker, S. J., Global numbers of infection and disease burden of soil transmitted helminth infections in 2010. *Parasit Vectors* **2014**, *7*, 37.

6. Global Burden of Disease Study, C., Global, regional, and national incidence, prevalence, and years lived with disability for 301 acute and chronic diseases and injuries in 188 countries, 1990-2013: a systematic analysis for the Global Burden of Disease Study 2013. *Lancet* **2015,** *386* (9995), 743-800.

7. Hotez, P. J.; Bethony, J.; Bottazzi, M. E.; Brooker, S.; Buss, P., Hookworm: "the great infection of mankind". *PLoS medicine* **2005,** *2* (3), e67.

8. Brooker, S.; Bethony, J.; Hotez, P. J., Human hookworm infection in the 21st century. *Advances in parasitology* **2004,** *58,* 197-288.

9. Sakti, H.; Nokes, C.; Hertanto, W. S.; Hendratno, S.; Hall, A.; Bundy, D. A.; Satoto, Evidence for an association between hookworm infection and cognitive function in Indonesian school children. *Tropical medicine & international health : TM & IH* **1999,** *4* (5), 322-34.

10. Bundy, D. A.; Chan, M. S.; Savioli, L., Hookworm infection in pregnancy. *Transactions of the Royal Society of Tropical Medicine and Hygiene* **1995,** *89* (5), 521-2.

11. Traub, R. J., Ancylostoma ceylanicum, a re-emerging but neglected parasitic zoonosis. *Int J Parasitol* **2013,** *43* (12-13), 1009-15.

12. George, S.; Kaliappan, S. P.; Kattula, D.; Roy, S.; Geldhof, P.; Kang, G.; Vercruysse, J.; Levecke, B., Identification of Ancylostoma ceylanicum in children from a tribal community in Tamil Nadu, India using a semi-nested PCR-RFLP tool. *Trans R Soc Trop Med Hyg* **2015,** *109* (4), 283-5.

13. Phosuk, I.; Intapan, P. M.; Thanchomnang, T.; Sanpool, O.; Janwan, P.; Laummaunwai, P.; Aamnart, W.; Morakote, N.; Maleewong, W., Molecular detection of Ancylostoma duodenale, Ancylostoma ceylanicum, and Necator americanus in humans in northeastern and southern Thailand. *Korean J Parasitol* **2013,** *51* (6), 747-9.

14. Thompson, R. C., Neglected zoonotic helminths: Hymenolepis nana, Echinococcus canadensis and Ancylostoma ceylanicum. *Clin Microbiol Infect* **2015,** *21* (5), 426-32.

15. Liu, Y.; Zheng, G.; Alsarakibi, M.; Zhang, X.; Hu, W.; Lin, L.; Tan, L.; Luo, Q.; Lu, P.; Li, G., The zoonotic risk of Ancylostoma ceylanicum isolated from stray dogs and cats in Guangzhou, South China. *Biomed Res Int* **2014,** *2014,* 208759.

16. Prociv, P.; Croese, J., Human eosinophilic enteritis caused by dog hookworm Ancylostoma caninum. *Lancet (London, England)* **1990,** *335* (8701), 1299-302.

17. Blackwell, V.; Vega-Lopez, F., Cutaneous larva migrans: clinical features and management of 44 cases presenting in the returning traveller. *The British journal of dermatology* **2001,** *145* (3), 434-7.

18. Cox, F. E., History of human parasitology. *Clin Microbiol Rev* **2002,** *15* (4), 595-612.

19. Ferreira, L. F.; Araujo, A., On hookworms in the Americas and trans-Pacific contact. *Parasitol Today* **1996,** *12* (11), 454; author reply 454.

20. Maldonado, A. E., Hookworm disease: Puerto Rico's secret killer. *P R Health Sci J* **1993,** *12* (3), 191-6.

21. Bleakley, H., Disease and Development: Evidence from Hookworm Eradication in the American South. *Q J Econ* **2007,** *122* (1), 73-117.

22. Stiles, C. W., A new species of hookworm (Uncinaria americana) parasitic in man. *Am Med* **1902,** *3* 777-778.

23. Stoll, N. R., On endemic hookworm, where do we stand today? Exp Parasitol. **1962,** *12* 241-51.

24. Dubini, A., Nuovo verme intestinale umano Ancylostoma duodenale, constitutente un sesto genere dei nematoidei proprii dell'uomo. . *Ann Univ Med Milano* **1843,** *106,* 5-13.

25. Schad, G. A.; Chowdhury, A. B.; Dean, C. G.; Kochar, V. K.; Nawalinski, T. A.; Thomas, J.; Tonascia, J. A., Arrested development in human hookworm infections: an adaptation to a seasonally unfavorable external environment. *Science (New York, N.Y.)* **1973,** *180* (4085), 502-4.

26. Brooker, S.; Bethony, J.; Hotez, P. J., Human hookworm infection in the 21st century. *Adv Parasitol* **2004,** *58,* 197-288.

27. Kojima, S., [Wakana disease]. *Ryoikibetsu Shokogun Shirizu* **1999,** (24 Pt 2), 437-8.

28. Nawalinski, T. A.; Schad, G. A., Arrested development in Ancylostoma duodenale: course of a self-induced infection in man. *Am J Trop Med Hyg* **1974,** *23* (5), 895-8.

29. Hoagland, K. E.; Schad, G. A., Necator americanus and Ancylostoma duodenale: life history

parameters and epidemiological implications of two sympatric hookworms of humans. *Experimental parasitology* **1978,** *44* (1), 36-49.

30. Plamer, E. D.; J., Course of egg output over a 15-year period in a case of experimentally induced necatoriasis americanus. 1955; Vol. 4 p756-757.

31. Yu, S. H.; Jiang, Z. X.; Xu, L. Q., Infantile hookworm disease in China. A review. *Acta tropica* **1995,** *59* (4), 265-70.

32. Hawdon, J. M.; Hotez, P. J., Hookworm: developmental biology of the infectious process. *Current opinion in genetics & development* **1996,** *6* (5), 618-23.

33. Zhan, B.; Hotez, P. J.; Wang, Y.; Hawdon, J. M., A developmentally regulated metalloprotease secreted by host-stimulated Ancylostoma caninum third-stage infective larvae is a member of the astacin family of proteases. *Molecular and biochemical parasitology* **2002,** *120* (2), 291-6.

34. Asojo, O. A.; Goud, G.; Dhar, K.; Loukas, A.; Zhan, B.; Deumic, V.; Liu, S.; Borgstahl, G. E. O.; Hotez, P. J., X-ray structure of Na-ASP-2, a pathogenesis-related-1 protein from the nematode parasite, Necator americanus, and a vaccine antigen for human hookworm infection. *Journal of molecular biology* **2005,** *346* (3), 801-14.

35. Cappello, M.; Vlasuk, G. P.; Bergum, P. W.; Huang, S.; Hotez, P. J., Ancylostoma caninum anticoagulant peptide: a hookworm-derived inhibitor of human coagulation factor Xa. *Proceedings of the National Academy of Sciences of the United States of America* **1995,** *92* (13), 6152-6.

36. Stanssens, P.; Bergum, P. W.; Sci, U. S. A., Anticoagulant repertoire of the hookworm Ancylostoma caninum. *Proc Natl Acad* **1996,** *93*, 2149-2154.

37. Ma, D.; Francischetti, I. M.; Ribeiro, J. M.; Andersen, J. F., The structure of hookworm platelet inhibitor (HPI), a CAP superfamily member from Ancylostoma caninum. *Acta Crystallogr F Struct Biol Commun* **2015,** *71* (Pt 6), 643-9.

38. Del Valle, A.; Jones, B. F.; Harrison, L. M.; Chadderdon, R. C.; Cappello, M., Isolation and molecular cloning of a secreted hookworm platelet inhibitor from adult Ancylostoma caninum. *Mol Biochem Parasitol* **2003,** *129* (2), 167-77.

39. Chadderdon, R. C.; Cappello, M., The hookworm platelet inhibitor: functional blockade of integrins GPIIb/IIIa (alphaIIbbeta3) and GPIa/IIa (alpha2beta1) inhibits platelet aggregation and adhesion in vitro. *J Infect Dis* **1999,** *179* (5), 1235-41.

40. Roche, M.; Layrisse, M.; J., The nature and causes of "hookworm anemia". *Am Med Hyg* **1996,** *15* 1031-1102.

41. Don, T. A.; Jones, M. K.; Smyth, D.; O'Donoghue, P.; Hotez, P.; Loukas, A., A pore-forming haemolysin from the hookworm, Ancylostoma caninum. *International journal for parasitology* **2004,** *34* (9), 1029-35.

42. Williamson, A. L.; Lecchi, P.; Turk, B. E.; Choe, Y.; Hotez, P. J.; McKerrow, J. H.; Cantley, L. C.; Sajid, M.; Craik, C. S.; Loukas, A., A multi-enzyme cascade of hemoglobin proteolysis in the intestine of blood-feeding hookworms. *The Journal of biological chemistry* **2004,** *279* (34), 35950-7.

43. Gupta, M. C.; Basu, A. K.; Tandon, B. N., Gastrointestinal protein loss in hookworm and roundworm infections. *Am J Clin Nutr* **1974,** *27* (12), 1386-9.

44. Chu, D.; Bungiro, R. D.; Ibanez, M.; Harrison, L. M.; Campodonico, E.; Jones, B. F.; Mieszczanek, J.; Kuzmic, P.; Cappello, M., Molecular characterization of Ancylostoma ceylanicum Kunitz-type serine protease inhibitor: evidence for a role in hookworm-associated growth delay. *Infect Immun* **2004,** *72* (4), 2214-21.

45. Gaze, S.; Bethony, J. M.; Periago, M. V., Immunology of experimental and natural human hookworm infection. *Parasite Immunol* **2014,** *36* (8), 358-66.

46. Pritchard, D. I.; Quinnell, R. J.; Slater, A. F.; McKean, P. G.; Dale, D. D.; Raiko, A.; Keymer, A. E., Epidemiology and immunology of Necator americanus infection in a community in Papua New Guinea: humoral responses to excretory-secretory and cuticular collagen antigens. *Parasitology* **1990,** *100 Pt 2*, 317-26.

47. Palmer, D. R.; Bradley, M.; Bundy, D. A., IgG4 responses to antigens of adult Necator americanus: potential for use in large-scale epidemiological studies. *Bulletin of the World Health Organization* **1996,** *74* (4), 381-6.

48. Segura, M.; Su, Z.; Piccirillo, C.; Stevenson, M. M., Impairment of dendritic cell function by excretory-secretory products: a potential mechanism for nematode-induced immunosuppression. *Eur J Immunol* **2007,** *37* (7), 1887-904.

49. Ricci, N. D.; Fiuza, J. A.; Bueno, L. L.; Cancado, G. G.; Gazzinelli-Guimaraes, P. H.; Martins, V. G.; Matoso, L. F.; de Miranda, R. R.; Geiger, S. M.; Correa-Oliveira, R.; Gazzinelli, A.; Bartholomeu, D. C.; Fujiwara, R. T., Induction of CD4(+)CD25(+)FOXP3(+) regulatory T cells during human hookworm infection modulates antigen-mediated lymphocyte proliferation. *PLoS Negl Trop Dis* **2011,** *5* (11), e1383.

50. Dondji, B.; Bungiro, R. D.; Harrison, L. M.; Vermeire, J. J.; Bifulco, C.; McMahon-Pratt, D.; Cappello, M., Role for nitric oxide in hookworm-associated immune suppression. *Infect Immun* **2008,** *76* (6), 2560-7.

51. Chow, S. C.; Brown, A.; Pritchard, D., The human hookworm pathogen Necator americanus induces apoptosis in T lymphocytes. *Parasite Immunol* **2000,** *22* (1), 21-9.

52. Quinnell, R. J.; Bethony, J.; Pritchard, D. I., The immunoepidemiology of human hookworm infection. *Parasite Immunol* **2004,** *26* (11-12), 443-54.

53. Albonico, M.; Smith, P. G.; Ercole, E.; Hall, A.; Chwaya, H. M.; Alawi, K. S.; Savioli, L., Rate of reinfection with intestinal nematodes after treatment of children with mebendazole or albendazole in a highly endemic area. *Transactions of the Royal Society of Tropical Medicine and Hygiene* **1995,** *89* (5), 538-41.

54. Nacher, M.; Singhasivanon, P.; Yimsamran, S.; Manibunyong, W.; Thanyavanich, N.; Wuthisen, R.; Looareesuwan, S., Intestinal helminth infections are associated with increased incidence of Plasmodium falciparum malaria in Thailand. *J Parasitol* **2002,** *88* (1), 55-8.

55. Kumar, S.; Pritchard, D. I., Skin penetration by ensheathed third-stage infective larvae of Necator americanus, and the host's immune response to larval antigens. *International journal for parasitology* **1992,** *22* (5), 573-9.

56. Hotez, P. J.; Diemert, D.; Bacon, K. M.; Beaumier, C.; Bethony, J. M.; Bottazzi, M. E.; Brooker, S.; Couto, A. R.; Freire Mda, S.; Homma, A.; Lee, B. Y.; Loukas, A.; Loblack, M.; Morel, C. M.; Oliveira, R. C.; Russell, P. K., The Human Hookworm Vaccine. *Vaccine* **2013,** *31 Suppl 2*, B227-32.

57. Bottazzi, M. E., The human hookworm vaccine: recent updates and prospects for success. *J Helminthol* **2015,** *89* (5), 540-4.

58. Pearson, M. S.; Jariwala, A. R.; Abbenante, G.; Plieskatt, J.; Wilson, D.; Bottazzi, M. E.; Hotez, P. J.; Keegan, B.; Bethony, J. M.; Loukas, A., New tools for NTD vaccines: A case study of quality control assays for product development of the human hookworm vaccine Na-APR-1M74. *Hum Vaccin Immunother* **2015,** *11* (5), 1251-7.

59. Howitt, M. R.; Lavoie, S.; Michaud, M.; Blum, A. M.; Tran, S. V.; Weinstock, J. V.; Gallini, C. A.; Redding, K.; Margolskee, R. F.; Osborne, L. C.; Artis, D.; Garrett, W. S., Tuft cells, taste-chemosensory cells, orchestrate parasite type 2 immunity in the gut. *Science* **2016,** *351* (6279), 1329-33.

60. Maxwell, C.; Hussain, R.; Nutman, T. B.; Poindexter, R. W.; Little, M. D.; Schad, G. A.; Ottesen, E. A., The clinical and immunologic responses of normal human volunteers to low dose hookworm (Necator americanus) infection. *Am J Trop Med Hyg* **1987,** *37* (1), 126-34.

61. White, C. J.; Maxwell, C. J.; Gallin, J. I., Changes in the structural and functional properties of human eosinophils during experimental hookworm infection. *J Infect Dis* **1986,** *154* (5), 778-83.

62. Yoshida, Y.; Nakanishi, Y.; Mitani, W.; J., Experimental studies on the infection mode of Ancylostoma duodenale and Necator americanus to the definitive host. *Japanese* **1958,** *7*, 102-112.

63. Schad, G. A.; Anderson, R. M., Predisposition to hookworm infection in humans. *Science (New York, N.Y.)* **1985,** *228* (4707), 1537-40.

64. Quinnell, R. J.; Griffin, J.; Nowell, M. A.; Raiko, A.; Pritchard, D. I., Predisposition to hookworm infection in Papua New Guinea. *Trans R Soc Trop Med Hyg* **2001,** *95* (2), 139-42.

65. Albonico, M.; Stoltzfus, R. J.; Savioli, L.; Tielsch, J. M.; Chwaya, H. M.; Ercole, E.; Cancrini, G., Epidemiological evidence for a differential effect of hookworm species, Ancylostoma duodenale or Necator americanus, on iron status of children. *International journal of epidemiology* **1998,** *27*

(3), 530-7.

66.   Stoltzfus, R. J.; Dreyfuss, M. L.; Chwaya, H. M.; Albonico, M., Hookworm control as a strategy to prevent iron deficiency. *Nutrition reviews* **1997,** *55* (6), 223-32.

67.   Stoltzfus, R. J.; Chwaya, H. M.; Tielsch, J. M.; Schulze, K. J.; Albonico, M.; Savioli, L., Epidemiology of iron deficiency anemia in Zanzibari schoolchildren: the importance of hookworms. *The American journal of clinical nutrition* **1997,** *65* (1), 153-9.

68.   Stoltzfus, R. J.; Albonico, M.; Chwaya, H. M.; Savioli, L.; Tielsch, J.; Schulze, K.; Yip, R., Hemoquant determination of hookworm-related blood loss and its role in iron deficiency in African children. *The American journal of tropical medicine and hygiene* **1996,** *55* (4), 399-404.

69.   Crosby, W. H., Whatever became of chlorosis? *JAMA* **1987,** *257* (20), 2799-800.

70.   Hotez, P. J., Hookworm disease in children. *The Pediatric infectious disease journal* **1989,** *8* (8), 516-20.

71.   Stephenson, L. S.; Latham, M. C.; Kurz, K. M.; Kinoti, S. N.; Brigham, H., Treatment with a single dose of albendazole improves growth of Kenyan schoolchildren with hookworm, Trichuris trichiura, and Ascaris lumbricoides infections. *The American journal of tropical medicine and hygiene* **1989,** *41* (1), 78-87.

72.   World Development Report. 1993.

73.   van Mens, S. P.; Aryeetey, Y.; Yazdanbakhsh, M.; van Lieshout, L.; Boakye, D.; Verweij, J. J., Comparison of real-time PCR and Kato smear microscopy for the detection of hookworm infections in three consecutive faecal samples from schoolchildren in Ghana. *Trans R Soc Trop Med Hyg* **2013,** *107* (4), 269-71.

74.   Phuphisut, O.; Yoonuan, T.; Sanguankiat, S.; Chaisiri, K.; Maipanich, W.; Pubampen, S.; Komalamisra, C.; Adisakwattana, P., Triplex polymerase chain reaction assay for detection of major soil-transmitted helminths, Ascaris lumbricoides, Trichuris trichiura, Necator americanus, in fecal samples. *Southeast Asian J Trop Med Public Health* **2014,** *45* (2), 267-75.

75.   Albonico, M.; Crompton, D. W.; Savioli, L., Control strategies for human intestinal nematode infections. *Advances in parasitology* **1999,** *42,* 277-341.

76.   DeClercq, D.; Sacko, M.; J., Failure of mebendazole in treatment of human hookworm infections in the southern region of Mali. *Am Med Hyg* **1997,** *57* 25-30.

77.   Steinmann, P.; Utzinger, J.; Du, Z. W.; Jiang, J. Y.; Chen, J. X.; Hattendorf, J.; Zhou, H.; Zhou, X. N., Efficacy of single-dose and triple-dose albendazole and mebendazole against soil-transmitted helminths and Taenia spp.: a randomized controlled trial. *PLoS One* **2011,** *6* (9), e25003.

78.   Soukhathammavong, P. A.; Sayasone, S.; Phongluxa, K.; Xayaseng, V.; Utzinger, J.; Vounatsou, P.; Hatz, C.; Akkhavong, K.; Keiser, J.; Odermatt, P., Low efficacy of single-dose albendazole and mebendazole against hookworm and effect on concomitant helminth infection in Lao PDR. *PLoS Negl Trop Dis* **2012,** *6* (1), e1417.

79.   Keiser, J.; Utzinger, J., Efficacy of current drugs against soil-transmitted helminth infections: systematic review and meta-analysis. *JAMA* **2008,** *299* (16), 1937-48.

80.   Brooker, S.; Peshu, N.; Warn, P. A.; Mosobo, M.; Guyatt, H. L.; Marsh, K.; Snow, R. W., The epidemiology of hookworm infection and its contribution to anaemia among pre-school children on the Kenyan coast. *Transactions of the Royal Society of Tropical Medicine and Hygiene* **1999,** *93* (3), 240-6.

81.   Christian, P.; Khatry, S. K.; West, K. P., Antenatal anthelmintic treatment, birthweight, and infant survival in rural Nepal. *Lancet (London, England)* **2004,** *364* (9438), 981-3.

82.   Albonico, M.; Engels, D.; Savioli, L., Monitoring drug efficacy and early detection of drug resistance in human soil-transmitted nematodes: a pressing public health agenda for helminth control. *International journal for parasitology* **2004,** *34* (11), 1205-10.

83.   Ndibazza, J.; Muhangi, L.; Akishule, D.; Kiggundu, M.; Ameke, C.; Oweka, J.; Kizindo, R.; Duong, T.; Kleinschmidt, I.; Muwanga, M.; Elliott, A. M., Effects of deworming during pregnancy on maternal and perinatal outcomes in Entebbe, Uganda: a randomized controlled trial. *Clin Infect Dis* **2010,** *50* (4), 531-40.

84.   Torp-Pedersen, A.; Jimenez-Solem, E.; Andersen, J. T.; Broedbaek, K.; Torp-Pedersen, C.; Poulsen, H. E., Exposure to mebendazole and pyrvinium during pregnancy: a Danish nationwide cohort

study. *Infect Dis Obstet Gynecol* **2012,** *2012,* 769851.

85.   Fennell, B.; Naughton, J.; Barlow, J.; Brennan, G.; Fairweather, I.; Hoey, E.; McFerran, N.; Trudgett, A.; Bell, A., Microtubules as antiparasitic drug targets. *Expert Opin Drug Discov* **2008,** *3* (5), 501-18.

86.   Von Samson-Himmelstjerna, G.; Blackhall, W. J.; McCarthy, J. S.; Skuce, P. J., Single nucleotide polymorphism (SNP) markers for benzimidazole resistance in veterinary nematodes. *Parasitology* **2007,** *134* (Pt 8), 1077-86.

87.   Zheng, Q.; Chen, Y.; Zhang, H. B.; Chen, J. X.; Zhou, X. N., The control of hookworm infection in China. *Parasit Vectors* **2009,** *2* (1), 44.

88.   Humphries, D. L.; Stephenson, L. S.; Pearce, E. J.; The, P. H.; Dan, H. T.; Khanh, L. T., The use of human faeces for fertilizer is associated with increased intensity of hookworm infection in Vietnamese women. *Transactions of the Royal Society of Tropical Medicine and Hygiene* **1997,** *91* (5), 518-20.

89.   Anderson, R.; Truscott, J.; Hollingsworth, T. D., The coverage and frequency of mass drug administration required to eliminate persistent transmission of soil-transmitted helminths. *Philos Trans R Soc Lond B Biol Sci* **2014,** *369* (1645), 20130435.

90.   Chan, M. S.; Bradley, M.; Bundy, D. A., Transmission patterns and the epidemiology of hookworm infection. *International journal of epidemiology* **1997,** *26* (6), 1392-400.

91.   Bartsch, S. M.; Hotez, P. J.; Hertenstein, D. L.; Diemert, D. J.; Zapf, K. M.; Bottazzi, M. E.; Bethony, J. M.; Brown, S. T.; Lee, B. Y., Modeling the economic and epidemiologic impact of hookworm vaccine and mass drug administration (MDA) in Brazil, a high transmission setting. *Vaccine* **2016,** *34* (19), 2197-206.

92.   Lee, B. Y.; Bacon, K. M.; Bailey, R.; Wiringa, A. E.; Smith, K. J., The potential economic value of a hookworm vaccine. *Vaccine* **2011,** *29* (6), 1201-10.

20. *Strongyloides stercoralis*
(Bavay 1876)

Introduction

Strongyloides stercoralis is a parasitic nematode with a worldwide distribution, and is particularly prevalent throughout tropical and subtropical regions, as well as temperate climates. In Sub-Saharan Africa, South East Asia (e.g. Cambodia), parts of the Caribbean and in South America, prevalence rates in many areas are higher than 20%.[1] In North America, it occurs frequently among immigrants, in parts of Appalachia and in patients at long-term care facilities.[2-4] Because of the difficulty in establishing a definitive diagnosis, and because the parasite may cause long-lasting asymptomatic infections, the true global prevalence of human strongyloidiasis is unknown. Estimates indicate that there may be as many as 100 million cases/year.[2, 5]

Reservoir hosts play an important part in this nematode's biology, with dogs and non-human primates able to harbor strongyloides.[6] There have been numerous outbreaks of strongyloidiasis among animal handlers.[7] *S. stercoralis* can also reproduce as a free-living nematode in soil. In this case, the L3 larva of that phase retains its ability to infect mammalian hosts. This qualifies *S. stercoralis* as one of the most environmentally adaptable nematode infections of humans.

A second form of human strongyloidiasis, caused by *S. fuelleborni kellyi*, has been described in infants living in Papua New Guinea, and in Sub-Saharan Africa.[8, 9] Children with this infection can develop a special clinical syndrome called swollen belly syndrome (SBS).[10] This condition is associated with a high rate of mortality. In some rural villages, the prevalence of *S. fuelleborni* may reach nearly 100% during the early years of life, then it declines in older children and adults.[11]

Historical Information

Clinical infection with *Strongyloides stercoralis* was first described by Arthur Bavay and Louis Normand in 1876, while they were working together in Toulon, France.[12, 13] Their patients were French army personnel, newly arrived from Cochin, Indochina (modern day southern Vietnam); thus the term for strongyloidal enteritis, "Cochin China diarrhea." Bavay recovered numerous larvae of a species of nematode that had not been previously described from the stool of these patients, and named it *Anguillula stercoralis*.[14]

Max Askanazy described the pathology of strongyloidiasis, and the life cycle was reported by Friedrich Fuelleborn.[15, 16] Fuelleborn conducted experiments in dogs and learned that infective larvae penetrate unbroken skin. In 1928, Masao Nishigoii described autoinfection with *S. stercoralis*, and also showed that infected dogs made

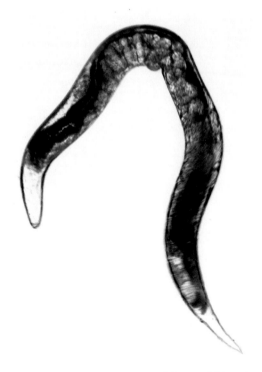

Figure 20.1. Free-living adult of *Strongyloides stercoralis*. This stage occurs in soil only. 600 μm.

Strongyloides stercoralis

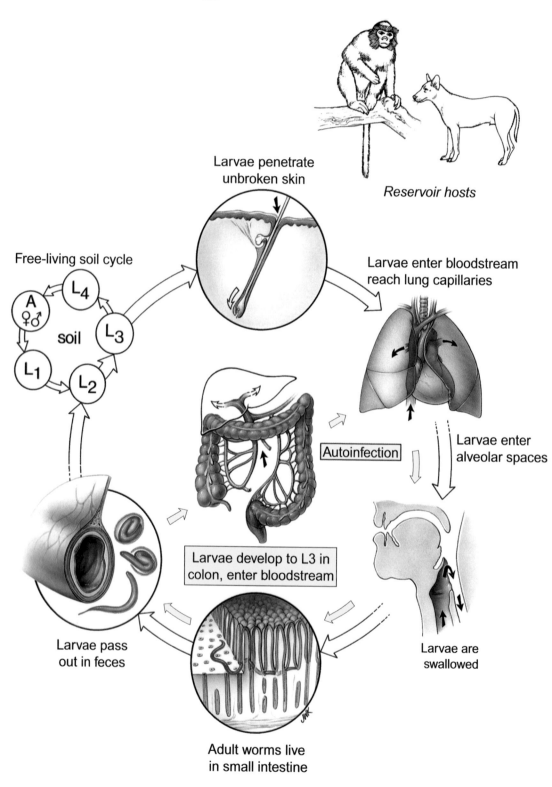

Reservoir hosts

Larvae penetrate
unbroken skin

Larvae enter bloodstream
reach lung capillaries

Free-living soil cycle

A ♀♂

L4

L3

soil

L1

L2

Autoinfection

Larvae enter
alveolar spaces

Larvae develop to L3 in
colon, enter bloodstream

Larvae pass
out in feces

Larvae are
swallowed

Adult worms live
in small intestine

constipated with morphine and bismuth subnitrate passed infective L3 larvae, rather than non-infective L2 larvae.[17] In addition, he noted that the number of larvae passed by these animals increased, so long as constipation was maintained. These studies preceded the clinical description of autoinfection now known to also occur in humans.

Life Cycle

Strongyloides stercoralis exists both as a free-living (Fig. 20.1) and as a parasitic nematode (Fig. 20.2a). The parasitic adult female is about 2 mm long and 35 μm wide. The parasitic worm lives embedded within a row of columnar epithelial cells in the small intestine (Fig. 20.2b), usually in the region of the duodenum and proximal jejunum. Adult worms may live for up to 5 years. Reproduction is by parthenogenesis during this portion of the life cycle, with release of eggs into lamina propria.[18]

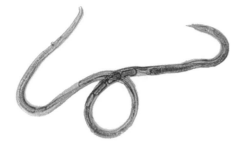

Figure 20.2a. Parasitic female of *S. stercoralis*. 2.5 mm x 35 μm. Courtesy L. Ash and T. Orihel.

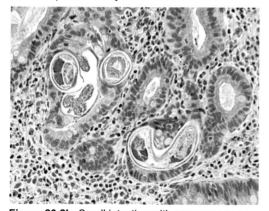

Figure 20.2b. Small intestine with numerous sections of a parasitic female *S. stercoralis*.

The embryonated eggs hatch rapidly into L1 larvae, which emerge into the lumen of the small intestine. Larvae proceed to the colon where they molt once, becoming L2 (rhabditiform) larvae that can then be deposited in soil with feces. Alternatively, they may molt into L3 (filariform) larvae while still within the lumen of the colon, burrow into the mucosa, and enter the circulation directly or through the perianal skin. This process is known as autoinfection.[19] Free-living phase L2 larvae require warm, moist, sandy, or loamy soil for the next developmental phase of the cycle to take place. In the proper soil, and under optimal environmental conditions, they develop to free-living adult worms. This occurs by four successive molts. In contrast to the parthenogenic portion of the life cycle in the mammalian host, adult worms of both sexes are found during the free-living phase in soil.[18] They mate, and the female produces embryonated eggs that hatch and develop into L2 larvae (Fig. 20.3) that may either mature into adults, continuing the free-living life cycle, or molt to become L3 larvae. The L3 larva can infect humans and other susceptible hosts. When conditions become unfavorable for the continuation of the free-living phase (e.g., lack of nutrition, low moisture) more L2 larvae transform into the infective L3 stage[20] that can remain in soil for several

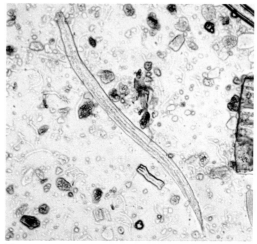

Figure 20.3. L2 larva of *S. stercoralis*. 580 μm x 15 μm.

days. When the L3 larvae encounter a suitable host, they penetrate the skin (Fig. 20.4.) and begin the parasitic phase of the infection. L3 larvae can also "swim" in aquatic environments, giving them a greater range in which to find a host, as compared to hookworm L3 larvae, which cannot do so. If L3 larvae fail to locate a host within 3 days, they expend all their stored glycogen and die.

Parasitic Phase (Homogonic Life Cycle)

The L3 larva enters the host through the skin, a process facilitated by the release of a protease by the parasite.[21] Upon entry into the host, the immature worm probably enters a venule and/or lymphatic vessel before being carried through the afferent circulation to the right heart, pulmonary artery, and pulmonary capillaries. The larva ruptures into the alveolar space, actively crawls up the respiratory tree, passes through the trachea into the pharynx, crosses the epiglottis, and is swallowed. *S. stercoralis* may not always

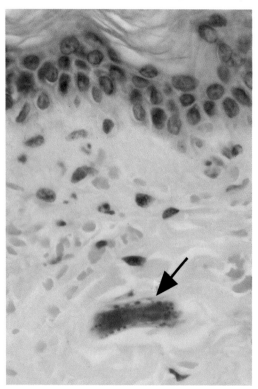

Figure 20.4. Filariform (L3) larva (arrow) of *S. stercoralis* in cutaneous layer of skin.

migrate through the lungs to reach the intestinal tract.[22] The larva undergoes a final molt in the small intestine and becomes the parasitic parthenogenic female. Egg production begins within 25-30 days after the initial infection.

Autoinfection, Hyperinfection, and Disseminated Infection

In some patients, L2 larvae develop within the colon to the infective L3 stage.[23] The infective larvae may reenter the circulation before they migrate through the lungs and are swallowed. This process is referred to as autoinfection, and allows the parasite to remain inside the same host for many years. Low levels of autoinfection are thought to be common, and may occur during a primary infection.[24] In debilitated, malnourished, or immunocompromised patients, autoinfection can amplify, leading to hyperinfection characterized by a large increase in the worm burden. *S. stercoralis* is one of the few parasitic nematodes infecting humans that can increase its numbers within the same individual (the other being *Capillaria philippinensis* (see Fig. 26.1)). Hyperinfection can also lead to disseminated infection, characterized by the presence of various stages of larvae at ectopic sites, including the central nervous system.

Vertical Transmission

The mode of transmission of *S. fuelleborni* infection leading to swollen belly syndrome is unknown, although the high incidence of this parasite in infants has led to the speculation that it is transmitted through mothers' milk. In support of this notion, the larvae of *S. fuelleborni* have been demonstrated in mammary secretions.[25]

Cellular and Molecular Pathogenesis

Parasitic females induce essentially no damage to the mucosa of the small intestine, but do elicit local inflammation. In some experimental studies, T-cell function appears to be necessary for the development of resistance to strongyloides infection, and may reflect the same immune cascade elicited by tuft cells in the small intestine.[20, 26] Impairment of T-cell function has been proposed as the basis by which subsets of infected individuals fail to regulate the number of worms in their small intestines, developing strongyloides hyperinfection and disseminated infection. This is evident in patients with immunosuppression due to malignancy, Human T-cell lymphotropic virus type 1 (HTLV-1) infection, alcoholism, malnutrition, corticosteroids, and cytotoxic medications.[19, 27-30] Despite a few reports of disseminated strongyloides in patients with HIV/AIDS, the significantly higher-than-expected incidence of hyperinfection and disseminated strongyloides infections has not been seen in HIV-1-infected patients.[31-33] Speculation focuses on the fact that hyperinfection occurs in response to elevated steroid levels in patients at risk for these conditions.[31, 32] The steroid effect may be mediated by their ability to suppress eosinophilia, interfere with lymphocyte activation, or have a direct impact on the parasitic larvae that accelerates their maturation into invasive L3 larvae while still within the colon of the infected patient.[20]

There is an association between HTLV-1 infection and strongyloidiasis.[20] This has been observed on the islands of Okinawa and Jamaica.[34-36] The basis for this association is unknown, although it is suggested that patients with HTLV-1 may have selective deficits in parasite-specific antibodies, including IgE and induced T-cell tolerance for strongyloides due to HTLV-1 tropism for regulatory T-cells.[36, 37] Severe strongyloidiasis has also been described in an IgA-deficient patient, but a causal connection between IgA deficiency and strongyloides is unclear.[36]

In cases of hyperinfection or disseminated infection, penetrating L3 larvae often carry enteric microorganisms in their gut tract that

they fed upon during their life as L2 larvae. As they develop further, they regurgitate these microbes throughout the tissues of the host, often leading to local infection/bacteremia, followed by general sepsis.[38] Such clinical sequelae are frequently fatal.[39]

Clinical Disease

Following infection of immunocompetent individuals there may be no prominent symptoms or a watery, mucosal diarrhea, the degree of which varies with the intensity of the infection. The majority of infected patients display no symptoms following infection, and peripheral eosinophilia may be the only evidence of acute infection.[40, 41] Some individuals may report skin reactions, commonly called ground itch, due to penetration of the skin by the infecting L3 larvae.[42] The rash of ground itch is characteristically on the feet. In the approximately 25% of symptomatic patients, states of alternating diarrhea and constipation, abdominal discomfort, vomiting and epigastric pain that worsens with eating have been reported.[40, 43] Although these symptoms typically last for about six weeks, some individuals may have persistent symptoms for years.[44] Children with *S. stercoralis* may develop a syndrome characterized by anorexia, cachexia, chronic diarrhea, fat and protein malabsorption, and abdominal distension. They can have impaired growth, which is reversible after specific anthelminthic chemotherapy.[45] Infants with swollen belly syndrome from *S. fuelleborni* may present acutely, but usually without fever and diarrhea.[8, 9] Instead, these children develop abdominal ascites as a result of protein loss, which can accumulate to the point of causing respiratory embarrassment.

During the migratory phase of the infection, symptoms may resemble those described for ascariasis and hookworm disease (e.g., pneumonitis), although in the absence of disseminated infection, pulmonary symptoms are not usually prominent. More commonly, pulmonary strongyloidiasis is characterized by asymptomatic circulating eosinophilia.[46] Migration of larvae through the skin gives rise to a serpiginous, creeping urticarial eruption, a condition known as *larva currens*.[47] Larvae have been observed to migrate through the skin as fast as 5-15 cm per hour, leaving intense red pruritic streaks on the abdomen or lateral thighs.[43] Strongyloidiasis may also present with a petechial purpuric rash (peri-umbilical parasitic thumbprint purpura) that is commonly present on the anterior abdomen or lateral thighs.[43, 48, 49]

Hyperinfection and Disseminated Infection

Clinical symptoms are exaggerated if hyperinfection is superimposed on an already chronic infection. Massive invasion by strongyloides larvae due to hyperinfection has an impressive presentation as acute enteritis, with severe diarrhea and ulcerating disease of the small and large intestine. These patients often have secondary bacterial enterocolitis that can result in a paralytic ileus, and bacterial invasion that results in metastatic abscesses and bacterial meningitis. During disseminated infection, the larvae themselves may enter the central nervous system with the development of gram-negative meningitis from enteric pathogens, and in some cases secondary abscesses.[50-53] Pulmonary invasion is also exaggerated during disseminated infection, and can lead to a clinical presentation of pneumonia, pulmonary embolism, intrapulmonary hemorrhage, or acute respiratory failure.[54]

Diagnosis

Strongyloides infection should be considered in any patient with unexplained gastrointestinal symptoms, with or without eosinophilia, and an appropriate exposure history.[55] Identification of the larvae in stool samples is the definitive method of diagnosis. Because few organisms are intermittently released into the stool, the sensitivity of a standard single stool examination is less than 50 percent, and even as low as 30% by some estimates.[2, 56, 57] As few as 50 L2 larva are released per day by each adult strongyloides. Compare this reproductive output with that of ascaris, which produces more than 200,000 eggs per day. It is highly recommended that a large quantity of stool (e.g., multiple samples on multiple days) must be made available, and all of it should be processed by a sedimentation method to concentrate the larvae, greatly improving the chances for seeing the organisms on microscopic examination (Figs. 20.3, 20.6). Even when sedimentation techniques are used, low-grade infections are usually missed, and a rigorous search with multiple stool examinations must be carried out before a patient can be declared free of the infection. *S. stercoralis* larvae can be differentiated from those of hookworm (Fig. 20.5) by two characteristics. The L2 larva of *S. stercoralis* has a short buccal cavity (Fig. 20.6), while the L3 larva has a notched tail (Fig. 20.7). Laboratories that are comfortable with handling the organism can enhance the sensitivity of their stool examinations by plating out a fecal pat on an agar plate and detecting the tracks of bacteria dragged along by migrating larvae. Alternatively, some laboratories can amplify the number of strongyloides larvae

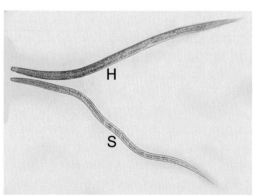

Figure 20.5. Filariform (L3) larvae. H = Hookworm and S = *Strongyloides*. Courtesy L. Ash and T. Orihel.

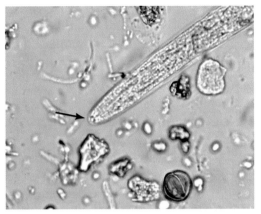

Figure 20.6. Buccal cavity (arrow) of the rhabditiform (L2) larva of *S. stercoralis*. Compare with Figure 19. 8.

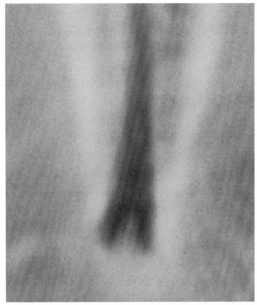

Figure 20.7. Notched tail of filariform larva of *S. stercoralis,* Hookworm L3 larva has a pointed tail.

by mixing the stool with bone charcoal and incubating the preparation under conditions that permit the heterogonic life cycle to take place (coproculture).[58, 59]

In patients with hyperinfection or disseminated infection, the yield of strongyloides larvae may be increased by recovering them from duodenal fluid.[57] Typically this is done through flexible endoscopy; intestinal biopsy is also a useful adjunct (Fig. 20.2b). During disseminated infections, it is possible to identify the parasite from sputum and bronchoalveolar lavage fluid.[19] Several different serological tests include ELISA for immunoglobulin G (IgG) are available, but their sensitivities and specificities can vary significantly.[60-62] Despite their limitations, serologic testing is currently the diagnostic method of choice. Immunological approaches for detecting parasite-specific antibodies in serum by indirect enzyme-linked immuosorbent assays (ELISA) can achieve diagnostic sensitivity around 85% but have a lower specificity primarily because of cross reactivity with other helminths. PCR assays are under development, including multiplex quantitative PCR assays to simultaneously diagnosis parasite co-infections.[63]

Treatment

While thiabendazole was administered in the past for uncomplicated infection, ivermectin has fewer side effects and has replaced it as the drug of choice.[64-68] Albendazole is an alternative drug, but is less effective than ivermectin.[69]

For patients with hyperinfection and disseminated disease the ideal treatment is unknown, but usually ivermectin is extended to between 5 days and several weeks and often albendazole is added.[64, 65, 70-72] Treatment efficacy can be monitored based on patient response and repeated stool examinations.[73] In some cases of severe infection veterinary parenteral preparations of ivermectin have been used successfully in the treatment of disseminated strongyloidiais.[74, 75] Intensive supportive therapy, including antimicrobial agents, is often required in patients with hyperinfection from *S. stercoralis*, as well as parenteral nutrition to compensate for extensive protein and lipid losses. *S. fuelleborni* infection is treated successfully with thiabendazole.[76]

Prevention and Control

Disease risk may be greatly reduced by

wearing shoes in endemic areas.[77] Reservoir hosts include dogs and primates, most notably chimpanzees. As mentioned, a small outbreak of human strongyloidiasis that originated in dogs has been described.[7] However, the role of primates as a foci of human infection in rural tropical areas is doubtful. Animal care personnel at research institutions are at high risk for acquiring strongyloidiasis. Newly-arrived primates intended for use in investigative research protocols are first kept in isolation and routinely treated with ivermectin to prevent the spread of this nematode parasite. Other even more serious pathogens have been introduced to this group of employees in past years, such as Marburg virus and Ebola virus. Quarantine is the best way of making sure that these serious pathogens do not cause in-house epidemics, such as the one that occurred at Hoechst in Marburg, Germany in 1967.[78]

Custodial institutions can be a foci of infection, and consequently screening and treating patients can prevent spread.[79] Efforts to diagnose and screen individuals who harbor *S. stercoralis* are sometimes carried out among patients who are candidates for immunosuppressive therapy.[5] Treatment of pregnant women or those who are infected and of childbearing age would reduce transmammary transmission of *S. fuelleborni*, although many of the available antihelminthic medications are relatively contraindicated during pregnancy. Currently strongyloidiasis is not targeted for mass drug administration, as are ascariasis, trichuriasis, hookworm, lymphatic filariasis, and onchocerciasis. Given the widespread use of albendazole and ivermectin for this purpose, it is conceivable that strongyloidiasis is also now being treated as a collateral parasitic infection, or possibly it could be added as a sixth helminthiasis in a newly designed global de-worming program.[80]

References

1. WHO Strongyloides. http://www.who.int/intestinal_worms/epidemiology/strongyloidiasis/en/ (accessed 9/2/2016).
2. Genta, R. M.; Weesner, R.; Douce, R. W.; Huitger-O'Connor, T.; Walzer, P. D., Strongyloidiasis in US veterans of the Vietnam and other wars. *JAMA* **1987,** *258* (1), 49-52.
3. Russell, E. S.; Gray, E. B.; Marshall, R. E.; Davis, S.; Beaudoin, A.; Handali, S.; McAuliffe, I.; Davis, C.; Woodhall, D., Prevalence of Strongyloides stercoralis antibodies among a rural Appalachian population--Kentucky, 2013. *Am J Trop Med Hyg* **2014,** *91* (5), 1000-1.
4. Centers for Disease, C.; Prevention, Notes from the field: strongyloides infection among patients at a long-term care facility--Florida, 2010-2012. *MMWR Morb Mortal Wkly Rep* **2013,** *62* (42), 844.
5. Genta, R. M., Global prevalence of strongyloidiasis: critical review with epidemiologic insights into the prevention of disseminated disease. *Reviews of infectious diseases* **1989,** *11* (5), 755-67.
6. Goncalves, A. L.; Machado, G. A.; Goncalves-Pires, M. R.; Ferreira-Junior, A.; Silva, D. A.; Costa-Cruz, J. M., Evaluation of strongyloidiasis in kennel dogs and keepers by parasitological and serological assays. *Vet Parasitol* **2007,** *147* (1-2), 132-9.
7. Georgi, J. R.; Sprinkle, C. L., A case of human strongyloidosis apparently contracted from asymptomatic colony dogs. *Am J Trop Med Hyg* **1974,** *23* (5), 899-901.
8. Ashford, R. W.; Vince, J. D.; Gratten, M. J.; Miles, W. E., Strongyloides infection associated with acute infantile disease in Papua New Guinea. *Transactions of the Royal Society of Tropical Medicine and Hygiene* **1978,** *72* (5), 554.
9. Barnish, G.; Ashford, R. W., Strongyloides cf. fuelleborni and hookworm in Papua New Guinea: patterns of infection within the community. *Transactions of the Royal Society of Tropical Medicine and Hygiene* **1989,** *83* (5), 684-8.
10. Vince, J. D.; Ashford, R. W.; Gratten, M. J.; Bana-Koiri, J., Strongyloides species infestation in young infants of papu, New Guinea: association with generalized oedema. *P N G Med J* **1979,** *22*

(2), 120-7.

11. Ashford, R. W.; Vince, J. D.; Gratten, M. A.; Bana-Koiri, J., Strongyloides infection in a mid-mountain Papua New Guinea community: results of an epidemiological survey. *P N G Med J* **1979**, *22* (2), 128-35.

12. Bavay, A.; R., C., Sur l'anguillule stercorale. *Sci Paris* **1876**, *83*, 694-696.

13. Normand, L. A.; R., C., Sur la maladie dite diarrhie de Cochinchine. *Sean Acad Sci* **1876**, *83* 316-318.

14. Darling, S. T., Strongyloides Infections in Man and Animals in the Isthmian Canal Zone. *J Exp Med* **1911**, *14* (1), 1-24.

15. Askanazy, M., Uber Art und Zweck der Invasion der Anguillula intestinalis in die Darmwand. *Zbl Bakt* **1900**, *27* 569-578.

16. Fuelleborn, F., Untersuchungen uber den Infektionsweg bei Strongyloides und Ankylostomum und die Biologie diesen Parasiten. *Arch Schiffs Trop* **1914**, *18* 26-80.

17. Nishigoii, M., On various factors influencing the development of Strongyloides stercoralis and autoinfection. *Taiwan Sgakkai Zassi* **1928**, *27*, 1-56.

18. Streit, A., Reproduction in Strongyloides (Nematoda): a life between sex and parthenogenesis. *Parasitology* **2008**, *135* (3), 285-94.

19. Keiser, P. B.; Nutman, T. B., Strongyloides stercoralis in the Immunocompromised Population. *Clin Microbiol Rev* **2004**, *17* (1), 208-17.

20. Genta, R. M., Dysregulation of strongyloidiasis: a new hypothesis. *Clinical microbiology reviews* **1992**, *5* (4), 345-55.

21. McKerrow, J. H.; Brindley, P., Strongyloides stercoralis: identification of a protease whose inhibition prevents larval skin invasion. *Exp Parasitol* **1990**, *70* 134-143.

22. Schad, G. A.; Aikens, L. M.; Smith, G., Strongyloides stercoralis: is there a canonical migratory route through the host? *J Parasitol* **1989**, *75* (5), 740-9.

23. Shekamer, J. H.; Neva, F. A.; Finn, D. R.; J., Persistent strongyloidiasis in an immunodeficent patient. *Am Med Hyg* **1982**, *31* 746-751.

24. Schad, G. A.; Smith, G.; Megyeri, Z.; Bhopale, V. M.; Niamatali, S.; Maze, R., Strongyloidcs stercoralis: an initial autoinfective burst amplifies primary infection. *Am J Trop Med Hyg* **1993**, *48* (5), 716-25.

25. Brown, R. C.; Girardeau, H. F., Transmammary passage of Strongyloides sp. larvae in the human host. *Am J Trop Med Hyg* **1977**, *26* (2), 215-9.

26. Howitt, M. R.; Lavoie, S.; Michaud, M.; Blum, A. M.; Tran, S. V.; Weinstock, J. V.; Gallini, C. A.; Redding, K.; Margolskee, R. F.; Osborne, L. C.; Artis, D.; Garrett, W. S., Tuft cells, taste-chemosensory cells, orchestrate parasite type 2 immunity in the gut. *Science* **2016**, *351* (6279), 1329-33.

27. Safdar, A.; Malathum, K.; Rodriguez, S. J.; Husni, R.; Rolston, K. V., Strongyloidiasis in patients at a comprehensive cancer center in the United States. *Cancer* **2004**, *100* (7), 1531-6.

28. Carvalho, E. M.; Da Fonseca Porto, A., Epidemiological and clinical interaction between HTLV-1 and Strongyloides stercoralis. *Parasite Immunol* **2004**, *26* (11-12), 487-97.

29. Marques, C. C.; da Penha Zago-Gomes, M.; Goncalves, C. S.; Pereira, F. E., Alcoholism and Strongyloides stercoralis: daily ethanol ingestion has a positive correlation with the frequency of Strongyloides larvae in the stools. *PLoS Negl Trop Dis* **2010**, *4* (6), e717.

30. Buonfrate, D.; Requena-Mendez, A.; Angheben, A.; Munoz, J.; Gobbi, F.; Van Den Ende, J.; Bisoffi, Z., Severe strongyloidiasis: a systematic review of case reports. *BMC Infect Dis* **2013**, *13*, 78.

31. Lucas, S. B., Missing infections in AIDS. *Transactions of the Royal Society of Tropical Medicine and Hygiene* **1990**, *84 Suppl 1*, 34-8.

32. Robinson, R. D., Parasitic infections associated with HIV/AIDS in the Caribbean. *Bulletin of the Pan American Health Organization* **1995**, *29* (2), 129-37.

33. Viney, M. E.; Brown, M.; Omoding, N. E.; Bailey, J. W.; Gardner, M. P.; Roberts, E.; Morgan, D.; Elliott, A. M.; Whitworth, J. A., Why does HIV infection not lead to disseminated strongyloidiasis? *J Infect Dis* **2004**, *190* (12), 2175-80.

34.   Dixon, A. C.; Yanagihara, E. T.; Kwock, D. W.; Nakamura, J. M., Strongyloidiasis associated with human T-cell lymphotropic virus type I infection in a nonendemic area. *The Western journal of medicine* **1989,** *151* (4), 410-3.

35.   Arakaki, T.; Kohakura, M.; Asato, R.; Ikeshiro, T.; Nakamura, S.; Iwanaga, M., Epidemiological aspects of Strongyloides stercoralis infection in Okinawa, Japan. *The Journal of tropical medicine and hygiene* **1992,** *95* (3), 210-3.

36.   Neva, F. A.; Murphy, E. L.; Gam, A.; N.; J., Antibodies to Strongyloides stercoralis in healthy Jamaican carriers of HTLV-1. **1989,** *320*, 252-3.

37.   Montes, M.; Sanchez, C.; Verdonck, K.; Lake, J. E.; Gonzalez, E.; Lopez, G.; Terashima, A.; Nolan, T.; Lewis, D. E.; Gotuzzo, E.; White, A. C., Jr., Regulatory T cell expansion in HTLV-1 and strongyloidiasis co-infection is associated with reduced IL-5 responses to Strongyloides stercoralis antigen. *PLoS Negl Trop Dis* **2009,** *3* (6), e456.

38.   Gorman, S. R.; Craven, D. E., Images in clinical medicine. Strongyloides stercoralis hyperinfection. *N Engl J Med* **2008,** *359* (11), e12.

39.   Geri, G.; Rabbat, A.; Mayaux, J.; Zafrani, L.; Chalumeau-Lemoine, L.; Guidet, B.; Azoulay, E.; Pene, F., Strongyloides stercoralis hyperinfection syndrome: a case series and a review of the literature. *Infection* **2015,** *43* (6), 691-8.

40.   Valerio, L.; Roure, S.; Fernandez-Rivas, G.; Basile, L.; Martinez-Cuevas, O.; Ballesteros, A. L.; Ramos, X.; Sabria, M.; North Metropolitan Working Group on Imported, D., Strongyloides stercoralis, the hidden worm. Epidemiological and clinical characteristics of 70 cases diagnosed in the North Metropolitan Area of Barcelona, Spain, 2003-2012. *Trans R Soc Trop Med Hyg* **2013,** *107* (8), 465-70.

41.   Gonzalez, A.; Gallo, M.; Valls, M. E.; Munoz, J.; Puyol, L.; Pinazo, M. J.; Mas, J.; Gascon, J., Clinical and epidemiological features of 33 imported Strongyloides stercoralis infections. *Trans R Soc Trop Med Hyg* **2010,** *104* (9), 613-6.

42.   Bailey, M. S.; Thomas, R.; Green, A. D.; Bailey, J. W.; Beeching, N. J., Helminth infections in British troops following an operation in Sierra Leone. *Trans R Soc Trop Med Hyg* **2006,** *100* (9), 842-6.

43.   Greaves, D.; Coggle, S.; Pollard, C.; Aliyu, S. H.; Moore, E. M., Strongyloides stercoralis infection. *BMJ* **2013,** *347*, f4610.

44.   Vadlamudi, R. S.; Chi, D. S.; Krishnaswamy, G., Intestinal strongyloidiasis and hyperinfection syndrome. *Clin Mol Allergy* **2006,** *4*, 8.

45.   Leung, V. K.; Liew, C. T.; Sung, J. J., Strongyloidiasis in a patient with IgA deficiency. *Tropical gastroenterology : official journal of the Digestive Diseases Foundation* **1995,** *16* (4), 27-30.

46.   Burke, J. A., Strongyloidiasis in childhood. *American journal of diseases of children (1960)* **1978,** *132* (11), 1130-6.

47.   Berk, S. L.; Verghese, A.; Alvarez, S.; Hall, K.; Smith, B., Clinical and epidemiologic features of strongyloidiasis. A prospective study in rural Tennessee. *Archives of internal medicine* **1987,** *147* (7), 1257-61.

48.   Ribeiro, L. C.; Rodrigues Junior, E. N.; Silva, M. D.; Takiuchi, A.; Fontes, C. J., [Purpura in patient with disseminated strongiloidiasis]. *Rev Soc Bras Med Trop* **2005,** *38* (3), 255-7.

49.   Weiser, J. A.; Scully, B. E.; Bulman, W. A.; Husain, S.; Grossman, M. E., Periumbilical parasitic thumbprint purpura: strongyloides hyperinfection syndrome acquired from a cadaveric renal transplant. *Transpl Infect Dis* **2011,** *13* (1), 58-62.

50.   Cho, J. Y.; Kwon, J. G.; Ha, K. H.; Oh, J. Y.; Jin, M. I.; Heo, S. W.; Lee, G. H.; Cho, C. H., [A case of steroid-induced hyperinfective strongyloidiasis with bacterial meningitis]. *Korean J Gastroenterol* **2012,** *60* (5), 330-4.

51.   Sasaki, Y.; Taniguchi, T.; Kinjo, M.; McGill, R. L.; McGill, A. T.; Tsuha, S.; Shiiki, S., Meningitis associated with strongyloidiasis in an area endemic for strongyloidiasis and human T-lymphotropic virus-1: a single-center experience in Japan between 1990 and 2010. *Infection* **2013,** *41* (6), 1189-93.

52.   Shimasaki, T.; Chung, H.; Shiiki, S., Five cases of recurrent meningitis associated with chronic strongyloidiasis. *Am J Trop Med Hyg* **2015,** *92* (3), 601-4.

53. Zammarchi, L.; Montagnani, F.; Tordini, G.; Gotuzzo, E.; Bisoffi, Z.; Bartoloni, A.; De Luca, A., Persistent strongyloidiasis complicated by recurrent meningitis in an HTLV seropositive Peruvian migrant resettled in Italy. *Am J Trop Med Hyg* **2015**, *92* (6), 1257-60.

54. Newberry, A. M.; Williams, D. N.; Stauffer, W. M.; Boulware, D. R.; Hendel-Paterson, B. R.; Walker, P. F., Strongyloides hyperinfection presenting as acute respiratory failure and gram-negative sepsis. *Chest* **2005**, *128* (5), 3681-4.

55. Arsic-Arsenijevic, V.; Dzamic, A.; Dzamic, Z.; Milobratovic, D.; Tomic, D., Fatal Strongyloides stercoralis infection in a young woman with lupus glomerulonephritis. *J Nephrol* **2005**, *18* (6), 787-90.

56. Siddiqui, A. A.; Berk, S. L., Diagnosis of Strongyloides stercoralis infection. *Clin Infect Dis* **2001**, *33* (7), 1040-7.

57. Jones, C. A.; Abadie, S. H., Studies in human strongyloidiasis. II. A comparison of the efficiency of diagnosis by examination of feces and duodenal fluid. *Am J Clin Pathol* **1954**, *24* (10), 1154-8.

58. Costa-Cruz, J. M.; Bullamah, C. B.; Goncalves-Pires Mdo, R.; Campos, D. M.; Vieira, M. A., Cryo-microtome sections of coproculture larvae of Strongyloides stercoralis and Strongyloides ratti as antigen sources for the immunodiagnosis of human strongyloidiasis. *Rev Inst Med Trop Sao Paulo* **1997**, *39* (6), 313-7.

59. Attia, M. M.; El-Ridi, A. M.; Taha, M., Some observations on coproculture of Strongyloides stercoralis. *J Egypt Soc Parasitol* **1982**, *12* (1), 103-6.

60. van Doorn, H. R.; Koelewijn, R.; Hofwegen, H.; Gilis, H.; Wetsteyn, J. C.; Wismans, P. J.; Sarfati, C.; Vervoort, T.; van Gool, T., Use of enzyme-linked immunosorbent assay and dipstick assay for detection of Strongyloides stercoralis infection in humans. *J Clin Microbiol* **2007**, *45* (2), 438-42.

61. Von Kuster, L. C.; Genta, R. M., Cutaneous manifestations of stron-gyloidiasis. *Arch Dermatol* **1988**, *124*, 1826-1830.

62. Buonfrate, D.; Sequi, M.; Mejia, R.; Cimino, R. O.; Krolewiecki, A. J.; Albonico, M.; Degani, M.; Tais, S.; Angheben, A.; Requena-Mendez, A.; Munoz, J.; Nutman, T. B.; Bisoffi, Z., Accuracy of five serologic tests for the follow up of Strongyloides stercoralis infection. *PLoS Negl Trop Dis* **2015**, *9* (2), e0003491.

63. Cimino, R. O.; Jeun, R.; Juarez, M.; Cajal, P. S.; Vargas, P.; Echazu, A.; Bryan, P. E.; Nasser, J.; Krolewiecki, A.; Mejia, R., Identification of human intestinal parasites affecting an asymptomatic peri-urban Argentinian population using multi-parallel quantitative real-time polymerase chain reaction. *Parasit Vectors* **2015**, *8*, 380.

64. Neva, F. A., Biology and immunology of human strongyloidiasis. *J Infect Dis* **1986**, *153* (3), 397-406.

65. Naquira, C.; Jimenez, G.; Guerra, J. G.; Bernal, R.; Nalin, D. R.; Neu, D.; Aziz, M., Ivermectin for human strongyloidiasis and other intestinal helminths. *Am J Trop Med Hyg* **1989**, *40* (3), 304-9.

66. Lyagoubi, M.; Datry, A.; Mayorga, R.; Brucker, G.; Hilmarsdottir, I.; Gaxotte, P.; Neu, D.; Danis, M.; Gentilini, M., Chronic persistent strongyloidiasis cured by ivermectin. *Transactions of the Royal Society of Tropical Medicine and Hygiene* **1992**, *86* (5), 541.

67. Wijesundera, M. D.; Sanmuganathan, P. S.; R., Ivermectin therapy in chronic strongyloidiasis. *Trans Trop Med Hyg 291* **1994**, *86*

68. Gann, P. H.; Neva, F. A.; Gam, A. A., A randomized trial of single- and two-dose ivermectin versus thiabendazole for treatment of strongyloidiasis. *J Infect Dis* **1994**, *169* (5), 1076-9.

69. Muennig, P.; Pallin, D.; Challah, C.; Khan, K., The cost-effectiveness of ivermectin vs. albendazole in the presumptive treatment of strongyloidiasis in immigrants to the United States. *Epidemiol Infect* **2004**, *132* (6), 1055-63.

70. Segarra-Newnham, M., Manifestations, diagnosis, and treatment of Strongyloides stercoralis infection. *Ann Pharmacother* **2007**, *41* (12), 1992-2001.

71. Mejia, R.; Nutman, T. B., Screening, prevention, and treatment for hyperinfection syndrome and disseminated infections caused by Strongyloides stercoralis. *Curr Opin Infect Dis* **2012**, *25* (4), 458-63.

72. Boggild, A. K.; Libman, M.; Greenaway, C.; McCarthy, A. E., CATMAT statement on disseminated strongyloidiasis: Prevention, assessment and management guidelines. *Can Comm Dis*

Rep **2016**, *42*, 12-19.

73.   Schar, F.; Hattendorf, J.; Khieu, V.; Muth, S.; Char, M. C.; Marti, H. P.; Odermatt, P., Strongyloides stercoralis larvae excretion patterns before and after treatment. *Parasitology* **2014**, *141* (7), 892-7.

74.   Barrett, J.; Newsholme, W., Subcutaneous ivermectin use in the treatment of severe Strongyloides stercoralis infection: two case reports and a discussion of the literature-authors' response. *J Antimicrob Chemother* **2016**.

75.   Buonfrate, D.; Gobbi, F.; Bisoffi, Z., Comment on: Subcutaneous ivermectin use in the treatment of severe Strongyloides stercoralis infection: two case reports and a discussion of the literature. *J Antimicrob Chemother* **2016**.

76.   Barnish, G.; Barker, J., An intervention study using thiabendazole suspension against Strongyloides fuelleborni-like infections in Papua New Guinea. *Trans R Soc Trop Med Hyg* **1987**, *81* (1), 60-3.

77.   Yori, P. P.; Kosek, M.; Gilman, R. H.; Cordova, J.; Bern, C.; Chavez, C. B.; Olortegui, M. P.; Montalvan, C.; Sanchez, G. M.; Worthen, B.; Worthen, J.; Leung, F.; Ore, C. V., Seroepidemiology of strongyloidiasis in the Peruvian Amazon. *Am J Trop Med Hyg* **2006**, *74* (1), 97-102.

78.   Slenczka, W.; Klenk, H. D., Forty years of marburg virus. *J Infect Dis* **2007**, *196 Suppl 2*, S131-5.

79.   Nair, D., Screening for Strongyloides infection among the institutionalized mentally disabled. *J Am Board Fam Pract* **2001**, *14* (1), 51-3.

80.   Krolewiecki, A. J.; Lammie, P.; Jacobson, J.; Gabrielli, A. F.; Levecke, B.; Socias, E.; Arias, L. M.; Sosa, N.; Abraham, D.; Cimino, R.; Echazu, A.; Crudo, F.; Vercruysse, J.; Albonico, M., A public health response against Strongyloides stercoralis: time to look at soil-transmitted helminthiasis in full. *PLoS Negl Trop Dis* **2013**, *7* (5), e2165.

21. *Trichinella spiralis*

(Railliet 1896)

Introduction

The genus *Trichinella* has 12 recognized species and genotypes with different geographical distributions and all are capable of infecting humans [1-9] The identified trichinella species include; *T. spiralis, T. britovi, T. pseudospiralis, T. papua, T. native, T. nelson, T. murrelli, T. zambabwensis, and T. patagoniensis.*[1, 10-12] Members of the genus *Trichinella* are able to infect a broad spectrum of mammalian hosts, making them one of the world's most widely distributed group of nematode infections. *Trichinella* spp. are members of the family Trichurata and are genetically related to *Trichuris trichiura* and *Capillaria* spp.. *Trichinella* spp. constitute an unusual group of organisms in the phylum Nematoda, in that they all live a part of their lives as intracellular parasites. All species of trichinella are transmitted by ingestion of raw or undercooked infected meats.

Trichinellosis is the name given to the diseases caused by the *Trichinella* spp.. Currently, prevalence of trichinellosis is low within the United States, occurring mostly as scattered outbreaks, less often involving pork consumption and more often involving poorly cooked game with the majority of human cases being due to *Trichinella spiralis* and *T. murrelli.*[9, 13-15] The domestic pig is the main reservoir host for *T. spiralis*. This species is significantly higher in prevalence in people living in certain parts of Europe, Asia, and Southeast Asia than in the United States. It is now considered endemic in Japan and China. A large outbreak of trichinellosis occurred in Lebanon in 1997, infecting over 200 people.[16] *Trichinella spiralis* infection in humans has been reported from Korea for the first time.[17] In contrast, trichinella infections in wildlife within the United States are now thought to be largely due to *T. murrelli.*[18]

An outbreak of *T. pseudospiralis* in Thailand was reported.[19] This species can also infect birds of prey. Foci have also been described in Sweden, the Slovak Republic and Tasmania (Australia).[20-22] *Trichinella paupae,* similar in biology to *T. pseudospiralis*, has been described in wild and domestic pigs in Papua New Guinea.[11]

Humans can also be infected with *T. nativa* and *T. britovi.*[23, 24] Reservoir hosts for *T. nativa* include sled dogs, walruses, and polar bears. *T. britovi* is the sylvatic form of trichinellosis throughout most of Asia and Europe. There are numerous reports in the literature of infections with this parasite in fox, raccoon, dog, opossum, domestic and wild dogs, and cats.

T. nelsoni is restricted to mammals in Equatorial Africa, such as hyenas and the large predatory cats.[25] Occasionally people acquire infection with *T. nelsoni.*[26] Most animals in the wild, regardless of their geographic location, acquire trichinella by scavenging. *T. zimbabwensis* infects crocodiles and mammals in Africa, and is a non-encapsulate species that has been associated with pansteatitis outbreaks in crocodile populations in many areas of Sub-Saharan Africa.[11, 27] *T. pseudospiralis* has been isolated from the Tasmanian Devil, but not from humans living in that part of Australia.[22]

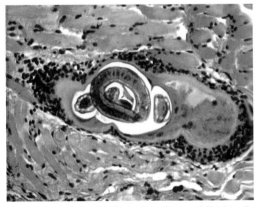

Figure 21.1. Infective first stage larva of *Trichinella spiralis* in its Nurse cell in muscle tissue. The worm measures 1mm x 36 µm.

Historical Information

In 1821, the encysted larva was recognized in muscle but was not associated with disease in humans.[28] In 1835, a medical student at St. Bartholomew's Hospital in London by the name of James Paget discovered the worm in humans.[29] Richard Owen, the director of the British Museum of Natural History, also saw the worms in muscle tissue derived from the same cadaver from which Paget obtained his muscle biopsy. The report of this discovery was published by Owen.[28] Both Rudolf Virchow and Friedrich Zenker, in 1859 and 1860, discovered the adult trichinella worms.[30] Zenker was the first to recognize that eating raw pork could result in infection of humans with trichinella.[31]

Life Cycle

There is both a domestic as well as a sylvatic cycle for trichinella. The domestic cycle involves animals such as pigs and horses, and the sylvatic cycle involves a very broad range of wild animals, including wild boar, bear, moose, cougars, crocodiles, foxes, birds and walruses.[32] In both cycles, infection is initiated by ingesting raw or undercooked meats harboring the nurse cell-larva complex (Fig. 21.1). Larvae are released from muscle tissue by digestive enzymes in the stomach, and then locate to the upper two-thirds of the small intestine. The outermost cuticular layer (epicuticle) becomes partially digested.[33, 34] This enables the parasite to receive environmental cues and to then select an infection site within the small intestine.[35] The immature parasites penetrate the columnar epithelium at the base of the villus. They live within a row of these cells, and are considered intra-multi-cellular organisms (Figs. 21.2, 21.7).[36]

Larvae molt four times in rapid succession over a 30-hour period, developing into adults. The female measures 3 mm in length by 36 μm in diameter (Fig. 21.3), while the male measures 1.5 mm in length by 36 μm in

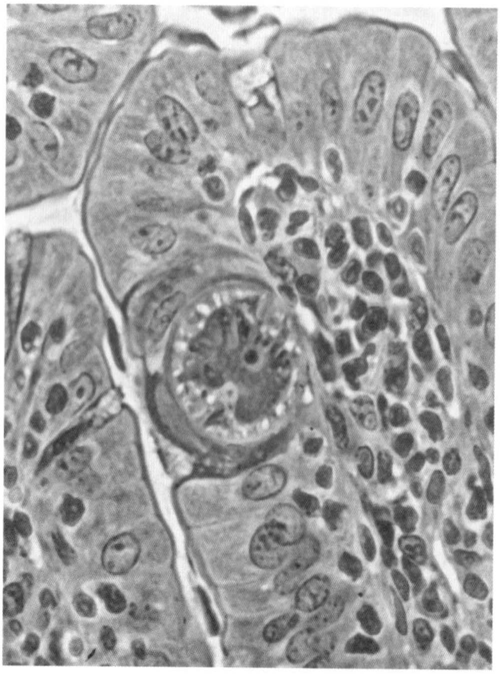

Figure 21.2. Adult *T. spiralis in situ*. Small intestine of experimentally infected mouse. The worm is embedded within the cytoplasm of the columnar cells.

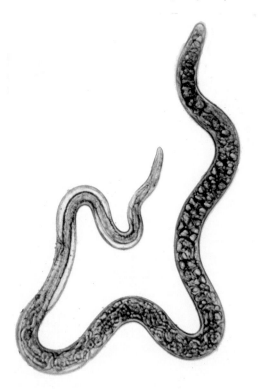

Figure 21.3. Adult female *T. spiralis*. 3 mm x 36 μm. Note fully formed larvae in uterus.

Trichinella spiralis

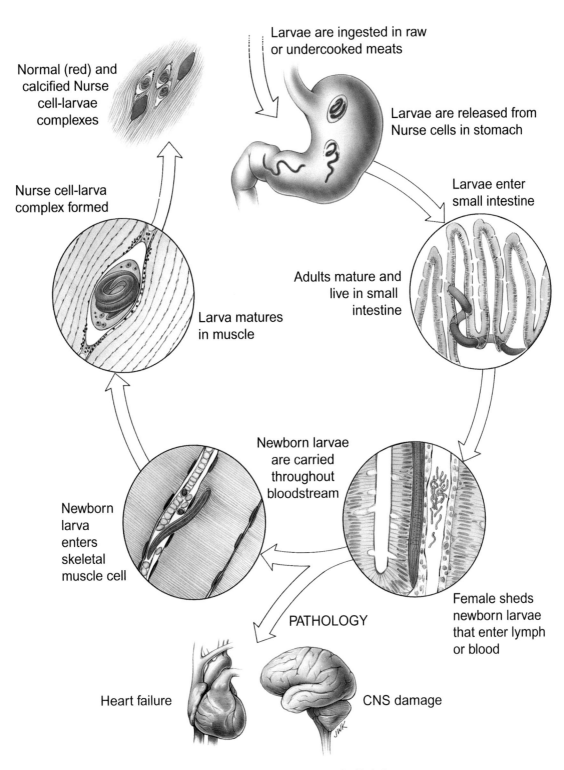

Larvae are ingested in raw or undercooked meats

Larvae are released from Nurse cells in stomach

Larvae enter small intestine

Normal (red) and calcified Nurse cell-larvae complexes

Nurse cell-larva complex formed

Larva matures in muscle

Adults mature and live in small intestine

Newborn larva enters skeletal muscle cell

Newborn larvae are carried throughout bloodstream

Female sheds newborn larvae that enter lymph or blood

PATHOLOGY

Heart failure

CNS damage

diameter (Fig. 21.4).

Patency occurs within five days after mating. Adult females produce live offspring — newborn larvae (Fig. 21.5) —that measure 0.08 mm long by 7 μm in diameter. The female produces offspring for as long as host immunity does not develop.[37] Eventually, acquired, protective responses interfere with the overall process of embryogenesis and creates physiological conditions in the local area of infection which forces the adult parasites to egress and relocate further down the intestinal tract. Expulsion of worms from the host is the final expression of immunity, and may take several weeks.

The newborn larva is the only stage of the parasite that possesses a sword-like stylet, located in its oral cavity. It uses it to create an entry hole in potential host cells. Larvae enter the lamina propria in this fashion, and penetrate into either the mesenteric lymphatics or into the bloodstream. Most newborn larvae enter the general circulation, and become dis-

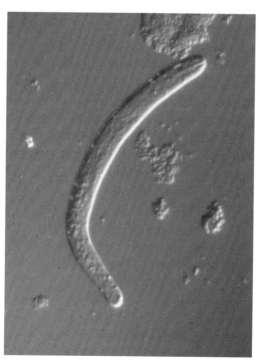

Figure 21.5. Newborn larva of *T. spiralis*. 70 x 7 μm.

tributed throughout the body.

Migrating newborns leave capillaries and enter cells (Fig. 21.6). There appears to be no tropism for any particular cell type. Once inside a cell, they can either remain or leave, depending upon environmental cues (yet to be determined) received by the parasite. Most cell types die as the result of invasion. Skeletal muscle cells are an exception.[38] Not only do the parasites remain inside them after invasion, they induce a remarkable series of changes, causing the fully differentiated muscle cell to transform into one that supports the growth and development of the larva (Figs 21.8, 21.9). This process is termed Nurse cell formation.[39] Parasite and host cell develop in a coordinated fashion. *T. spiralis* is infective by the 14th day of infection, but the worm continues to grow in size through day 20.[40] The significance of this precocious behavior has yet to be appreciated.

Parasites inside cells other than striated muscle cells fail to induce Nurse cells, and either reenter the general circulation or die. Nurse cell formation results in an intimate and

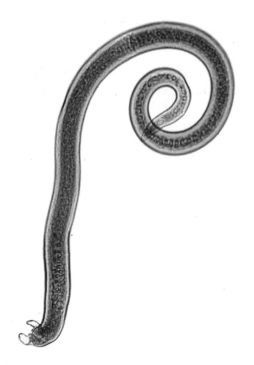

Figure 21. 4. Adult male *T. spiralis*. Note claspers on tail (lower end). 1.5mm x 36 μm.

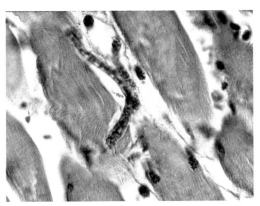

Figure 21.6. Newborn larva of *T. spiralis* entering muscle cell.

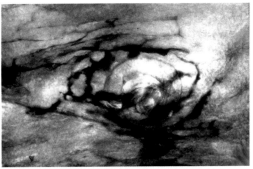

Figure 21.8. Nurse cell-parasite complex of *T. spiralis, in situ*. Infected mouse was injected with India ink to visualize circulatory rete.

permanent association between the worm and its intracellular niche. At the cellular level, myofilaments, and other related muscle cell components, become replaced over a 14-16 day period by whorls of smooth membranes and clusters of dysfunctional mitochondria. The net result is that the host cell switches from an aerobic to an anaerobic metabolism.[41] Host cell nuclei enlarge and divide,[42] amplifying the host's genome within the Nurse cell cytoplasm.[43] The Nurse cell-parasite complex can live for as long as the host remains alive. Most do not, and are calcified within several months after forming. In order for the life cycle to continue, an infected host must die and be eaten by another mammal. Scavenging is a common behavior among most wild mammals, and this helps to ensure the maintenance of *T. spiralis* and its relatives in their respective host species.

Cellular and molecular pathogenesis

The enteral (intestinal) phase includes larval stages L1 through L4, and the immature and reproductive adult stages. In humans, this phase can last up to 3 weeks or more. Developing worms damage columnar epithelium, depositing shed cuticula there. Later in the infection, at the onset of production of newborns, local inflammation, consisting of infiltration by eosinophils, neutrophils, and lymphocytes, intensifies in the local area. Villi flatten and become somewhat less absorbent, but not enough to result in malabsorption syndrome.

When larvae penetrate into the lymphatic circulation or bloodstream, a bacteremia due to enteric flora may result, and cases of death due to sepsis have been reported. While trichinella can induce polymicrobial bacteremia through violation of the gastrointestinal mucosal barrier, the excretory-secretory products of trichinella may be protective

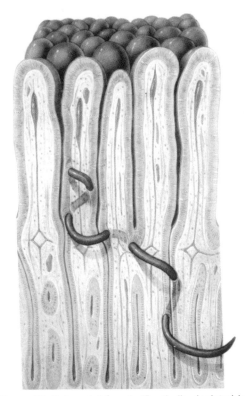

Figure 21. 7. An adult female *T. spiralis,* depicted *in situ*. Drawing by J. Karapelou.

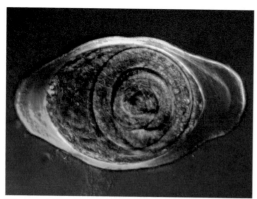

Figure 21.9. Nurse cell-parasite complex. Phase interference. Photo by E. Gravé.

against an overly robust host response by restraining MyD88 signaling via the mannose receptor.[44] Loss of wheat germ agglutinin receptors along the entire small intestine occurs.[45] The myenteric electric potential is interrupted during the enteral phase, and as the result, gut motility slows down.[45]

The parenteral phase of infection induces most of the pathological consequences. It is dose-dependent and is attributable directly to the migrating newborn larvae as they randomly penetrate cells (e.g., brain, liver, kidney, heart) in their search for striated skeletal muscle cells (Fig. 21.6). Cell death is the usual result of these events. The more penetration events there are, the more severe the resulting pathology. The result during heavy infection is a generalized edema. Proteinuria may ensue. Cardiomyopathies and central nervous system abnormalities are also common in those experiencing moderate to heavy infection.[1]

Experimental infections in immunologically-defined strains of rodents have shown that the total number of muscle larvae produced was dependent upon numerous factors related to the immune capabilities of a given strain. Induction of IL-4, and IL-13, as well as production of eosinophils and IgE antibodies appear to be essential for limiting production of newborn larvae and for the expulsion of adult worms.[46, 47] While host factors may lead to expulsion of adult worms and

limiting their production of newborn larvae, these same factors, IL-4, IL-13, and the influx of eosinophils to infected muscle cells appears to be essential for maturation of the Nurse-cell complex.[48] TNF-induced nitric oxide (NO) production is, however, not one of the effector mechanisms, since knockout mice unable to produce NO expelled their parasites in a normal fashion in the absence of local gut damage.[49] In NO+ mice, expulsion of adults was accompanied by cellular pathology surrounding the worms. Local production of nitric oxide during the development of inflammation may be a contributing factor to the development of intestinal pathology during infection with trichinella.

Clinical Disease

The presentation of the disease varies over time, and, as a result, resembles a wide variety of clinical conditions.(Fig. 21.10).[1, 50] Trichinellosis is often misdiagnosed for that reason. The severity of disease is dose-dependent, making the diagnosis based solely on symptoms difficult, at best. In severe cases, death may ensue. There are signs and symptoms that should alert the physician to include trichinellosis into the differential diagnosis.

While light infection with trichinella can pass unnoticed with minimal or no identifiable symptoms, heavy infection with a large number of viable larvae presents as a distinct two-stage syndrome.[7] The first few days of the infection are characterized by the gastrointestinal stage with gastroenteritis associated with secretory diarrhea, abdominal pain, and vomiting.[51] This phase is transitory, and abates within 10 days after ingestion of infected tissue. A history of eating raw or undercooked meats helps to rule in this parasitic infection. Others who also ate the same meats and are suffering similarly reinforces the suspicion of trichinellosis. Unfortunately, most clinicians opt for a food poisoning scenario at this juncture.

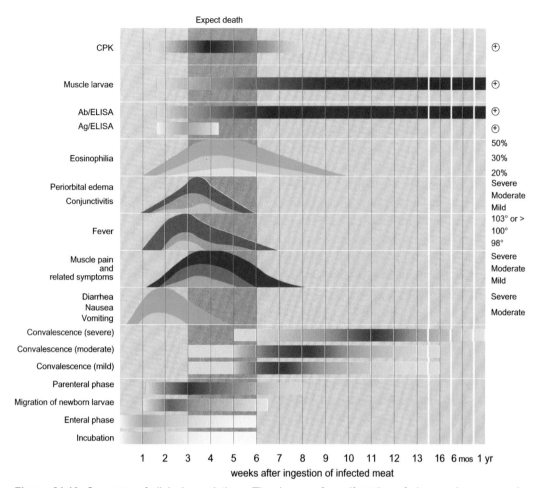

Figure 21.10. Summary of clinical correlations. The degree of manifestation of signs and symptoms is dependent upon the dose of larvae ingested. The stages of the parasite and the signs and symptoms associated with them are shown in the same colors.

The parenteral phase begins approximately one week after infection and may last several weeks. Typically, the patient has fever and myalgia, bilateral periorbital edema, and petechial hemorrhages, which are seen most clearly in the subungual region, but are also observable in the conjunctivae and other mucosal sites.[52] Muscle tenderness can be readily detected. Laboratory studies reveal a moderately elevated white blood cell count (12,000-15,000 cells/mm³), and a circulating eosinophilia ranging from 5% to as high as 50%.[53, 54]

Larvae penetrating tissues other than skeletal muscle may give rise to serious sequelae. In many cases of moderate to severe infec-

tion, cardiovascular involvement may lead to myocarditis, but this aspect of the infection has been overrated as a clinical feature typical of most infections with this parasite, since most instances encountered by the clinician are of the mild variety.[55] Electrocardiographic (ECG) changes can occur during this phase, even in the absence of symptoms. Parasite invasion of the diaphragm and the accessory muscles of respiration may result in dyspnea.[56] Neuro-trichinellosis occurs in association with invasion of the central nervous system.[57] In up to 25% of patients with heavy infection, meningitis and encephalitis can develop with edema, infarcts, and hemorrhage in fatal cases.[58, 59] The convalescent phase follows the acute phase, during which time many, but not all, Nurse cell-parasite complexes are destroyed.

Two clinical presentations have been described for *T. nativa* infections resulting from the ingestion of infected polar bear or walrus meat; a classic myopathic form, and a second form that presents as a persistent diarrheal illness. The second form is thought to represent a secondary infection in previously sensitized individuals.[60] It is apparent that not only the amount of ingested larvae but also the species of trichinella and the status of the infected host impact the clinical presentation.[61]

Diagnosis

Definitive diagnosis depends upon finding the Nurse cell-parasite complex in muscle biopsy by microscopic examination (Fig 21.1), or detection of trichinella–specific DNA by PCR.[62] PCR is sensitive and specific for detecting small numbers of larvae in muscle tissue, but is rarely used in the clinical setting[52] Real-time PCR has been developed and is used in surveillance studies of wildlife trichinella infection.[63]

Muscle biopsy can be negative, even in the heaviest of infections, due to sampling errors and as a consequence it is recommended that one biopsy a symptomatic muscle, preferentially a more proximal muscle such as the deltoid, near the tendinous insertion to improve sensitivity.[1] In addition, the larvae may be at an early stage of their development, making them inconspicuous, even to experienced pathologists. Serological tests are available with confirmation with a Western blot.[64] Serological tests begin to show positive results within two weeks. ELISA can detect antibodies in some patients as early as 12 days after infection. Muscle enzymes, such as creatine phosphokinase (CPK) and lactic dehydrogenase (LDH), are released into the circulation causing an increase in their serum levels.

A rising, plateauing and falling level of circulating eosinophils throughout the infection period is not direct proof of infection, but armed with this information and an exposure history, the clinician could treat the patient presumptively. It is helpful to remember that wild mammals can also be sources of infection. Outbreaks of trichinellosis have been traced to hunters and the recipients of their kills.[65-67]

Treatment

While many case of trichinella infection may be mild or even asymptomatic and easily managed with analgesics and antipyretics, more significant infections are usually managed with a combination of antihelminthic therapy and corticosteroids.[52] Since larvae may still be burrowing through the gastrointestinal tract when patients present with symptoms, treatment with albendazole or mebendazole may be beneficial. Treatment with mebendazole early in the course of infection has been associated with decreased muscle pain and muscle inflammation.[68] Once muscle invasion has occurred, treatment with these agents will not succeed in destroying encysted larvae.[69] Anti-inflammatory corticosteroids, particularly prednisolone, are recommended if the diagnosis is secure.[1, 49] The myopathic phase is treated in conjunction with antipyretics and analgesics (aspirin, acetaminophen), and should be continued until the fever and allergic signs recede. Because of their immunosuppressive potential, steroids should be administered with caution.

Prevention and control

Within the last 10 years, outbreaks of trichinellosis in the United States have been rare and sporadic in nature.[13-15, 70] Most have been associated with the ingestion of raw or undercooked meats from game animals, and not from commercial sources.[13-15] This represents a shift in the epidemiology of outbreaks compared to 20-30 years ago, when commercial sources of infected pork were much more common than today. Pigs raised on individual farms, as compared with commercial farm operations, are more likely to be fed uncooked garbage, and acquire the infection. This is because feeding unprocessed garbage containing meat scraps is against federally mandated regulations. In the past 10 years, small farms have, in the main, been bought up and replaced with larger so-called "factory" farms, in which upwards of 10,000 pigs can be managed with a minimum of labor. Enforcement of laws governing the running of large production facilities is a full-time activity, and has been key in reducing the spread of diseases infecting livestock and humans alike.[70]

As already mentioned, top carnivores such as bear, fox, cougar, and the like often become infected. Hunters sharing their kill with others are best warned to cook all meat thoroughly. Herbivores can harbor the infection as well, since most plant eaters occasionally ingest meat when the opportunity arises. Epidemics due to eating raw horsemeat have been reported from France, Italy, and Poland.[71]

Meat inspection is nonexistent in the United States with respect to trichinella. In Europe, the countries participating in the common market employ several strategies for examining meat for muscle larvae. Most serve to identify pools of meat samples from given regions. If they are consistently negative, then a trichinella-free designation is applied to that supply of meat. Rare outbreaks occur, despite this rigorous system of inspection.

Trichinellosis due to *Trichinella spiralis* derived from pork can be prevented by either cooking meat thoroughly at 58.5° C for 10 minutes or by freezing it at -20° C for three days. Freezing is not always effective with meat from other animals or for other species of trichinella. For example, trichinella in bears and raccoons may survive at temperatures below freezing.[72]. *Trichinella nativa* was found to survive for up to 34 months in frozen muscles of grizzly bear and up to 5 years frozen at -18⁰ C in the muscles of carnivores[5]. It appears that freeze tolerance of encapsulated trichinella muscle larva is largely determined by *Trichinella* spp. but may also be dependent on aspects of host tissue[73-75]. Thorough cooking achieving an internal temperature of 58.5° C for 10 minutes is the only way to render all meats safe from all *Trichinella* species.

References

1.   Bruschi, F.; Murrell, K. D., New aspects of human trichinellosis: the impact of new Trichinella species. *Postgraduate medical journal* **2002,** *78* (915), 15-22.
2.   Rombout, Y. B.; Bosch, S.; Van Der Giessen, J. W., Detection and identification of eight Trichinella genotypes by reverse line blot hybridization. *Journal of clinical microbiology* **2001,** *39* (2), 642-6.
3.   Zarlenga, D. S.; Chute, M. B.; Martin, A.; Kapel, C. M., A multiplex PCR for unequivocal differentiation of all encapsulated and non-encapsulated genotypes of Trichinella. *International journal for parasitology* **1999,** *29* (11), 1859-67.
4.   Appleyard, G. D.; Zarlenga, D.; Pozio, E.; Gajadhar, A. A., Differentiation of Trichinella genotypes by polymerase chain reaction using sequence-specific primers. *The Journal of parasitology* **1999,** *85* (3), 556-9.
5.   Pozio, E.; Zarlenga, D. S., Recent advances on the taxonomy, systematics and epidemiology of Trichinella. *International journal for parasitology* **2005,** *35* (11-12), 1191-204.
6.   Murrell, K. D.; Lichtenfels, R. J.; Zarlenga, D. S.; Pozio, E., The systematics of the genus Trichinella with a key to species. *Veterinary parasitology* **2000,** *93* (3-4), 293-307.

7.   Murrell, K. D.; Bruschi, F., Clinical trichinellosis. *Prog Clin Parasitol* **1994,** *4,* 117-50.
8.   Murrell, K. D.; Pozio, E., Trichinellosis: the zoonosis that won't go quietly. *Int J Parasitol* **2000,** *30* (12-13), 1339-49.
9.   Korhonen, P. K.; Pozio, E.; La Rosa, G.; Chang, B. C.; Koehler, A. V.; Hoberg, E. P.; Boag, P. R.; Tan, P.; Jex, A. R.; Hofmann, A.; Sternberg, P. W.; Young, N. D.; Gasser, R. B., Phylogenomic and biogeographic reconstruction of the Trichinella complex. *Nat Commun* **2016,** *7,* 10513.
10.   Pozio, E., Foodborne and waterborne parasites. *Acta Microbiol Pol* **2003,** *52 Suppl*, 83-96.
11.   Pozio, E.; Foggin, C. M.; Marucci, G.; La Rosa, G.; Sacchi, L.; Corona, S.; Rossi, P.; Mukaratirwa, S., Trichinella zimbabwensis n.sp. (Nematoda), a new non-encapsulated species from crocodiles (Crocodylus niloticus) in Zimbabwe also infecting mammals. *International journal for parasitology* **2002,** *32* (14), 1787-99.
12.   Krivokapich, S. J.; Pozio, E.; Gatti, G. M.; Prous, C. L.; Ribicich, M.; Marucci, G.; La Rosa, G.; Confalonieri, V., Trichinella patagoniensis n. sp. (Nematoda), a new encapsulated species infecting carnivorous mammals in South America. *Int J Parasitol* **2012,** *42* (10), 903-10.
13.   Wilson, N. O.; Hall, R. L.; Montgomery, S. P.; Jones, J. L., Trichinellosis surveillance--United States, 2008-2012. *Morbidity and mortality weekly report. Surveillance summaries* **2015,** *64 Suppl 1*, 1-8.
14.   Greene, Y. G.; Padovani, T.; Rudroff, J. A.; Hall, R.; Austin, C.; Vernon, M.; Centers for Disease, C.; Prevention, Trichinellosis caused by consumption of wild boar meat - Illinois, 2013. *MMWR. Morbidity and mortality weekly report* **2014,** *63* (20), 451.
15.   Moorehead, A.; Grunenwald, P. E.; Deitz, V. J.; Schantz, P. M.; J., Trichinellosis in the United States, : declining but not gone. *Am Med Hyg 6669* **1999,** *60,* 1991-1996.
16.   Haim, M.; Efrat, M.; Wilson, M.; Schantz, P. M.; Cohen, D.; Shemer, J., An outbreak of Trichinella spiralis infection in southern Lebanon. *Epidemiology and infection* **1997,** *119* (3), 357-62.
17.   Sohn, W. M.; Kim, H. M.; Chung, D. I.; Yee, S. T., The first human case of Trichinella spiralis infection in Korea. *The Korean journal of parasitology* **2000,** *38* (2), 111-5.
18.   Pozio, E.; La Rosa, G., Trichinella murrelli n. sp: etiological agent of sylvatic trichinellosis in temperate areas of North America. *The Journal of parasitology* **2000,** *86* (1), 134-9.
19.   Jongwutiwes, S.; Chantachum, N.; Kraivichian, P.; Siriyasatien, P.; Putaporntip, C.; Tamburrini, A.; La Rosa, G.; Sreesunpasirikul, C.; Yingyourd, P.; Pozio, E., First outbreak of human trichinellosis caused by Trichinella pseudospiralis. *Clinical infectious diseases : an official publication of the Infectious Diseases Society of America* **1998,** *26* (1), 111-5.
20.   Pozio, E.; Christensson, D.; Stéen, M.; Marucci, G.; La Rosa, G.; Bröjer, C.; Mörner, T.; Uhlhorn, H.; Agren, E.; Hall, M., Trichinella pseudospiralis foci in Sweden. *Veterinary parasitology* **2004,** *125* (3-4), 335-42.
21.   Hurnikova, Z.; Snabel, V., First record of Trichinella pseudospiralis in the Slovak Republic found in domestic focus. *Vet Parasitol* **2005,** *128,* 91-8.
22.   Obendorf, D. L.; Handlinger, J. H.; Mason, R. W.; Clarke, K. P.; Forman, A. J.; Hooper, P. T.; Smith, S. J.; Holdsworth, M., Trichinella pseudospiralis infection in Tasmanian wildlife. *Australian veterinary journal* **1990,** *67* (3), 108-10.
23.   Pozio, E.; Kapel, C. M., Trichinella nativa in sylvatic wild boars. *Journal of helminthology* **1999,** *73* (1), 87-9.
24.   Pozio, E.; Miller, I.; Järvis, T.; Kapel, C. M.; La Rosa, G., Distribution of sylvatic species of Trichinella in Estonia according to climate zones. *The Journal of parasitology* **1998,** *84* (1), 193-5.
25.   La Rosa, G.; Pozio, E., Molecular investigation of African isolates of Trichinella reveals genetic polymorphism in Trichinella nelsoni. *International journal for parasitology* **2000,** *30* (5), 663-7.
26.   Mukaratirwa, S.; La Grange, L.; Pfukenyi, D. M., Trichinella infections in animals and humans in sub-Saharan Africa: a review. *Acta Trop* **2013,** *125* (1), 82-9.
27.   La Grange, L. J.; Govender, D.; Mukaratirwa, S., The occurrence of Trichinella zimbabwensis in naturally infected wild crocodiles (Crocodylus niloticus) from the Kruger National Park, South Africa. *J Helminthol* **2013,** *87* (1), 91-6.
28.   Cox, F. E., History of human parasitology. *Clin Microbiol Rev* **2002,** *15* (4), 595-612.
29.   Owens, R., Description of a microsopic entozoon infesting the muscles of the human body. *London*

Med. Gaz. **1835**, *16*, 125-127.

30. Virchow, R., Recherches sur le developpement de la trichina spiralis (ce ver devient adulte dans l'intestin du chien). *C. R. Seanc. Acad. Sci.* **1859**, *49*, 660-662.

31. Zenker, F. A., Ueber die Trichinen-krankheit des Menschen. *Arch. Pathol. Anat. Physiol. Klin. Med.* **1860**, *18*, 561-572.

32. Pozio, E., Factors affecting the flow among domestic, synanthropic and sylvatic cycles of Trichinella. *Vet Parasitol* **2000**, *93* (3-4), 241-62.

33. Stewart, G. L.; Despommier, D. D.; Burnham, J.; Raines, K. M., Trichinella spiralis: behavior, structure, and biochemistry of larvae following exposure to components of the host enteric environment. *Experimental parasitology* **1987**, *63* (2), 195-204.

34. Modha, J.; Roberts, M. C.; Robertson, W. M.; Sweetman, G.; Powell, K. A.; Kennedy, M. W.; Kusel, J. R., The surface coat of infective larvae of Trichinella spiralis. *Parasitology* **1999**, *118 (Pt 5)*, 509-22.

35. Despommier, D., Behavioral cues in migration and location of parasitic nematodes, with special emphasis on Trichinella spiralis. 1982; p 110-126.

36. Wright, K. A., Trichinella spiralis: an intracellular parasite in the intestinal phase. *The Journal of parasitology* **1979**, *65* (3), 441-5.

37. Howitt, M. R.; Lavoie, S.; Michaud, M.; Blum, A. M.; Tran, S. V.; Weinstock, J. V.; Gallini, C. A.; Redding, K.; Margolskee, R. F.; Osborne, L. C.; Artis, D.; Garrett, W. S., Tuft cells, taste-chemosensory cells, orchestrate parasite type 2 immunity in the gut. *Science* **2016**, *351* (6279), 1329-33.

38. Despommier, D. D., Trichinella spiralis and the concept of niche. *J Parasitol* **1993**, *79* (4), 472-82.

39. Despommier, D. D., How does Trichinella spiralis make itself at home? *Parasitology today (Personal ed.)* **1998**, *14* (8), 318-23.

40. Despommier, D.; Aron, L.; Turgeon, L., Trichinella spiralis: growth of the intracellular (muscle) larva. *Experimental parasitology* **1975**, *37* (1), 108-16.

41. Despommier, D. D.; Campbell, W. C., Trichinella and trichinellosis. 1983; p 75-152.

42. Despommier, D.; Symmans, W. F.; Dell, R., Changes in nurse cell nuclei during synchronous infection with Trichinella spiralis. *The Journal of parasitology* **1991**, *77* (2), 290-5.

43. Jasmer, D. P., Trichinella spiralis infected skeletal muscle cells arrest in G2/M and cease muscle gene expression. *The Journal of cell biology* **1993**, *121* (4), 785-93.

44. Du, L.; Liu, L.; Yu, Y.; Shan, H.; Li, L., Trichinella spiralis excretory-secretory products protect against polymicrobial sepsis by suppressing MyD88 via mannose receptor. *Biomed Res Int* **2014**, *2014*, 898646.

45. Castro, G. A.; Bullock, G. R.; Campbell, W. C., Pathophysiology of the gastrointestinal Phase. 1983; p 209-241.

46. Finkelman, F. D.; Shea-Donohue, T.; Morris, S. C.; Gildea, L.; Strait, R.; Madden, K. B.; Schopf, L.; Urban, J. F., Interleukin-4- and interleukin-13-mediated host protection against intestinal nematode parasites. *Immunological reviews* **2004**, *201*, 139-55.

47. Bell, R. G., The generation and expression of immunity to Trichinella spiralis in laboratory rodents. *Advances in parasitology* **1998**, *41*, 149-217.

48. Huang, L.; Beiting, D. P.; Gebreselassie, N. G.; Gagliardo, L. F.; Ruyechan, M. C.; Lee, N. A.; Lee, J. J.; Appleton, J. A., Eosinophils and IL-4 Support Nematode Growth Coincident with an Innate Response to Tissue Injury. *PLoS Pathog* **2015**, *11* (12), e1005347.

49. Lawrence, C. E.; Paterson, J. C.; Wei, X. Q.; Liew, F. Y.; Garside, P.; Kennedy, M. W., Nitric oxide mediates intestinal pathology but not immune expulsion during Trichinella spiralis infection in mice. *Journal of immunology (Baltimore, Md. : 1950)* **2000**, *164* (8), 4229-34.

50. Pozio, E.; Gomez Morales, M. A.; Dupouy-Camet, J., Clinical aspects, diagnosis and treatment of trichinellosis. *Expert review of anti-infective therapy* **2003**, *1* (3), 471-82.

51. Kalia, N.; Hardcastle, J.; Keating, C.; Grasa, L.; Keating, C.; Pelegrin, P.; Bardhan, K. D.; Grundy, D., Intestinal secretory and absorptive function in Trichinella spiralis mouse model of postinfective gut dysfunction: role of bile acids. *Gut* **2008**, *57* (1), 41-9.

52. Gottstein, B.; Pozio, E.; Nockler, K., Epidemiology, diagnosis, treatment, and control of

trichinellosis. *Clin Microbiol Rev* **2009**, *22* (1), 127-45, Table of Contents.

53. Bruschi, F.; Korenaga, M.; Watanabe, N., Eosinophils and Trichinella infection: toxic for the parasite and the host? *Trends Parasitol* **2008**, *24* (10), 462-7.

54. Vu Thi, N.; Trung, D. D.; Litzroth, A.; Praet, N.; Nguyen Thu, H.; Nguyen Thu, H.; Nguyen Manh, H.; Dorny, P., The hidden burden of trichinellosis in Vietnam: a postoutbreak epidemiological study. *Biomed Res Int* **2013**, *2013*, 149890.

55. Lazarevic, A. M.; Neskovic, A. N.; J., Low incidence of cardiac abnormalities in treated trichinosis: a prospective study of 62 patients from a single-source outbreak. *Am* **1999**, *107*, 18-23.

56. Compton, S. J.; Celum, C. L.; Lee, C.; Thompson, D.; Sumi, S. M.; Fritsche, T. R.; Coombs, R. W., Trichinosis with ventilatory failure and persistent myocarditis. *Clin Infect Dis* **1993**, *16* (4), 500-4.

57. Bruschi, F.; Brunetti, E.; Pozio, E., Neurotrichinellosis. *Handb Clin Neurol* **2013**, *114*, 243-9.

58. Gelal, F.; Kumral, E.; Vidinli, B. D.; Erdogan, D.; Yucel, K.; Erdogan, N., Diffusion-weighted and conventional MR imaging in neurotrichinosis. *Acta Radiol* **2005**, *46* (2), 196-9.

59. Mawhorter, S. D.; Kazura, J. W., Trichinosis of the central nervous system. *Semin Neurol* **1993**, *13* (2), 148-52.

60. MacClean, J. D.; Poirier, L.; J., Epidemiologic and serologic definition of primary and secondary trichinosis in the arctic. *Dis* **1992**, *165*, 908-912.

61. Kociecka, W., Trichinellosis: human disease, diagnosis and treatment. *Vet Parasitol* **2000**, *93* (3-4), 365-83.

62. Wu, Z.; Nagano, I.; Pozio, E.; Takahashi, Y., Polymerase chain reaction-restriction fragment length polymorphism (PCR-RFLP) for the identification of Trichinella isolates. *Parasitology* **1999**, *118 (Pt 2)*, 211-8.

63. Cuttell, L.; Corley, S. W.; Gray, C. P.; Vanderlinde, P. B.; Jackson, L. A.; Traub, R. J., Real-time PCR as a surveillance tool for the detection of Trichinella infection in muscle samples from wildlife. *Vet Parasitol* **2012**, *188* (3-4), 285-93.

64. Moskwa, B.; Bien, J.; Cabaj, W.; Korinkova, K.; Koudela, B.; Stefaniak, J., The comparison of different ELISA procedures in detecting anti-Trichinella IgG in human infections. *Vet Parasitol* **2009**, *159* (3-4), 312-5.

65. Mmwr, Centers for Disease Control and Prevention (CDC). Trichinellosis associated with bear meat-New York and Tennessee. *MMWR* **2004**, *53*, 606-10.

66. Garcia, E.; Mora, L., First record of human trichinosis in Chile associated with consumption of wild boar (Sus scrofa). . *Mem Inst Oswaldo Cruz* **2005**, *100:17-8*, 17-8.

67. Rah, H.; Chomel, B. B.; Follmann, E. H.; Kasten, R. W.; Hew, C. H.; Farver, T. B.; Garner, G. W.; Amstrup, S. C., Serosurvey of selected zoonotic agents in polar bears (Ursus maritimus). *The Veterinary record* **2005**, *156* (1), 7-13.

68. Watt, G.; Saisorn, S.; Jongsakul, K.; Sakolvaree, Y.; Chaicumpa, W., Blinded, placebo-controlled trial of antiparasitic drugs for trichinosis myositis. *J Infect Dis* **2000**, *182* (1), 371-4.

69. Pozio, E.; Sacchini, D.; Sacchi, L.; Tamburrini, A.; Alberici, F., Failure of mebendazole in the treatment of humans with Trichinella spiralis infection at the stage of encapsulating larvae. *Clin Infect Dis* **2001**, *32* (4), 638-42.

70. Roy, S. L.; Lopez, A. S.; Schantz, P. M., Trichinellosis surveillance--United States, 1997-2001. *Morbidity and mortality weekly report. Surveillance summaries (Washington, D.C. : 2002)* **2003**, *52* (6), 1-8.

71. Murrell, K. D.; Djordjevic, M.; Cuperlovic, K.; Sofronic, L.; Savic, M.; Damjanovic, S., Epidemiology of Trichinella infection in the horse: the risk from animal product feeding practices. *Veterinary parasitology* **2004**, *123* (3-4), 223-33.

72. Kapel, C. M.; Pozio, E.; Sacchi, L.; Prestrud, P., Freeze tolerance, morphology, and RAPD-PCR identification of Trichinella nativa in naturally infected arctic foxes. *The Journal of parasitology* **1999**, *85* (1), 144-7.

73. Kapel, C. M.; Pozio, E.; Sacchi, L.; Prestrud, P., Freeze tolerance, morphology, and RAPD-PCR identification of Trichinella nativa in naturally infected arctic foxes. *The Journal of parasitology* **1999**, *85* (1), 144-7.

74. Lacour, S. A.; Heckmann, A.; Mace, P.; Grasset-Chevillot, A.; Zanella, G.; Vallee, I.; Kapel, C. M.; Boireau, P., Freeze-tolerance of Trichinella muscle larvae in experimentally infected wild boars. *Veterinary parasitology* **2013,** *194* (2-4), 175-8.

75. Theodoropoulos, G.; Kapel, C. M.; Webster, P.; Saravanos, L.; Zaki, J.; Koutsotolis, K., Infectivity, predilection sites, and freeze tolerance of Trichinella spp. in experimentally infected sheep. *Parasitology research* **2000,** *86* (5), 401-5.

22. Lymphatic Filariae

Wuchereria bancrofti
(Cobbold 1877)

Brugia malayi
(Brug 1927)

Introduction

There are three species of vector-born nematodes that cause lymphatic filariais in humans; *Wuchereria bancrofti, Brugia malayi*, and *Brugia timori*.[1] These are thread-like nematodes whose adult stage lives within the lumen of lymphatic vessels.[2] More than 100 million people in Southeast Asia, Africa, and the Americas are infected with some form of filariasis, with more than 90 percent due to *W. bancrofti* infection.[3, 4] Of these, approximately 40 million suffer from clinical disease. Only about 10 to 20 million people are infected with *B. malayi,* while *B. timori* is a minor filarial parasite largely restricted to the islands of Timor and Flores in southeastern Indonesia.[5] Elephantiasis, a disfiguring disease caused by blockage of

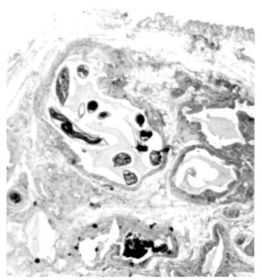

Figure 22.1. Adults of *Wuchereria bancrofti* in lymphatic vessels.

the lymphatic vessels, affects large numbers of individuals living in endemic areas. The worms are ovoviviparous, and their larvae are called microfilariae. Lymphatic filariasis (LF) is transmitted by culicine and anophelene species of mosquitoes.

Humans are the only host for *W. bancrofti*. The infection is widely distributed in the tropics, especially in South Asia, Africa (including Egypt), and tropical regions of the Americas. The major vectors are culicine mosquitoes in most urban and semi-urban areas, anophelines in rural areas of Africa and elsewhere, and Aedes species in the Pacific islands. With the exception of the South Pacific, most of the *W. bancrofti* strains are nocturnal, referring to the periodicity with which the microfilariae appear in the peripheral circulation.

Infection with *B. malayi*, on the other hand, is a zoonosis, with both feline and monkey reservoirs. *Mansonia* spp. serve as the major mosquito vector, although anophelines are also sometimes involved in transmission. *B. malayi* infections occur in India, Malaysia, and other parts of Southeast Asia. There are other minor members of the genus *Brugia* that cause disease in humans, including *B. timori* on the Indonesian islands of Timor and Flores, and accidental zoonotic brugia infections (e.g., *B. beaveri* and *B. lepori*) that occur sporadically in the United States.[6, 7]

A major global effort is underway to eliminate LF by the year 2020, based on the successes of reducing the age-adjusted prevalence by approximately one-half over the last twenty years.[8-10] (https://www.neglecteddiseases.gov/about/index.html) The term 'elimination' refers to the reduction of disease incidence to zero or close to zero, with a requirement for ongoing control efforts.[11] The strategy for LF elimination relies on interrupting mosquito transmission by mass administration of combination therapy in endemic regions in order to reduce the

Wuchereria bancrofti

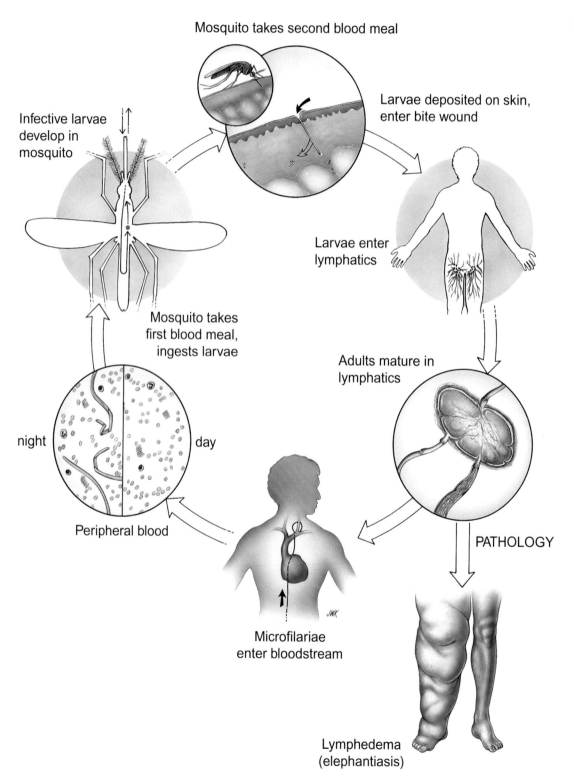

Mosquito takes second blood meal

Infective larvae develop in mosquito

Larvae deposited on skin, enter bite wound

Larvae enter lymphatics

Mosquito takes first blood meal, ingests larvae

Adults mature in lymphatics

night   day

Peripheral blood

PATHOLOGY

Microfilariae enter bloodstream

Lymphedema (elephantiasis)

number of microfilariae circulating in the bloodstream of infected individuals.

Historical Information

In 1863, Jean-Nicolas Demarquay, a French surgeon described microfilariae of wuchereria in hydrocele fluid.[12] In 1866, Otto Wucherer described the microfilariae in urine in Brazil.[13] In 1872, a Scottish physician working in Calcutta, Timothy Lewis, confirmed the presence of the microfilariae in urine as well as blood and recognized the connection with the severe lymphedema and deformities known as elephantiasis.[14, 15] In 1877, Spencer Cobbold wrote a description of the adult worm and named the worm *Filaria bancrofti* in honor of Joseph Bancroft, the surgeon who had investigated the causes of hydrocele and lymphatic disease in Australia.[15, 16] Lewis described the adult worm in India that same year.[17] In 1878, Patrick Manson completed the description of the life cycle while working in Amoy (now called Xiamen) along the Chinese coast in Fujian Province.[18] Today, lymphatic filariasis has been largely eradicated from China. Manson first demonstrated that mosquitoes were intermediate hosts for the parasite. For two decades, Manson maintained that infection was acquired when individuals drank water contaminated with larvae released from dead or dying mosquitoes. Eventually, he came to accept the concept that larvae were transmitted by the bite of mosquitoes. Filariasis may, in fact, be a water-borne disease under some circumstances, since experimental infections can be induced by the oral route.[19]

One of the most important developments in the history of LF control was the discovery by Francis Hawking (father of Stephen Hawking) and others that it is possible to reduce the prevalence of LF through mass treatment, or in some cases to fortify the salt with diethylcarbamazine citrate (DEC) to affected populations.[20, 21] During the 1970s and 1980s, Chinese parasitologists thought that it was possible to dramatically scale up this process to the national level. This was achieved primarily through fortification of regional salt supplies with DEC. The LF life cycle was discovered in China and LF was first eliminated there as well. The accomplishments of the Chinese provided proof-of-principle that it might be possible to eliminate LF worldwide through similar measures.

Life Cycle

Adult worms occupy the lumen of lymphatic vessels (Fig. 22.1), and have been found at all sites within the lymphatic circulation. Most commonly, they live in the lymphatics of the lower and upper extremities and male genitalia. Adult wuchereria females are 0.3-1cm in length while the adult wuchereria males are about half this length. Adult brugia females are smaller, measuring 0.4-0.55cm in length, with adult brugia males being less than half this length. After mating, the female worm releases 10,000 or more offspring per day. Instead of releasing eggs, the worms release L1 larvae (microfilariae). Each microfilaria (Figs. 22.2, 22.3) measures approximately 270 μm by 10 μm and contains nuclei that characteristically do not extend to the tip of the tail. Another distinguishing feature is that the microfilaria is encased in a sheath comprised of chitin, a remnant of its eggshell.

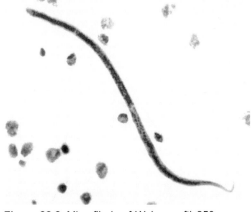

Figure 22.2. Microfilaria of *W. bancrofti.* 250 μm

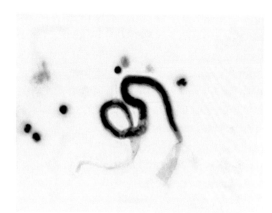

Figure 22.3. Microfilaria of *Brugia malayi*. 220 µm

Microfilariae migrate from the lymphatic circulation into the bloodstream. They are typically present in large numbers in the peripheral blood only at night (between 10 pm and 6 am) in most endemic areas of the world. During the day, the microfilariae aggregate in the capillaries of the lungs when activity of the host is increased (i.e., during strenuous exercise). Nocturnal periodicity can be a result of the microfilaria's penchant for low oxygen tension, at which time they are found in the peripheral blood stream, or it may reflect subtle pH changes in the pulmonary venous circulation during sleep.[22] Experiments in which sleep habits of infected volunteers were reversed also reversed the periodicity of microfilariae. The diurnal periodicity pattern characteristic of the South Pacific strain has not been satisfactorily explained. Microfilariae live for about 1.5 years, and must be ingested by a mosquito to continue their life cycle.

W. bancrofti is transmitted by a wide variety of mosquito genera and species, the most important being *Culex pipiens quinquefasciatus*, *Culex pipiens pipiens*, *Anopheles gambiae*, and *A. polynesiensis*. *Aedes aegypti*, the yellow fever mosquito, can also transmit the infection in some of the Pacific Islands. Ingested microfilariae penetrate the stomach wall of the female mosquito and locate to the thoracic flight muscles. There, they undergo three molts, developing into L3 larvae and become infective after 10-20 days of growth and development in the insect muscle tissue.

Infective L3 larvae locate to the biting mouthparts, and are deposited onto the skin adjacent to the bite wound during consumption of a subsequent blood meal. When the mosquito withdraws her mouthparts, larvae crawl into the open wound. Immature worms migrate through the subcutaneous tissues to the lymphatic vessels, and come to rest near the draining lymph nodes of each of those vessels. The worms slowly develop into mature adults in about 1 year, and soon after copulation, begin shedding microfilariae. The longevity of adults, measured by the continuous production of microfilariae, is estimated at 5-8 years. Infections lasting 40 years have been reported.[23]

The adult and larval stages of *B. malayi* resemble those of *W. bancrofti*. The life cycles of the two species of filariae are similar, although animal reservoirs occur for some members of the genus *Brugia*. The sub-periodic strain of *B. malayi* is a zoonosis acquired from forest monkeys and other wild animals, and transmitted through the bite of *Mansonia* spp. mosquitoes.[6]

Cellular and Molecular Pathogenesis

The pathogenesis of lymphangitis leading to elephantiasis has not been fully explained. It may result from a sequence of host-mediated immunopathologic events that occur in response to dead and dying adults within the lymphatics (Fig. 22.4). In contrast, living adult worms or the microfilariae are believed to suppress these responses, and typically adult worms do not trigger an inflammatory response.[24, 25] The processes associated with lymphangitis and elephantiasis can take years to develop, and are not commonly seen in children. Exactly how living worms and microfilariae suppress the host inflammatory response is being explored. It has been noted that microfilariae produce prostaglandin E2,

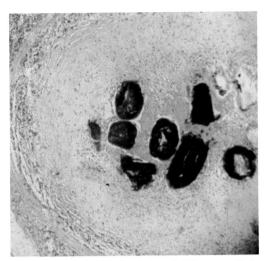

Figure 22.4. Calcified adults of *W. bancrofti* in blocked lymphatic vessel.

a modulatory agent for leukocytes, and adult worms secrete anti-mitotic and immunosuppressive substances.[26] Adult worms can also influence host immune responses through the release of small RNA-containing exosome-like vesicles that influence host immune cell gene expression.[27]

When dead and dying adult worms relinquish control of the host's defense mechanisms, a series of inflammatory reactions result causing alterations of the walls of the lymphatics. After an intense lymphocytic infiltration, the lumen of the vessel eventually closes, and the remnants of the adult worms calcify. The blockage of lymphatic circulation continues in heavily infected individuals until most major lymph channels are occluded, causing lymphedema in the affected region of the body. In addition, hypertrophy of smooth muscle tissue occurs in the area immediately surrounding the site of involvement. Individuals can develop complications, such as the development of new hydroceles when treated with agents that kill adult filarial worms.[28]

The process of lymphatic blockage is a protracted one and results from repeated infections. Consequently, individuals visiting endemic areas for short periods usually do not develop lymphedema.

Not all patients with chronic exposure of infective larvae of *W. bancrofti* develop overt clinical disease. It is unclear why, despite relatively equal levels of exposure, some infected residents remain largely asymptomatic, but with evidence of microfilaremia, whereas other individuals progress to advanced clinical disease comprised of lymphangitis and elephantiasis. Frequently, patients with advanced clinical disease do not have evidence of circulating microfilariae, while patients with elevated levels of circulating microfilaria are often asymptomatic.[29] Differences in host cytokine patterns have been noted among these different groups of patients. It has been suggested that different populations are prone to either Th2 or Th1 biases in their cellular inflammatory responses.[24, 30, 31] Growing evidence suggests that there is host genetic variability that accounts for the different range of clinical manifestations seen among patients with similar exposures.[32, 33]

There is a complex relationship between the host and the parasite, and there is often a complex pathologic sequence of events leading to lymphangitis, lymphedema and elephantiasis. While much inflammation occurs once adults have died, there is evidence from ultrasound studies conducted in LF-endemic areas that the living adult filarial worms induce important pathologic changes, including lymphatic dilatation, which may lead to subsequent chronic lymphatic changes. Secondary bacterial and fungal infections contribute significantly to the chronic pathology of elephantiasis, as well as being significant complications for patients with full-blown elephantiasis. Adult *W. bancrofti* worms harbor bacterial symbionts of the genus *Wolbachia*. Adult *W. bancrofti* depend on these symbionts for their survival, and antibiotics that target them exhibit an anthelminthic effect. Further, wolbachia contain endotoxin-like molecules and evidence suggests that these molecules may contribute to the inflammatory responses seen to dead and dying worms. Wolbachia plays a major role in the pathogenesis of filarial disease. Some of the progression of clinical disease appears to be due to immune responses triggered by the wolbachia endosymbiont.[34-37]

Clinical Disease

There is a spectrum of clinical manifestations resulting from *W. bancrofti* or *B. malayi* infections, ranging from asymptomatic infection to advanced elephantiasis.

Asymptomatic Infection (Lymphatic Dilatation)

The majority of residents living in an endemic area do not manifest strong inflammatory responses to their filarial parasite load. They are noted to be asymptomatic even though they have circulating microfilariae. Some of these so-called asymptomatic patients have been observed to exhibit subtle pathology when examined more closely by ultrasound or radionuclide studies.[38] The central event in the pathogenesis of more advanced disease may begin at this stage when dilatation of the lymphatic vessels begins to occur. Dilatation initiates a subsequent series of events that results in the chronic clinical manifestations of LF, including lymphedema and hydrocele.[39] In some cases, the dilated vessels rupture to produce chyluria and chylocele.

Acute Lymphadenitis and Filarial Fevers

Death of the adult worm causes the next step in the progression of disease by producing an acute inflammatory response that is manifested as acute lymphadenitis. In endemic areas, this occurs frequently during the patient's adolescent years, and is manifested with fevers and painful swellings over the lymph nodes.[40] This typically occurs in the inguinal area. Episodes of painful swellings can last up to a week and commonly recur. Secondary bacterial infections may also result. Acute filarial lymphadenitis is exacer-

bated by secondary bacterial infections.

Some individuals who have travelled to and spent several months in endemic areas can also develop acute lymphadenitis, but the pathogenesis of this process occurs by a poorly understood process. This phenomenon was described in the 1940s among American troops returning from war in the Pacific theatre.[41]

Elephantiasis

A subset of patients with acute lymphangitis and filarial fevers will go on to develop lymphedema of the arms, legs, breasts and genitalia leading to elephantiasis (Fig 22.5.). During these inflammatory processes, the skin becomes doughy and exhibits some degree of pitting, though it is rather firm. As the inflammatory reaction continues, the area becomes firmer still, and pitting disappears. There is substantial spread of the inflammation into the subcutaneous tissue and consequent loss

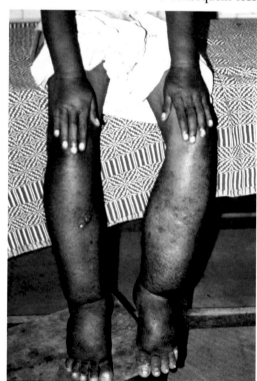

Figure 22.5 Patient suffering from long-term infection with *W. bancrofti*. Most adult worms have died and calcified, blocking all lymphatic drainage from the groin. The result is elephantiasis of both legs.

of elasticity of the overlying skin. Characteristically, and in contrast to cellulitis caused by some bacteria, filarial cellulitis shows no demarcation line between the affected and the healthy skin. In bancroftian filariasis, the legs are more likely to be involved than are the upper extremities, and the lower portions of the legs are more involved than the upper ones. The scrotum is frequently affected in the form of hydroceles and may become gigantic, weighing up to 10 kg; much larger scrotums have been described in rare cases.

Tropical Pulmonary Eosinophilia (TPE)

TPE develops in some individuals with filarial infections. This syndrome, which occurs frequently in southern India, particularly in young adult men, is characterized by high levels of serum immunoglobulin E (IgE), nocturnal asthma with interstitial infiltrates on chest radiographs, fatigue, weight loss, and circulating eosinophilia.[42] Left untreated, TPE can progress to chronic restrictive lung disease. Diethylcarbamazine is highly effective in these patients. The pathogenesis of this syndrome is related to local immune responses to microfilariae in the pulmonary vasculature, and results in eosinophil accumulation in the lung with the release of cytotoxic eosinophil products (e.g., major basic protein and eosinophil cationic protein).[42]

Diagnosis

Lymphatic filariasis should be suspected in an individual who resides in an endemic region, is beyond the first decade of life, and has lymphedema in the extremities or genitalia. Definitive diagnosis has traditionally depended upon microscopically observing the characteristic microfilariae in the blood (Figs. 22.2, 22.3, C.46 – C.53). Occasionally, infection is so heavy that microfilariae can be observed on a thin blood smear stained with Giemsa. In lighter infections, methods include filtering blood onto a 0.45μm pore sized nucleopore filter, then staining it with Giemsa solution. In the case of very light infection, 1 ml of blood is preserved in 9 ml of 1% formalin and then concentrated by centrifugation (Knott test; see Appendix B). The pellet contains red blood cell ghosts and microfilariae. Stained smears of the pellet are then examined microscopically. Because of the nocturnal periodicity of some strains, it is best to draw blood during the customary hours of sleep (usually between 22:00 and 02:00 hours).

Antigen tests that detect circulating *W. bancrofti* antigens have been developed which are more sensitive than microscopy, can be used for daytime testing, and can give a quantitative result correlating with adult worm burden.[43-45] These are available in the form of ELISA test or an immunochromatographic card.[46] The card-based assay, which recognizes an adult worm 200 kDa antigen, has a sensitivity of 96-100 percent and a specificity approaching 100 percent.[47] The ELISA also has a sensitivity approaching 100 percent in microfilaremic patients. For both assays, the circulating filarial antigen remains diurnally constant, so that blood for diagnosis can be collected during the day. PCR-based tests have been developed, but while used to monitor filarial infection in mosquitos, are currently not routinely used in clinical practice.[48]

Serological tests that detect levels of human IgG directed against the worms that cause lymphatic filariasis have been developed and are in use clinically. These serve as rapid tests that can aid in the diagnosis of this disease but detect exposure rather than confirm current infection.[49-51]

Increasingly, ultrasound has provided an important noninvasive modality for monitoring the efficacy of antifilarial drugs.[34] Ultrasound examination of the lymphatic vessels of the spermatic cord of infected men results in a distinctive sign, known as the "filarial dance sign" reflective of nests of live worms in the lymphatics.[52] Adult worm death following treatment with DEC can be subsequently followed.

Treatment

It is recommended that all patients be treated, because even patients with so-called asymptomatic infection may have abnormal lymphatics, and there is increasing evidence that early treatment may prevent subsequent lymphatic damage and may reverse early lymphatic dysfunction.[53] It is critical that, prior to treatment, co-infection with *Loa Loa* with a high *Loa Loa* microfilarial load is ruled out, due to the risk of severe adverse events if treatment is given to such patients.[54] For treatment of mono-infected patients, diethylcarbamazine (DEC) has both macrofilaricidal (adult worm) and microfilaricidal properties, and is the treatment of choice for such patients. In many regions it is given in a dose of 6 mg/kg/day for 12 consecutive days for a total of 72 mg/kg body weight.[34, 55] For *W. bancrofti* infections, this results in at least a 90% decrease in microfilaremia within one month. DEC decreases the incidence of filarial lymphangitis, and in some cases reverses existing lymphatic damage. The addition of doxycycline for 4-6 weeks may be beneficial based on evidence demonstrating macrofilaricidal activity and reduced pathology.[56-58] In men, the efficacy of treatment can be monitored by serial ultrasound examinations (see above), and by serial blood sampling.[34] Since DEC is only partially effective against the adult worm, repeat treatments are often required. This is often done every 6-12 months.[34] Recent data has suggested that single dose treatment with 6 mg/kg of DEC has comparable macrofilaricidal and long-term microfilaricidal therapy. Some clinicians have suggested that single-dose treatment can be repeated every 6-12 months.[34] DEC is associated with fever (probably resulting from disintegration of a few of the adult worms),

occasional nausea and vomiting, and fleeting skin rashes. Ivermectin, a drug effective for therapy of onchocerciasis, also kills microfilariae of *W. bancrofti*, but it appears to have no macrofilaricidal properties. Ivermectin and albendazole, a drug that also does not kill adult filarial worms, have been used in mass drug campaigns and dose reduce microfilarial blood levels and decreases transmission.[59]

Aside from the use of anthelminthic drugs, there are several treatment modalities that help to improve the chronic sequelae of LF, including lymphedema and elephantiasis. Both conditions, when they occur in the leg, are reversible with a hygienic regimen that includes prevention of secondary bacterial infections by prompt antibiotic treatment of acute bacterial attacks, aggressive treatment of skin lesions including those caused by candida and other fungi, and physiotherapy.[34] Treatment of secondary bacterial infections has been identified as a critical treatment modality for worsening lymphedema and elephantiasis. Hydrocele drainage without corrective surgery, while it does provide relief, is often associated with reaccumulation of fluid.[60] For certain affected areas, (e.g., the scrotum) corrective surgical interventions may be required.[61] Surgical techniques have been developed that can, in most cases, alleviate hydroceles and greatly improve the morbidity associated with the scrotal and other morbidity associated with filarial infections.[62]

Prevention and Control

Patent microfilaremia is first detected in children 5 to 10 years old who live in endemic regions.[6] Transplacental immunity and breast-feeding may limit the intensity of infection in younger individuals. The prevalence of microscopically confirmed infection gradually increases up to the age of 30-40 years.

The frequency of exposure to third-stage larvae by vectors is the most important determinant in the community prevalence of filariasis.[63] Prevention depends upon control of mosquito vectors, which, unfortunately, has had limited success because mosquitoes develop resistance to insecticides. Insect-treated bed nets have been effective in reducing transmission in areas where anopheline mosquitos transmit the disease.[64] Urbanization of vast areas of tropical Asia has resulted in a concomitant rise in the prevalence of both *W. bancrofti* and *B. malayi* varieties of filariasis, carried by mosquitoes that breed in non-sylvatic habitats.

In 1997, the World Health Assembly passed a resolution calling on its member states to undertake a global elimination program for LF. The major strategy for LF elimination is based on two principles: 1) to interrupt transmission of infection and 2) to alleviate and prevent the suffering and disability caused by LF. To interrupt transmission, it is essential to reduce the levels of microfilariae in the blood for a sustainable period. This is achieved by administering a yearly, single-dose, 2-drug regimen.[65] For most countries, the recommended drugs are DEC (6 mg/kg) and albendazole (400 mg).[65, 66] The goal of this approach is to provide annual treatment with this drug combination, although in some countries DEC-fortified salt is used.

However, in many parts of Sub-Saharan Africa (and Yemen as well) where there is epidemiological overlap with onchocerciasis, the toxicities caused by DEC in people with these conditions necessitate substituting ivermectin (200 mcg/kg). Such populations would receive ivermectin or albendazole.[64, 66] A period of 5 years of annual treatments is currently recommended. To date, the number of serious adverse events from LF control mass chemotherapy has been remarkably low. In some areas, a treatment regimen comprised of daily DEC-fortified salt is used. A Global Program to Eliminate LF (GPELF) in collaboration with the WHO is leading these efforts.

To alleviate suffering and decrease the disability caused by LF, the major strategy has been to decrease secondary bacterial and fungal infections of the affected limbs and genitals. This includes meticulous local hygiene, judicious use of antibiotics, physiotherapy and health education.

References

1.   Knopp, S.; Steinmann, P.; Hatz, C.; Keiser, J.; Utzinger, J., Nematode infections: filariases. *Infect Dis Clin North Am* **2012,** *26* (2), 359-81.
2.   Nelson, G. S., Current concepts in parasitology. Filariasis. *The New England journal of medicine* **1979,** *300* (20), 1136-9.
3.   Global programme to eliminate lymphatic filariasis: progress report for 2012. *Wkly Epidemiol Rec* **2013,** *88* (37), 389-99.
4.   Global programme to eliminate lymphatic filariasis. *Wkly Epidemiol Rec* **2010,** *85* (38), 365-72.
5.   Taylor, M. J.; Hoerauf, A.; Bockarie, M., Lymphatic filariasis and onchocerciasis. *Lancet* **2010,** *376* (9747), 1175-85.
6.   Nanduri, J.; Kazura, J. W., Clinical and laboratory aspects of filariasis. *Clinical microbiology reviews* **1989,** *2* (1), 39-50.
7.   Baird, J. K.; Alpert, L. I.; Friedman, R.; Schraft, W. C.; Connor, D. H., North American brugian filariasis: report of nine infections of humans. *The American journal of tropical medicine and hygiene* **1986,** *35* (6), 1205-9.
8.   Molyneux, D. H.; Bradley, M.; Hoerauf, A.; Kyelem, D.; Taylor, M. J., Mass drug treatment for lymphatic filariasis and onchocerciasis. *Trends in parasitology* **2003,** *19* (11), 516-22.
9.   Molyneux, D. H.; Zagaria, N., Lymphatic filariasis elimination: progress in global programme development. *Ann Trop Med Parasitol 96 Suppl 2* **2003,** S15-40.
10. Global Burden of Disease Study, C., Global, regional, and national incidence, prevalence, and

years lived with disability for 301 acute and chronic diseases and injuries in 188 countries, 1990-2013: a systematic analysis for the Global Burden of Disease Study 2013. *Lancet* **2015,** *386* (9995), 743-800.

11. Hotez, P. J.; Remme, J. H. F.; Buss, P.; Alleyne, G.; Morel, C.; Breman, J. G., Combating tropical infectious diseases: report of the Disease Control Priorities in Developing Countries Project. *Clinical infectious diseases : an official publication of the Infectious Diseases Society of America* **2004,** *38* (6), 871-8.

12. Demarquay, M., Note sur une tumeur des bourses contenant un liquide laiteux (galactocele de Vidal) et refermant des petits etres vermiformes que l'on peut considerer comme des helminths hematoides a l'etat d'embryon. Gaz Med Pans. **1863,** *18*, 665-667.

13. Wucherer, O. E., Sobre a molestia vulgarmente denominada oppilacao ou cancaco. *Gaz. Med. Bahia* **1866,** *1*, 27-29, 39-41, 52-54, 63-64.

14. Lewis, T. R., On a haematozoon inhabiting human blood, its relation to chyluria and other diseases. *8th Annual Report of the Sanitary Commission Government of India. Sanitary Commission Government of India, Calcutta.* **1872**, 241-266.

15. Cox, F. E., History of human parasitology. *Clin Microbiol Rev* **2002,** *15* (4), 595-612.

16. Cobbold, T. S., Discovery of the adult representative of microscopic filariae. *Lancet* **1877,** *2* 70-71.

17. Lewis, T., Filaria sanguinis hominis (mature form), found in a bloodclot in naevoid elephantiasis of the scrotum. *Lancet* **1877,** *2*, 453-455.

18. Manson, P., Further Observations on Filaria sanguinis hominis. *Medical Reports, China Imperial Maritime Customs Shanghai no 14 pp* **1878**, 1-26.

19. Gwadz, R. W.; Chernin, E., Oral transmission of Brugia pahangi to Jirds (Meriones unguiculatus). *Nature* **1972,** *239* (5374), 524-5.

20. Hawking, F.; Marques, R. J., Control of Bancroftian filariasis by cooking salt medicated with diethylcarbamazine. *Bull World Health Organ* **1967,** *37* (3), 405-14.

21. Hawking, F., A review of progress in the chemotherapy and control of filariasis since 1955. *Bull World Health Organ* **1962,** *27*, 555-68.

22. Hawking, F.; Pattanayak, S.; Sharma, H. L., The periodicity of microfilariae. XI. The effect of body temperature and other stimuli upon the cycles of Wuchereria bancrofti, Brugia malayi, B. ceylonensis and Dirofilaria repens. *Transactions of the Royal Society of Tropical Medicine and Hygiene* **1966,** *60* (4), 497-513.

23. Carme, B.; Laigret, J., Longevity of Wuchereria bancrofti var. pacifica and mosquito infection acquired from a patient with low level parasitemia. *The American journal of tropical medicine and hygiene* **1979,** *28* (1), 53-5.

24. Ottesen, E. A., The Wellcome Trust Lecture. Infection and disease in lymphatic filariasis: an immunological perspective. *Parasitology* **1992,** *104 Suppl*, S71-9.

25. King, C. L.; Kumaraswami, V.; Poindexter, R. W.; Kumari, S.; Jayaraman, K.; Alling, D. W.; Ottesen, E. A.; Nutman, T. B., Immunologic tolerance in lymphatic filariasis. Diminished parasite-specific T and B lymphocyte precursor frequency in the microfilaremic state. *J Clin Invest* **1992,** *89* (5), 1403-10.

26. Liu, L. X.; Buhlmann, J. E.; Weller, P. F., Release of prostaglandin E2 by microfilariae of Wuchereria bancrofti and Brugia malayi. *The American journal of tropical medicine and hygiene* **1992,** *46* (5), 520-3.

27. Zamanian, M.; Fraser, L. M.; Agbedanu, P. N.; Harischandra, H.; Moorhead, A. R.; Day, T. A.; Bartholomay, L. C.; Kimber, M. J., Release of Small RNA-containing Exosome-like Vesicles from the Human Filarial Parasite Brugia malayi. *PLoS Negl Trop Dis* **2015,** *9* (9), e0004069.

28. Hussein, O.; El Setouhy, M.; Ahmed, E. S.; Kandil, A. M.; Ramzy, R. M.; Helmy, H.; Weil, G. J., Duplex Doppler sonographic assessment of the effects of diethylcarbamazine and albendazole therapy on adult filarial worms and adjacent host tissues in Bancroftian filariasis. *Am J Trop Med Hyg* **2004,** *71* (4), 471-7.

29. Dissanayake, S., In Wuchereria bancrofti filariasis, asymptomatic microfilaraemia does not progress to amicrofilaraemic lymphatic disease. *Int J Epidemiol* **2001,** *30* (2), 394-9.

30. Almeida, A. B.; de Silva, M. C. M.; J., The presence or absence of active infection, not clinical

status, is most closely associated with cytokine responses in lymphatic filariasis. *Dis 1453* **1996**, *173*.

31. Piessens, W. F.; McGreevy, P. B.; Piessens, P. W.; McGreevy, M.; Koiman, I.; Saroso, J. S.; Dennis, D. T., Immune responses in human infections with Brugia malayi: specific cellular unresponsiveness to filarial antigens. *The Journal of clinical investigation* **1980**, *65* (1), 172-9.

32. Lammie, P. J.; Cuenco, K. T.; Punkosdy, G. A., The pathogenesis of filarial lymphedema: is it the worm or is it the host? *Ann N Y Acad Sci* **2002**, *979*, 131-42; discussion 188-96.

33. Choi, E. H.; Nutman, T. B.; Chanock, S. J., Genetic variation in immune function and susceptibility to human filariasis. *Expert Rev Mol Diagn* **2003**, *3* (3), 367-74.

34. Taylor, M. J., A new insight into the pathogenesis of filarial disease. *Current molecular medicine* **2002**, *2* (3), 299-302.

35. Taylor, M. J., Wolbachia in the inflammatory pathogenesis of human filariasis. *Ann N Y Acad Sci* **2003**, *990*, 444-9.

36. Tamarozzi, F.; Wright, H. L.; Johnston, K. L.; Edwards, S. W.; Turner, J. D.; Taylor, M. J., Human filarial Wolbachia lipopeptide directly activates human neutrophils in vitro. *Parasite Immunol* **2014**, *36* (10), 494-502.

37. Turner, J. D.; Langley, R. S.; Johnston, K. L.; Gentil, K.; Ford, L.; Wu, B.; Graham, M.; Sharpley, F.; Slatko, B.; Pearlman, E.; Taylor, M. J., Wolbachia lipoprotein stimulates innate and adaptive immunity through Toll-like receptors 2 and 6 to induce disease manifestations of filariasis. *J Biol Chem* **2009**, *284* (33), 22364-78.

38. Freedman, D. O.; de Almeida Filho, P. J.; Besh, S.; Maia e Silva, M. C.; Braga, C.; Maciel, A., Lymphoscintigraphic analysis of lymphatic abnormalities in symptomatic and asymptomatic human filariasis. *The Journal of infectious diseases* **1994**, *170* (4), 927-33.

39. Addiss, D. G.; Dreyer, G.; Nutman, T. B., Treatment of lymphatic filariasis. Vol. 2000, p 151-199.

40. Pani, S. P.; Yuvaraj, J.; Vanamail, P.; Dhanda, V.; Michael, E.; Grenfell, B. T.; Bundy, D. A., Episodic adenolymphangitis and lymphoedema in patients with bancroftian filariasis. *Transactions of the Royal Society of Tropical Medicine and Hygiene* **1995**, *89* (1), 72-4.

41. Huntington, R. W.; Fogel, R. H.; Eichold, S.; Dickson, J. G., Filariasis Among American Troops in a South Pacific Island Group. *Yale J Biol Med* **1944**, *16* (5), 529-538 1.

42. Ottesen, E. A.; Nutman, T. B., Tropical pulmonary eosinophilia. *Annual review of medicine* **1992**, *43*, 417-24.

43. El-Moamly, A. A.; El-Sweify, M. A.; Hafez, M. A., Using the AD12-ICT rapid-format test to detect Wuchereria bancrofti circulating antigens in comparison to Og4C3-ELISA and nucleopore membrane filtration and microscopy techniques. *Parasitol Res* **2012**, *111* (3), 1379-83.

44. Rocha, A.; Braga, C.; Belem, M.; Carrera, A.; Aguiar-Santos, A.; Oliveira, P.; Texeira, M. J.; Furtado, A., Comparison of tests for the detection of circulating filarial antigen (Og4C3-ELISA and AD12-ICT) and ultrasound in diagnosis of lymphatic filariasis in individuals with microfilariae. *Mem Inst Oswaldo Cruz* **2009**, *104* (4), 621-5.

45. Wattal, S.; Dhariwal, A. C.; Ralhan, P. K.; Tripathi, V. C.; Regu, K.; Kamal, S.; Lal, S., Evaluation of Og4C3 antigen ELISA as a tool for detection of bancroftian filariasis under lymphatic filariasis elimination programme. *J Commun Dis* **2007**, *39* (2), 75-84.

46. Cunningham, J.; Hasker, E.; Das, P.; El Safi, S.; Goto, H.; Mondal, D.; Mbuchi, M.; Mukhtar, M.; Rabello, A.; Rijal, S.; Sundar, S.; Wasunna, M.; Adams, E.; Menten, J.; Peeling, R.; Boelaert, M.; Network, W. T. V. L. L., A global comparative evaluation of commercial immunochromatographic rapid diagnostic tests for visceral leishmaniasis. *Clin Infect Dis* **2012**, *55* (10), 1312-9.

47. Well, G. J.; Jam, D. C.; Santhanam, S.; J., A monoclonal antibody-based enzyme immunoassay for detecting parasite antigenemia in Bancroftian filariasis. *Dis* **1987**, *156*, 350-355.

48. Wijegunawardana, A. D.; Gunawardane, N. S.; Hapuarachchi, C.; Manamperi, A.; Gunawardena, K.; Abeyewickrama, W.; Latif, B., Evaluation of PCR-ELISA as a tool for monitoring transmission of Wuchereria bancrofti in District of Gampaha, Sri Lanka. *Asian Pac J Trop Biomed* **2013**, *3* (5), 381-7.

49. Steel, C.; Golden, A.; Kubofcik, J.; LaRue, N.; de Los Santos, T.; Domingo, G. J.; Nutman, T. B., Rapid Wuchereria bancrofti-specific antigen Wb123-based IgG4 immunoassays as tools for

surveillance following mass drug administration programs on lymphatic filariasis. *Clin Vaccine Immunol* **2013**, *20* (8), 1155-61.

50. Steel, C.; Kubofcik, J.; Ottesen, E. A.; Nutman, T. B., Antibody to the filarial antigen Wb123 reflects reduced transmission and decreased exposure in children born following single mass drug administration (MDA). *PLoS Negl Trop Dis* **2012**, *6* (12), e1940.

51. Kubofcik, J.; Fink, D. L.; Nutman, T. B., Identification of Wb123 as an early and specific marker of Wuchereria bancrofti infection. *PLoS Negl Trop Dis* **2012**, *6* (12), e1930.

52. Mand, S.; Marfo-Debrekyei, Y.; Dittrich, M.; Fischer, K.; Adjei, O.; Hoerauf, A., Animated documentation of the filaria dance sign (FDS) in bancroftian filariasis. *Filaria J* **2003**, *2* (1), 3.

53. Moore, T. A.; Reynolds, J. C.; Kenney, R. T.; Johnston, W.; Nutman, T. B., Diethylcarbamazine-induced reversal of early lymphatic dysfunction in a patient with bancroftian filariasis: assessment with use of lymphoscintigraphy. *Clin Infect Dis* **1996**, *23* (5), 1007-11.

54. Bhalla, D.; Dumas, M.; Preux, P. M., Neurological manifestations of filarial infections. *Handb Clin Neurol* **2013**, *114*, 235-42.

55. Kazura, J. W.; Guerrant, R. L.; Walker, D. H.; Weller, P. F., Filariasis. In: Tropical Infectious Diseases, Principles, Pathogens, & Practice, Volume 2 (eds). Churchill Livingstone, pp. **1999**, 852-60.

56. Mand, S.; Debrah, A. Y.; Klarmann, U.; Batsa, L.; Marfo-Debrekyei, Y.; Kwarteng, A.; Specht, S.; Belda-Domene, A.; Fimmers, R.; Taylor, M.; Adjei, O.; Hoerauf, A., Doxycycline improves filarial lymphedema independent of active filarial infection: a randomized controlled trial. *Clin Infect Dis* **2012**, *55* (5), 621-30.

57. Mand, S.; Pfarr, K.; Sahoo, P. K.; Satapathy, A. K.; Specht, S.; Klarmann, U.; Debrah, A. Y.; Ravindran, B.; Hoerauf, A., Macrofilaricidal activity and amelioration of lymphatic pathology in bancroftian filariasis after 3 weeks of doxycycline followed by single-dose diethylcarbamazine. *Am J Trop Med Hyg* **2009**, *81* (4), 702-11.

58. Taylor, M. J.; Hoerauf, A., A new approach to the treatment of filariasis. *Current opinion in infectious diseases* **2001**, *14* (6), 727-31.

59. Dembele, B.; Coulibaly, Y. I.; Dolo, H.; Konate, S.; Coulibaly, S. Y.; Sanogo, D.; Soumaoro, L.; Coulibaly, M. E.; Doumbia, S. S.; Diallo, A. A.; Traore, S. F.; Diaman Keita, A.; Fay, M. P.; Nutman, T. B.; Klion, A. D., Use of high-dose, twice-yearly albendazole and ivermectin to suppress Wuchereria bancrofti microfilarial levels. *Clin Infect Dis* **2010**, *51* (11), 1229-35.

60. Freeman, C. D.; Klutman, N. E.; Lamp, K. C., Metronidazole. A therapeutic review and update. *Drugs* **1997**, *54* (5), 679-708.

61. Capuano, G. P.; Capuano, C., Surgical management of morbidity due to lymphatic filariasis: the usefulness of a standardized international clinical classification of hydroceles. *Trop Biomed* **2012**, *29* (1), 24-38.

62. Addiss, D. G.; Brady, M. A., Morbidity management in the Global Programme to Eliminate Lymphatic Filariasis: a review of the scientific literature. *Filaria J* **2007**, *6*, 2.

63. Piessens, W. F.; Partono, F., Host-vector-parasite relationships in human filariasis. *Semin Infect Dis* **1980**, *3* 131-152.

64. Global Programme to Eliminate Lymphatic Filariasis. *Wkly Epidemiol Rec* **2006**, *81* (22), 221-32.

65. Kazura, J.; Greenberg, J.; Perry, R.; Weil, G.; Day, K.; Alpers, M., Comparison of single-dose diethylcarbamazine and ivermectin for treatment of bancroftian filariasis in Papua New Guinea. *The American journal of tropical medicine and hygiene* **1993**, *49* (6), 804-11.

66. Sabesan, S., Albendazole for mass drug administration to eliminate lymphatic filariasis. *Lancet Infect Dis* **2006**, *6* (11), 684-5.

23. *Onchocerca volvulus*
(Leuckart 1893)

Introduction

Onchocerca volvulus is a vector-borne, filarial nematode parasite. The adult worm lives in the subcutaneous tissues. Its offspring, microfilariae, migrate and induce injury to a variety of anatomical sites contiguous with that tissue. There are no reservoir hosts for *Onchocerca volvulus*, the usual species responsible for human disease.[1] The black fly, *Simulium* spp., is the vector of *O. volvulus*. This filarial parasite occurs mostly in West and Central Africa, except for foci in Yemen in the Middle East, while in the Americas this disease is rapidly being eliminated with the exception of foci among indigenous populations living on the Brazil-Venezuela border. Onchocerciasis used to be the major cause of blindness throughout Sub-Saharan Africa, often affecting more than 50% of the inhabitants of towns and villages in endemic areas.[2] River blindness is now the second-leading infectious cause of blindness in the world with approximately half a million people being blind due to *Onchocerca volvulus*.[3] The

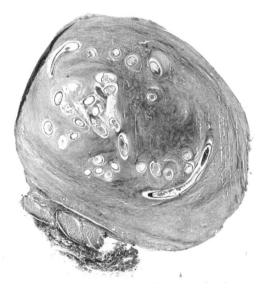

Figure 23.1. Cross section of nodule (onchocercoma) induced by *Onchocerca volvulus*. Numerous sections of adult worms are seen. 2.5 cm in diam.

disease also causes a disfiguring dermatitis (Onchocercia skin disease) that at one time was second only to polio as a cause of long-term disability in endemic areas. *O. volvulus* was once so prevalent that people could not live in many places along riverbanks.[4]

Vector control, together with a program of donation and administration of the Merck drug ivermectin (Mectizan) have resulted in dramatic reductions in the incidence and prevalence of this disease. For instance, between 1974 and 2002, the Onchocerciasis Control Program (OCP) halted transmission in 11 West African countries (Benin, Burkina Faso, Cote d'Ivoire, Ghana, Guinea, Guinea-Bissau, Mali, Niger, Senegal, Sierra Leone and Togo), and prevented an estimated 600,000 cases of blindness. It has been further estimated that 18 million children born in the OCP area are now free from the risk of river blindness, and approximately 25 million hectares (1 hectare = 2.5 acres) of land have now been rendered free of the disease.[5]

Current estimates indicate that approximately 17 million people remain infected worldwide, with 99 percent or more living in Sub-Saharan Africa. Since 1995, an African initiative, the African Programme for Onchocerciasis Control (APOC), a partnership under the leadership of the World Bank, the World Health Organization (WHO), the United Nations Development Programme (UNDP), and the Food and Agriculture Organization (FAO) of the United Nations, has coordinated the annual mass treatment of ivermectin in 19 countries and has had a highly cost effective impact on controlling this disease (see book dedication).[6] This organization has built on the previous successes of the OCP, and there is optimism that onchocerciasis might be eliminated in the coming decades. APOC aims to extend its reach to all to the remaining 19 endemic countries in Central and East Africa (Angola, Burundi, Cameroon, Central African Republic, Chad, Democratic Republic of Congo, Equatorial

Onchocerca volvulus

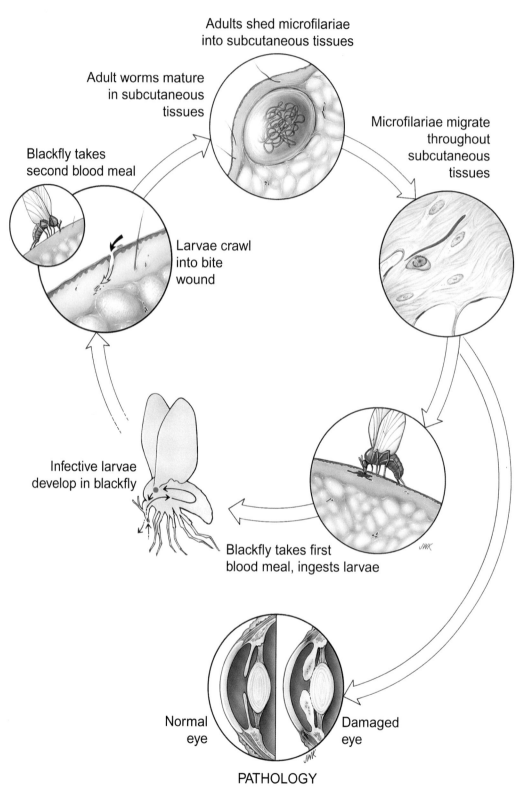

Adults shed microfilariae into subcutaneous tissues

Adult worms mature in subcutaneous tissues

Microfilariae migrate throughout subcutaneous tissues

Blackfly takes second blood meal

Larvae crawl into bite wound

Infective larvae develop in blackfly

Blackfly takes first blood meal, ingests larvae

Normal eye

Damaged eye

PATHOLOGY

Guinea, Ethiopia, Gabon, Kenya, Liberia, Malawi, Mozambique, Nigeria, Rwanda, Sudan, Tanzania and Uganda).[5, 6] Similarly the Onchocerciasis Elimination Program for the Americas (OEPA) is working to eliminate river blindness in Latin America as well as South America.[7] Currently, thanks in large part to the efforts of the OEPA, active transmission is limited to two foci in Venezuela and Brazil.[7] Elimination of this disease is so close to being achieved that the World Health Organization has recently issued guidelines for when to stop mass treatment programs and for verifying the elimination of the parasite from a given geographic region.[8]

Historical Information

In 1874, John O'Neill, an Irish naval surgeon, discovered microfilaria in skin snips of individuals in Ghana.[9] Credit for the first description of *Onchocerca volvulus* is given to Rudolf Leuckart who recounted his discovery of the parasite to Patrick Manson, who, in turn, published the full description in 1893, giving Leuckart full credit.[10] Onchocerciasis in Latin America was not reported until 1917, when Rodolfo Robles found ocular disease associated with the presence of nodules on the forehead of a small boy.[11] He dissected the nodule and found that it contained the adult worms. Later Robles described the anatomy of the worm, the pathology of the disease, and the epidemiology of the infection. Moreover, he suspected that the black fly was the vector, which was later proved by Donald Blacklock in 1927.[12]

Life Cycle

Adult females measure 20 to 80 cm in length and 0.3 cm in width, while the male measures 3 to 5 cm in length. Both sexes lie entwined about each other, locating to subcutaneous fibrous nodules, onchocercomas (Fig. 23.1), which vary in size depend-

ing on the number of adult worms in them. The male worms are able to migrate between nodules to fertilize different females, likely in response to chemoattractants released by female worms.[13] Some nodules are so small that they cannot be palpated.[14] Microfilariae are produced within the nodules, and leave these sites to migrate throughout the subcutaneous tissues (Figs. 23.2, 23.3). Only female black flies (Fig. 38.5) acquire the larvae while taking a blood meal as males do not feed on blood. The black fly injects anticoagulants creating a blood meal from which it ingests blood and microfilariae.[15] The immature worms penetrate the insect's hemocele and the muscle fibers of the flight wing bundles in the thorax. After 6-8 days of development, during which the larvae molt twice, the now infective L3 larvae leave the muscles, enter the cavity of the proboscis, and are deposited on the skin when the fly bites. Larvae enter the bite wound after the fly withdraws its biting mouthparts. The immature parasites invade the subcutaneous tissues with the aid of a protease and take up residence there.[16] After completing their development, they mate. There is a pre-patent period of 10-12 months after initial infection before the female worms

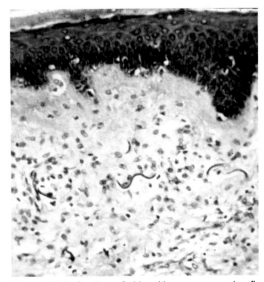

Figure 23.2. Section of skin with numerous microfilariae of *O. volvulus*.

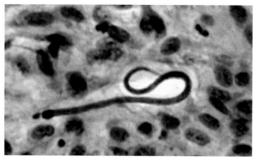

Figure 23.3. Higher magnification of a microfilaria of *O. volvulus* in skin. 310 μm x 7 μm.

start to produce microfilariae. Adults produce hundreds to thousands of microfilariae during their life span of 8-10 years (about 700 microfilariae per day). Growth and molting of worms in the subcutaneous tissues induces formation of the fibrous nodules and also elicits an angiogenic response, resulting in the production of a network of vessels, the function of which is presumably to supply nutrients to the parasites and carry away metabolic wastes.[17, 18] A similar angiogenic response is induced by the Nurse cell-parasite complex of *Trichinella spiralis*.[19]

Cellular and Molecular Pathogenesis

Onchocerca larvae migrate through the tissues with the aid of macromolecules that promote tissue degradation, angiogenesis, and plasmin-mediated proteolysis.[16-18, 20] *O. volvulus* has impressive immunomodulatory properties, with the capacity to bias host responses to a Th2-type pattern. By this mechanism, host-cell-mediated Th1-type immunity is suppressed leading to impaired responses to PPD skin testing for tuberculosis, tetanus, and other vaccinations, and increased susceptibility to intercurrent infections with lepromatous leprosy.[21-23] Down regulation of the host immune response is thought to be induced by excretory-secretory products of *O. volvulus*, such as secretory omega-class glutathione transferase 3 (OvGST).[24]

The degree of pathogenesis varies directly with the intensity of infection and the degree of host responsiveness to dying adult worms and microfilariae and their secretions. The release of wolbachia endosymbiont bacteria-derived antigens upon the death of the filariae are thought to play an essential role in triggering the destruction caused by the host's innate immune cells.[25, 26] Dead microfilariae induce inflammatory reactions that become more severe as the infection persists; this point is important when considering therapy. The lesions, primarily involving the skin and the eyes, occur as a consequence of cell-mediated immunity to parasite antigens. Individuals with the most vigorous cell-mediated immune responses develop the most severe manifestations.[2, 20, 27] The magnitude of the immunopathologic response significantly influences the severity of clinical onchodermatitis.[27, 28] Host mast cells play an important role in this phenomenon.[28]

The major ocular lesions occur in the cornea to produce a keratitis.[29] In this case, the keratitis results from an accumulation of punctate opacities in the cornea arising from immune-mediated damage resulting from reaction to microfilariae in the eye. This is a Th2-dependent process with a heavy reliance on host IL-4, as well as neutrophil recruitment to the corneal stroma.[29, 30] While corneal pathology appears to be in response to both wolbachia and microfilarial antigens, the skin reactions appear to be mainly if not exclusively due to filarial antigens.[31] In the skin, this leads to pruritus and angioedema.

The pathogenesis of onchocerciasis is dependent on the number of worms infecting an individual as well as certain host factors. Polymorphisms in the *FcyRIIa* gene that impact binding affinities of immunoglobulin subclasses have been correlated with clinical outcomes.[27] Genome-wide association studies have detected genetic variants associated with disease.[32] Hyperreactive response that trigger the skin manifestation known as *sowda* have been linked to variants of the IL-13 gene that lead to elevated levels of IgE and overly exuberant immune responses.[33]

Subcutaneous nodules, the other hallmark of clinical onchocerciasis, vary in size from barely discernable to approximately 5 cm in diameter. Nodules develop over an 18-month period depending on the number of adult worms in each. The number of nodules also varies, from an occasional one to several hundred, occupying large areas of subcutaneous tissue. In the latter instance, black flies biting such individuals may actually expire due to the overwhelming nature of the infection in their flight wing muscles. Those areas in which peripheral lymphatics converge (e.g., occiput, suboccipital areas, intercostal spaces, axilla, and iliac crests) have the highest predilection for nodules. The body regions most affected differ according to geographic locales. In Africa, the nodules predominate in the lower part of the body, whereas in Central America they tend to be found more often in the upper portions of the body. This difference is related to the biting habits of the vector insects, and the styles of clothing worn by the inhabitants of each endemic area.

O. volvulus, like *Wuchereria bancrofti*, contain bacterial symbionts of the genus *Wolbachia*. These are rickettsia-like organisms that are found in the body wall, in oocytes, and in all embryonic stages, including microfialriae.[34] The wolbachia symbionts are believed to be essential for nematode fertility and are transmitted transovarially to the next worm generation, in a manner similar to mitochondria.[35] Wolbachia also contains endotoxin-like products that are proinflammatory. This has led to the hypothesis that the bacterial symbionts contribute significantly to the skin and eye pathology of *O. volvulus*-infected patients.[34, 35]

Clinical Disease

Clinical onchocerciasis includes dermatitis, eye lesions, onchocercomas, and systemic disease.

Onchodermatitis

The major skin manifestations of onchocerciasis are papular (acute and chronic), lichenified (*sowda*), atrophy (hanging groin), and depigmentation (leopard skin).[36-38] Mild infection (less than five nodules per infected individual) is usually asymptomatic. In contrast, moderate to severe infection (ten or more nodules, with many in the head and neck region) produce correspondingly more serious and more numerous symptoms. In acute papular onchodermatitis there are pruritic papules, vesicles and pustules mainly on the buttocks and shoulders.[39] In chronic papular the papules are slightly larger and symmetrically distributed in these same areas but may also involve the waist and display hyperpigmentation. Lichenified skin manifestations tend to be geographically limited to areas such as the Sudan and Yemen and are named for the dark color to the plaques from the Arabic word for dark.[40, 41] There have been rare descriptions of this occurring outside these geographical confines including cases in the New World.[42, 43] Skin atrophy may develop from loss of skin elasticity and the skin may take on the appearance of tissue paper in areas around the waist, buttocks, and upper legs.[36, 37] Hanging groin can be associated with intense pruritus and the development of hernias.[44, 45] Leopard skin is a manifestation with dermal hypopigmentation that has gained some attention as a low-tech means of rapidly estimating endemicity of onchocerciasis, but tends to only develop in older individuals.[4, 46, 47] Occasionally, the pruritus of onchodermatitis is intense and disabling. It is alleged that occasional suicides result from the extreme discomfort associated with it.[2] A reported manifestation in Central American children who are infected involves facial lesions that are reddish in color, described as *erysipelas de la costa*.[48]

Lymphadenopathy

Lymph node involvement in Africa is usually found in the inguinal and femoral nodes, whereas in the American tropics it is in the head and neck.[2]

Ocular Lesions

Ocular manifestations of onchocerciasis include keratitis (punctate and sclerosing), iritis, uveitis, optic atrophy, optic neuritis, cataracts and chorioretinitis with the major cause of blindness being corneal blindness.[49] All parts of the eye are affected in chronic, long-term infections. Initially, there may be conjunctivitis, with irritation, lacrimation, and photophobia, a reaction analogous to the dermatitis in response to dead microfilariae. In general the ocular manifestations appear to be the result of damage due to immune cells that are triggered by antigens from microfilaria and the wolbachia endosymbiont. The cornea initially may display the punctate lesions of keratitis. Slit-lamp examination reveals motile or dead microfilariae in the conjunctiva. A long-standing infection produces sclerosis and vascularization. Sclerosing keratitis of the cornea is the leading cause of blindness due to onchocerciasis, and develops over a 20- to 30-year period.[49] Onchocercal blindness peaks in those between 30 and 40 years of age; individuals most responsible for taking care of their families. There is little evidence suggesting that sclerosing keratitis can be reversed sufficiently to restore vision once it has developed.[50] The anterior chamber is also invaded, and microfilariae can be seen with a slit lamp. Finally, there may be iritis, iridocyclitis, and secondary glaucoma. Invasion of the posterior segment of the eye causes optic neuritis and papillitis; the choroid and the retina can also be involved, although it remains unclear if this is due to a direct effect of the parasite or an immune response due to molecular mimicry.

Nodding Syndrome

In recent years a new neurological disorder known as 'nodding syndrome' has emerged among school-aged children and adolescents living in some onchocerciasis-endemic areas, especially in Uganda and in neighboring countries.[51] Although nodding syndrome has not been directly linked to onchocerciasis an epidemiological association has been noted.[52] Children with nodding syndrome exhibit periods of seizures and unresponsiveness comprised of multiple head nods and lack of responsiveness, as well as long-term mental disabilities. The etiology of nodding syndrome is under investigation.

Diagnosis

Because of its highly focal distribution, a travel history is critical in order to entertain a clinical suspicion of onchocerciasis. A definitive diagnosis can be made by examining a skin snip. This involves the bloodless removal of a 2-5 mm^2 piece of skin with a corneoscleral punch, a small beveled needle, or a disposable razor blade from an area thought to have the highest levels of microfilaria. In Africa, the specimen should be obtained from the lower part of the body, and in Central America from the upper part. The skin should be alcohol-cleansed, elevated with a needle, and cut with a scalpel blade. Next, a preferably bloodless piece should be placed in warm physiological saline and examined microscopically for motile microfilariae within 10 minutes. A representative sample of skin can be weighed and the number of microfilariae per milligram of tissue calculated as an index of the intensity of infection. In addition, the piece of skin can be pressed against a dry microscope slide, and the impression stained with Giemsa solution and examined microscopically for microfilariae (Fig. 23.4). When performed it is recommended that 6 snips be taken to increase sensitivity. Unfortunately, although skin snip microscopy has excellent specificity approaching 100%, it is only sensitive enough to make the diagnosis in less than half of cases even with multiple skin snips.[53] Histologic sections of a subcu-

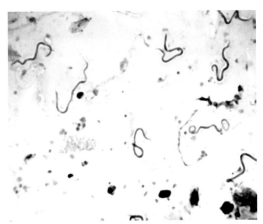

Figure 23.4. Impression smear of a skin snip from a patient heavily infected with *O. volvulus*. Microfilariae were visualized with Giemsa stain.

taneous nodule (Fig. 23.2, 23.3) may also reveal microfilariae. The sensitivity of skin snips was improved by PCR amplification, but this approach still requires the collection of skin tissue specimens.[54, 55] Highly sensitive and specific rapid serological tests have been developed, but are not in wide use and can not reliably distinguish between past versus current active infection in endemic areas.[56] Both urine and a tear antigen dipstick assay have been developed with high sensitivities, but as yet are not commercially available. The Mazzotti Test is a provocative challenge test using a 50 mg dose of diethylcarbamazine (DEC). Within 3 hours after treatment, patients with *O. volvulus* infection will develop pruritus. In heavily infected patients, the Mazzotti reaction can be severe and may exacerbate the ocular pathology in a patient. As an alternative, some physicians perform a type of patch test by applying DEC to a small region in order to elicit a local Mazzotti-like reaction.[57]

Ultrasound has been used to visualize adult worms in nodules as well as to monitor their viability following the initiation of therapy.[58]

Treatment

Ivermectin is the drug of choice for onchocerciasis. Ivermectin inhibits the release of microfilariae from the female and can reduce microfilarial counts by up to 90% within one week.[59] A single oral dose of 150 mcg/kg administered every 6 months can slow or reverse the progression of both ocular and cutaneous diseases.[60] The drug is available through the Mectizan® Donation Program established in 1988 by Merck & Co. Ivermectin does not kill the adult worms encased in a nodule. Therefore, repeat dosing is necessary to suppress the release of microfilariae for the entire 10-17 year life span of the adult worms. In some patients more frequent interval dosing is required in order to suppress pruritus. Community-wide chemotherapy can interrupt transmission of onchocerciasis.[61, 62] The major toxicity of ivermectin is generally not from the drug itself but rather from its ability to increase the antigen load from dead and dying parasites, leading to fever, angioedema and pruritus. These symptoms usually occur within 24 hours of treatment. In those patients with concurrent *Loa loa* infection, ivermectin can elicit severe reactions, including encephalopathy and consequently it is essential to evaluate the patients in areas endemic for *Loa loa* for co-infection.[63] This point is especially critical in areas such as West and Central Africa, where there is epidemiologic overlap between the two helminth infections. In Latin America, the surgical removal of palpable subcutaneous nodules has led to successful resolution of the infection in some instances.

The possible role of wolbachia endosymbionts in the inflammatory processes that caused eye and skin changes in *O. volvulus* infection, as well as their role in embryogenesis and parasite fertility, has led to the suggestion that antibiotics could have a therapeutic activity for patients with onchocerciasis.[64] Prolonged administration of doxycycline (200 mg/day for 4-6 weeks) was shown to interrupt *O. volvulus* embryogenesis.[34]

Prevention and Control

Onchocerca volvulus distribution follows that of the dipteran vectors. Black flies breed in fast-running water of mountainous streams in regions of Africa and South and Central America, and they have a fairly long flight range. Thus, onchocerciasis can be found several miles from the nearest endemic breeding site. Because much of the coffee of the world is grown on mountainous hillsides, the prevalence of onchocerciasis among workers on coffee plantations is high. The OCP was launched in 1974, with a primary emphasis on reducing black fly larval vector populations with DDT and other insecticides.[65] With the increasing availability of ivermectin, the OCP has increasingly focused on control using this drug as an agent of mass chemotherapy.[66]

In Africa, efforts to control onchocerciasis are currently being conducted by APOC.[5] Critical to the success of APOC is the Merck Mectizan Donation Program (MMDP), one of the first and largest public private partnerships devoted to a neglected disease. The Merck MDP was launched in 1987 when Roy Vagelos, then CEO of Merck made an historic announcement that his company would donate Mectizan® to anyone who needed it, for as long as it was needed.[5, 66] The MDP works closely with the Carter Center and the Task Force for Child Survival and Development, both Atlanta-based non-governmental organizations, for this purpose. To date, the Merck MDP has donated more than 300 million treatments worth over $450 million.[5]

APOC works with the organizations previously involved with the OCP, as well as Merck, the governments of 19 developing countries, 27 donor countries, at least 30 NGOs, and more than 80,000 rural Africa communities. This is done by coordinating with the ministries and NGOs to deliver Mectizan along with existing national health systems of the participating African countries. To accomplish its mission, APOC has implemented a novel system of community-directed treatment programs. It is likely that the sight of more than 500,000 people has been saved so far. In addition, the community-based health systems created by APOC are expected to provide a framework for additional pro-poor health interventions including those that target other neglected diseases such as soil-transmitted helminth infections, schistosomiasis, and trachoma.

The African Program for Onchocerciasis Control (APOC) and the Onchocerciasis Elimination Program for the Americas (OEPA) have been successful in coordinating efforts to greatly reduce the transmission of this parasite throughout the world with only limited areas of active transmission occurring.[5-7] Working with the Carter Center the number of people at risk for onchocerciasis continues to decline. APOC has reached the end of its lifespan and as of this writing plans are in discussions for a new generation of control programs possibly integrated with intestinal helminth infections, schistosomiasis, lymphatic filariasis and trachoma

As a complementary approach to onchocerciasis control, there have been some efforts to develop recombinant vaccines.[66, 67] This program known as TOVA (The Onchocerciasis Vaccine for Africa) includes the development of a vaccine that containing two antigens, Ov-103 and Ov-RAL-2, shows promise in laboratory animals.[68-71] Work to create an onchocerca vaccine continues with the hope that even if this vaccine is not completely protective it will substantially impact endemic areas by reducing host microfilarial loads in children and adolescents.[70, 72]

References

1. Otranto, D.; Dantas-Torres, F.; Cebeci, Z.; Yeniad, B.; Buyukbabani, N.; Boral, O. B.; Gustinelli, A.; Mounir, T.; Mutafchiev, Y.; Bain, O., Human ocular filariasis: further evidence on the zoonotic role of Onchocerca lupi. *Parasit Vectors* **2012,** *5*, 84.
2. Greene, B. M., Modern medicine versus an ancient scourge: progress toward control of onchocerciasis. *The Journal of infectious diseases* **1992,** *166* (1), 15-21.
3. Kapoor, U.; Sharma, V.; Chittoria, R. S., Onchocercoma in a United Nations Peacekeeper. *Med J Armed Forces India* **2015,** *71* (Suppl 1), S104-6.
4. Abanobi, O. C.; Edungbola, L. D.; Nwoke, B. E.; Mencias, B. S.; Nkwogu, F. U.; Njoku, A. J., Validity of leopard skin manifestation in community diagnosis of human onchocerciasis infection. *Appl Parasitol* **1994,** *35* (1), 8-11.
5. Levine, R.; Proven, S.; Case, H.; Washington, D. C., The What Works Working Group. *Millions in Global Onchocerciasis in SubSaharan Africa Center for Global Development pp* **2004,** *6* 57-64.
6. Coffeng, L. E.; Stolk, W. A.; Zoure, H. G.; Veerman, J. L.; Agblewonu, K. B.; Murdoch, M. E.; Noma, M.; Fobi, G.; Richardus, J. H.; Bundy, D. A.; Habbema, D.; de Vlas, S. J.; Amazigo, U. V., African Programme For Onchocerciasis Control 1995-2015: model-estimated health impact and cost. *PLoS Negl Trop Dis* **2013,** *7* (1), e2032.
7. Centers for Disease, C.; Prevention, Progress toward elimination of onchocerciasis in the Americas - 1993-2012. *MMWR Morb Mortal Wkly Rep* **2013,** *62* (20), 405-8.
8. WHO, Guidelines for Stopping Mass Drug Administration and Verifying Elimination of Human Onchocerciasis: Criteria and Procedures. Geneva, 2016.
9. O'Neill, J., On the presence of a filaria in "crawcraw." *Lancet* **1875,** *1*, 265-266.
10. Manson, P.; Davidson, A. H., Filaria volvuloxus. 1893; Vol. 1016
11. Robles, R., Enfermidad nueva en Guatemala. *Juventud Med* **1917,** *17* 97-115.
12. Blacklock, D. B., THE INSECT TRANSMISSION OF ONCHOCERCA VOLVULUS (LEUCKART, 1893): THE CAUSE OF WORM NODULES IN MAN IN AFRICA. *British medical journal* **1927,** *1* (3446), 129-33.
13. Schulz-Key, H.; Karam, M., Periodic reproduction of Onchocerca volvulus. *Parasitol Today* **1986,** *2* (10), 284-6.
14. Duke, B. O., The population dynamics of Onchocerca volvulus in the human host. *Tropical medicine and parasitology : official organ of Deutsche Tropenmedizinische Gesellschaft and of Deutsche Gesellschaft fur Technische Zusammenarbeit (GTZ)* **1993,** *44* (2), 61-8.
15. Burnham, G., Onchocerciasis. *Lancet* **1998,** *351* (9112), 1341-6.
16. Lackey, A.; James, E. R.; Sakanari, J. A.; McKerrow, J. H., Extracellular proteases of Onchocerca volvulus. *Exp Parasitol* **1993,** *68*, 176-185.
17. Tawe, W.; Pearlman, E.; Unnasch, T. R.; Lustigman, S., Angiogenic activity of Onchocerca volvulus recombinant proteins similar to vespid venom antigen 5. *Molecular and biochemical parasitology* **2000,** *109* (2), 91-9.
18. Higazi, T. B.; Pearlman, E.; Whikehart, D. R.; Unnasch, T. R., Angiogenic activity of an Onchocerca volvulus Ancylostoma secreted protein homologue. *Molecular and biochemical parasitology* **2003,** *129* (1), 61-8.
19. Capo, V.; Despommier, D. D.; Polvere, R. I.; J., Trichinella spiralis: vascular endothelial growth factor is up-regulated within the Nurse cell during early phase of its formation. **1998,** *84* 209-214.
20. Jolodar, A.; Fischer, P.; Bergmann, S.; Büttner, D. W.; Hammerschmidt, S.; Brattig, N. W., Molecular cloning of an alpha-enolase from the human filarial parasite Onchocerca volvulus that binds human plasminogen. *Biochimica et biophysica acta* **2003,** *1627* (2-3), 111-20.
21. Rougemont, A.; Boisson-Pontal, M. E.; Pontal, P. G.; Gridel, F.; Sangare, S., Tuberculin skin tests and B.C.G. vaccination in hyperendemic area of onchocerciasis. *Lancet (London, England)* **1977,** *1* (8006), 309.
22. Cooper, P. J.; Espinel, I.; Wieseman, M.; Paredes, W.; Espinel, M.; Guderian, R. H.; Nutman, T. B., Human onchocerciasis and tetanus vaccination: impact on the postvaccination antitetanus antibody response. *Infection and immunity* **1999,** *67* (11), 5951-7.

23. Prost, A.; Nebout, M.; Rougemont, A., Lepromatous leprosy and onchocerciasis. *British medical journal* **1979,** *1* (6163), 589-90.

24. Liebau, E.; Hoppner, J.; Muhlmeister, M.; Burmeister, C.; Luersen, K.; Perbandt, M.; Schmetz, C.; Buttner, D.; Brattig, N., The secretory omega-class glutathione transferase OvGST3 from the human pathogenic parasite Onchocerca volvulus. *FEBS J* **2008,** *275* (13), 3438-53.

25. Brattig, N. W., Pathogenesis and host responses in human onchocerciasis: impact of Onchocerca filariae and Wolbachia endobacteria. *Microbes Infect* **2004,** *6* (1), 113-28.

26. Hise, A. G.; Daehnel, K.; Gillette-Ferguson, I.; Cho, E.; McGarry, H. F.; Taylor, M. J.; Golenbock, D. T.; Fitzgerald, K. A.; Kazura, J. W.; Pearlman, E., Innate immune responses to endosymbiotic Wolbachia bacteria in Brugia malayi and Onchocerca volvulus are dependent on TLR2, TLR6, MyD88, and Mal, but not TLR4, TRIF, or TRAM. *J Immunol* **2007,** *178* (2), 1068-76.

27. Ali, M. M.; Baraka, O. Z.; AbdelRahman, S. I.; Sulaiman, S. M.; Williams, J. F.; Homeida, M. M.; Mackenzie, C. D., Immune responses directed against microfilariae correlate with severity of clinical onchodermatitis and treatment history. *The Journal of infectious diseases* **2003,** *187* (4), 714-7.

28. Cooper, P. J.; Schwartz, L. B.; Irani, A.-M.; Awadzi, K.; Guderian, R. H.; Nutman, T. B., Association of transient dermal mastocytosis and elevated plasma tryptase levels with development of adverse reactions after treatment of onchocerciasis with ivermectin. *The Journal of infectious diseases* **2002,** *186* (9), 1307-13.

29. Pearlman, E.; Lass, J. H.; Bardenstein, D. S.; Kopf, M.; Hazlett, F. E.; Diaconu, E.; Kazura, J. W., Interleukin 4 and T helper type 2 cells are required for development of experimental onchocercal keratitis (river blindness). *The Journal of experimental medicine* **1995,** *182* (4), 931-40.

30. Gentil, K.; Pearlman, E., Gamma interferon and interleukin-1 receptor 1 regulate neutrophil recruitment to the corneal stroma in a murine model of Onchocerca volvulus keratitis. *Infect Immun* **2009,** *77* (4), 1606-12.

31. Timmann, C.; Abraha, R. S.; Hamelmann, C.; Buttner, D. W.; Lepping, B.; Marfo, Y.; Brattig, N.; Horstmann, R. D., Cutaneous pathology in onchocerciasis associated with pronounced systemic T-helper 2-type responses to Onchocerca volvulus. *Br J Dermatol* **2003,** *149* (4), 782-7.

32. Timmann, C.; van der Kamp, E.; Kleensang, A.; Konig, I. R.; Thye, T.; Buttner, D. W.; Hamelmann, C.; Marfo, Y.; Vens, M.; Brattig, N.; Ziegler, A.; Horstmann, R. D., Human genetic resistance to Onchocerca volvulus: evidence for linkage to chromosome 2p from an autosome-wide scan. *J Infect Dis* **2008,** *198* (3), 427-33.

33. Hoerauf, A.; Kruse, S.; Brattig, N. W.; Heinzmann, A.; Mueller-Myhsok, B.; Deichmann, K. A., The variant Arg110Gln of human IL-13 is associated with an immunologically hyper-reactive form of onchocerciasis (sowda). *Microbes Infect* **2002,** *4* (1), 37-42.

34. Hoerauf, A.; Büttner, D. W.; Adjei, O.; Pearlman, E., Onchocerciasis. *BMJ (Clinical research ed.)* **2003,** *326* (7382), 207-10.

35. Keiser, P. B.; Reynolds, S. M.; Awadzi, K.; Ottesen, E. A.; Taylor, M. J.; Nutman, T. B., Bacterial endosymbionts of Onchocerca volvulus in the pathogenesis of posttreatment reactions. *The Journal of infectious diseases* **2002,** *185* (6), 805-11.

36. Bari, A. U., Clinical spectrum of onchodermatitis. *J Coll Physicians Surg Pak* **2007,** *17* (8), 453-6.

37. Murdoch, M. E., Onchodermatitis. *Curr Opin Infect Dis* **2010,** *23* (2), 124-31.

38. Murdoch, M. E.; Hay, R. J.; Mackenzie, C. D.; Williams, J. F.; Ghalib, H. W.; Cousens, S.; Abiose, A.; Jones, B. R., A clinical classification and grading system of the cutaneous changes in onchocerciasis. *Br J Dermatol* **1993,** *129* (3), 260-9.

39. Lazarov, A.; Amihai, B.; Sion-Vardy, N., Pruritus and chronic papular dermatitis in an Ethiopian man. Onchocerciasis (chronic papular onchodermatitis). *Arch Dermatol* **1997,** *133* (3), 382-3, 385-6.

40. Siddiqui, M. A.; al-Khawajah, M. M., The black disease of Arabia, Sowda-onchocerciasis. New findings. *Int J Dermatol* **1991,** *30* (2), 130-3.

41. Richard-Lenoble, D.; al Qubati, Y.; Toe, L.; Pisella, P. J.; Gaxotte, P.; al Kohlani, A., [Human onchocerciasis and "sowda" in the Republic of Yemen]. *Bull Acad Natl Med* **2001,** *185* (8), 1447-59; discussion 1459-61.

42. Somorin, A. O., Sowda onchocerciasis in Nigeria. *Cent Afr J Med* **1982,** *28* (10), 253-6.
43. Schwartz, D. A.; Brandling-Bennett, A. D.; Figueroa, H.; Connor, D. H.; Gibson, D. W., Sowda-type onchocerciasis in Guatemala. *Acta Trop* **1983,** *40* (4), 383-9.
44. Nelson, G. S., Hanging groin and hernia complications of onchocerciasis. *Trans R Soc Trop Med Hyg* **1958,** *52* (3), 272-5.
45. Niamba, P.; Gaulier, A.; Taieb, A., Hanging groin and persistent pruritus in a patient from Burkina Faso. *Int J Dermatol* **2007,** *46* (5), 485-6.
46. Fuglsang, H., "Leopard skin" and onchocerciasis. *Trans R Soc Trop Med Hyg* **1983,** *77* (6), 881.
47. Edungbola, L. D.; Alabi, T. O.; Oni, G. A.; Asaolu, S. O.; Ogunbanjo, B. O.; Parakoyi, B. D., 'Leopard skin' as a rapid diagnostic index for estimating the endemicity of African onchocerciasis. *Int J Epidemiol* **1987,** *16* (4), 590-4.
48. Goldman, L.; Figueroa Ortiz, L., Types of dermatitis in American onchocerciasis. *Arch Derm Syphilol* **1946,** *53,* 79-93.
49. Babalola, O. E., Ocular onchocerciasis: current management and future prospects. *Clin Ophthalmol* **2011,** *5,* 1479-91.
50. Thylefors, B., Ocular onchocerciasis. *Bull World Health Organ* **1978,** *56* (1), 63-73.
51. Colebunders, R.; Hendy, A.; Mokili, J. L.; Wamala, J. F.; Kaducu, J.; Kur, L.; Tepage, F.; Mandro, M.; Mucinya, G.; Mambandu, G.; Komba, M. Y.; Lumaliza, J. L.; van Oijen, M.; Laudisoit, A., Nodding syndrome and epilepsy in onchocerciasis endemic regions: comparing preliminary observations from South Sudan and the Democratic Republic of the Congo with data from Uganda. *BMC Res Notes* **2016,** *9* (1), 182.
52. Idro, R.; Opar, B.; Wamala, J.; Abbo, C.; Onzivua, S.; Mwaka, D. A.; Kakooza-Mwesige, A.; Mbonye, A.; Aceng, J. R., Is nodding syndrome an Onchocerca volvulus-induced neuroinflammatory disorder? Uganda's story of research in understanding the disease. *Int J Infect Dis* **2016,** *45,* 112-7.
53. Boatin, B. A.; Toe, L.; Alley, E. S.; Nagelkerke, N. J.; Borsboom, G.; Habbema, J. D., Detection of Onchocerca volvulus infection in low prevalence areas: a comparison of three diagnostic methods. *Parasitology* **2002,** *125* (Pt 6), 545-52.
54. Boatin, B. A.; Toé, L.; Alley, E. S.; Nagelkerke, N. J. D.; Borsboom, G.; Habbema, J. D. F., Detection of Onchocerca volvulus infection in low prevalence areas: a comparison of three diagnostic methods. *Parasitology* **2002,** *125* (Pt 6), 545-52.
55. Bradley, J. E.; Unnasch, T. R., Molecular approaches to the diagnosis of onchocerciasis. *Advances in parasitology* **1996,** *37,* 57-106.
56. Udall, D. N., Recent updates on onchocerciasis: diagnosis and treatment. *Clin Infect Dis* **2007,** *44* (1), 53-60.
57. Kilian, H. D., The use of a topical Mazzotti test in the diagnosis of onchocerciasis. *Tropical medicine and parasitology : official organ of Deutsche Tropenmedizinische Gesellschaft and of Deutsche Gesellschaft fur Technische Zusammenarbeit (GTZ)* **1988,** *39* (3), 235-8.
58. Mand, S.; Marfo-Debrekyei, Y.; Debrah, A.; Buettner, M.; Batsa, L.; Pfarr, K.; Adjei, O.; Hoerauf, A., Frequent detection of worm movements in onchocercal nodules by ultrasonography. *Filaria J* **2005,** *4* (1), 1.
59. Greene, B. M.; Taylor, H. R.; Cupp, E. W.; Murphy, R. P.; White, A. T.; Aziz, M. A.; Schulz-Key, H.; D'Anna, S. A.; Newland, H. S.; Goldschmidt, L. P., Comparison of ivermectin and diethylcarbamazine in the treatment of onchocerciasis. *The New England journal of medicine* **1985,** *313* (3), 133-8.
60. Burnham, G., Ivermectin treatment of onchocercal skin lesions: observations from a placebo-controlled, double-blind trial in Malawi. *The American journal of tropical medicine and hygiene* **1995,** *52* (3), 270-6.
61. Taylor, H. R.; Pacqué, M.; Muñoz, B.; Greene, B. M., Impact of mass treatment of onchocerciasis with ivermectin on the transmission of infection. *Science (New York, N.Y.)* **1990,** *250* (4977), 116-8.
62. Cupp, E. W.; Ochoa, J. O.; Collins, R. C.; Cupp, M. S.; Gonzales-Peralta, C.; Castro, J.; Zea-Flores, G., The effects of repetitive community-wide ivermectin treatment on transmission of

Onchocerca volvulus in Guatemala. *The American journal of tropical medicine and hygiene* **1992,** *47* (2), 170-80.

63.   Chippaux, J. P.; Ernould, J. C.; Gardon, J.; Gardon-Wendel, N.; Chandre, F.; Barberi, N., Ivermectin treatment of loiasis. *Transactions of the Royal Society of Tropical Medicine and Hygiene* **1992,** *86* (3), 289.

64.   Hoerauf, A.; Mand, S.; Volkmann, L.; Büttner, M.; Marfo-Debrekyei, Y.; Taylor, M.; Adjei, O.; Büttner, D. W., Doxycycline in the treatment of human onchocerciasis: Kinetics of Wolbachia endobacteria reduction and of inhibition of embryogenesis in female Onchocerca worms. *Microbes and infection / Institut Pasteur* **2003,** *5* (4), 261-73.

65.   Omura, S.; Crump, A., The life and times of ivermectin - a success story. *Nature reviews. Microbiology* **2004,** *2* (12), 984-9.

66.   Peters, D. H.; Phillips, T., Mectizan Donation Program: evaluation of a public-private partnership. *Tropical medicine & international health : TM & IH* **2004,** *9* (4), A4-15.

67.   Lustigman, S.; James, E. R.; Tawe, W.; Abraham, D., Towards a recombinant antigen vaccine against Onchocerca volvulus. *Trends in parasitology* **2002,** *18* (3), 135-41.

68.   Nutman, T. B., Future directions for vaccine-related onchocerciasis research. *Trends in parasitology* **2002,** *18* (6), 237-9.

69.   MacDonald, A. J.; Tawe, W.; Leon, O.; Cao, L.; Liu, J.; Oksov, Y.; Abraham, D.; Lustigman, S., Ov-ASP-1, the Onchocerca volvulus homologue of the activation associated secreted protein family is immunostimulatory and can induce protective anti-larval immunity. *Parasite immunology* **2004,** *26* (1), 53-62.

70.   Hotez, P. J.; Bottazzi, M. E.; Zhan, B.; Makepeace, B. L.; Klei, T. R.; Abraham, D.; Taylor, D. W.; Lustigman, S., The Onchocerciasis Vaccine for Africa--TOVA--Initiative. *PLoS Negl Trop Dis* **2015,** *9* (1), e0003422.

71.   Arumugam, S.; Wei, J.; Liu, Z.; Abraham, D.; Bell, A.; Bottazzi, M. E.; Hotez, P. J.; Zhan, B.; Lustigman, S.; Klei, T. R., Vaccination of Gerbils with Bm-103 and Bm-RAL-2 Concurrently or as a Fusion Protein Confers Consistent and Improved Protection against Brugia malayi Infection. *PLoS Negl Trop Dis* **2016,** *10* (4), e0004586.

72.   Makepeace, B. L.; Babayan, S. A.; Lustigman, S.; Taylor, D. W., The case for vaccine development in the strategy to eradicate river blindness (onchocerciasis) from Africa. *Expert Rev Vaccines* **2015,** *14* (9), 1163-5.

24. *Loa loa*
(Cobbold 1864)

Introduction

Loa loa is a filarial nematode infection acquired in Central and West Africa, where it infects millions of individuals in the areas endemic for this pathogen.[1] In some hyperendemic regions, prevalence may be as high as 40%.[1, 2] Loiasis is an emerging infection in areas where the establishment of rubber plantations has altered the rainforest ecology.[3] Increasingly, *L. loa* infection is seen in returning travelers who spend long periods of time in rural Africa. This includes a diverse array of people with unique occupational exposures, such as anthropologists and individuals involved in ecotourism.[4] The overwhelming concern for loiasis patients is the severe and adverse reaction in a small percentage of individuals who are recipients of mass drug administration for onchocerciasis. The adult worm lives in subcutaneous tissues. Its main vectors are dipteran flies of the genus *Chrysops* (the deer fly).

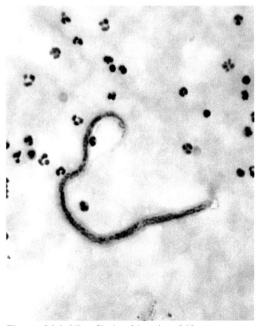

Figure 24.1. Microfilaria of *Loa loa*. 240 μm

Historical Information

In 1770, M. Mongin, a French surgeon, described a worm passing though the eye of a woman in Santo Domingo, in the Caribbean, and his unsuccessful attempt to remove it.[5] In 1778, Francois Guyot, a French ship's surgeon, successfully removed a worm from one of the slaves in transit from West Africa to the Americas.[6] In 1890, Stephen McKenzie, an ophthalmologist, found microfilaria and sent them to Patrick Manson suggesting that they might be the larvae of *Loa loa*.[7] In 1895, Douglas Argyll-Robertson published the first complete description of the worm and the clinical presentation of the infection.[8] The woman from whom he removed two adult worms (one of each sex) had lived in Old Calabar (a port city in the area of Africa that is now Nigeria). Swellings in her arms accompanied her infections, and he was the first to describe these swellings in detail.[6] In 1910, Patrick Manson, along with his colleague George Low, suggested that the swellings were directly connected with infections due to *Loa loa*.[9, 10] These inflammatory lesions are still referred to as Calabar swellings. In 1913, Robert Leiper, described two species of dipterans, *Chrysops dimidiata and C. silacae,* as the vectors of *L. loa*.[11]

Life Cycle

Female adults measure 0.5 mm wide and 60 mm long; the males are 0.4 mm by 32 mm.[12] Adult worms deposit microfilariae (Fig. 24.1), while they wander throughout the subcutaneous tissues. There is an interval of 6-12 months between the initial bite by an infected fly and the appearance of microfilaria in the blood. Microfilariae (80 μm long by 7 μm in diameter) penetrate capillaries and enter the bloodstream, where they circulate until they become ingested in a blood meal by a *Chrysops* spp.. These flies are commonly called deer flies, horse flies, yellow

Loa loa

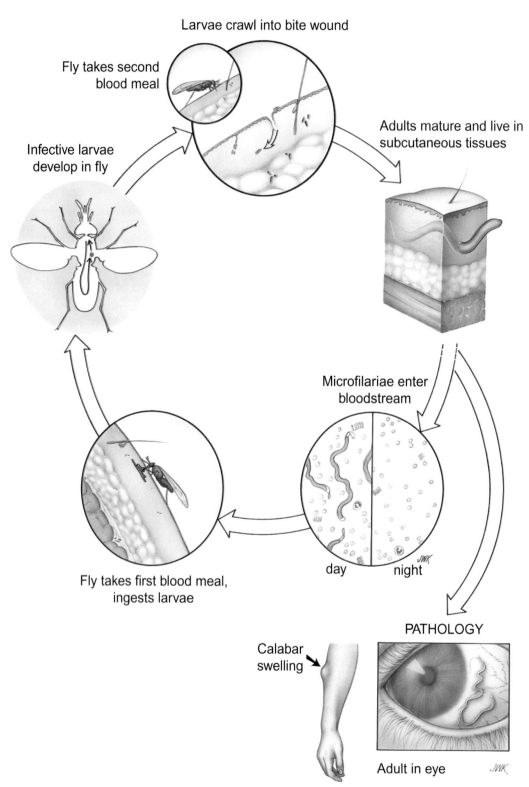

Larvae crawl into bite wound

Fly takes second
blood meal

Infective larvae
develop in fly

Adults mature and live in
subcutaneous tissues

Microfilariae enter
bloodstream

day   night

Fly takes first blood meal,
ingests larvae

PATHOLOGY

Calabar
swelling

Adult in eye

flies, stouts, mango flies, or mangrove flies.[12-14] *L. loa* microfilariae exhibit diurnal periodicity that coincides with the feeding habits of chrysops.[15] Larvae penetrate the stomach of the fly, and locate to the fat body. Eight to ten days later, the infective L3 larvae migrate to the cavity of the biting mouthparts, and are released into the bite wound when the fly takes another blood meal. The larvae, now in the subcutaneous tissues of the host, develop slowly into adults within 1-4 years. Mature worms mate, and the females begin depositing microfilariae. The adult worms can live in the tissues for up to 17-years.[16]

Cellular and Molecular Pathogenesis

In most cases, neither the adult worms in the subcutaneous tissues or the microfilariae in the bloodstream cause any direct pathologic changes. In individuals native to and living in endemic areas there is evidence for immune tolerance with high levels of circulating microfilaria, low levels of filarial-specific IgG, and few if any clinical symptoms.[17] In temporary residents there can be peripheral eosinophilia, high levels of filarial specific IgG, eosinophil activation and degranulation, and localized subcutaneous edema.[17, 18] The Calabar swellings are usually restricted to visitors to endemic areas and are not typically seen in residents who live for many years in these same regions.[19, 20] The visitors to endemic areas with exuberant immune responses develop swellings as a local inflammatory reaction in response to migrating adult worms and/or released microfilariae. It is presumed to result from a robust IgE and IL-5 production in response to secretions from the adults, or from those of the microfilariae that are released inside the female adult parasite during their development. Upregulation of IL-5 results in circulating eosinophilia.[21, 22] A third group of infected individuals who neither have circulating microfilariae nor Calabar swellings, while still living in hyperendemic areas, are suspected to have developed protective sterilizing immunity early on in their lives.[23, 24] Unlike other filarial nematodes, there is currently no evidence that *L. loa* contains wolbachia symbionts, based on extensive investigations employing light microscopy, electron microscopy, and PCR.[25, 26]

Clinical Disease

The clinical manifestations of loaisis include Calabar swellings, eye symptoms, encephalitis, cardiomyopathy, renal disease, arthritis, and lymphadenitis. Calabar swellings are 10-20 cm non-erythematous, angioedematous swellings that last for a few days. They occur most typically on the extremities and the face, particularly in the periorbital region. The angioedema is often preceded by pain and itching. Recurrences are common. The occasional passage of an adult worm across the subconjunctival space of the eye is perhaps the most disturbing aspect of *L. loa* to most infected individuals. Patients with more serious complications, including cardiomyopathy, nephropathy, and pleural effusions, have been reported.[20] The most serious and life threatening reactions result after patients are exposed to antihelminthic medications. Some complications occur only after administration of diethylcarbamazine. These sequelae may result from immune complex deposition. Encephalitis has also been described in patients with very high levels of microfilariae, including microfilariae in the cerebrospinal fluid.[23] Most of these individuals have received diethylcarbamazine or ivermectin while suffering from elevated levels of microfilariae in the blood, and the syndrome probably occurs as part of host immune responses.[27] While less common in patients with low levels of microfilariae in the blood, neurological symptoms have been seen with treatment initiation.[28] A rare cardiac condition known as endomyocardial fibrosis may result from eosinophilic infiltration of the myocardium in response to *L. loa*.[29]

Significant differences in the clinical presentation of loiasis occur among long-term visitors to endemic areas, in contrast to people native to these areas.[21] People living in endemic regions are often asymptomatic, despite high levels of circulating microfilaria, whereas visitors and expatriates suffer from a variety of allergic responses, such as frequent episodes of angioedema, Calabar swellings, hypereosinophilia, and hyper-gammaglobulinemia. This disorder is sometimes referred to as the "hyper-responsive syndrome" of loiasis, reflecting elevated humoral and cell-mediated immune responses to the parasite.[20]

Diagnosis

Patients returning from West or Central Africa with localized angioedema or a worm beneath the conjunctiva should be suspected of having loiasis. The Calabar swellings should be clinically differentiated from other causes of angioedema, including C1 inhibitor deficiency.[30] Definitive diagnosis is by identifying the microfilariae microscopically in a thin blood smear stained with either Giemsa or Wright's solution. Among the distinguishing features of *L. loa* microfilariae (Figs. C.50, C.51) are their diurnal periodicity, the presence of a sheath, and three or more terminal nuclei.[24] With the diurnal periodicity it is important to draw blood for this test during the middle of the day and employ a concentration technique such as the Knott's test (using formalin), or nucleopore filtration.[31] Since visitors to endemic areas often have low levels of circulating microfilariae, serology can be useful in this population.[30, 32, 33] Anti-loa antibodies of the IgG_4 immunoglobulin subclass may be a reliable marker of infection.[30] This includes IgG_4 antibodies against the loa recombinant antigen L1-SXP-1.[34] There is also a PCR that has been developed to detect microfilariae in blood.[33, 35] Real-time PCR

was developed and then adapted for loop-mediated isothermal amplification (LAMP) as a point of care test.[36, 37]

Since levels of circulating microfilariae are critical in decisions regarding treatment, a group has repurposed an automated handheld cell counter as a point of care test to assess microfilarial levels.[38] Alternatively, new blood and urine *L. loa*- specific biomarker tests have been developed.[39, 40]

Treatment

The first step in treatment of *Loa loa* infection is based on levels of circulating microfilariae. If levels are greater than 2,500 microfilariae/ml, then an attempt should be made to lower these levels. This may be accomplished through apheresis or several weeks of treatment with albendazole.[24, 41, 42] Once the levels of microfilariae are below 2,500 microfilariae/ml diethylcarbamazine (DEC) for 21 days may be administered. The drug destroys all stages of the infecting parasite. The full dose of the drug is not typically started on the first day of treatment. Instead, it is given in a graded manner, beginning with a test dose on day 1 and then increasing the dose to full dose by day four. This is done to reduce the likelihood of treatment-associated complications, including encephalopathy, that occur as a consequence of mass destruction of loa microfilariae.[28] These iatrogenic complications of loiasis are rare when the microfilarial concentration in blood is less than 2,500 mf/ml at initiation of therapy.[24] Antihistamines or corticosteroids may be required to decrease allergic reactions during treatment. In up to 50% of patients, DEC treatment may need to be repeated several times in order to effect a cure.[43] Adult worms in the eye can be removed surgically. Since they tend not to cause any pathology it is not a required part of curative therapy. Alternatives to DEC include albendazole that can effectively reduce the numer of circulating microfilariae by acting directing on adult worms. Ivermectin is not a preferred agent for the treatment of loaisis and can be associated with significant morbidity if given to patients with high levels of circulating microfilariae. Weekly chemoprophylaxis with DEC given in a dose of 300 mg is effective in preventing loiasis among long-term visitors but is not currently recommended for short-term visitors to endemic areas.[43]

Prevention and Control

In hyperendemic regions of Central Africa, 95% of the population have antibodies to *L. loa* antigen by the age of two years.[41] In the Chailu Mountains in the Democratic Republic of Congo, 19% of the native populations are microfilaremic, and more than 50% of the adults have reported sub-conjunctival migrations of an adult worm. Mass or targeted chemotherapy with diethylcarbamazine may reduce transmission in these areas.[44, 45] Spraying mango groves with insecticides, particularly DDT, remains an effective method for controlling populations of the vector, since resistance to this insecticide in chrysops has not yet developed.

Widespread use of mass drug administration in Sub-Saharan Africa for purposes of controlling lymphatic filariasis and onchocerciasis has raised concerns about *L. loa* co-infections. The potential complications of unmonitored DEC treatment of loiasis and the risk of encephalopathy are major reasons why this agent is not used routinely. Even the alternative combination of ivermectin and albendazole poses some risk. Loa encephalopathy is associated with ivermectin treatment of individuals with loa microfilaremia > 30,000 mf/ml blood, with most of the cases of ivermectin-induced encephalopathy occurring in Cameroon.[45] In order to reduce the risks associated with ivermectin in this region, albendazole has been evaluated as a possible first-line measure to gradually lower microfilariae burdens.[46, 47] The recent development of blood and urine tests to detect loa antigen may represent a future breakthrough in detecting loiasis patients targeted for mass drug administration to combat lymphatic filariasis or onchocerciasis.[39]

References

1. Zoure, H. G.; Wanji, S.; Noma, M.; Amazigo, U. V.; Diggle, P. J.; Tekle, A. H.; Remme, J. H., The geographic distribution of Loa loa in Africa: results of large-scale implementation of the Rapid Assessment Procedure for Loiasis (RAPLOA). *PLoS Negl Trop Dis* **2011,** *5* (6), e1210.

2. Noireau, F.; Carme, B.; Apembet, J. D.; Gouteux, J. P., Loa loa and Mansonella perstans filariasis in the Chaillu mountains, Congo: parasitological prevalence. *Transactions of the Royal Society of Tropical Medicine and Hygiene* **1989,** *83* (4), 529-34.

3. Rodhain, F., [Hypotheses on the dynamic ecology of Loa infections]. *Bulletin de la Societe de pathologie exotique et de ses filiales* **1980,** *73* (2), 182-91.

4. Thompson, C.; Cy, A.; Boggild, A. K., Chronic symptomatic and microfilaremic loiasis in a returned traveller. *CMAJ* **2015,** *187* (6), 437.

5. Mongin, Sur un ver trouve´ sous la conjunctive a` Maribarou, isle Saint-Dominique. *J. Med. Chir. Pharm* **1770,** *32,* 338-339.

6. Cox, F. E., History of human parasitology. *Clin Microbiol Rev* **2002,** *15* (4), 595-612.

7. Manson, P., The Filaria sanguinis hominis major and minor, two new species of haematozoa. *Lancet* **1891,** *i,* 4-8.

8. Argyll-Robertson, D.; Soc, U. K., Case of Filaria loa in which the parasite was removed from under the conjunctiva. *Trans Ophthalmol* **1895,** *15,* 137-167.

9. Low, G. C., Discussion of Manson, P. On the nature and origin of Calabar swellings. *Trans. R. Soc. Trop. Med. Hyg* **1910,** *3,* 251-253.

10. Manson, P., On the nature and origin of Calabar swellings. *Trans. R. Soc. Trop. Med. Hyg* **1910,** *3,*

244-251.

11. Leiper, R. T., Report of the Helminthologist for the Half Year Ending 30 April, . Report of the Advisory Commission on Tropical Diseases Research Fund. **1913**, 1913-1914.

12. Padgett, J. J.; Jacobsen, K. H., Loiasis: African eye worm. *Trans R Soc Trop Med Hyg* **2008,** *102* (10), 983-9.

13. Horvath, G.; Majer, J.; Horvath, L.; Szivak, I.; Kriska, G., Ventral polarization vision in tabanids: horseflies and deerflies (Diptera: Tabanidae) are attracted to horizontally polarized light. *Naturwissenschaften* **2008,** *95* (11), 1093-100.

14. Baldacchino, F.; Desquesnes, M.; Mihok, S.; Foil, L. D.; Duvallet, G.; Jittapalapong, S., Tabanids: neglected subjects of research, but important vectors of disease agents! *Infect Genet Evol* **2014,** *28*, 596-615.

15. Duke, B. O. L.; J., Studies of the biting habits of Chrysops. *Trop Med Parasitol* **1955,** *49*.

16. Eveland, L. K.; Yermakov, V.; Kenney, M., Loa loa infection without microfilaraemia. *Transactions of the Royal Society of Tropical Medicine and Hygiene* **1975,** *69* (3), 354-5.

17. Herrick, J. A.; Metenou, S.; Makiya, M. A.; Taylar-Williams, C. A.; Law, M. A.; Klion, A. D.; Nutman, T. B., Eosinophil-associated processes underlie differences in clinical presentation of loiasis between temporary residents and those indigenous to Loa-endemic areas. *Clin Infect Dis* **2015,** *60* (1), 55-63.

18. Olness, K.; Franciosi, R. A.; Johnson, M. M.; Freedman, D. O., Loiasis in an expatriate American child: diagnostic and treatment difficulties. *Pediatrics* **1987,** *80* (6), 943-6.

19. Nutman, T. B.; Miller, K. D.; Mulligan, M.; Ottesen, E. A., Loa loa infection in temporary residents of endemic regions: recognition of a hyperresponsive syndrome with characteristic clinical manifestations. *The Journal of infectious diseases* **1986,** *154* (1), 10-8.

20. Nutman, T. B.; Reese, W.; Poindexter, R. W.; Ottesen, E. A., Immunologic correlates of the hyperresponsive syndrome of loiasis. *The Journal of infectious diseases* **1988,** *157* (3), 544-50.

21. Kilon, A. D.; Massougbodji, A.; J., Loiasis in endemic and non-endemic populations: immunologically mediated differences in clinical presentation. *Dis* **1991,** *163*, 1318-1325.

22. Limaye, A. P.; Abrams, J. S.; Silver, J. E.; Ottesen, E. A.; Nutman, T. B., Regulation of parasite-induced eosinophilia: selectively increased interleukin 5 production in helminth-infected patients. *The Journal of experimental medicine* **1990,** *172* (1), 399-402.

23. Kilon, A. D.; Einstein, E. M., Pulmonary involvement in loiasis. *Am Rev Respir Dis* **1992,** *145*, 961-963.

24. Kilon, A. D.; Nutman, T. B.; Guerrant, R. L.; Walker, D. H.; Weller, P. F., Loiasis and Mansonella infections In: Tropical Infectious Diseases, Principles, Pathogens, and Practice. *Vol 2 eds Churchill Livingstone Pubs New York pp* **1999**, 861-872.

25. Grobusch, M. P.; Kombila, M.; Autenrieth, I.; Mehlhorn, H.; Kremsner, P. G., No evidence of Wolbachia endosymbiosis with Loa loa and Mansonella perstans. *Parasitology research* **2003,** *90* (5), 405-8.

26. Brouqui, P.; Fournier, P. E.; Raoult, D., Doxycycline and eradication of microfilaremia in patients with loiasis. *Emerg Infect Dis* **2001,** *7* (3 Suppl), 604-5.

27. Gardon, J.; Gardon-Wendel, N.; Demanga, N.; Kamgno, J.; Chippaux, J. P.; Boussinesq, M., Serious reactions after mass treatment of onchocerciasis with ivermectin in an area endemic for Loa loa infection. *Lancet* **1997,** *350* (9070), 18-22.

28. Carme, B.; Boulesteix, J.; Boutes, H.; Puruehnce, M. F., Five cases of encephalitis during treatment of loiasis with diethylcarbamazine. *The American journal of tropical medicine and hygiene* **1991,** *44* (6), 684-90.

29. Andy, J. J.; Bishara, F. F.; Soyinka, O. O.; Odesanmi, W. O., Loasis as a possible trigger of African endomyocardial fibrosis: a case report from Nigeria. *Acta tropica* **1981,** *38* (2), 179-86.

30. Akue, J. P.; Egwang, T. G.; Devaney, E., High levels of parasite-specific IgG4 in the absence of microfilaremia in Loa loa infection. *Tropical medicine and parasitology : official organ of Deutsche Tropenmedizinische Gesellschaft and of Deutsche Gesellschaft fur Technische Zusammenarbeit (GTZ)* **1994,** *45* (3), 246-8.

31. Mak, J. W., Recent advances in the laboratory diagnosis of filariasis. *Malays J Pathol* **1989,** *11*,

1-5.

32. Toure, F. S.; Egwang, T. G.; Millet, P.; Bain, O.; Georges, A. J.; Wahl, G., IgG4 serology of loiasis in three villages in an endemic area of south-eastern Gabon. *Trop Med Int Health* **1998,** *3* (4), 313-7.

33. Toure, F. S.; Mavoungou, E.; Deloron, P.; Egwang, T. G., [Comparative analysis of 2 diagnostic methods of human loiasis: IgG4 serology and nested PCR]. *Bull Soc Pathol Exot* **1999,** *92* (3), 167-70.

34. Klion, A. D.; Vijaykumar, A.; Oei, T.; Martin, B.; Nutman, T. B., Serum immunoglobulin G4 antibodies to the recombinant antigen, Ll-SXP-1, are highly specific for Loa loa infection. *The Journal of infectious diseases* **2003,** *187* (1), 128-33.

35. Nutman, T. B.; Zimmerman, P. A.; Kubofcik, J.; Kostyu, D. D., A universally applicable diagnostic approach to filarial and other infections. *Parasitology today (Personal ed.)* **1994,** *10* (6), 239-43.

36. Drame, P. M.; Fink, D. L.; Kamgno, J.; Herrick, J. A.; Nutman, T. B., Loop-mediated isothermal amplification for rapid and semiquantitative detection of Loa loa infection. *J Clin Microbiol* **2014,** *52* (6), 2071-7.

37. Fernandez-Soto, P.; Mvoulouga, P. O.; Akue, J. P.; Aban, J. L.; Santiago, B. V.; Sanchez, M. C.; Muro, A., Development of a highly sensitive loop-mediated isothermal amplification (LAMP) method for the detection of Loa loa. *PLoS One* **2014,** *9* (4), e94664.

38. Bennuru, S.; Pion, S. D.; Kamgno, J.; Wanji, S.; Nutman, T. B., Repurposed automated handheld counter as a point-of-care tool to identify individuals 'at risk' of serious post-ivermectin encephalopathy. *PLoS Negl Trop Dis* **2014,** *8* (9), e3180.

39. Geary, T. G., A Step Toward Eradication of Human Filariases in Areas Where Loa Is Endemic. *MBio* **2016,** *7* (2).

40. Drame, P. M.; Meng, Z.; Bennuru, S.; Herrick, J. A.; Veenstra, T. D.; Nutman, T. B., Identification and Validation of Loa loa Microfilaria-Specific Biomarkers: a Rational Design Approach Using Proteomics and Novel Immunoassays. *MBio* **2016,** *7* (1), e02132-15.

41. Ottesen, E. A., Filarial infections. *Infectious disease clinics of North America* **1993,** *7* (3), 619-33.

42. Kilon, A. D.; Massougbodji, A.; J., Albendazole in human loiasis: Results of a double-blind, placebo-controlled trial. *Dis 202* **1993,** *168*.

43. Kilon, A. D.; Ottesen, E. A.; Nutman, T. B.; J., Effectiveness of diethylcarbamazine in treating loiasis acquired by expatriate visitors to endemic regions: long-term follow-up. *Dis 602* **1994,** *169.*

44. Nutman, T. B.; Miller, K. D.; Mulligan, M.; Reinhardt, G. N.; Currie, B. J.; Steel, C.; Ottesen, E. A., Diethylcarbamazine prophylaxis for human loiasis. Results of a double-blind study. *The New England journal of medicine* **1988,** *319* (12), 752-6.

45. Molyneux, D. H.; Bradley, M.; Hoerauf, A.; Kyelem, D.; Taylor, M. J., Mass drug treatment for lymphatic filariasis and onchocerciasis. *Trends in parasitology* **2003,** *19* (11), 516-22.

46. Tabi, T.-E.; Befidi-Mengue, R.; Nutman, T. B.; Horton, J.; Folefack, A.; Pensia, E.; Fualem, R.; Fogako, J.; Gwanmesia, P.; Quakyi, I.; Leke, R., Human loiasis in a Cameroonian village: a double-blind, placebo-controlled, crossover clinical trial of a three-day albendazole regimen. *The American journal of tropical medicine and hygiene* **2004,** *71* (2), 211-5.

47. Tsague-Dongmo, L.; Kamgno, J.; Pion, S. D. S.; Moyou-Somo, R.; Boussinesq, M., Effects of a 3-day regimen of albendazole (800 mg daily) on Loa loa microfilaraemia. *Annals of tropical medicine and parasitology* **2002,** *96* (7), 707-15.

25. *Dracunculus medinensis*
(Linnaeus 1758)

Introduction

Dracunculus medinensis (the 'Guinea worm'), sometimes referred to as "the fiery serpent", used to occur throughout Central Africa, Yemen, India, Pakistan, and, to a lesser extent, Latin America. In 1986, the World Health Assembly adopted a resolution calling for the eradication of dracunculiasis as part of its initiative to control water-born infections.[1] At that time, there were an estimated 3.5 million cases in 20 countries. However, through an extraordinary global eradication campaign spearheaded by a coalition that included the World Health Organization (WHO), Centers for Disease Control and Prevention (CDC), and the Carter Center in Atlanta, Georgia, as well as other agencies, the prevalence of Guinea worm infection has fallen dramatically. These efforts have been so successful that in 2014 the total number of reported cases had decreased from over 3 million to just 126.[2-4]

Most of the remaining cases occur in the southern region of the Sudan where civil conflict and war has limited the access of public health interventions. Even in the Sudan former President Jimmy Carter was able to negotiate a several month long cease-fire to allow eradication efforts to continue.[5, 6] As

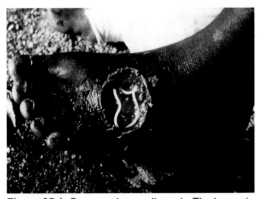

Figure 25.1. *Dracunculus medinensis*. The large circular blister, from which the worm is emerging, will heal leaving a disfiguring scar.

the result, there is some optimism that the last case of Guinea worm infection could be eradicated by the coming decade, some thirty years after the world was declared free from smallpox.

Infection with *D. medinensis* disfigures the skin and subcutaneous tissues with unsightly scars, and can result in serious secondary bacterial infections. Like other neglected diseases, Guinea worm has promoted poverty in developing countries. Humans are the primary and in most areas only reservoir for *D. medinensis*. There has been significant confusion regarding the existence of other animal reservoirs due to the presence of different dracunculids in cats, dogs, monkeys, horses, cattle, raccoons, foxes and other animals.[7] There is some evidence *D. medinensis* can, in fact, infect dogs. The presence of Guinea worm in dogs in Chad may possibly be sustaining transmission in that country.[7-9]

Historical Information

The first descriptions of *Dracunculus medinensis* infection can be found in papyrus dating back to 1500 BC.[10] *Dracunculus medinensis* worms have been found in Egyptian mummies.[11] One of the most recognizable features of *Dracunculus medinensis* is the treatment for this infection, which involves removal of the adult female worm by slowly wrapping it around a stick to extract the worm. The Guinea worm is thought by many to be the serpent depicted on the Rod of Asclepius which has come down as a symbol of the many involved in the healing arts.[12] Dracunculiasis is described in the Bible as the fiery serpents that afflicted the Israelites.[13] In 1819, Carl Rudolphi described adult female *D. medinensis* worms containing larvae. In 1838, D. Forbes, a British officer serving in India, described *D. medinensis* in water. In 1849, George Busk published on Guinea worm and suggested that humans become infected through the skin when they are

Dracunculus medinensis

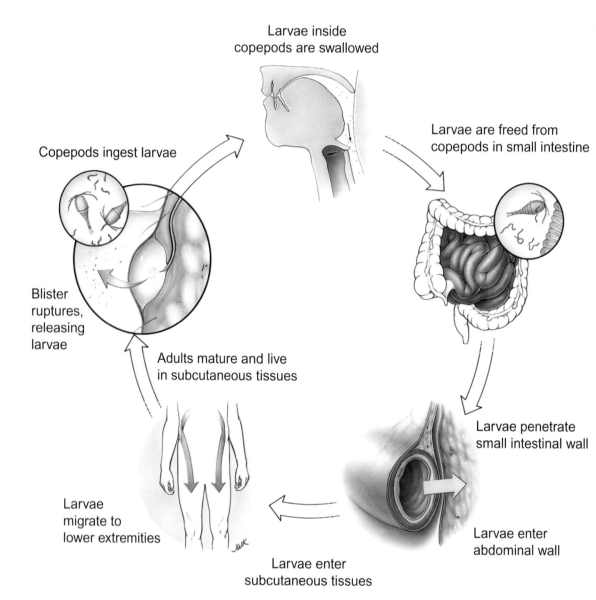

Larvae inside
copepods are swallowed

Larvae are freed from
copepods in small intestine

Copepods ingest larvae

Blister
ruptures,
releasing
larvae

Adults mature and live
in subcutaneous tissues

Larvae penetrate
small intestinal wall

Larvae enter
abdominal wall

Larvae
migrate to
lower extremities

Larvae enter
subcutaneous tissues

exposed to water containing the contagion.[14] In 1863, Henry Bastian provided the first formal description of the anatomy of *D. medinensis.*[15] In 1870, seven years later, Aleksej Fedchenko reported a partial outline of its life cycle, in which he recognized a crustacean, cyclops, as the intermediate host.[16] Cyclops, commonly called water fleas, is the most common genera of freshwater copepods. In 1913, the Indian bacteriologist Dyneshvar Turkhud pieced together all the crucial steps in the life cycle, and fulfilled the requirements of Koch's postulates for this infection when he infected human volunteers by having them ingest infected cyclops. He established that infection occurs through ingestion of water contaminated with infected copepods, and not through direct contact between the skin and contaminated water.[17]

Life Cycle

The female adult parasite is long and thin, measuring more than 100 cm by 1.5 mm. The smaller male typically measures 40 mm by 0.4 mm. Some members of the species are red in color, but the reason for this is not known.[18] Adult worms live in the subcutaneous tissues, usually in the lower extremities. Members of both sexes have acutely curved tails that serve to anchor them in the tissues. Humans, usually in drinking water, swallow copepods infected with L3 larva. The copepods are digested in the small intestine, releasing the infective immature worms. The L3 larvae penetrate the wall of the small intestine, and migrate within the connective tissues for up to a year, during which time they molt twice and mature to adults. Approximately one year after ingestion of an infected copepod, the fertilized female Guinea worm finishes her migration to the subcutaneous tissues and induces the formation of a papule that evolves into a fluid-filled vesicle or blister. This vesicle forms in such a way that it surrounds the worm's anterior vulva. The vesicles usually develop in the lower extremity, particularly the foot, but can also develop in a number of other locations.[19] A severe burning sensation develops at the location of this vesicle, prompting the afflicted individual to submerge the limb or foot into water in an attempt to find relief from the pain.[12] When the vesicle comes in contact with freshwater, it ruptures, inducing the worm to undergo prolapse of its uterus. Motile L1 larvae are released into the vulvar cavity, and then into the water.[20] Larvae are ingested by copepods of many genera, including cyclops, mesocyclops, and thermocyclops. The larvae rapidly penetrate the hemocele of the crustacean and develop within 2-3 weeks into infective L3 larvae. The life cycle is completed when a human host ingests these infected crustaceans. In other disease-endemic countries, particularly Chad, dogs may serve as an important reservoir.[8, 9]

Cellular and Molecular Pathogenesis

During a primary infection, there are no apparent host responses to the presence of the worm during its maturation process. If worms do not complete their migration and die, they may either disintegrate or become calcified. This causes disease if the calcification event happens to occur near a joint. At the conclusion of a successful migration, the worm secretes a toxin that induces local inflammation, leading to a papule that evolves into a blister and ultimately results in the formation of an ulcer. Just prior to formation of the blister, infected individuals can develop systemic symptoms including fever, nausea, vomiting and diarrhea.[21] Ulcers occur most frequently on the lower part of the body (legs and feet), but can also locate on the upper extremities and the trunk. Patients can become sensitized to secretions of the worm, with the consequent allergic reactions of urticaria and pruritus. Anaphylactic reactions have also been reported. If left untreated, ulcers often become secondarily infected, leading to tetanus, gangrene, and even death. Historically, about 1% of the cases worldwide were fatal due largely to bacterial super-infection and death from septicemia.[22]

Clinical Disease

Multiple cutaneous blisters and ulcers are characteristic manifestations of infection with *Dracunculus medinensis*. Allergic reactions usually occur in advance of the rupture of the blister, or with attempts to remove the worm. Dracunculiasis is not usually a fatal disease, but it causes substantial disability (3-10 weeks) in nearly half of the affected individuals. In Nigeria, dracunculiasis was responsible for 25% of the absenteeism in infected school children.[23] Secondary bacterial infections are common, with cellulitis spreading along the track of the worm. In some cases, ankylosing of joints, arthritis, or contractures can develop, and lead to permanent disability.[23] At one time in Nigeria, it was estimated that Guinea worm infection in adults resulted in an average of 100 days of work lost per year.[24]

Diagnosis

Definitive diagnosis is by locating the head of the adult worm in the skin lesion and/or identifying the larvae that are released into freshwater. Radiographs may reveal calcifications corresponding to the adult worms in the subcutaneous tissues. There is a reliable ELISA test for *D. medinensis*, but its availability is limited.[25]

Treatment

The time-honored therapy involves winding the worm on a thin stick until it is totally extracted (Fig. 24.1). This must be done slowly to insure that the worm does not break.

Surgical removal of the worms has been effective, but may exaggerate allergic reactions. Mebendazole treatment or use of other antihelminthic therapy of dracunculiasis is not recommended.[26] Wound care and pain management are important components of the care of patients with dracunculiasis.

Prevention and Control

Successful eradication of dracunculiasis has been possible because; 1. there is no human carrier state (beyond a 1-year incubation period), 2. there are few if any significant animal reservoirs, 3. transmission is seasonal, 4. cases are easily detected by observing individuals with protruding worms, 5. the methods for controlling transmission are relatively simple.[27, 28] Recently, however it has been noted that the dog may serve as an animal reservoir for Guinea worm in Chad, a complication that could thwart global eradication efforts.[8, 9]

The major approaches to Guinea worm prevention and eradication include; 1. filtering drinking water through finely-woven cloth in order to mechanically remove copepods, or drinking water through filter straws, 2. treating contaminated water with a larvicide known as temephos (ABATE®), 3. health education to prevent infected individuals from entering drinking water sources when Guinea worms are emerging, and 4. providing clean water from wells.[2] The successes of this approach have resulted in international acclaim, and in large measure reflect extraordinary disease control efforts by the WHO and CDC, together with advocacy efforts personally championed by former President Jimmy Carter, Dr. Donald Hopkins, Dr. Ernesto Ruiz-Tiben and the staff of the Carter Center. Guinea worm eradication may be the most impressive accomplishment ever achieved by a former U.S. President.

References

1. Despommier, D. D., People, parasites, and plowshares : learning from our body's most terrifying invaders. Columbia University Press: 2014; p xxi, 213 pages.
2. Mmwr, Centers for Disease Control and Prevention (CDC). Progress toward eradication of drancunculiasis, . Mortal Wkly Rep : 871-2. **2004**, *53* (37), 2002-2003.
3. Hopkins, D. R.; Ruiz-Tiben, E.; Eberhard, M. L.; Roy, S. L., Progress Toward Global Eradication of Dracunculiasis, January 2014-June 2015. *MMWR Morb Mortal Wkly Rep* **2015**, *64* (41), 1161-5.
4. Al-Awadi, A. R.; Al-Kuhlani, A.; Breman, J. G.; Doumbo, O.; Eberhard, M. L.; Guiguemde, R. T.; Magnussen, P.; Molyneux, D. H.; Nadim, A., Guinea worm (Dracunculiasis) eradication: update on progress and endgame challenges. *Trans R Soc Trop Med Hyg* **2014**, *108* (5), 249-51.
5. Implementation of health initiatives during a cease fire-Sudan, . MMWR. **1995**, *44*, 433-436.
6. Imported dracunculiasis-United States, and . MMWR 209. **1998**, *47*.
7. Bimi, L.; Freeman, A. R.; Eberhard, M. L.; Ruiz-Tiben, E.; Pieniazek, N. J., Differentiating Dracunculus medinensis from D. insignis, by the sequence analysis of the 18S rRNA gene. *Ann Trop Med Parasitol* **2005**, *99* (5), 511-7.
8. Callaway, E., Dogs thwart effort to eradicate Guinea worm. *Nature* **2016**, *529* (7584), 10-1.
9. Eberhard, M. L.; Ruiz-Tiben, E.; Hopkins, D. R.; Farrell, C.; Toe, F.; Weiss, A.; Withers, P. C., Jr.; Jenks, M. H.; Thiele, E. A.; Cotton, J. A.; Hance, Z.; Holroyd, N.; Cama, V. A.; Tahir, M. A.; Mounda, T., The peculiar epidemiology of dracunculiasis in Chad. *Am J Trop Med Hyg* **2014**, *90* (1), 61-70.
10. Cox, F. E., History of human parasitology. *Clin Microbiol Rev* **2002**, *15* (4), 595-612.
11. Nunn, J. F.; Tapp, E., Tropical diseases in ancient Egypt. *Trans R Soc Trop Med Hyg* **2000**, *94* (2), 147-53.
12. Awofeso, N., Towards global Guinea worm eradication in 2015: the experience of South Sudan. *Int J Infect Dis* **2013**, *17* (8), e577-82.
13. Kuchenmeister, F., Animal and vegetable parasites. *The Sydenham Society, London, United Kingdom.* **1857**.
14. Busk, G., Observations on the Structure and Nature of the Filaria medinensis, or Guinea Worm. *Trans. Microsc. Soc.* **1864**, *2*, 65-80.
15. Bastian, H. C., On the structure and the nature of Dracunculus, or Guinea worm. *Trans Linn Soc* **1863**, *24*, 101-134.
16. Fedehenko, A. P., Concerning the structure and reproduction of the guinea worm (Filaria medinensis, L). Izv Imper Obscuh Liubit Estes *Anthrop Ethnog* **1870**, *8*, 71-81.
17. Turkhud, D. A.; Major, W., Report of the Bombay Bacteriological Laboratory for the Year. *Report presented by Glen Liston Government Central Press Bombay pp* **1914**, 14-16.
18. Eberhard, M. L.; Rab, M. A.; Dilshad, M. N., Red Dracunculus medinensis. *Am J Trop Med Hyg* **1989**, *41* (4), 479-81.
19. Karam, M.; Tayeh, A., Dracunculiasis eradication. *Bull Soc Pathol Exot* **2006**, *99* (5), 377-85.
20. Ruiz-Tiben, E.; Hopkins, D. R.; Ruebush, T. K.; Kaiser, R. L., Progress toward the eradication of dracunculiasis (Guinea worm disease). *Emerg Infect Dis* **1995**, *1* (2), 58-60.
21. Greenaway, C., Dracunculiasis (guinea worm disease). *CMAJ* **2004**, *170* (4), 495-500.
22. Cairncross, S.; Muller, R.; Zagaria, N., Dracunculiasis (Guinea worm disease) and the eradication initiative. *Clin Microbiol Rev* **2002**, *15* (2), 223-46.
23. Llegbodu, V. A.; Oladele, K. O.; Wise, R. A.; J., Impact of guinea worm disease on children in Nigeria. *Am Med Hyg* **1986**, *35*, 962-964.
24. Kale, O. O., The clinico-epidemiological profile of guinea worm in the Ibadan district of Nigeria. *The American journal of tropical medicine and hygiene* **1977**, *26* (2), 208-14.
25. Klicks, M. M.; Rao, C. K.; J., Development of a rapid ELISA for early sero-diagnosis of dracunculosis. *Dis* **1984**, *16*, 287-294.
26. Chippaux, J. P., Mebendazole treatment of dracunculiasis. *Transactions of the Royal Society of Tropical Medicine and Hygiene* **1991**, *85* (2), 280.
27. Hopkins, D. R.; Ruiz-Tiben, E., Strategies for dracunculiasis eradication. *Bulletin of the World*

Health Organization **1991,** *69* (5), 533-40.

28.   Hopkins, D. R.; Foege, W. H., Guinea worm disease (letter to the editor). *Science* **1981**, 212-495.

26. Nematode Infections of Minor Medical Importance

Several nematode infections of low to moderate prevalence present with serious clinical consequences wherever they occur, and deserve mention. Table 26.1 lists their geographic distribution, major pathologic effects, modes of infection, methods of diagnosis, and therapies. A brief description of those preceded by an asterisk is given in the text below.

Mansonella ozzardi
(Manson 1897)

Mansonella ozzardi is a filarial infection found throughout South and Central America and the Caribbean islands, especially Haiti. In some highly endemic regions, up to 70% of the population may harbor circulating microfilariae.[1-5] Vectors include biting midges and black flies of the genus *Simulium*.[6] Adult worms locate to the visceral adipose tissue, the peritoneal or thoracic cavities, or even the lymphatics. Microfilariae are non-periodic and possess a characteristic sharp tail. They can be found circulating in the bloodstream. This infection may produce allergic-type symptoms, such as urticaria and lymphadenopathy, although it usually results in asymptomatic eosinophilia. The infection has been implicated as a possible cause of chronic arthritis. Diagnosis depends upon finding the microfilariae on a stained blood smear, or in a skin sample. Ivermectin is the treatment of choice for *M. ozzardi* infection and has been shown to significantly reduce the number of circulating microfilariae and reduce symptoms.[7-10] Neither diethylcarbamazine nor benzimidazoles are effective against *M. ozzardi*.[8, 11]

Mansonella perstans
(Manson 1891)

Mansonella perstans is a filarial parasite found in Africa, and in northeastern South America and parts of the Caribbean. It is transmitted from person to person by biting midges. In Africa, gorillas and chimpanzees may be significant reservoirs. High infection prevalence rates were recently reported from rural Senegal.[12] The adults live free in serous cavities such as the pleural, pericardial, or peritoneal cavities, where they produce microfilariae that circulate in blood. *M. perstans* infection is usually asymptomatic, but it is known to cause painless nodules in the conjunctiva with swelling of the eyelids in Africa, where it is known as the Ugandan eye worm or Kampala eye worm.[13] The organism may also result in symptoms that are similar to *Loa loa* infection, such as angioedema and Calabar swellings. Microfilariae of *M. perstans* may be observed in peripheral blood, and can be demonstrated by examination of a stained blood smear or by the Knott test. Most standard antihelminthic therapies have been ineffective for *M. perstans*.[14-16] The discovery that this filarial parasite harbors wolbachia endosymbionts suggested that doxycycline might be an effective treatment option.[17-19] Subsequent use of doxycycline has proven to be a highly effective therapy.[20] Co-infections with *M. perstans* do not appear to significantly alter post-treatment reaction profiles to single-dose ivermectin/albendazole for patients with lymphatic filariasis.[21]

Mansonella streptocerca
(Macfie and Corson 1922)

Mansonella streptocerca is a filarial parasite with a distribution restricted to tropical rainforests in Central Africa. Adult worms locate to the subcutaneous tissues, as do microfilariae.[22, 23] Biting midges are its vectors. The major clinical manifestation of this infection is a pruritic dermatitis with hypopigmented macules that may resemble onchocerciasis. There is often an associated axillary or inguinal lymphadenopathy. Diagnosis is made by microscopically identifying microfilariae in specimens of skin or impression smears made from them. A nested polymerase chain reaction test has been developed that can aid in detection of the microfilariae in skin biopsy specimens.[24] Microfilariae must be differentiated from those of *Onchocerca volvulus*, usually by attempting to identify the characteristic hook-shaped tail, which is sometimes referred to as a "shepherd's crook."[25] Diethylcarbamazine is the drug of choice, but it may exacerbate pruritus; in which case, anti-inflammatory agents and antihistamines may be necessary. Although ivermectin may also be effective, especially against microfilariae, but not against adult worms, there are some concerns about side-effects.[26, 27]

Dirofilaria immitis
(Leidy 1856)

and other *Dirofilaria* spp.

Dirofilaria immitis, the dog heartworm, is an accidental parasite of humans, usually infecting the lungs where it produces solitary nodules. The pulmonary lesion probably results from a dead worm being washed into the pulmonary artery from the right ventricle, followed by embolization to the lung.[28] These nodules are frequently diagnosed on chest radiographs as a "coin lesion" that mimics lung carcinoma. The diagnosis of pulmonary dirofilariasis is usually made after finding a calcified worm in a granuloma in the resected lesion. This parasite is transmitted by the bite of an infected mosquito, and is not transmitted directly from person to person or dog to person.[29] There is concern that climate change is driving an increase in the incidence of *Dirofilaria* spp. in animals as well as humans.[29] A number of cases have been

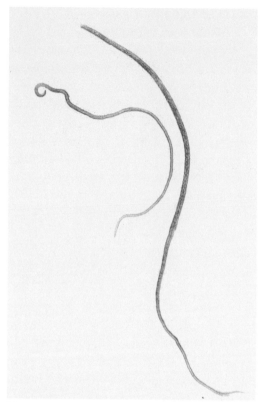

Figure 26.1 Adults of *Capillaria philippinensis*. The female is 3 mm x 45 μm, and the male is 2.5 mm x 30 μm.

identified in the United States, particularly in Texas, Florida, and Louisiana, but this pathogen has now spread as far north as Alaska.[28, 30] The seroprevalence in humans or other animals can be estimated by immunodiagnostic tests using either excretory-secretory products or somatic antigen from the adult worm.[31] *Dirofilaria tenuis*, a parasite of raccoons and related *Dirofilaria* spp., cause zoonotic subcutaneous infections in humans that result in discrete nodules.[32] The diagnosis is typically established when the parasite is noted in a histopathologic section of tissue. Some patients have eosinophilia.

Capillaria hepatica
(Bancroft 1893)

Capillaria hepatica is a parasite of rodents, particularly the rat, that can on rare occasion infect humans.[33] Human cases have

Table 26.1. Nematode infections of minor importance

Parasite	Geographic distribution	Major pathologic consequences	Mode of infection	Diagnosis
Capillaria hepatica	Worldwide	Necrotic lesions in liver	Oral route	Biopsy
*Capillaria philippinensis	Philippines	Malabsorption syndrome, diarrhea	Oral route	Stool examination for larvae and eggs
Dioctophyma renale	North and South America, China	Complete destruction of kidneys	Oral route	Urine examination for eggs
*Mansonella perstans	Central and South America, Africa	None	Bite of infected midge	Blood smear or Knott test for microfilariae
*Mansonella streptocerca	Africa	Pruritic dermatitis	Bite of infected midge	Impression smear of skin snip for microfilariae
*Mansonella ozzardi	Central and South America, Caribbean	Chronic arthritis	Bite of infected midge	Blood smear or Knott test for microfilariae
Oesophagostomum bifurcum	West Africa	Intestinal nodules	Oral route	Stool examination for eggs
Syngamus laryngeus	South America, Caribbean, Philippines	Asthma, hemoptysis	Unknown	Sputum or stool examination for eggs
Ternidens diminutus	Africa	Iron-deficiency anemia	Unknown	Stool examination for eggs
Trichostrongylus spp.	Worldwide	Anemia	Oral route	Stool examination for eggs

*Discussed in the text.

been reported in Asia, South America, North America, Eastern and Western Europe.[33, 34] Adult worms live and lay eggs in the liver parenchyma within a syncytium. These eggs are not released into the environment until the infected animal dies or is eaten by a predator. Once released into the environment, eggs embryonate and become infective for another host. Infective eggs are ingested, and hatch in the small intestine. Eventually, larvae mature to adults and reach the liver. After mating, they begin to lay eggs, completing the life cycle. The liver serves as the source of nourishment for adults. If enough parasites are present, the host may suffer liver failure and die. Rarely this pathogen can be transmitted to humans if they accidentally ingest embryonated eggs in contaminated water or undercooked infected animals. Diagnosis had required liver biopsy and the visualization of adults or eggs in the samples, but now serological testing is available.[35] Often the disease is unsuspected and discovered only at autopsy or incidentally

through liver biopsy. Alternatively, it can present with abdominal lymphadenopathy and eosinophilia.[36] Occasionally, patients may be asymptomatic and pass *C. hepatica* eggs in their stools, but this is felt to be passage through the intestinal tract of ingested eggs, as true infection does not result in egg release into the feces. (Fig. C.55) Numerous treatment regimens, including disophenol (2-6-diiodo-4-nitrophenol), albendazole and prednisone have been used successfully in management of this infection.[37-39]

Capillaria philippinensis
(Chitwood, Valesquez, and Salazar 1968)

The genus *Capillaria* has four members capable of infecting humans; *C. philippinensis, C. hepatica, C. plica,* and *C. aerophila.*[40] Only *C. philippinensis* is a significant regional public health problem. Infection with *C. philippinensis* occurs mainly in parts of Thailand

and the Philippines, where infection can lead to death.[41] A number of deaths were associated with an outbreak of chronic gastroenteritis in central Luzon. Cases have also been reported in Japan, Taiwan, and Korea and the infection has emerged recently in Egypt.[42]

Adult worms resemble those of *Trichinella spiralis* in both size (Fig. 26.1) and general biology. Like trichinella and trichuris, the adults have an attenuated anterior end with an esophagus surrounded by a row of secretory cells called stichocytes.[40] The worms locate to the intracellular compartment of the columnar epithelium of the small intestine, and deposit living larvae there, which are infectious within the same host. In this respect, its biology mimics the auto-infectious cycle of *Strongyloides stercoralis*. In contrast, there is no evidence that patients harboring *C. philippinensis* are immunosuppressed. As infection progresses, the patient first begins passing embryonated, then unembryonated eggs in the stools.

Capillaria philippinensis is most likely a parasite of waterfowl that feed on fish and crustaceans, which are the intermediate hosts for this nematode. Humans become infected by eating raw or undercooked infected fish or shrimp. In the Philippines, ingestion of "jumping salad," which consists of vegetables and a variety of live aquatic animals including shrimp, is thought to be a common source of this infection. *C. philippinensis* infection has also emerged in Egypt. The clinical disease consists of a rampant diarrhea associated with malaise, anorexia, and vomiting. Patients frequently develop a protein-losing enteropathy and malabsorption of fats and carbohydrates, which, in turn, leads to a wasting syndrome. Patients who are ill for more than several months without treatment develop profound electrolyte imbalance.[40] Death results from cachexia, heart failure, and secondary bacterial infections. The mortality rate approaches 10% in some endemic areas. Numerous *C. philippinensis* worms

can be identified at all stages in the lumen, and in the intestinal mucosa at autopsy. As many as 200,000 worms have been recovered in 1 liter of bowel fluid, a consequence of auto-infection.[40]

Diagnosis depends upon finding eggs or larvae in feces, or detecting the parasite on biopsy of the small intestine.[43] They are usually present in patients presenting with abdominal pain, diarrhea, and weight loss.[40] Eggs bear some resemblance to those of *Trichuris trichiura* (Fig. C.58).

Mebendazole or albendazole are effective treatments for *Capillaria philippinensis*.[40] Albendazole is preferable, as the drug appears to act on larvae as well as adult worms, and relapses have not yet been reported.[41, 42] Because of the risk of auto-infection, all infected patients should be treated.

During the epidemic in central Luzon, the lagoons were contaminated with bed sheets soiled with feces from infected patients.[40] This situation helped to propagate the life cycle in fish and other intermediate hosts. Avoidance of raw or undercooked fish and crustaceans is recommended to prevent infection. Cultural eating habits are, however, extremely difficult to change.

Oesophagostomum bifurcum
(Creplin 1849)

Oesophagostomum bifurcum is a nematode mostly infecting non-human primates in Africa and Asia. In northern Togo and northeastern Ghana, *O. bifurcum* infects up to 30% of these human populations, with an estimated 250,000 cases.[44-47] Sporadic cases have also been described in other parts of Africa, Asia and South America.[46] In these regions, adults 30-40 years of age have the highest prevalence. These nematodes are often called nodular worms because they cause nodule formation on the wall of the intestine. Adult worms produce about 5,000 eggs per day, which pass with feces and mature to infective L3 larvae in soil.[48] Eggs morphologically resemble those of hookworms. Humans are infected when they ingest infective larvae, which then penetrate the small intestinal wall and develop to adults. Some patients develop multi-nodular disease, while, in others, a single nodular mass develops.[45] The nodules in male patients are larger than the ones in females.[45] The nodular disease of oesophagostomum infection often presents as an abdominal mass, which can be painful, and mimics a surgical abdomen. Often the mass is asymptomatic. As a result, the infection is frequently diagnosed at biopsy, although ultrasound is also of great value.[49] Fecal examination is the diagnostic method of choice in individual patients, while PCR has been developed and is used in prevalence studies.[50] Pyrantel pamoate is the recommended drug for treating infections due to *O. bifurcum*, and

albendazole is also effective.[51] Surgical resection of the nodules is sometimes necessary.

Ternidens diminutus

Ternidens diminutus is a nematode infection of humans that resembles *O. bifurcum*. Ternidens eggs resemble hookworm eggs, so that *T. diminutus* is sometimes referred to as "the false hookworm."[52] It is primarily a parasite of non-human primates, but has been demonstrated to cause human infections in Zambia, Zimbabwe, Tanzania and Asia.[53, 54] *T. diminutus* can result in colonic ulcerations and nodular lesions, but there are usually few symptoms. Both pyrantel pamoate and thiabendazole have been used to treat patients, and other benzimidazoles may also be effective.[52, 55, 56]

References

1. Marinkelelle, C. J.; German, E., Mansonelliasis in the Comiasria del Vaupes of Colombia. *Trop Geogr Med 101* **1970**, *22*

2. Raccurt, C. P.; Brasseur, P.; Ciceron, M.; Boncy, J., Epidemiologic survey of Mansonella ozzardi in Corail, Haiti. *Am J Trop Med Hyg* **2014**, *90* (6), 1167-9.

3. Veggiani Aybar, C. A.; Dantur Juri, M. J.; Zaidenberg, M. O., Mansonella ozzardi in Neotropical region of Argentina: Prevalence through time (1986-2010). *Acta Trop* **2016**, *153*, 1-6.

4. Medeiros, J. F.; Py-Daniel, V.; Barbosa, U. C.; Izzo, T. J., Mansonella ozzardi in Brazil: prevalence of infection in riverine communities in the Purus region, in the state of Amazonas. *Mem Inst Oswaldo Cruz* **2009**, *104* (1), 74-80.

5. Raccurt, C. P.; Brasseur, P.; Boncy, J., Mansonelliasis, a neglected parasitic disease in Haiti. *Mem Inst Oswaldo Cruz* **2014**, *109* (6), 709-11.

6. Nathan, M. B.; Tikasingh, E. S.; Munroe, P., Filariasis in Amerindians of western Guyana with observations on transmission of Mansonella ozzardi by a Simulium species of the amazonicum group. *Tropenmedizin und Parasitologie* **1982**, *33* (4), 219-22.

7. Krolewiecki, A. J.; Cajal, S. P.; Villalpando, C.; Gil, J. F., Ivermectin-related adverse clinical events in patients treated for Mansonella ozzardi infections. *Rev Argent Microbiol* **2011**, *43* (1), 48-50.

8. Basano Sde, A.; Fontes, G.; Medeiros, J. F.; Aranha Camargo, J. S.; Souza Vera, L. J.; Parente Araujo, M. P.; Pires Parente, M. S.; Mattos Ferreira Rde, G.; Barreto Crispim, P.; Aranha Camargo, L. M., Sustained clearance of Mansonella ozzardi infection after treatment with ivermectin in the Brazilian Amazon. *Am J Trop Med Hyg* **2014**, *90* (6), 1170-5.

9. Nutman, T. B.; Nash, T. E.; Ottesen, E. A., Ivermectin in the successful treatment of a patient with Mansonella ozzardi infection. *J Infect Dis* **1987**, *156* (4), 662-5.

10. Nutman, T. B.; Nash, T. E.; Ottesen, E. A.; J., Ivermectin in the successful treatment of a patient with Mansonella ozzardi infection. *Dis 662* **1997**, *156*.

11. Bartholomew, C. F.; Nathan, M. B.; Tikasingh, E. S., The failure of diethylcarbamazine in the

treatment of Mansonella ozzardi infections. *Trans R Soc Trop Med Hyg* **1978,** *72* (4), 423-4.

12. Bassene, H.; Sambou, M.; Fenollar, F.; Clarke, S.; Djiba, S.; Mourembou, G.; L, Y. A.; Raoult, D.; Mediannikov, O., High Prevalence of Mansonella perstans Filariasis in Rural Senegal. *Am J Trop Med Hyg* **2015,** *93* (3), 601-6.

13. Baird, J. K.; Neafie, R. C.; Connor, D. H., Nodules in the conjunctiva, bung-eye, and bulge-eye in Africa caused by Mansonella perstans. *The American journal of tropical medicine and hygiene* **1988,** *38* (3), 553-7.

14. Wahlgren, M.; Frolov, I., Treatment of Dipetalonema perstans infections with mebendazole. *Transactions of the Royal Society of Tropical Medicine and Hygiene* **1983,** *77* (3), 422-3.

15. Gardon, J.; Kamgno, J.; Gardon-Wendel, N.; Demanga, N.; Duke, B. O. L.; Boussinesq, M., Efficacy of repeated doses of ivermectin against Mansonella perstans. *Transactions of the Royal Society of Tropical Medicine and Hygiene* **2002,** *96* (3), 325-6.

16. Van den Enden, E.; Van Gompel, A.; Vervoort, T.; Van der Stuyft, P.; Van den Ende, J., Mansonella perstans filariasis: failure of albendazole treatment. *Annales de la Societe belge de medecine tropicale* **1992,** *72* (3), 215-8.

17. Gehringer, C.; Kreidenweiss, A.; Flamen, A.; Antony, J. S.; Grobusch, M. P.; Belard, S., Molecular evidence of Wolbachia endosymbiosis in Mansonella perstans in Gabon, Central Africa. *J Infect Dis* **2014,** *210* (10), 1633-8.

18. Keiser, P. B.; Coulibaly, Y.; Kubofcik, J.; Diallo, A. A.; Klion, A. D.; Traore, S. F.; Nutman, T. B., Molecular identification of Wolbachia from the filarial nematode Mansonella perstans. *Mol Biochem Parasitol* **2008,** *160* (2), 123-8.

19. Grobusch, M. P.; Kombila, M.; Autenrieth, I.; Mehlhorn, H.; Kremsner, P. G., No evidence of Wolbachia endosymbiosis with Loa loa and Mansonella perstans. *Parasitol Res* **2003,** *90* (5), 405-8.

20. Coulibaly, Y. I.; Dembele, B.; Diallo, A. A.; Lipner, E. M.; Doumbia, S. S.; Coulibaly, S. Y.; Konate, S.; Diallo, D. A.; Yalcouye, D.; Kubofcik, J.; Doumbo, O. K.; Traore, A. K.; Keita, A. D.; Fay, M. P.; Traore, S. F.; Nutman, T. B.; Klion, A. D., A randomized trial of doxycycline for Mansonella perstans infection. *N Engl J Med* **2009,** *361* (15), 1448-58.

21. Keiser, P. B.; Coulibaly, Y. I.; Keita, F.; Traore, D.; Diallo, A.; Diallo, D. A.; Semnani, R. T.; Doumbo, O. K.; Traore, S. F.; Klion, A. D.; Nutman, T. B., Clinical characteristics of post-treatment reactions to ivermectin/albendazole for Wuchereria bancrofti in a region co-endemic for Mansonella perstans. *The American journal of tropical medicine and hygiene* **2003,** *69* (3), 331-5.

22. Okelo, G. B.; Kyobe, J.; Gatiri, G., Mansonella streptocerca in the Central African Republic. *Trans R Soc Trop Med Hyg* **1988,** *82* (3), 464.

23. Fischer, P.; Bamuhiiga, J.; Buttner, D. W., Occurrence and diagnosis of Mansonella streptocerca in Uganda. *Acta Trop* **1997,** *63* (1), 43-55.

24. Fischer, P.; Buttner, D. W.; Bamuhiiga, J.; Williams, S. A., Detection of the filarial parasite Mansonella streptocerca in skin biopsies by a nested polymerase chain reaction-based assay. *Am J Trop Med Hyg* **1998,** *58* (6), 816-20.

25. Orihel, T. C.; J., The tail of the Mansonella streptocerca microfilaria. *Am Med Hyg 1278* **1978,** *33*.

26. Fischer, P.; Tukesiga, E.; Büttner, D. W., Long-term suppression of Mansonella streptocerca microfilariae after treatment with ivermectin. *The Journal of infectious diseases* **1999,** *180* (4), 1403-5.

27. Fischer, P.; Bamuhiiga, J.; Buttner, D. W., Treatment of human Mansonella streptocerca infection with ivermectin. *Trop Med Int Health* **1997,** *2* (2), 191-9.

28. Asimacopoulos, P. J.; Katras, A.; Christie, B., Pulmonary dirofilariasis. The largest single-hospital experience. *Chest* **1992,** *102* (3), 851-5.

29. Simon, F.; Morchon, R.; Gonzalez-Miguel, J.; Marcos-Atxutegi, C.; Siles-Lucas, M., What is new about animal and human dirofilariosis? *Trends Parasitol* **2009,** *25* (9), 404-9.

30. Diaz, J. H.; Risher, W. H., Risk factors for human heartworm infections (dirofilariasis) in the South. *J La State Med Soc* **2015,** *167* (2), 79-86.

31. Akao, N.; Kondo, K.; Fujita, K., Immunoblot analysis of Dirofilaria immitis recognized by infected humans. *Annals of tropical medicine and parasitology* **1991,** *85* (4), 455-60.

32. Orihel, T. C.; Helentjaris, D.; Alger, J., Subcutaneous dirofilariasis: single inoculum, multiple worms. *The American journal of tropical medicine and hygiene* **1997**, *56* (4), 452-5.

33. Li, C. D.; Yang, H. L.; Wang, Y., Capillaria hepatica in China. *World J Gastroenterol* **2010**, *16* (6), 698-702.

34. Wang, Z.; Lin, X.; Wang, Y.; Cui, J., The emerging but neglected hepatic capillariasis in China. *Asian Pac J Trop Biomed* **2013**, *3* (2), 146-7.

35. Juncker-Voss, M.; Prosl, H.; Lussy, H.; Enzenberg, U.; Auer, H.; Nowotny, N., Serological detection of Capillaria hepatica by indirect immunofluorescence assay. *J Clin Microbiol* **2000**, *38* (1), 431-3.

36. Sharma, R.; Dey, A. K.; Mittal, K.; Kumar, P.; Hira, P., Capillaria hepatica infection: a rare differential for peripheral eosinophilia and an imaging dilemma for abdominal lymphadenopathy. *Ann Parasitol* **2015**, *61* (1), 61-4.

37. McQuown, A. L.; J., Capillaria hepatica: reported genuine and spurious cases. *Am Med Hyg* **1950**, *30*, 761-767.

38. Nabi, F.; Palaha, H. K.; Sekhsaria, D.; Chiatale, A., Capillaria hepatica infestation. *Indian Pediatr* **2007**, *44* (10), 781-2.

39. Pereira, V. G.; Mattosinho Franca, L. C., Successful treatment of Capillaria hepatica infection in an acutely ill adult. *Am J Trop Med Hyg* **1983**, *32* (6), 1272-4.

40. Cross, J. H., Intestinal capillariasis. *Clinical microbiology reviews* **1992**, *5* (2), 120-9.

41. el-Karaksy, H.; el-Shabrawi, M.; Mohsen, N.; Kotb, M.; el-Koofy, N.; el-Deeb, N., Capillaria philippinensis: a cause of fatal diarrhea in one of two infected Egyptian sisters. *Journal of tropical pediatrics* **2004**, *50* (1), 57-60.

42. Bair, M.-J.; Hwang, K.-P.; Wang, T.-E.; Liou, T.-C.; Lin, S.-C.; Kao, C.-R.; Wang, T.-Y.; Pang, K.-K., Clinical features of human intestinal capillariasis in Taiwan. *World journal of gastroenterology : WJG* **2004**, *10* (16), 2391-3.

43. Limsrivilai, J.; Pongprasobchai, S.; Apisarnthanarak, P.; Manatsathit, S., Intestinal capillariasis in the 21st century: clinical presentations and role of endoscopy and imaging. *BMC Gastroenterol* **2014**, *14*, 207.

44. Polderman, A. M.; Krepel, H. P.; Baeta, S.; Blotkamp, J.; Gigase, P., Oesophagostomiasis, a common infection of man in northern Togo and Ghana. *The American journal of tropical medicine and hygiene* **1991**, *44* (3), 336-44.

45. Storey, P. A.; Steenhard, N. R.; Van Lieshout, L.; Anemana, S.; Magnussen, P.; Polderman, A. M., Natural progression of Oesophagostomum bifurcum pathology and infection in a rural community of northern Ghana. *Transactions of the Royal Society of Tropical Medicine and Hygiene* **2001**, *95* (3), 295-9.

46. Bogers, J. J.; Storey, P. A.; Faile, G.; Hewitt, E.; Yelifari, L.; Polderman, A.; Van Marck, E. A., Human oesophagostomiasis: a histomorphometric study of 13 new cases in northern Ghana. *Virchows Archiv : an international journal of pathology* **2001**, *439* (1), 21-6.

47. Ziem, J. B.; Olsen, A.; Magnussen, P.; Horton, J.; Agongo, E.; Geskus, R. B.; Polderman, A. M., Distribution and clustering of Oesophagostomum bifurcum and hookworm infections in northern Ghana. *Parasitology* **2006**, *132* (Pt 4), 525-34.

48. Kepel, H. P.; Polderman, A. M.; J., Egg production of Oesophagostomum bifurcum, a locally common parasite of humans in Togo. *Am Med Hyg* **1992**, *46*, 469-472.

49. Storey, P. A.; Spannbrucker, N.; Agongo, E. A.; van Lieshout, L.; Zeim, J. P.; Magnussen, P.; Polderman, A. M.; Doehring, E., Intraobserver and interobserver variation of ultrasound diagnosis of Oesophagostomum bifurcum colon lesions. *The American journal of tropical medicine and hygiene* **2002**, *67* (6), 680-3.

50. Verweij, J. J.; Pit, D. S.; van Lieshout, L.; Baeta, S. M.; Dery, G. D.; Gasser, R. B.; Polderman, A. M., Determining the prevalence of Oesophagostomum bifurcum and Necator americanus infections using specific PCR amplification of DNA from faecal samples. *Trop Med Int Health* **2001**, *6* (9), 726-31.

51. Ziem, J. B.; Kettenis, I. M. J.; Bayita, A.; Brienen, E. A. T.; Dittoh, S.; Horton, J.; Olsen, A.; Magnussen, P.; Polderman, A. M., The short-term impact of albendazole treatment on

Oesophagostomum bifurcum and hookworm infections in northern Ghana. *Annals of tropical medicine and parasitology* **2004,** *98* (4), 385-90.

52.   Bradley, M., Rate of expulsion of Necator americanus and the false hookworm Ternidens deminutus Railliet and Henry 1909 (Nematoda) from humans following albendazole treatment. *Transactions of the Royal Society of Tropical Medicine and Hygiene* **1990,** *84* (5), 720.

53.   Kilala, C. P., Ternidens deminutus infecting man in Southern Tanzania. *East Afr Med J* **1971,** *48* (11), 636-45.

54.   Hemsrichart, V., Ternidens deminutus infection: first pathological report of a human case in Asia. *J Med Assoc Thai* **2005,** *88* (8), 1140-3.

55.   Goldsmid, J. M.; Saunders, C. R., Preliminary trial using pyrantal pamoate for the treatment of human infections with Teernidens deminutus. *Transactions of the Royal Society of Tropical Medicine and Hygiene* **1972,** *66* (2), 375-6.

56.   Goldsmid, J. M., Thiabendazole in the treatment of human infections with Ternidens deminutus (Nematoda). *S Afr Med J* **1972,** *46* (30), 1046-7.

27. Aberrant Nematode Infections

Many nematodes are zoonotic and only occasionally infect humans. These "aberrant" nematodes are incapable of maturing to adult parasites in the human body. Cutaneous larva migrans (CLM) and visceral larva migrans (VLM) are two diseases caused by this type of parasite. The nematodes causing CLM and VLM and the clinical manifestations of these diseases are listed in Tables 27.1 and 27.2. Although the number of nematode species resulting in aberrant infections is large, this chapter emphasizes only the most important ones, as defined by the seriousness of the diseases they induce.

Cutaneous Larva Migrans (CLM)

CLM (Table 27.1) has a worldwide distribution. It is caused by larvae of the dog and cat hookworms *Ancylostoma braziliense*, and *Uncinaria stenocephala* completing their life cycle in animal hosts, similar to the way human hookworms behave. Zoonotic transmission from the dog hookworm *Ancylostoma caninum* also occurs in humans, but disease from this parasite usually causes eosinophilic enteritis rather than CLM (see The Hookworms). Other less common nematodes may also be responsible for CLM, including a raccoon-transmitted *Strongyloides procyonis* that results in "duck hunter's itch." The L3 larvae (Fig. 27.1) of *A. braziliense* survive in sandy, moist soils for several days. These larvae are especially common on beaches in Southeast Asia, the Caribbean, and Puerto Rico, where dogs and cats are permitted to wander the beaches and freely defecate. In the U.S., CLM occurs occasionally along the Gulf and Atlantic coasts of Florida and the beaches of the Carolinas. In the human host, infection begins when the L3 larvae penetrate unbroken skin, but fail to receive the proper environmental cues. Rather than going further in their life cycle,

instead they migrate laterally in the deeper layers of the epidermis (Fig. 27.2), and can survive there for about 10 days.[1, 2]

An intense inflammatory reaction, associated with itching in the affected areas, develops within days after the larvae enter the dermis. The secretions of the larvae, which consist of hydrolytic enzymes, provoke this inflammatory reaction. The serpiginous lesions known as "creeping eruption" are evident after an incubation period of one week. Secondary bacterial infections caused by scratching are common. In one review of CLM patients seen at a travelers' clinic, 39 percent of the lesions appeared on the feet, 18 percent on the buttocks, 16 percent on the abdomen, and the remainder were on the lower legs, arms, and face.[3] In another review of patients with CLM seen at a travelers' clinic in Munich, 73% of the lesions were found on the lower extremities, with the buttocks and anogenital region (13%) and trunk and upper extremities (7% each) affected less frequently.[4] Some patients with CLM manifest eosinophilia or elevated IgE, but laboratory findings generally play little or no role in establishing a diagnosis of CLM.[4] The treatment of choice for CLM is oral antihelminthic therapy. A single dose of ivermectin (200 μg/kg once, sometimes repeated) is considered more effective than a single dose of albendazole, but repeated treatments of albendazole (400 mg daily for 5–7 days) are comparable. Some investigators recom-

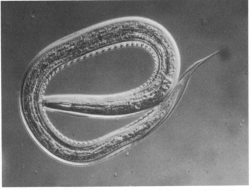

Figure 27.1. Third stage larva of *Ancylostoma braziliense*. Photo E. Gravé

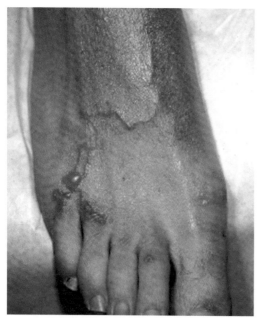

Figure 27.2. "Creeping eruption" on the foot of a patient who stepped on an infective larva of *A. braziense*. Courtesy G. Zalar.

mend a 3-day course of albendazole (400 mg daily). Topical thiabendazole in a concentration of 10% to 15% 3 times daily for 5–7 days is an alternative treatment.[5] Cryotherapy with liquid nitrogen can cause blistering and ulceration of the skin and for this reason many experts recommend that this should not be performed[6].

Visceral Larva Migrans (VLM)

Toxocara canis
(Johnston 1916)

Toxocara cati
(Brumpt 1927)

Besides *Enterobius vermicularis* (pinworm), toxocariasis may be the most common helminth infection in the United States. Seroprevalence in many areas of the United States and Mexico often exceed 20 percent, especially among some African American populations living in poverty.[7, 8] The true burden of disease resulting from this large number

of infections is poorly characterized[7]. Visceral larva migrans (VLM) and ocular larva migrans (OLM) are typically caused by *Toxocara canis* and *T. cati*. Aberrant migration of larvae through the viscera (Table 27.2) results in a far more serious condition than cutaneous larva migrans. Human infection with *Toxocara* spp. was first described by Helenor Wilder in 1950, who discovered a larva within a retinal granuloma of a child.[9] In 1952, Paul Beaver and colleagues reported on a series of children who had a high circulating eosinophilia, and suffered severe multisystem disease cause by *T. canis* and *T. cati* larvae.[10] Both *T. canis* and *T. cati* have a life cycle in their respective hosts resembling that of ascaris in humans. Toxocara adults (Fig. 27.3) are smaller than those of ascaris, but are similar to them regarding nutritional requirements and physiologic behavior.[11] Since the discovery of VLM and OLM, some investigators have found that a significant percentage of children may suffer a so-called "covert" form of the disease in which patients do not have the full-blown syndrome of VLM, but more subtle manifestations including pulmonary dysfunction, or cognitive deficits leading to developmental delays.[12-14]

In humans, infection begins with ingestion of embryonated toxocara eggs (Fig. 27.4). This commonly occurs where children are playing on sandboxes and in playgrounds contaminated with toxocara eggs. This situation is especially common in poor neighborhoods where stray dogs and cats are widespread. Pathology results when larvae hatch in the small intestine, penetrate into the mesenteric blood vessels and migrate throughout the body, invading all organs. There is controversy as to whether these are L2 or L3 larvae. The degree of host damage varies with the tissues invaded; the liver, lungs, and central nervous system (CNS - Fig. 27.5), including the eyes, are the organ systems most seriously affected. Ultimately, after

Table 27.1. Cutaneous larva migrans: clinical manifestations

Organism	Predominant location in body	Major pathologic consequences	Diagnosis
Ancylostoma braziliense	Skin	Urticaria, serpiginous lesion	Biopsy
Uncinaria stenocephala	Skin	Urticaria, serpiginous lesion	Biopsy
Strongyloides procyonis	"Duck-hunter's itch"	Urticaria	Biopsy
Dirofilaria conjunctivae	Palpebral conjunctivae,	Abscess formation subcutaneous tissues	Biopsy
Dirofilaria repens	Subcutaneous tissues	Fibrotic, painless nodule formation	Biopsy
Anatrichosoma cutaneum	Subcutaneous tissues	Serpiginous lesions	Biopsy
Rhabditis niellyi	Skin	Papule, urticaria	Biopsy
Lagochilascaris minor	Subcutaneous tissues around head and neck	Abscess formation	
Gnathostoma spingerum	Subcutaneous tissues	Abscess formation	Biopsy, ELISA
Thelazia callipaeda	Conjunctival sac, corneal conjunctiva	Paralysis of lower eyelid muscles, ectropion, fibrotic scarring	Ophthalmoscopic examination of conjunctiva

ELISA: enzyme-linked immunosorbent assay.

Table 27.2. Visceral larva migrans: clinical manifestations

Organism	Predominant location in body	Major pathologic consequences	Diagnosis
Toxocara cati	Viscera, eye	Blindness	ELISA or RIA
Toxocara canis	Viscera, eye	Blindness	ELISA or RIA
Baylisascaris procyonis	Meninges	Meningoencephalitis	CSF examination
Angiostrongylus cantonensis	Meninges	Meningoencephalitis	CSF examination
Angiostrongylus costaricensis	Mesenteric arterioles	Peritonitis	Biopsy
Anisakis spp.	Stomach wall	Granuloma	Biopsy
Phocanema spp.	Stomach wall	Granuloma	Biopsy
Terranova spp.	Stomach wall	Granuloma	Biopsy
Oesophagostonum stephanostomum var. *thomasi*	Small and large intestinal wall	Granuloma	Biopsy
Gnathostoma spingerum	Striated muscles, subcutaneous tissues, brain, small intestinal wall	Abscess, meningoencephalitis	Biopsy, ELISA
Dirofilaria immitis	Lung, heart	Granuloma in lung	Biopsy

ELISA: enzyme-linked immunosorbent assay; RIA: radioimmunoassay; CSF: cerebrospinal fluid

weeks to months of migration, the larvae die, followed by marked delayed-type and immediate-type hypersensitivity responses. These inflammatory responses manifest as eosinophilic granulomas. The immediate hypersensitivity responses to dead and dying larvae in the viscera, including the lungs, liver, and brain, result in VLM. In the eye, the larvae causing OLM can affect the retina, where the larval tracks and granulomas are sometimes mistaken for retinoblastoma (Fig. 27.6.). As a result of this similarity, unnecessary enucle-

ation has been carried out in some cases. In many cases, the granuloma itself was responsible for the loss of sight.[15, 16]

Epidemiologic evidence suggests that ocular disease tends to occur in the absence of systemic involvement and vice versa, which has led to the proposal that the two manifestations of this infection be reclassified as ocular larva migrans and visceral larva migrans.[17] There may be strains of *T. canis* with specific tropisms. Alternatively, VLM may reflect the consequences of a host

Toxocara canis and Toxocara cati

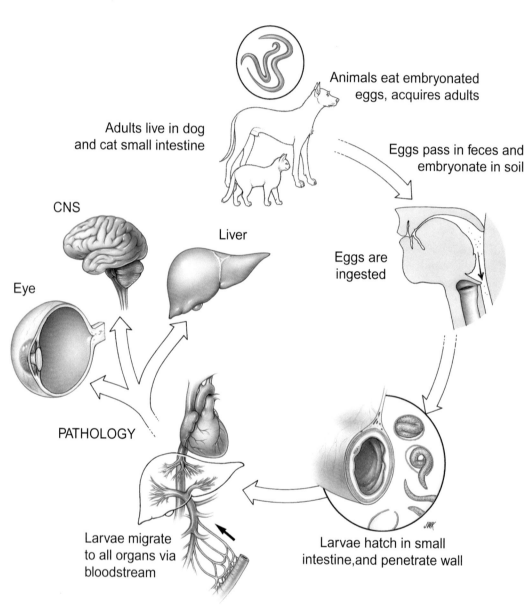

Animals eat embryonated eggs, acquires adults

Adults live in dog and cat small intestine

Eggs pass in feces and embryonate in soil

CNS

Liver

Eggs are ingested

Eye

PATHOLOGY

Larvae migrate to all organs via bloodstream

Larvae hatch in small intestine, and penetrate wall

Parasitic Diseases 6th Ed. Parasites Without Borders wwww.parasiteswithoutborders.com

inflammatory response to repeated waves of migrating larvae through the viscera, whereas ocular larva migrans occurs in individuals who have not been previously sensitized.[11]

VLM and Covert Toxocariasis

Visceral larva migrans (VLM) is mainly a disease of young children (<5 years of age).[18, 19] It presents with fever, enlargement of the liver and spleen, lower respiratory symptoms (particular bronchospasm, resembling asthma), eosinophilia sometimes approaching 70%, and hypergammaglobulinemia of immunoglobulin M (IgM) and IgG classes. Myocarditis, nephritis, and involvement of the CNS have been described. CNS involvement can lead to seizures, neuropsychiatric symptoms, or an encephalopathy. *T. canis* can

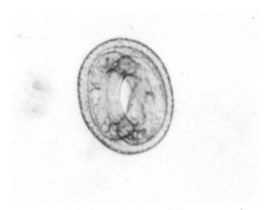

Figure 27.4. Embryonated egg of *Toxocara canis*.

also be associated with a eosinophilic meningoencephalitis.[20] There has been an increasing appreciation that more subtle clinical manifestations might also arise as a result of larval migrations. So-called "covert toxocariasis" ranges in spectrum from asymptomatic infection to larvae migrating in specific target organs.[21-23] Covert toxocariasis is felt to be due to chronic exposure.[24] In the lungs, larval migrations may result in asthma; *T. canis* has been suggested as an environmental risk factor for asthma among some inner-city populations.[25-27] In the brain, *T. canis* has been implicated as one of the causes of "idiopathic" seizure disorders, and infection is significantly more prevalent in children with mental disabilities, including non-institutionalized children.[13, 14, 28, 29] Toxocariasis has also been linked to functional intestinal disorders, arthritis and skin rashes.[22, 25, 30, 31] There is a concern that the cases of *Toxocara* spp. identified through serological testing may be associated with long term cognitive consequences. Measurable reductions in scores on cognitive tests have been demonstrated when comparing children with serological evidence of Toxocara infection to those without.[13] Longitudinal studies to confirm these findings are still needed, but concern has been raised that the impact of this disease goes far beyond the cases brought to medical attention by symptoms. The full clinical spectrum of disease of covert toxocariasis has yet to be explored.[14]

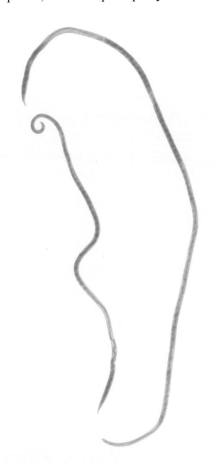

Figure 27.3. Adults of *Toxocara canis*. The female is 9 cm, the male is 6 cm.

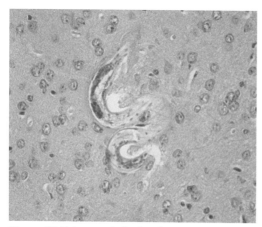

Figure 27.5. Larvae in brain of mouse experimentally infected with *T. canis*.

OLM

Ocular larva migrans (OLM) usually occurs in older children (5-10 years old), and typically presents as unilateral vision impairment that is sometimes accompanied by strabismus.[30] In temperate climates, such as in the UK, it is estimated that the prevalence of OLM may be as high as 9.7 cases per 100,000 persons.[32] The most serious consequence of the infection is invasion of the retina, leading to granuloma formation, which occurs typically peripherally, or in the posterior pole. These granulomas drag the retina and create a distortion, heteropia, or detachment of the macula.[33] The degree of visual acuity impairment depends upon the specific area involved, and blindness is common. Ocular larva migrans can also cause diffuse endopthalmitis or papillitis; secondary glaucoma can follow. In some cases these lesions have been visualized on ophthalmic examination, and due to their visual similarities with retinoblastoma there is the risk of unnecessary enucleation of the infected eye.[34-37]

Diagnosis

Any pediatric age patient with an unexplained febrile illness and eosinophilia should be suspected of having VLM. Hepatosplenomegaly and evidence of multisystem disease and history of pica make the diagnosis of VLM more likely. Similarly, OLM should be suspected in any child with unilateral vision loss and strabismus. Diagnostic tests for VLM are primarily immunological.[38] The precipitin test is subject to cross-reactions with common antigens of the larvae and blood group substance A. The recommended test for toxocariasis detects IgG against excretory-secretory antigens derived from toxocara L2 larvae. A toxocara ELISA is available through the Center for Disease Control and Prevention (CDC), and is estimated to be 78% sensitive and 92% specific when using the appropriate cutoff.[39, 40] Newer diagnostics are also under development including those that use recombinant antigens in place of parasite natural products.[41, 42] Stool examinations of infected individuals is not helpful, as these aberrant nematodes do not complete their life cycle in humans, so no eggs are produced.

Other indicators include hypergammaglobulinemia and an elevated isohemoagglutin titer. A constellation of clinical disease described above, a history of pica, eosinophilia, and positive serology strongly point to the diagnosis. Liver biopsy may reveal a granuloma surrounding a larva, but a successful diagnosis using this approach is fortuitous at best, and not recommended. Ocular larva migrans is diagnosed primarily on the basis of clinical criteria during an ophthalmologic

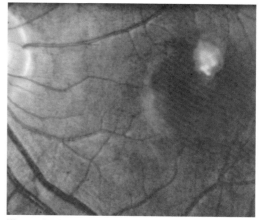

Figure 27.6 Granuloma in retina of patient with OLM. The lesion consists largely of eosinophils.

examination. The immunodiagnostic tests used for VLM are not as reliable for OLM. In one study, only 45% of patients with clinically diagnosed OLM had titers high enough to be classified as positive.[43]

Treatment

While there is limited reliable evidence-based guidance with regard to treatment, *Toxocara canis* and *Toxocara cati* can be treated with albendazole 400mg oral 2x/day for a total of 5 days (Adult and Pediatric Dose).[31] The other commonly used drug, mebendazole, is poorly absorbed outside the gastrointestinal tract, although some success has been reported in patients who ingest 1 g or more of this agent for a 21 day course[44]. Symptomatic treatment, including administration of corticosteroids, has been helpful for suppressing intense manifestations of the infection. OLM is treated either by surgery (vitrectomy), anthelminthic chemotherapy, and/ or corticosteroids.[45-48] In the case of ocular involvement with active ocular inflammation, the role of antihelminthic therapy is unclear, owing to the lack of knowledge regarding the intraophthalmic pharmacokinetics and pharmacodynamics, and the impact of therapy on outcomes.

The toxocara group of parasites is common in young pets. For example, young puppies often harbor these worms, since the infection can be congenitally acquired. Having a litter of puppies in the home has been identified as a significant risk factor.[45] While *Toxocara* spp. are able to cause death in puppies, death is rare in human infection. Children with pica are at risk of ingesting embryonated eggs from soil. Adult patients who have been institutionalized for mental retardation are also at risk.[46] Treatment of dogs and control of their feces are major control measures for this disease. Toxocariasis is an understudied and underreported disease. Through scattered serological surveys, there is increasing evidence that it is one of the most common helminthic diseases in temperate climates of North America and Europe, including some large inner-city urban areas, as well as in Brazil and elsewhere.[7, 49-53]

Baylisascaris procyonis
(Sprent, 1968)

Baylisascaris procyonis, the raccoon ascarid, causes visceral larva migrans and neural larva migrans in humans when they accidentally ingest embryonated eggs that are shed in sylvatic environs, as well as in peri-domestic environs, in which suburban dwellings permit accessiblity to raccoons, such as attics and rain gutters.[38, 40, 43] Although it is rare, the pathological consequences of infection with the larva of *B. procyonis* is generally more severe than that caused by *T. canis*. Neural larva migrans can result in neurodevastation, even with anthelminthic chemotherapy and steroids.[54] The large, developing larvae (up to 2 mm.) cause considerable mechanical damage.[54] Larvae migrating through brain tissue can result in eosinophilic meningitis associated with high mortality (Fig. 27.7). Neural larva migrans is associated with ocular disease characterized by retinitis and multiple choroidal infiltrates.[55]

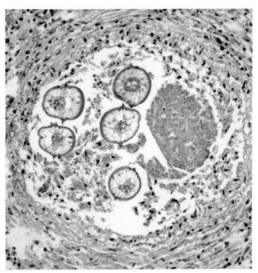

Figure 27.7. Larvae of *B. procyonis* in brain of child who died of VLM.

Since antibodies to *B. procyonis* antigens do not cross-react with *T. canis*, the excretory and secretory products of *B. procyonis* have been examined as a possible species-specific immunodiagnostic reagent.[56] Although a serological test has been developed for *Baylisascaris procyonis* that has high sensitivity and specificity, most human cases have been diagnosed at autopsy. There are but a few cases diagnosed to date, so there is little overall experience with anthelminthic therapy for baylisascariasis, but good outcomes have been reported with high dose albendazole 25-50mg/kg/day in divided doses started promptly and continued for 10-20 days with concomitant steroids[57-59]

Angiostrongylus cantonensis
(Chen 1935)

Angiostrongylus costaricensis
(Morera and Cespedes 1971)

Angiostrongylus cantonensis infection occurs in Southeast Asia, the Philippine Islands, Taiwan, and both North and South Pacific islands. Human infection was first described in Taiwan when larvae of the parasite were isolated from the CSF of a child. Infected rodents, but not human cases, have also been reported from East Africa. A survey of wharf rats in New Orleans revealed a high rate of infection, although none had been detected several years prior to that study.[51] Acquisition of human infection depends upon the locale and the nutritional habits of the specific population. A case in Hawaii resulted from ingestion of a raw slug given for a traditional medicinal purpose. In Tahiti, epidemics have resulted from consumption of raw freshwater prawns (i.e., shrimp-like crustaceans), and elsewhere, other invertebrates (e.g., planarians) either consumed directly or in vegetation.

Rats are the definitive host for *Angiostrongylus* spp. Angiostrongylus infect a number of species of wild rats including the common wharf rat, *Rattus norvegicus*. These worms live and lay eggs in the pulmonary arteries of rats. The released eggs move through the capillaries in the lung, and then penetrate into the alveolar spaces. From the alveolar spaces, the larvae migrate up the respiratory tree and are swallowed, ultimately to pass out of the rat in feces.[60] *Angiostrongylus cantonensis* larvae incubate in the soil before being consumed by a variety of mollusks and crustaceans.[61-64] Humans are infected when they inadvertently consume the larval stages of *Angiostrongylus cantonensis* present in uncooked snails, slugs, or raw vegetables contaminated with secretions from these invertebrates. *Angiostrongylus costaricensis* larvae are generally restricted to infecting only one invertebrate host, the slug. In most cases, the specific slug is *Vaginulus plebius*. Human infection results when they accidently ingest these slugs, or food contaminated with its secretions.

Most cases of human infection with *Angiostrongylus* spp. result in failure of the worm to complete its life cycle. Once in a human host, the larvae often migrate to the brain or rarely to the lungs, as has been observed in infants and small children. These nematodes die surrounded by an eosinophil-rich inflammatory infiltrate.[65] The pattern of clinical presentation varies with each species of Angiostrongylus. *Angiostrongylus cantonensis* L3 larvae usually migrate to the meningeal capillaries, where dying larvae trigger eosinophilic inflammation resulting in eosinophilic meningoencephalitis. Part of the pathology can involve vascular thrombosis and aneurysms. *Angiostrongylus cantonensis* is the most common cause of eosinophilic meningitis outside of the developed world, and should be considered in the differential of travelers returning from endemic areas.[65]

Individuals infected with *Angiostrongylus costaricensis* present with fever, bitemporal or frontal headache, and meningismus. Vomiting is reported in the majority of cases, as are migrating painful paresthesias.[66] Painful paraesthesias often persist for weeks to months along with headaches. Although an eosinophilic meningitis is characteristic on cerebral spinal fluid examination, focal lesions are usually not present on head CT or MRI. This can be useful in distinguishing the disease from other etiologies, such as *Gnathostoma spinigerum* and neurocysticercosis.[67] The natural course of the disease without treatment is for resolution of symptoms in 1-2 weeks. Disease duration and severity may be worse in children.

Diagnosis of *Angiostrongylus* spp. is based on clinical presentation, as serological testing is not widely available. Confirmation of suspected cases has been achieved using post treatment serological testing in concert with research laboratories.[66]

With the self-limiting nature of this disease, treatment often focuses on symptoms rather than on antihelmith therapy. Although animal models have supported the use of antihelminthic therapy trials, efficacy in human infection has not been demonstrated, and there are reports that antihelminthic therapy may lead to more serious disease.[68-70] Serial lumbar punctures and analgesics are the usual approaches to therapy.

Widespread education about the proper cooking of food and vegetable washing, as well as the control of mollusks and planarians in vegetable gardens, can reduce the incidence of infections.[50]

Gnathostoma spinigerum
(Owen 1838)

Gnathostoma spinigerum is a nematode parasite in various mammals, including cats, dogs, and the mongoose. The intermediate hosts include; 1. copepods in the genus *Cyclops*, and 2. snakes, frogs, fish, and birds. Gnathostomiasis in humans is prevalent throughout Mexico, Thailand, and Asia. In Mexico, infections are commonly acquired in and around Acapulco.[54, 59, 71]

Female adults are 25-54 mm in length, while males measure 11-25 mm. Adults live coiled in the wall of the small intestine in their definitive hosts. Eggs pass in feces and hatch in water, releasing larvae that are ingested by macroinvertebrate crustaceans. Fish, snakes, and birds eat infected crustaceans and the infective stage for humans then develops within them. When humans eat these infected vertebrates the larvae invade the small intestinal tissue. The worms leave the SI and migrate into the deep tissues.[72-74]

Although the disease is likely asymptomatic in most cases; skin manifestations can include cutaneous larva migrans, panniculitis, and subcutaneous swellings. Invasion of the CNS can occur with peripheral eosinophilia as well as eosinophilic meningitis, with radicular pain and paresthesias due to larval migration. *Gnathostoma spinigerum* is also able to invade the eye and result in an intraocular form of this disease.[75]

Previously the diagnosis of gnathostomiasis was limited to an appropriate travel history, clinical presentation and eosinophilia, but diagnostic tests have become available. ELISA and Western Blot aid in diagnosis, but these are only available at laboratories outside of the United States, and definitive diagnosis with isolation of the parasite is often not possible.[76]

Although this disease can be self-limited, therapy often involves a 21 day oral course of albendazole at a dose of 400mg once daily.[77] Ivermectin has been shown to be effective in several trials, and may serve as an alternate agent. It remains unclear as to the role of antihelminthic therapy in ocular and neurological disease where it may worsen symptoms. In some cases, surgical removal is employed.[54] Corticosteroids have been used in the treatment of patients with CNS manifestations. Relapses have been reported with either therapy.[66]

Anisakiasis and Related Illnesses

Anisakiasis in humans is caused by a number of species of nematode belonging to the genera *Anisakis, Phocanema, Terranova,* and *Contracoecum.* They infect sea mammals, particularly dolphins, whales, sea lions, and seals.[78] In these hosts, adults live in the lumen of the intestinal tract. Anasakid L1 larvae infect a number of crustacean species. L2, L3, and L4 larvae infect a wide variety of bottom-feeding fish.[79]

The adult worms of marine mammal ascarids embed in the gastric mucosa and pass unembryonated eggs out into the environment in the feces. The eggs embryonate and larvae mature inside the eggs until free-swimming larvae are released. Crustaceans, their first intermediate host, ingest these larvae. There they mature into the stage infective for fish, as well as squid, their second intermediate host. After being ingested, rather than staying in the fish or squid intestine, larvae migrate to the peritoneal cavity, where they grow up to 3cm in length. Upon the death of the cold-blooded vertebrate host, larvae migrate to their muscles where they may be ingested by marine warm-blooded predator/scavengers, and develop into adult worms. After mating and then embedding into the mucosa, adult female worms begin laying eggs. At this point, the life cycle is complete.[80]

Raw or undercooked saltwater fish, often in the form of sushi or sashimi, has become a popular style of cuisine throughout the world.[55, 56] When an infected piece of raw fish is eaten, the parasites in the muscle tissue are released by the enzymes in the stomach, or more rarely, into the small intestine. Tissue invasion is facilitated by release of parasite hydrolytic enzymes.[81, 82] Infected individuals often present with abdominal pain that can be severe, and can be confused with the symptoms of an acute gastric ulcer.[83] From ingestion to onset of symptoms is usually a matter of minutes to hours. Nausea, vomiting, abdominal distension, mild fever and diarrhea with blood and mucous in the stool can be part of the presentation.[84] If larvae are able to penetrate the mucosa, angioedema, urticarial and allergic symptoms can dominate the clinical presentation.[85]

All species of anasakid worms die within a few days in humans. Dead parasites provoke an eosinophilic granulomatous infiltration. Initially, infection may be asymptomatic, but soon thereafter vague upper abdominal pain may develop. Symptoms may mimic gastric ulcer.[83]

Definitive diagnosis and treatment is made by removal of the parasite. Sometimes the worms are expelled through coughing or vomiting, but at other times endoscopic removal or surgery for extraintestinal manifestations is necessary. Serologic tests using an antigen capture ELISA are available in some countries and have sensitivities reported near 100%.[86] PCR tests have been developed, but are not commercially available.[87, 88]

Thorough cooking or freezing of seafood prior to ingestion can prevent infection by anisakid nematodes. Most sushi restaurants in the U.S. and elsewhere now inspect pieces of raw fish carefully prior to serving them, and the FDA under food code 101 requires freezing prior to serving raw fish. Flash freezing in liquid nitrogen has become a popular way of processing fish destined for sushi restaurants. After a peak in the 1980s, the incidence of anisakiasis in Europe and North America due to the consumption of raw fish has been reduced to a few sporadic cases annually.[89]

References

1. Sulica, V. I.; Kao, G. F.; Berberian, B.; J., Histopathologic findings of cutaneous larva migrans. *Pathol 346* **1988,** *15.*

2. Bowman, D. D.; Montgomery, S. P.; Zajac, A. M.; Eberhard, M. L.; Kazacos, K. R., Hookworms of dogs and cats as agents of cutaneous larva migrans. *Trends in parasitology* **2010,** *26* (4), 162-7.

3. Blackwell, V.; Vega-Lopez, F., Cutaneous larva migrans: clinical features and management of 44 cases presenting in the returning traveller. *The British journal of dermatology* **2001,** *145* (3), 434-7.

4. Caumes, E., It's time to distinguish the sign 'creeping eruption' from the syndrome 'cutaneous larva migrans'. *Dermatology* **2006,** *213* (3), 179-81.

5. Albanese, G.; Venturi, C., Albendazole: a new drug for human parasitoses. *Dermatologic clinics* **2003,** *21* (2), 283-90.

6. Albanese, G.; Venturi, C.; Galbiati, G., Treatment of larva migrans cutanea (creeping eruption): a comparison between albendazole and traditional therapy. *International journal of dermatology* **2001,** *40* (1), 67-71.

7. Lee, R. M.; Moore, L. B.; Bottazzi, M. E.; Hotez, P. J., Toxocariasis in North America: a systematic review. *PLoS Negl Trop Dis* **2014,** *8* (8), e3116.

8. Won, K. Y.; Kruszon-Moran, D.; Schantz, P. M.; Jones, J. L., National seroprevalence and risk factors for Zoonotic Toxocara spp. infection. *Am J Trop Med Hyg* **2008,** *79* (4), 552-7.

9. Wilder, H. C., Nematode endophthalmitis. *Trans Am Acad Ophthalmol Otolaryngol* **1950,** *55* 99-104.

10. Beaver, P. C.; Snyde, C. H., Chronic eosinophilia due to visceral larva migrans. *Pediatrics* **1952,** *9* 7-19.

11. Despommier, D., Toxocariasis: clinical aspects, epidemiology, medical ecology, and molecular aspects. *Clinical microbiology reviews* **2003,** *16* (2), 265-72.

12. Walsh, M. G.; Haseeb, M. A., Toxocariasis and lung function: relevance of a neglected infection in an urban landscape. *Acta Parasitol* **2014,** *59* (1), 126-31.

13. Walsh, M. G.; Haseeb, M. A., Reduced cognitive function in children with toxocariasis in a nationally representative sample of the United States. *Int J Parasitol* **2012,** *42* (13-14), 1159-63.

14. Hotez, P. J., Neglected infections of poverty in the United States and their effects on the brain. *JAMA Psychiatry* **2014,** *71* (10), 1099-100.

15. Despommier, D., Toxocariasis: clinical aspects, epidemiology, medical ecology, and molecular aspects. *Clin Microbiol Rev* **2003,** *16* (2), 265-72.

16. Ahn, S. J.; Ryoo, N. K.; Woo, S. J., Ocular toxocariasis: clinical features, diagnosis, treatment, and prevention. *Asia Pac Allergy* **2014,** *4* (3), 134-41.

17. Glickman, L. I.; Schantz, P. M., Epidemiology and pathogenesis of zoonotic toxocariasis. *Epidemiol Rev* **1982,** *10,* 143-148.

18. Kazacos, K. R., Visceral and ocular larva migrans. *Seminars in veterinary medicine and surgery (small animal)* **1991,** *6* (3), 227-35.

19. Worley, G.; Green, J. A.; Frothingham, T. E.; Sturner, R. A.; Walls, K. W.; Pakalnis, V. A.; Ellis, G. S., Toxocara canis infection: clinical and epidemiological associations with seropositivity in kindergarten children. *The Journal of infectious diseases* **1984,** *149* (4), 591-7.

20. Xinou, E.; Lefkopoulos, A.; Gelagoti, M.; Drevelegas, A.; Diakou, A.; Milonas, I.; Dimitriadis, A. S., CT and MR imaging findings in cerebral toxocaral disease. *AJNR. American journal of neuroradiology* **2003,** *24* (4), 714-8.

21. Taylor, M. R.; Keane, C. T.; O'Connor, P.; Mulvihill, E.; Holland, C., The expanded spectrum of toxocaral disease. *Lancet (London, England)* **1988,** *1* (8587), 692-5.

22. Sharghi, N.; Schantz, P.; Hotez, P. J., Toxocariasis: An occult cause of childhood asthma, seizures, and neuropsychological deficit? . *Sem Pediatr Infect Dis* **2000,** *11* 257-60.

23. Nathwani, D.; Laing, R. B.; Currie, P. F., Covert toxocariasis--a cause of recurrent abdominal pain in childhood. *The British journal of clinical practice* **1992,** *46* (4), 271.

24. Minvielle, M. C.; Niedfeld, G.; Ciarmela, M. L.; De Falco, A.; Ghiani, H.; Basualdo, J. A., [Asthma and covert toxocariasis]. *Medicina* **1999,** *59* (3), 243-8.

25. Buijs, J.; Borsboom, G.; van Gemund, J. J.; Hazebroek, A.; van Dongen, P. A.; van Knapen, F.; Neijens, H. J., Toxocara seroprevalence in 5-year-old elementary schoolchildren: relation with allergic asthma. *American journal of epidemiology* **1994**, *140* (9), 839-47.

26. Tariq, S. M.; Matthews, S.; Stevens, M.; Ridout, S.; Hakim, E. A.; Hide, D. W., Epidemiology of allergic disorders in early childhood. *Pediatric pulmonology. Supplement* **1997**, *16*, 69.

27. Sharghi, N.; Schantz, P. M.; Caramico, L.; Ballas, K.; Teague, B. A.; Hotez, P. J., Environmental exposure to Toxocara as a possible risk factor for asthma: a clinic-based case-control study. *Clinical infectious diseases : an official publication of the Infectious Diseases Society of America* **2001**, *32* (7), E111-6.

28. Critchley, E. M.; Vakil, S. D.; Hutchinson, D. N.; Taylor, P., Toxoplasma, Toxocara, and epilepsy. *Epilepsia* **1982**, *23* (3), 315-21.

29. Kaplan, M.; Kalkan, A.; Hosoglu, S.; Kuk, S.; Ozden, M.; Demirdag, K.; Ozdarendeli, A., The frequency of Toxocara infection in mental retarded children. *Memorias do Instituto Oswaldo Cruz* **2004**, *99* (2), 121-5.

30. Konate, A.; Duhamel, O.; Basset, D.; Ayral, J.; Poirette, A.; Granier, P.; Ramdani, M.; Gislon, J., [Toxocariasis and functional intestinal disorders. Presentation of 4 cases]. *Gastroenterologie clinique et biologique* **1996**, *20* (10), 909-11.

31. Dinning, W. J.; Gillespie, S. H.; Cooling, R. J.; Maizels, R. M., Toxocariasis: a practical approach to management of ocular disease. *Eye (London, England)* **1988**, *2 (Pt 5)*, 580-2.

32. Good, B.; Holland, C. V.; Taylor, M. R. H.; Larragy, J.; Moriarty, P.; O'Regan, M., Ocular toxocariasis in schoolchildren. *Clinical infectious diseases : an official publication of the Infectious Diseases Society of America* **2004**, *39* (2), 173-8.

33. Small, K. W.; McCuen, B. W.; de Juan, E.; Machemer, R., Surgical management of retinal traction caused by toxocariasis. *American journal of ophthalmology* **1989**, *108* (1), 10-4.

34. Ota, K. V.; Dimaras, H.; Heon, E.; Gallie, B. L.; Chan, H. S., Radiologic surveillance for retinoblastoma metastases unexpectedly showed disseminated toxocariasis in liver, lung, and spinal cord. *Canadian journal of ophthalmology. Journal canadien d'ophtalmologie* **2010**, *45* (2), 185-6.

35. Ota, K. V.; Dimaras, H.; Heon, E.; Babyn, P. S.; Yau, Y. C.; Read, S.; Budning, A.; Gallie, B. L.; Chan, H. S., Toxocariasis mimicking liver, lung, and spinal cord metastases from retinoblastoma. *The Pediatric infectious disease journal* **2009**, *28* (3), 252-4.

36. Lopez-Velez, R.; Suarez de Figueroa, M.; Gimeno, L.; Garcia-Camacho, A.; Fenoy, S.; Guillen, J. L.; Castellote, L., [Ocular toxocariasis or retinoblastoma?]. *Enfermedades infecciosas y microbiologia clinica* **1995**, *13* (4), 242-5.

37. Van Nerom, P. R.; Gaudy, F.; Verstappen, A.; Carlier, Y., [Differential diagnosis between retinoblastoma and ocular toxocariasis]. *Journal francais d'ophtalmologie* **1987**, *10* (4), 279-82.

38. Schantz, P. M., Toxocara larva migrans now. *The American journal of tropical medicine and hygiene* **1989**, *41* (3 Suppl), 21-34.

39. Rubinsky-Elefant, G.; Hirata, C. E.; Yamamoto, J. H.; Ferreira, M. U., Human toxocariasis: diagnosis, worldwide seroprevalences and clinical expression of the systemic and ocular forms. *Annals of tropical medicine and parasitology* **2010**, *104* (1), 3-23.

40. Fong, M. Y.; Lau, Y. L., Recombinant expression of the larval excretory-secretory antigen TES-120 of Toxocara canis in the methylotrophic yeast Pichia pastoris. *Parasitol Res* **2003**, *92*, 173-6.

41. Anderson, J. P.; Rascoe, L. N.; Levert, K.; Chastain, H. M.; Reed, M. S.; Rivera, H. N.; McAuliffe, I.; Zhan, B.; Wiegand, R. E.; Hotez, P. J.; Wilkins, P. P.; Pohl, J.; Handali, S., Development of a Luminex Bead Based Assay for Diagnosis of Toxocariasis Using Recombinant Antigens Tc-CTL-1 and Tc-TES-26. *PLoS Negl Trop Dis* **2015**, *9* (10), e0004168.

42. Zhan, B.; Ajmera, R.; Geiger, S. M.; Goncalves, M. T.; Liu, Z.; Wei, J.; Wilkins, P. P.; Fujiwara, R.; Gazzinelli-Guimaraes, P. H.; Bottazzi, M. E.; Hotez, P., Identification of immunodominant antigens for the laboratory diagnosis of toxocariasis. *Trop Med Int Health* **2015**, *20* (12), 1787-96.

43. Schantz, P. M.; Meyer, D.; Glickman, L. T., Clinical, serologic, and epidemiologic characteristics of ocular toxocariasis. *The American journal of tropical medicine and hygiene* **1979**, *28* (1), 24-8.

44. Hotez, P. J.; Burg, F. D.; Wald, E. R.; Ingelfinger, J. R.; Polin, P. A., Toxocara canis. 1995.

45. Marmor, M.; Glickman, L.; Shofer, F.; Faich, L. A.; Rosenberg, C.; Cornblatt, B.; Friedman, S.,

Toxocara canis infection of children: epidemiologic and neuropsychologic findings. *American journal of public health* **1987,** *77* (5), 554-9.

46. Hummer, D.; Symon, K.; J., Seroepidemiologic study of toxocariasis and strongyloidiasis in institutionalized mentally retarded adults. *Am Med Hyg* **1992,** *46,* 278-281.

47. Sturchler, D.; Schubarth, P., Thiabendazole v albendazole in treatment of toxocariasis a clinical trial. *Ann Trop Med Parasitol* **1989,** *83* 473-478.

48. Sturchler, D.; Schubarth, P.; Gualzata, M.; Gottstein, B.; Oettli, A., Thiabendazole vs. albendazole in treatment of toxocariasis: a clinical trial. *Annals of tropical medicine and parasitology* **1989,** *83* (5), 473-8.

49. Gauthier, J. L.; Gupta, A.; Hotez, P.; Richardson, D. J.; Krause, P. J., Stealth parasites: the under appreciated burden of parasitic zoonoses in North America. 2001; p 1-21.

50. Hotez, P. J., Reducing the global burden of human parasitic diseases. *Comp Parasitol* **2002,** *69,* 140-45.

51. Anaruma Filho, F.; Chieffi, P. P., Human toxocariasis: incidence among residents in the outskirts of Campinas, State of Sao Paulo, Brazil. Rev Inst Med Trop Sao Paulo. **2003,** *45,* 293-4.

52. Fialho, P. M.; Correa, C. R., A Systematic Review of Toxocariasis: A Neglected but High-Prevalence Disease in Brazil. *Am J Trop Med Hyg* **2016.**

53. Borecka, A.; Klapec, T., Epidemiology of human toxocariasis in Poland - A review of cases 1978-2009. *Ann Agric Environ Med* **2015,** *22* (1), 28-31.

54. Kazacos, K. R.; Boyce, W. M.; J., Baylisascaris larva migrans. *VeMed Assoc* **1990,** *195,* 894-903.

55. Mets, M. B.; Noble, A. G.; Basti, S.; Gavin, P.; Davis, A. T.; Shulman, S. T.; Kazacos, K. R., Eye findings of diffuse unilateral subacute neuroretinitis and multiple choroidal infiltrates associated with neural larva migrans due to Bbaylisascaris procyonis. *American journal of ophthalmology* **2003,** *135* (6), 888-90.

56. Boyce, W. M.; Asai, D. J.; Wilder, J. K.; Kazacos, K. R., Physicochemical characterization and monoclonal and polyclonal antibody recognition of Baylisascaris procyonis larval excretory-secretory antigens. *The Journal of parasitology* **1989,** *75* (4), 540-8.

57. Peters, J. M.; Madhavan, V. L.; Kazacos, K. R.; Husson, R. N.; Dangoudoubiyam, S.; Soul, J. S., Good outcome with early empiric treatment of neural larva migrans due to Baylisascaris procyonis. *Pediatrics* **2012,** *129* (3), e806-11.

58. Pai, P. J.; Blackburn, B. G.; Kazacos, K. R.; Warrier, R. P.; Begue, R. E., Full recovery from Baylisascaris procyonis eosinophilic meningitis. *Emerging infectious diseases* **2007,** *13* (6), 928-30.

59. Gavin, P. J.; Kazacos, K. R.; Tan, T. Q.; Brinkman, W. B.; Byrd, S. E.; Davis, A. T.; Mets, M. B.; Shulman, S. T., Neural larva migrans caused by the raccoon roundworm Baylisascaris procyonis. *The Pediatric infectious disease journal* **2002,** *21* (10), 971-5.

60. Mackerras, M. J.; Sandars, D. F., Lifehistory of the rat lung-worm and its migration through the brain of its host. *Nature* **1954,** *173* (4411), 956-7.

61. Qvarnstrom, Y.; Sullivan, J. J.; Bishop, H. S.; Hollingsworth, R.; da Silva, A. J., PCR-based detection of Angiostrongylus cantonensis in tissue and mucus secretions from molluscan hosts. *Applied and environmental microbiology* **2007,** *73* (5), 1415-9.

62. Richards, C. S.; Merritt, J. W., Studies on Angiostrongylus cantonensis in molluscan intermediate hosts. *The Journal of parasitology* **1967,** *53* (2), 382-8.

63. Wallace, G. D.; Rosen, L., Studies on eosinophilic meningitis. V. Molluscan hosts of Angiostrongylus cantonensis on Pacific Islands. *The American journal of tropical medicine and hygiene* **1969,** *18* (2), 206-16.

64. Drozdz, J.; Doby, J. M.; Mandahl-Barth, G., [Study of the morphology and larval development of Angiostrongylus (Parastrongylus) dujardini Drozdz and Doby 1970, Nematoda: Metastrongyloiidea. Infestation of the molluscan intermediary hosts]. *Annales de parasitologie humaine et comparee* **1971,** *46* (3), 265-76.

65. Slom, T. J.; Cortese, M. M.; Gerber, S. I.; Jones, R. C.; Holtz, T. H.; Lopez, A. S.; Zambrano, C. H.; Sufit, R. L.; Sakolvaree, Y.; Chaicumpa, W.; Herwaldt, B. L.; Johnson, S., An outbreak of eosinophilic meningitis caused by Angiostrongylus cantonensis in travelers returning from the

Caribbean. *The New England journal of medicine* **2002**, *346* (9), 668-75.

66. Ramirez-Avila, L.; Slome, S.; Schuster, F. L.; Gavali, S.; Schantz, P. M.; Sejvar, J.; Glaser, C. A., Eosinophilic meningitis due to Angiostrongylus and Gnathostoma species. *Clinical infectious diseases : an official publication of the Infectious Diseases Society of America* **2009**, *48* (3), 322-7.

67. Lo Re, V., 3rd; Gluckman, S. J., Eosinophilic meningitis. *The American journal of medicine* **2003**, *114* (3), 217-23.

68. Hidelaratchi, M. D.; Riffsy, M. T.; Wijesekera, J. C., A case of eosinophilic meningitis following monitor lizard meat consumption, exacerbated by anthelminthics. *The Ceylon medical journal* **2005**, *50* (2), 84-6.

69. Sawanyawisuth, K.; Limpawattana, P.; Busaracome, P.; Ninpaitoon, B.; Chotmongkol, V.; Intapan, P. M.; Tanawirattananit, S., A 1-week course of corticosteroids in the treatment of eosinophilic meningitis. *The American journal of medicine* **2004**, *117* (10), 802-3.

70. Chotmongkol, V.; Wongjitrat, C.; Sawadpanit, K.; Sawanyawisuth, K., Treatment of eosinophilic meningitis with a combination of albendazole and corticosteroid. *The Southeast Asian journal of tropical medicine and public health* **2004**, *35* (1), 172-4.

71. Moore, D. A.; McCroddan, J.; Dekumyoy, P.; Chiodini, P. L., Gnathostomiasis: an emerging imported disease. *Emerging infectious diseases* **2003**, *9* (6), 647-50.

72. Maleewong, W.; Intapan, P. M.; Khempila, J.; Wongwajana, S.; Wongkham, C.; Morakote, N., Gnathostoma spinigerum: growth and development of third-stage larvae in vitro. *The Journal of parasitology* **1995**, *81* (5), 800-3.

73. Janwan, P.; Intapan, P. M.; Sanpool, O.; Sadaow, L.; Thanchomnang, T.; Maleewong, W., Growth and development of Gnathostoma spinigerum (Nematoda: Gnathostomatidae) larvae in Mesocyclops aspericornis (Cyclopoida: Cyclopidae). *Parasites & vectors* **2011**, *4*, 93.

74. Maleewong, W.; Intapan, P. M.; Ieamviteevanich, K.; Wongkham, C.; Morakote, N., Growth and development of Gnathostoma spinigerum early third-stage larvae in vitro. *Journal of helminthology* **1997**, *71* (1), 69-71.

75. Funata, M.; Custis, P.; de la Cruz, Z.; de Juan, E.; Green, W. R., Intraocular gnathostomiasis. *Retina* **1993**, *13* (3), 240-4.

76. Intapan, P. M.; Khotsri, P.; Kanpittaya, J.; Chotmongkol, V.; Sawanyawisuth, K.; Maleewong, W., Immunoblot diagnostic test for neurognathostomiasis. *The American journal of tropical medicine and hygiene* **2010**, *83* (4), 927-9.

77. Lv, S.; Zhang, Y.; Chen, S. R.; Wang, L. B.; Fang, W.; Chen, F.; Jiang, J. Y.; Li, Y. L.; Du, Z. W.; Zhou, X. N., Human angiostrongyliasis outbreak in Dali, China. *PLoS neglected tropical diseases* **2009**, *3* (9), e520.

78. Sorvillo, F.; Ash, L. R.; Berlin, O. G. W.; Morse, S. A., Baylisascaris procyonis: an emerging helminthic zoonosis. *Emerging infectious diseases* **2002**, *8* (4), 355-9.

79. Hochberg, N. S.; Hamer, D. H., Anisakidosis: Perils of the deep. *Clinical infectious diseases : an official publication of the Infectious Diseases Society of America* **2010**, *51* (7), 806-12.

80. Abollo, E.; Gestal, C.; Pascual, S., Anisakis infestation in marine fish and cephalopods from Galician waters: an updated perspective. *Parasitology research* **2001**, *87* (6), 492-9.

81. Lo Re, V.; Gluckman, S. J., Eosinophilic meningitis. *The American journal of medicine* **2003**, *114* (3), 217-23.

82. Takei, H.; Powell, S. Z., Intestinal anisakidosis (anisakiosis). *Annals of diagnostic pathology* **2007**, *11* (5), 350-2.

83. Morera, P., Life history and redescription of Angiostrongylus costaricensis Morera and Céspedes, 1971. *The American journal of tropical medicine and hygiene* **1973**, *22* (5), 613-21.

84. Nawa, Y.; Hatz, C.; Blum, J., Sushi delights and parasites: the risk of fishborne and foodborne parasitic zoonoses in Asia. *Clin Infect Dis* **2005**, *41* (9), 1297-303.

85. Lopez-Serrano, M. C.; Gomez, A. A.; Daschner, A.; Moreno-Ancillo, A.; de Parga, J. M.; Caballero, M. T.; Barranco, P.; Cabanas, R., Gastroallergic anisakiasis: findings in 22 patients. *Journal of gastroenterology and hepatology* **2000**, *15* (5), 503-6.

86. Lorenzo, S.; Iglesias, R.; Leiro, J.; Ubeira, F. M.; Ansotegui, I.; Garcia, M.; Fernandez de Corres, L., Usefulness of currently available methods for the diagnosis of Anisakis simplex allergy. *Allergy*

2000, *55* (7), 627-33.

87.   Chen, Q.; Yu, H. Q.; Lun, Z. R.; Chen, X. G.; Song, H. Q.; Lin, R. Q.; Zhu, X. Q., Specific PCR assays for the identification of common anisakid nematodes with zoonotic potential. *Parasitology research* **2008,** *104* (1), 79-84.

88.   Kim, D. Y.; Stewart, T. B.; Bauer, R. W.; Mitchell, M., Parastrongylus (=Angiostrongylus) cantonensis now endemic in Louisiana wildlife. *The Journal of parasitology* **2002,** *88* (5), 1024-6.

89.   Audicana, M. T.; Kennedy, M. W., Anisakis simplex: from obscure infectious worm to inducer of immune hypersensitivity. *Clinical microbiology reviews* **2008,** *21* (2), 360-79, table of contents.

VI. The Cestodes

The phylum Platyhelminthes includes the class Cestoidea (tapeworms), all of which are parasitic in the gut tracts of various vertebrate hosts. Tapeworms are flat, segmented worms, composed of a head (scolex), and a series of segments, known as proglottids. Together, all proglottids are referred to as the strobila. The scolex is the point of attachment between the host and the parasite. It may be equipped with suckers, hooks, or grooves, which aid in the attachment process. The scolex contains nerves terminating in ganglia, while the segments contain only nerves. The neck region of the scolex is metabolically active, and is the site in most tapeworms from which new proglottids form.

The tapeworm does not have a functional gut tract. Rather, the segments are enclosed in a specialized tegument, whose structure and function are directly related to nutrient acquisition. Evenly-spaced microvilli cover the entire surface of the tegument, underneath which lie mitochondria, vesicles (perhaps involved in tegument replacement), and related structures. The tapeworm obtains some of its nutrients by actively transporting them across the tegument. Each proglottid is able to absorb a wide variety of low-molecular-weight substrates, but its precise metabolic requirements have yet to be fully defined.

High levels of ATPase in the tegument are related to active transport, but may also help the worm resist digestion by the mammalian host. Inhibitors of tapeworm ATPase, such as niclosamide, cause disintegration of adult tapeworms by digestion in the presence of pancreatic secretions.

Each proglottid has two layers of muscle – longitudinal and transverse – enabling the segment to move. Two lateral branches of nerves innervate the worm, with perpendicular commissures branching out into the parenchyma of each segment. Segments are anatomically independent, but they are all connected by a common nervous system emanating from central ganglia located in the scolex. Osmoregulation and excretion of wastes is via a lateral pair of excretory tubules.

Mature proglottids possess both male and female sex organs, but self-mating within a segment is unusual. Typically, sperm are transferred between mature proglottids that lie next to each other. Gravid proglottids develop after mating, and contain hundreds to thousands of embryonated eggs. The gravid proglottids then detach from the parent organism and exit via the anus. In some species, proglottids exit intact, while in others, segments disintegrate before leaving the host. Eggs are usually passed embryonated, and contain a hexacanth larva referred to as an oncosphere. Eggs may remain viable in the external environment for weeks to months after being deposited in soil. Hatching occurs typically within the small intestine of the intermediate host. The oncosphere then penetrates the gut tract and lodges within the tissues, developing into the metacestode. This stage is ingested by the definitive host and transforms to the adult in the lumen of the small intestine.

Adult tapeworms do not cause significant pathology in the human intestine. Unlike adult nematodes or trematodes, the adult cestodes do not adversely impact childhood development. However, when humans serve as intermediate hosts, the cestodes become significant causes of global morbidity. For instance, neurocysticercosis caused by the larval stages of the pork tapeworm, *Taenia solium*, is a leading cause of neurologic disease; in many countries it is the leading cause of epilepsy.

28. *Taenia saginata*
(Goeze 1782)

Introduction

Taenia saginata belongs to the order Cyclophyllidea, and is one of the largest parasites infecting humans, often achieving lengths approaching 8-10 m. Like all other adult tapeworms, it lives in the lumen of the upper half of the small intestine. There are no reservoir hosts for *T. saginata*. This tapeworm occurs wherever cattle husbandry is prevalent, and where human excreta are not disposed of properly.[1, 2] It is commonly referred to as the beef tapeworm, although the adult sexual stage of the parasite lives exclusively in humans and should perhaps be more properly called the "human tapeworm". Endemic foci include vast regions of Sub-Saharan grasslands in Africa, particularly in Ethiopia, due to the common dietary prac-

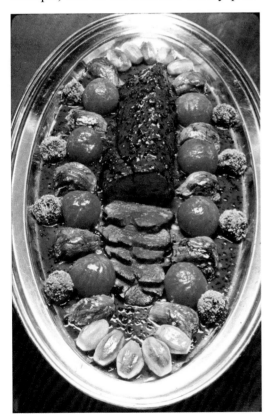
Figure 28.1. A rare beef tenderloin.

tice there of ingesting raw beef (*kitfo*), large portions of Northern Mexico, Argentina, and to a lesser extent, middle Europe. It is infrequently acquired in the United States, where most clinical cases are imported.

A third species, *Taenia asiatica*, infects people in Taiwan, Korea, China, Vietnam, and Indonesia.[3-5] Initially investigators felt that this organism should be considered a separate species (*T. asiatica*) from *T. saginata*, particularly since the intermediate host is porcine not bovine.[5, 6] With the introduction of molecular tools it became apparent that *T. asiatica* is a third species of the Taenia genus that infects humans.[7, 8] The full clinical spectrum of disease caused by *T. asiatica* is still not fully appreciated.

Historical Information

In 1683, Edward Tyson described several species of tapeworms, which he recovered from dogs.[9] Tyson is credited as the first person to recognize the head or scolex of these tapeworms.[10] In 1656, Félix Plater, a Swiss physician, wrote about the distinctions between *Taenia* spp. and *Diphyllobothrium latum* (then called *Lumbricus latus*).[11] Nicolas Andry de Boisregard is credited with the first report of *T. saginata* in 1700, but he didn't recognize that each proglottid was a separate unit, and did not distinguish this worm from other, similar tapeworms.[12] Johann Goeze was the first to describe the worm correctly, in 1782, in a larger treatise on helminthology, and suggested that *T. saginata* and *T. solium* adult worms were two different species.[13] In 1784, Goeze indicated that intermediate hosts in the life cycle of tapeworms were required when he noted that the scolices of tapeworms in humans resembled the cysts present in the muscles of pigs.[14] Carl Von Siebold, in 1850, speculated that "bladder worms" (i.e., cysticerci) could develop into adult tapeworms, or that perhaps they were only degenerated adults.[15] In 1861, Friedrich Kuchenmeister

Taenia saginata

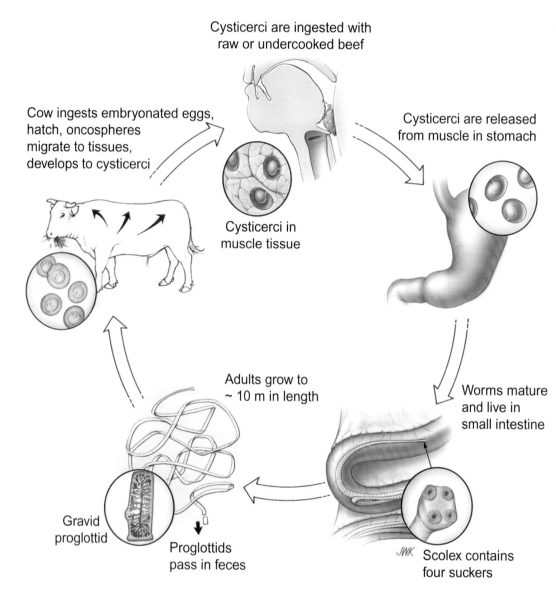

Cysticerci are ingested with
raw or undercooked beef

Cow ingests embryonated eggs,
hatch, oncospheres
migrate to tissues,
develops to cysticerci

Cysticerci are released
from muscle in stomach

Cysticerci in
muscle tissue

Adults grow to
~ 10 m in length

Worms mature
and live in
small intestine

Gravid
proglottid

Proglottids
pass in feces

Scolex contains
four suckers

Parasitic Diseases 6th Ed. Parasites Without Borders wwww.parasiteswithoutborders.com

fed meat from pigs containing tapeworm cysticerci to condemned prisoners, and then recovered the adult worms from these individuals intestines after their execution.[16] In 1863, Friedrich Leuckart reported on experiments showing that the proglottids of *T. saginata*, when fed to young calves, developed into cysticerci (metacestodes) in the animals' muscles.[17] In 1870, John Oliver, demonstrated that after human ingestion of measly beef, humans developed adult *T. saginata* infections, and further suggested that thorough cooking of infected meat would prevent infection with the adult tapeworm.[18]

Life Cycle

Infection begins when the cysticercus is ingested in raw or undercooked beef (Fig. 28.1). The cyst enters the small intestine and the wall of the cyst is digested away, freeing the worm inside. The parasite then everts its scolex and attaches to the intestinal wall with the aid of four sucker disks (Fig. 28.2). A mature adult tapeworm (Fig. 28.3) takes about three months to grow to full length. The developing proglottids (segments) extend down the small intestine, sometimes reaching the ileum. All adult tapeworms feed by

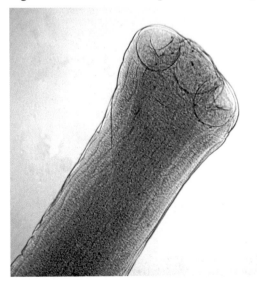

Figure 28.2. Scolex of *T. saginata*. Note four suckers.

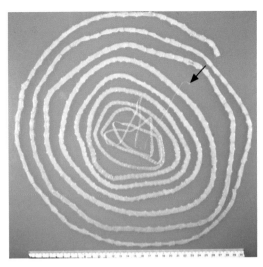

Figure 28.3. Adult *T. saginata*. Note the position of the scolex (arrow). Courtesy of U. Martin.

actively transporting nutrients (e.g., sugars, amino acids, nucleic acids) across their tegumental surface, since they have no digestive tract. Segments mature as they progress towards the terminal end of the worm. Terminal proglottids, gravid with hundreds of embryonated, infectious eggs, may detach from the colony, and may even actively migrate out the anus, where they may be deposited on the ground. Sometimes, whole ribbons of worms (20-30 segments) "escape" from an infected person.

A cow must then ingest a gravid segment, usually along with grass or hay, in order for the life cycle to continue. Eggs lying inside the lumen of the uterine branches of the proglottid are freed from the tapeworm tissue by the cow's digestive enzymes, stimulating the eggs to hatch in the small intestine (Fig. 28.5). The oncosphere (hexacanth or six-hooked larva) penetrates the intestinal wall, most likely aided by its hooks and peptidases that it secretes.[19] The larva enters the bloodstream and is passively carried throughout the body. Oncospheres can lodge in any one of a variety of tissues, depending upon where the circulation takes them. Mostly, they infect striated skeletal muscle tissue. There they encyst, and develop to the cysticercus (metacestode). This stage can live for several years before calcifying.

Cattle can experience disease due to the space-filling lesions created by cysticerci, especially if the cysts develop in sensitive areas (i.e., neurological tissues).[20] Usually they do not show signs of infection, since cattle are routinely slaughtered within several years of being born, and live cysticerci tend not to cause problems, even in neurological tissues (Chapter 32).

It is important to note that cattle cannot become infected with adult parasites if they accidentally ingest cysticerci. Similarly, humans cannot harbor the metacestode, since *Taenia saginata* eggs will only hatch in the stomachs of cows. There is no risk of invasive disease in humans from this parasite. This situation is in contrast to the significant health problem of cysticercosis due to the pork tapeworm, *Taenia solium*, in humans.

Most infected individuals harbor a single adult parasite, but there have been cases where numerous worms were recovered from a single infected individual. In these instances, the worms tend to be shorter due to crowding.[21]

Cellular and Molecular Pathogenesis

Taenia saginata occupies a large part of the lumen of the small intestine, but it is flexible and relatively fragile. Bowel obstruction does not occur. Adult worms are immunogenic, and specific serum antibodies are produced throughout the infection period, but local gut inflammatory responses are minimal.[22]

In cattle, immunity to reinfection develops locally in the small intestine, and is directed at newly arrived onchospheres. Challenge infection can be prevented by vaccination of cows with recombinant egg antigens.[22] Secretory IgA antibodies are thought to play a major role in this protective response, because colostrum from immune mothers protects sheep from invasion by oncospheres in experimental infections with closely related tapeworms.[23]

Clinical Disease

Most infections induce no symptoms, but some people may experience epigastric fullness. Rarely, postprandial nausea and vomiting occurs, and individual cases of jejunal perforation and Meckel's diverticulitis have been reported.[24, 25] Infection is usually first detected by noting proglottids in stool. Frequently, proglottids migrate out of the infected person overnight, and can be discovered in bedding or clothing the following morning. A somewhat disconcerting feature is that these proglottids move in a manner very similar to inchworms.

Diagnosis

One means of definitive diagnosis is by inspection of proglottids. Gravid proglottids can be fixed in 10% formaldehyde solution,

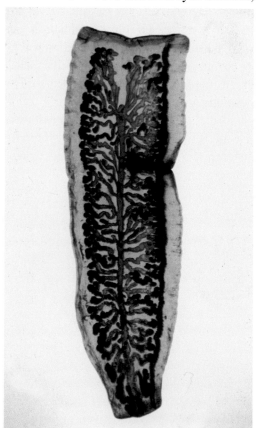

Figure 28.4. Gravid proglottid of *Taenia saginata*.

and the uterus injected with India ink, with the aid of a 26-gauge needle (Fig. 28.4). *T. saginata* proglottids have 12 or more branches on either side of the uterus.[26] In many modern labs these uterine branches are now visualized using hematoxyline-eosin staining techniques.[26] Eggs of *T. saginata* are occasionally found in stool, since most progottids usually pass out of the host intact. If an egg is seen on stool examination, the species cannot be determined on visual microscopy based on morphology, since all members of the family taeniidae produce visually identical ova. Upon acid-fast staining, occasionally the species can be distinguished, as fully-mature eggs of *T. saginata* have an acid-fast shell.[27, 28]

Adult worms remain in the intestine. Only proglottid segment pass in the stool. On the rare occasions that the scolex passes, such as after anti-parasitic therapy, it can be speciated. *T. saginata's* scolex has four lateral suckers but no hooks. The scolex of *T. solium* also has four suckers, but in addition, it has a double row of hooks.[26] Stool examination for eggs or proglottids is insensitive, since the passing of segments and eggs occurs only intermittentanly. Caution needs to be exercised by diagnostic parasitology technicians, because the eggs of *T. solium* are infectious for humans. An additional diagnostically relevant test is the sticky tape test (see: diagnosis for *Enterobius vermicularis*). When proglot-

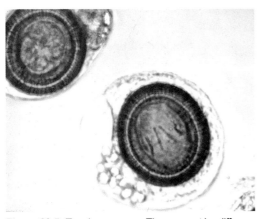

Figure 28.5. *Taenia* spp. eggs. They cannot be differentiated from eggs of other members of the taeniid family.

tids migrate out of the anus, they express eggs that remain on the perineum.

T. saginata eggs can also be differentiated from *T. solium* and *T. asiatica* eggs by PCR.[29-33] These molecular techniques have now advanced and loop-mediated isothermal amplification (LAMP) and multiplex PCR tests have become available.[34, 35] An ELISA test has been developed that detects soluble *T. saginata* antigens in stool samples (coproantigens) of infected humans.[36]

Treatment

Praziquantel (5-10 mg/kg) is effective for the treatment of *T. saginata* infection, and often allows recovery of the intact scolex, confirming cure of the patient.[37] Niclosamide is also effective in a single dose.[38, 39] Niclosamide inhibits the parasite's ATPase, thus preventing it from interfering with host digestive enzymes. The consequence of treatment is dissolution of the adult worm. A search for the scolex is futile. Quinacrine has also been reported to be effective for patients with niclosamide-resistant *T. saginata* infection, but it is not considered standard therapy.[40]

Prevention and Control

Preventing tapeworm infection in the community is through proper disposal of human feces, but has proven difficult in some parts of the world, since untreated human feces is widely used as fertilizer. Infection is fully prevented by cooking beef thoroughly, or by thoroughly freezing it prior to cooking. This is also not easily done, as people throughout the world enjoy eating rare or even raw beef. Meat inspection programs are effective in identifying contaminated meat, but inspection is not carried out in many endemic areas. A vaccine against the oncosphere of *T. saginata* for use in cattle has been developed and may prove useful in some endemic situations where vaccines are affordable.[22, 41] The development of an ELISA test that detects antibodies in cattle, specific for the cysticercus stage, will allow for efficient evaluation of control programs, especially where good public health practices are coupled with meat inspection at the abattoir.[42]

References

1.   Ito, A.; Wandra, T.; Li, T.; Dekumyoy, P.; Nkouawa, A.; Okamoto, M.; Budke, C. M., The present situation of human taeniases and cysticercosis in Asia. *Recent Pat Antiinfect Drug Discov* **2014,** *9* (3), 173-85.
2.   Silva, C. V.; Costa-Cruz, J. M., A glance at Taenia saginata infection, diagnosis, vaccine, biological control and treatment. *Infect Disord Drug Targets* **2010,** *10* (5), 313-21.
3.   Fan, P. C.; J., Annual economic loss caused by Taenia saginata asiatica Taeniasis in three endemic areas of east Asia. *Southeast Asian Med Public Health 28 Suppl* **1997,** *1* 217-21.
4.   McManus, D. P.; J., Molecular genetic variation in Echinococcus and Taenia: an update. *Southeast Asian Med Public Health 28 Suppl* **1997,** *1* 110-6.
5.   Ito, A.; Nakao, M.; Wandra, T., Human Taeniasis and cysticercosis in Asia. *Lancet (London, England)* **2003,** *362* (9399), 1918-20.
6.   Flisser, A.; Viniegra, A.-E.; Aguilar-Vega, L.; Garza-Rodriguez, A.; Maravilla, P.; Avila, G., Portrait of human tapeworms. *The Journal of parasitology* **2004,** *90* (4), 914-6.
7.   Galan-Puchades, M. T.; Fuentes, M. V., Lights and shadows of the Taenia asiatica life cycle and pathogenicity. *Trop Parasitol* **2013,** *3* (2), 114-9.
8.   Eom, K. S., What is Asian Taenia? *Parasitol Int* **2006,** *55 Suppl,* S137-41.
9.   Tyson, E., Lumbricus latus, or a discourse read before the Royal Society, of the joynted worm, wherein great many mistakes of former writers concerning it, are remarked; its natural history from more exact information is attempted; and the whole urged, as a difficulty against doctrine of univocal generation. *Philos Trans* **1683,** *13,* 113-144.
10.   Cox, F. E., History of human parasitology. *Clin Microbiol Rev* **2002,** *15* (4), 595-612.
11.   Plater, F., Praxeos Medicae Opus. *Basel* **1656.**
12.   Andry, N., De la Generation des Vers dans le Corps de l'Homme Paris. *1700.*
13.   Goeze, J. A. E.; Blankenburg, P. A., Versuch ciner Naturgeschichte der Eingeweiderwumer Thierischer Korper. *Pape* **1782.**
14.   Goeze, J. A. E., Neueste Entdeckung. Dass die Finnen im Schweinefleische keine Drusenkrankheit sondern wahre Blasenwurmer sind. Halle. **1784.**
15.   Siebold, C. T. E.; Z., Von Uber den Generationswechsel der Cestoden nebst einer Revision der Gattung Tetrarhynchus. *Zool* **1850,** *2* 198-253.
16.   Kuchenmeister, F., The Cysticercus cellulosus transformed within the organism of man into Taenia solium. *Lancet* **1861,** *i,* 39.
17.   Leuckart, R., Die menschlichen Parasiten und die von ihnen her ruhenden Krankheiten. *Em Handund Lehrbuch fur Naturforscher und Arzte C E Wintersche Verlagshandlung Leipzig* **1863.**
18.   Oliver, J. H., The importance of feeding the cattle and the thorough cooking of the meat, as the best preservatives against tapeworms. *Seventh Annual Report of the Sanitary Commissioner with the Government of India Calcutta pp* **1871,** 82-83.
19.   White, A. C.; Baig, S.; Robinson, P.; J., Taenia saginata oncosphere excretory/secretory peptidases. **1997,** *82* 7-10.
20.   Oryan, A.; Gaur, S. N.; Moghaddar, N.; Delavar, H., Clinico-pathological studies in cattle experimentally infected with Taenia saginata eggs. *Journal of the South African Veterinary Association* **1998,** *69* (4), 156-62.
21.   Despommier, D., People, Parasites, and Plowshares. 2014.
22.   Lightowlers, M. W.; Rolfe, R.; Gauci, C. G., Taenia saginata: vaccination against cysticercosis in cattle with recombinant oncosphere antigens. *Experimental parasitology* **1996,** *84* (3), 330-8.
23.   Gemmell, M. A.; Blundell-Hasell, S. K.; Macnamara, F. N., Immunological responses of the

mammalian host against tapeworm infections. IX. The transfer via colostrum of immunity to Taenia hydatigena. *Experimental parasitology* **1969,** *26* (1), 52-7.

24. Jongwutiwes, S.; Putaporntip, C.; Chantachum, N.; Sampatanukul, P., Jejunal perforation caused by morphologically abnormal Taenia saginata saginata infection. *The Journal of infection* **2004,** *49* (4), 324-8.

25. Chirdan, L. B.; Yusufu, L. M.; Ameh, E. A.; Shehu, S. M., Meckel's diverticulitis due to Taenia saginata: case report. *East African medical journal* **2001,** *78* (2), 107-8.

26. Mayta, H.; Talley, A.; Gilman, R. H.; Jimenez, J.; Verastegui, M.; Ruiz, M.; Garcia, H. H.; Gonzalez, A. E., Differentiating Taenia solium and Taenia saginata infections by simple hematoxylin-eosin staining and PCR-restriction enzyme analysis. *J Clin Microbiol* **2000,** *38* (1), 133-7.

27. Ide, L., To differentiate Taenia eggs. *J Clin Microbiol* **2012,** *50* (8), 2836; author reply 2837.

28. Jimenez, J. A.; Rodriguez, S.; Moyano, L. M.; Castillo, Y.; Garcia, H. H.; Cysticercosis Working Group in, P., Differentiating Taenia eggs found in human stools: does Ziehl-Neelsen staining help? *Trop Med Int Health* **2010,** *15* (9), 1077-81.

29. Gonzalez, L. M.; Montero, E.; R., Differential diagnosis of Taenia saginata and Taenia solium infections: from DNA probes to polymerase chain reaction. *Trans Trop Med Hyg 96 Suppl* **2002,** *1* S243-50.

30. Gonzalez, L. M.; Montero, E.; J., Differential diagnosis of Taenia saginata and Taenia solium infection by PCR. *Microbiol* **2000,** *38*, 737-44.

31. Rodriguez-Hidalgo, R.; Geysen, D.; Benítez-Ortiz, W.; Geerts, S.; Brandt, J., Comparison of conventional techniques to differentiate between Taenia solium and Taenia saginata and an improved polymerase chain reaction-restriction fragment length polymorphism assay using a mitochondrial 12S rDNA fragment. *The Journal of parasitology* **2002,** *88* (5), 1007-11.

32. Nunes, C. M.; Lima, L. G. F.; Manoel, C. S.; Pereira, R. N.; Nakano, M. M.; Garcia, J. F., Taenia saginata: polymerase chain reaction for taeniasis diagnosis in human fecal samples. *Experimental parasitology* **2003,** *104* (1-2), 67-9.

33. Gonzalez, L. M.; Montero, E., Differential diagnosis of Taenia saginata and Taenia saginata asiatica Taeniasis through PCR. *Diagn Microbiol Infect Dis* **2004,** *49*, 183-8.

34. Sako, Y.; Nkouawa, A.; Yanagida, T.; Ito, A., Loop-mediated isothermal amplification method for a differential identification of human Taenia tapeworms. *Methods Mol Biol* **2013,** *1039*, 109-20.

35. Nkouawa, A.; Sako, Y.; Li, T.; Chen, X.; Nakao, M.; Yanagida, T.; Okamoto, M.; Giraudoux, P.; Raoul, F.; Nakaya, K.; Xiao, N.; Qiu, J.; Qiu, D.; Craig, P. S.; Ito, A., A loop-mediated isothermal amplification method for a differential identification of Taenia tapeworms from human: application to a field survey. *Parasitol Int* **2012,** *61* (4), 723-5.

36. Deplazes, P.; Eckert, J.; Pawlowski, Z. S.; Machowska, L.; Gottstein, B., An enzyme-linked immunosorbent assay for diagnostic detection of Taenia saginata copro-antigens in humans. *Transactions of the Royal Society of Tropical Medicine and Hygiene* **1991,** *85* (3), 391-6.

37. Pawlowski, Z. S., Efficacy of low doses of praziquantel in taeniasis. *Acta Trop Basel* **1991,** *48*, 83-88.

38. Keeling, J. E. D., The chemotherapy of cestode infections. *Adv Chemother* **1978,** *3*, 109-152.

39. Vermund, S. H.; MacLeod, S.; Goldstein, R. G., Taeniasis unresponsive to a single dose of niclosamide: case report of persistent infection with Taenia saginata and a review of therapy. *Reviews of infectious diseases* **1986,** *8* (3), 423-6.

40. Koul, P. A.; Wahid, A.; Bhat, M. H.; Wani, J. I.; Sofi, B. A., Mepacrine therapy in niclosamide resistant taeniasis. *The Journal of the Association of Physicians of India* **2000,** *48* (4), 402-3.

41. Lightowlers, M. W.; Colebrook, A. L.; Gauci, C. G.; Gauci, S. M.; Kyngdon, C. T.; Monkhouse, J. L.; Vallejo Rodriquez, C.; Read, A. J.; Rolfe, R. A.; Sato, C., Vaccination against cestode parasites: anti-helminth vaccines that work and why. *Veterinary parasitology* **2003,** *115* (2), 83-123.

42. Onyango-Abuje, J. A.; Hughes, G.; Opicha, M.; Nginyi, K. M.; Rugutt, M. K.; Wright, S. H.; Harrison, L. J., Diagnosis of Taenia saginata cysticercosis in Kenyan cattle by antibody and antigen ELISA. *Veterinary parasitology* **1996,** *61* (3-4), 221-30.

29. *Taenia solium*
(Linnaeus 1758)

Introduction

Taenia solium belongs to the order Cyclophyllidea, and its occurrence is associated with the raising of pigs. It is commonly known as the pork tapeworm, although this worm only reaches sexual maturity as an adult in humans.[1, 2] In order to transmit *T. solium*, human feces, contaminated with the mature segments of the worm, must be a regular contaminant of the pigs' environment, and coincident with the habit of eating raw or undercooked pork products. These conditions exist in many parts of the world.

T. solium is a large tapeworm, often achieving lengths of more than 6 m. It lives in the lumen, attached to the wall of the small intestine. There are no reservoir hosts for this parasite.[3] Unlike the egg of *T. saginata*, the egg of *T. solium* can infect the human host, resulting in a condition called cysticercosis. This juvenile infection can be serious, even fatal, particularly if the larval tapeworm invades the CNS.[4, 5] Neurocysticercosis ranks among the most common causes of acquired epilepsy, worldwide.[6]

T. solium is endemic in most of South America (particularly in the Andean region and Brazil), Central America, Mexico, China, the Indian subcontinent and Southeast Asia, Sub-Saharan Africa (particularly, Burundi, Tanzania, Democratic Republic of Congo, and South Africa), and Eastern Europe.[7, 8] It is an issue worldwide due to the high number of imported cases seen even outside the endemic areas.[4, 5, 9] In some of these endemic regions up to 6 percent of the population may harbor *T. solium* adult tapeworms.[6] The highest prevalence of *T. solium* infection in the United States occurs among Hispanic populations in Southern California, New Mexico, and Texas. This is because of the large number of immigrants from some endemic areas mentioned above.[6, 10, 11] Among adult migrant workers in California, for instance, the sero-prevalence of *T. solium* is approximately 1-2 percent.[12, 13] In endemic regions, *T. solium* occurs more commonly in children and adolescents.[6] In addition to imported infections, it is believed that autochthonous transmission of *T. solium* infection also occurs in the US.[14] One estimate suggests that tens of thousands of cases occur in the U.S., but there is a need for better surveillance and disease detection in order to obtain a more precise estimate.[15]

In 2003, the Fifty-Sixth World Health Assembly highlighted the public health threat caused by *T. solium* and urged its member states to increase measures to control this infection.[10] In 2012, the World Health Organization (WHO), the Food and Agriculture Organization (FAO), and the UK Department for International Development (DFID), included *Taenia solium* among the 17 neglected zoonotic diseases that they felt could be targeted for effective control.[16, 17]

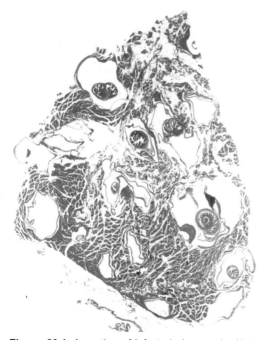

Figure 29.1. A section of infected pig muscle. Note numerous cysticerci.

Historical Information

The history of the different tapeworms is initially intertwined, as it was not until many years after their initial discovery that it was determined that these similar parasites were fundamentally different in terms of their morphology and host specificity.[18] In 1683, Edward Tyson described several tapeworms, which he recovered from dogs.[19] Tyson is credited as the first person to recognize the head or scolex of these tapeworms.[18] In 1656, Félix Plater, a Swiss physician, wrote about the distinctions between *Taenia* spp. and *Diphyllobothrium latum* (then called *Lumbricus latus*).[20] In 1782, Johann Goeze described the adult tapeworm, but it was Aristole who wrote about the cysticercus stage of the worm in the muscles of pigs.[21] There is no evidence that Goeze comprehended the relationship between the larval infection in the pig and the adult infection in humans. Cysticercosis in pigs was described by Philip Hartmann in 1688.[22] In 1861, Friedrich Kuchenmeister, fed meat from pigs containing tapeworm cysticerci to condemned prisoners and then recovered the adult worms from these individuals intestines 120 hours after death at autopsy.[23, 24]

Life Cycle

The phase of the life cycle that occurs in humans is dependent on whether a human ingests *T. solium* eggs or encapsulated cysticeri in undercooked meat. Intestinal infection in the human host begins following the ingestion of raw or undercooked pork that harbors the encapsulated cysticercus (i.e., juvenile) stage of the worm (Figs. 29.1, 29.2). The capsule is digested in the stomach freeing the juvenile parasite. Upon entering the small intestine, the worm everts its scolex and attaches to the intestinal wall with the aid of its four suckers and crown of hooklets. In an experimental infection of hamsters with onchospheres of *T. solium*, the attachment site

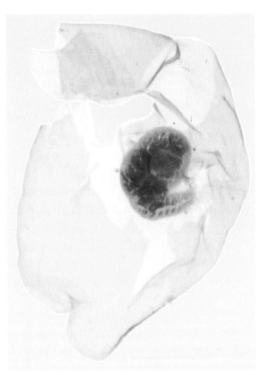

Figure 29.2. Isolated whole cysticercus of *Taenia solium*, measuring 2-5 mm in diameter.

in the gut tract was studied.[25] The hooklets penetrated the intestinal wall, while the four suckers all attached to cells of the surrounding villi. Host cell damage was observed in and around each sucker disk.

The intestinal phase of the life cycle of *T. solium* is very similar to that of *T. saginata*. The juvenile parasite develops to the adult (Fig. 29.3) in the small intestine over a three-month period, after which gravid (egg-laden) proglottids begin passing from the host. Adult *Taenia solium* scolices closely resemble the adult worm of *T. saginata*, except that *T. solium* scolex possesses two rows of hooklets, in addition to four sucker disks (Fig. 29.4). Usually, adult *T. solium* do not live in the human gastrointestinal tract for more than 5 years.[6] Humans are the only definitive host, and the adult of *T. solium* will not develop in the pig if it accidentally ingests cysticerci from contaminated pork scraps.

Unlike infection with *Taenia saginata*, the tissue phase of the life cycle can occur in humans, as well as in pigs following ingestion

Taenia solium

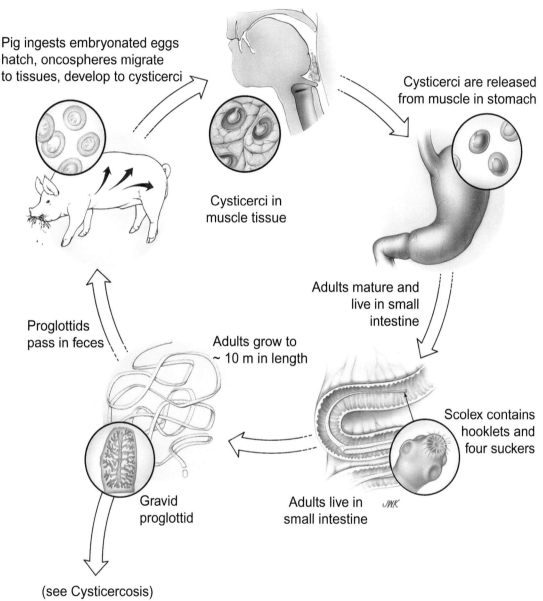

Cysticerci are ingested
with raw or undercooked pork

Pig ingests embryonated eggs
hatch, oncospheres migrate
to tissues, develop to cysticerci

Cysticerci are released
from muscle in stomach

Cysticerci in
muscle tissue

Adults mature and
live in small
intestine

Proglottids
pass in feces

Adults grow to
~ 10 m in length

Scolex contains
hooklets and
four suckers

Gravid
proglottid

Adults live in
small intestine

(see Cysticercosis)

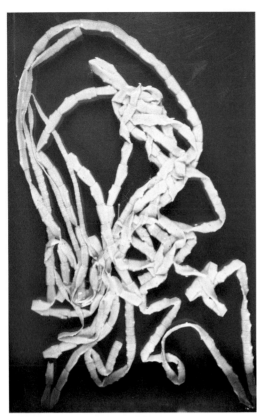

Figure 29.3. Whole adult *T. solium.* Arrow indicates scolex.

of embryonated *Taenia solium* eggs (Figs. 29.5, 29.6). When the egg is ingested, the larva (oncosphere) inside survives the gastric acid of the stomach and enters the small intestine. The egg hatches and the larva penetrates the intestinal wall and enters the bloodstream. Eventually, the oncosphere penetrates into one of many tissues (e.g., striated muscles, heart, brain, eye) and encysts there. The oncosphere rapidly differentiates into a cysticercus (Fig. 29.7), grows, develops, and creates a space-filling lesion within 2-3 months, typically measuring approximately 10 mm.[3] Cysticerci achieve maximum growth about three weeks after entering a given tissue, and then cease growing. In some cases, it is thought that humans auto-infect with the contaminated eggs of their own tapeworm. The frequency of *T. solium* auto-infection is not known, although it has been observed that up to 15 percent of patients with cysticercosis also harbor an adult *T. solium* tapeworm.[6]

Cellular and Molecular Pathogenesis

The adult parasite living in the intestinal lumen does not usually cause a significant host inflammatory response, but it does elicit the formation of humoral antibodies.[26] Infected pigs harboring the juvenile stage are less likely to become re-infected when they ingest more eggs, most likely because they are protected by immune responses directed against the oncosphere.[27] A similar situation exists between the cysticercus of *T. saginata* and cattle. The cDNAs encoding two *Taenia solium* glucose transporter molecules have been expressed in bacteria, and their fusion proteins identified and characterized.[28] One is on the tegumental surface of the adult worm (TGTP1) and the other is on the surface of the larva (TGTP2). Both molecules have the potential for being used as targets of vaccines aimed at preventing each stage from access-

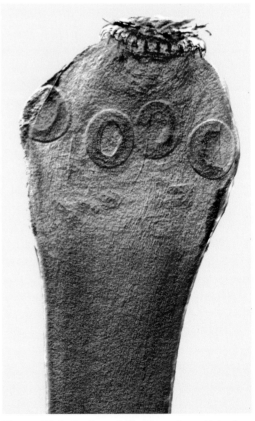

Figure 29.4. Scolex of *Taenia solium.* Note four suckers and hooks. Photo E. Gravé

Cysticercosis
(Taenia solium)

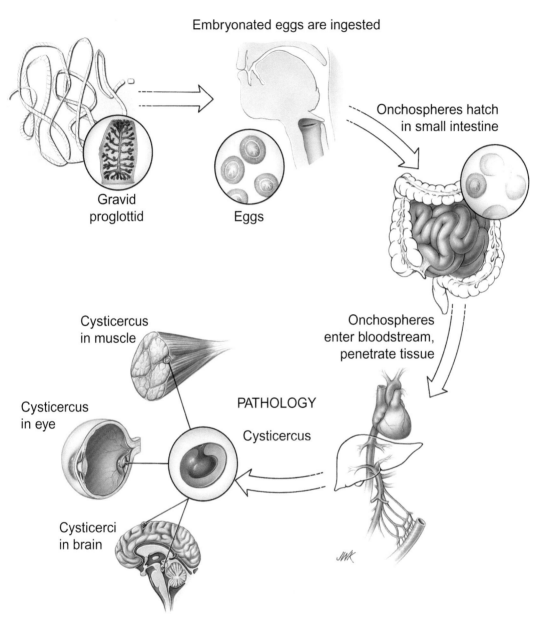

Embryonated eggs are ingested

Gravid proglottid

Eggs

Onchospheres hatch in small intestine

Onchospheres enter bloodstream, penetrate tissue

Cysticercus in muscle

Cysticercus in eye

PATHOLOGY

Cysticercus

Cysticerci in brain

Parasitic Diseases 6th Ed. Parasites Without Borders www.parasiteswithoutborders.com

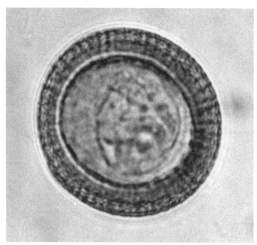

Figure 29.5. *Taenia* spp. egg. The species of tapeworm cannot be determined based on its morphology. Eggs measure 30-40 μm in diameter.

ing host glucose. Vaccines using recombinant *Taenia solium* oncosphere larval antigens TSOL18, TSOL45-1A and TSOL16 produced in *E. coli* have been studied with demonstrated efficacy in preventing infection in pigs, both under controlled experimental conditions and in field trials.[29, 30]

In the tissue phase, much of the pathological consequences are those of a space-occupying lesion and the inflammation that results upon death of the parasites.[31] Oncospheres that lodge in the CNS (Fig. 29.8) or brain (Fig. 29.9) develop with little immune response until the parasites start to die, triggering an intense immune response accompanied by edema, and in many cases, seizures.[32]

Oncospheres, other than those in the CNS, are presumably more susceptible to immune attack, but their rapid development to the cysticercus stage may account for the high rate of survival, at least during a primary infection. Cysticercus development is coincident with modulation of host immune responses, favoring expression of parasite immune evasion mechanisms that interfere with Th2-type protective immune responses.[32] Immunomodulatory substances have been identified and partially characterized; for example, *Taenia*statin, a protease inhibitor, and para-

myosin, which inhibit different aspects of the complement cascade.[33-35]

Ultimately, cysticerci die after several years and become calcified. Dying parasites release their suppressive hold on protective host immune responses, and antigens are released. When cellular reactions are present, they are in part due to the result of interleukin signaling from T cells. Specific IgM antibodies and NK+ cells are also present in these infiltrates.[36] An acute local inflammatory reaction follows, consisting of lymphocytes, plasma cells, and eosinophils, which may be clinically significant in neurocysticercosis.[32] This host inflammatory response around degenerating cysticerci, when it occurs in the brain, may be responsible for eliciting seizures and intracranial hypertension. Neuroimaging studies (CT with contrast or MRI) reveal the inflammation encircling the lesion, giving rise to the appearance of "ring-enhancement." In addition, cysticerci occurring in anatomically sensitive sites in the central nervous system can cause mass effect, or block the circulation of cerebrospinal fluid leading to hydrocephalus.[6]

Strong, protective immunity to invasion of tissues by oncospheres can be induced in a variety of animals, and these findings offer hope for developing a vaccine for use in pigs and possibly humans.[37]

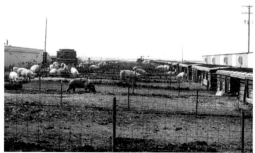

Figure 29.6. Commercial feedlot. This environment is frequently contaminated with human feces in many regions of the world where pigs are raised. Courtesy P. M. Schantz.

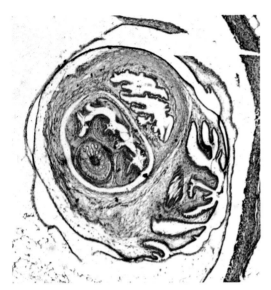

Figure 29.7. Cysticercus of *Taenia solium*.

Clinical Disease

Adult *T. solium* cause few symptoms other than perhaps epigastric fullness in some individuals. Patients are usually asymptomatic, and do not become aware of their infection until they discover the proglottids in stool, on the perianal skin, in clothing, or bed sheets. Some patients report abdominal pain, distension, diarrhea, and nausea, but there are no controlled studies to demonstrate their link with the presence of *T. solium* in the gut. These symptoms may be due to other causes.[6] Two patients with *T. solium* infection were reported to develop ascites, chronic diarrhea, and malabsorption, which resolved following anthelminthic therapy, but the connection to infection with *T. solium* is still unclear.[38]

Invasive disease has two major clinical presentations; extraneural (subcutaneous and intramuscular) cysticercosis and neurocysticercosis.[6] These two conditions are not mutually exclusive, as most of the patients with neurocysticercosis also have evidence for disease in other parts of the body.[6]

Extraneural cysticercosis is usually asymptomatic, but patients may notice painless subcutaneous nodules in the arms or chest, or small, discrete swellings of particu-lar muscles (Fig. 29.10), in which cysticerci have lodged.[39] After several months, the nodules become swollen and tender, presumably because of the host inflammatory response to the cysticerci. Subsequently, the nodules disappear. There may be geographic variation in this clinical presentation because subcutaneous cysticercosis is common in Asia and Africa, but rare in Latin America.[6] Ultimately, these lesions will calcify after death of the parasite. The calcifications can persist for years. Some patients with extraneural cysticercosis can also harbor cardiac cysticerci, which is usually also asymptomatic.[6]

Neurocysticercosis (cysticercosis in the central nervous system) is the most severe manifestation that follows the ingestion of *T. solium* eggs. The signs and symptoms vary greatly with the number and distribution of cysts (Figs. 29.8 – 29.13).[39] It often presents as a space-occupying lesion, and in many respects mimics a tumor.[31] Seizures, hydrocephalus, epilepsy, and focal neurologic abnormalities may be the presenting signs.[40] It has been estimated that seizures occur in 50-80 percent of patients with brain parenchymal cysts, which occur as a consequence of host inflammation around dead and degenerating parasites.[6, 41] In endemic regions, teen-

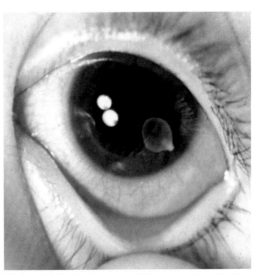

Figure 29.8 Cysticercus of *Taenia solium* floating free in the anterior chamber of the eye.

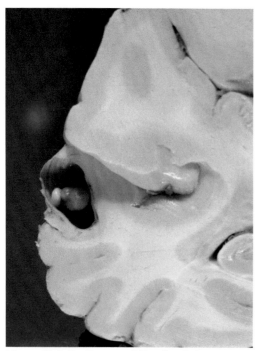

Figure 29.9. Cysticercus of *T. solium* in brain.

inflammation.[6]

Ophthalmic cysticercosis occurs in approximately 1-3 percent of all infections, and most typically manifests as intraocular cysts floating freely in the vitreous humor or the subretinal space. Patients complain of seeing shadows. Subsequent development of uveitis, retinitis, or choroidal atrophy can lead to visual loss.[6]

Diagnosis

Diagnosis of the adult phase can be made by identifying the taenia eggs by microscopy, by analysis of the gravid proglottids, or by recovery and identification of the scolex in feces. Overall, the sensitivity of stool microscopy is poor, and even then, *T. solium* eggs are morphologically indistinguishable from *T. saginata* eggs. A DNA dot blot test can differ-

age and young adults exhibit the highest rates of *T. solium* seizures.[6] These patients, especially females, can also develop an accompanying encephalitis.[6] Children immigrating to the United States from endemic areas may present with a solitary mass or multiple lesions and seizures.[42] Usually, with those suffering seizures, the cysticercus has begun to degenerate and in some cases started to calcify (Fig. 29.13).[43]

People still residing in endemic areas are often found to have more complex disease, and have a greater likelihood of presenting with multiple cysts, including cysts that locate in the subarachnoid space or the ventricles.[6] These patients present with elevated intracranial pressure, arachnoiditis, meningitis, encephalitis, or hydrocephalus.[44] They are also more likely to experience stroke.

There appear to be geographic differences in the presentation of clinical neurocysticercosis. In Asia, patients most commonly present with a single enhancing brain lesion, whereas in Latin America it is common to find multiple cysts without evidence of

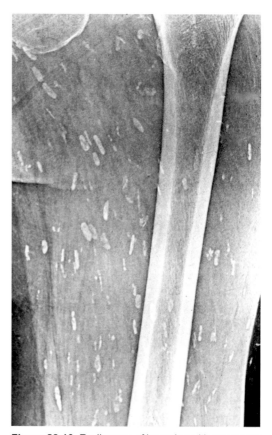

Figure 29.10. Radiogram of lower leg with numerous cysticerci of *Taenia solium*.

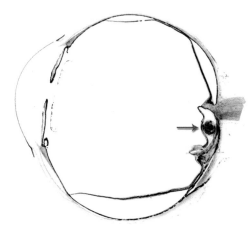

Figure 29.11. Cross section of whole eye with cysticercus of *T. solium* (arrow) in retina at the level of the optic nerve.

entiate *T. solium* from *T. saginata*.[45] Nucleic acid amplification tests as well as fecal antigen tests are now available for diagnosis and differentiation of *T. solium* eggs from *T. saginata*.[46-48] Perianal scraping with adhesive tape to trap eggs has been used to improve the sensitivity of microscopy, but this technique is not as effective for *T. solium* infection as it is for *T. saginata*.

Gravid proglottid segments should be fixed in 10% formaldehyde solution, and injected with India ink to fill the uterus. Proglottids of *T. solium* have less than 12 uterine branches per side (Fig. 29.14), compared to those of *T. saginata*, which have 12 or more (Fig. 28.4). These proglottid segments can also be prepared and viewed using standard hematoxylin and eosin staining. Extreme caution must be exercised when handling unfixed proglottids of *T. solium*, since the embryonated eggs are infectious.

Because of the distinct morphological features of the *T. solium* scolex compared with that of *T. saginata*, the gold standard of taeniasis diagnosis had traditionally been the recovery and visualization of this portion of the parasite. Polyethylene glycol salt purges to improve bowel cleaning significantly improves the likelihood of scolex recovery, but is not often used.[49]

ELISA performed on fecal extracts for antigen detection is sensitive (95 percent) and specific (99 percent).[50] Patients with adult tapeworms also produce antibodies detectable by immunoblot assay.[51] Serological assay is particularly useful for epidemiological studies.

Diagnosis of cysticercosis is usually based on imaging tests and criteria have been established.[6, 44, 52] Neuroimaging by CT or MRI is of critical importance in diagnosing neurocysticercosis. Ideally, both modalities are employed, combining the advantage of higher sensitivity of MRI with CT detection of calcium. Because it is often not practical to biopsy cysticerci, consulting a neuroradiologist is extremely helpful. On CT, the cysts appear as hypodense images containing a small hyperdense nodule that represents the parasite scolex. At times, calcium can also be observed. Inflammation surrounding dead and dying parasites will provide so-called

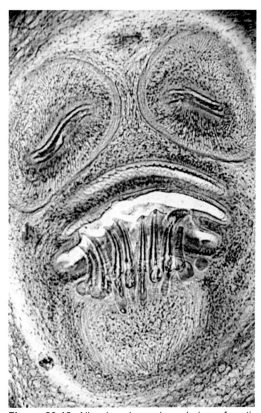

Figure 29.12. Alien invader: enlarged view of cysticercus from Figure 29.11.

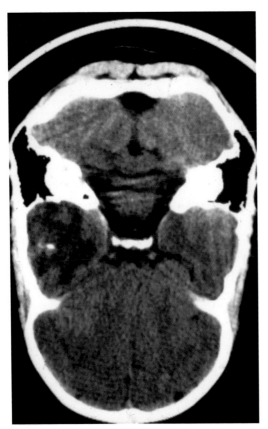

Figure 29.13. Radiogram of brain with calcified lesion due to infection with the metacestode of *T. solium*.

ring-enhancement in the presence of contrast media. In the natural history of neurocysticercosis, the dead and dying cysts calcify. MRI is more expensive but is becoming more available in developing countries, as it often provides a clearer image of the cysticercus, and has greater sensitivity for multiple lesions.[6]

Serologic testing provides important confirmatory data for patients with suspicious lesions on CT or MRI. Serological testing assays have improved, with a sensitivity of 98 percent and a specificity approaching 100 percent.[6, 53-55] For patients with a solitary lesion, the sensitivity is much lower, presumably because of the small amount of parasite antigen available to the host immune system. In an acute care setting, the ELISA requires considerable interpretation because antibody titers can remain high long after the death of the parasites.[6]

Treatment

Before initiation of treatment for any taenia infection, it is important to look for the presence of neurocysticercosis. Praziquantel is the drug of choice for adult *T. solium*, but its use must be tempered by the possibility that this treatment will also destroy occult cysticerci in the brain, and trigger central nervous system manifestations.[6] If neurocysticercosis has either been effectively ruled out or treated, then treatment of the intestinal worms can be given. Praziquantel is usually available in developing countries, particularly because of its use for global schistosomiasis control, and its proven success in Mexico in reducing the prevalence where taeniasis is endemic.[10] No purgatives should be used, because this increases the risk of regurgitating eggs into the stomach, initiating infection leading to cysticercosis.[56, 57] Niclosamide is an alternative for adult *T. solium* when praziquantel is unavailable (2 g orally in a single dose).[6, 58]

Treatment of neurocysticercosis is based

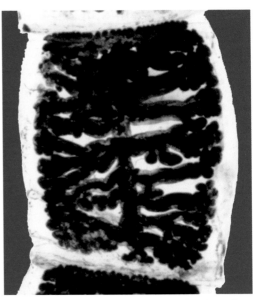

Figure 29.14 Gravid proglottid of *Taenia solium*. Uterus contains less than 12 lateral branches on each side.

on the number of lesions, the stage of these lesions, and their location. Lesions can be single or multiple. The lesions may be viable (vesicular stage), degenerate (the colloidal stage), collapsed (granular nodular stage), or nonviable (calcified).[59] The lesions can be either intraparenchymal or extraparenchymal (vesicular). Seizures most often occur in neurocysticercosis when the host inflammatory response is activated as parasites begin to die. In this situation, initiation of therapy can trigger edema with resultant seizure activity.[6] Increasingly, the complexities of the medical and surgical management of neurocysticercosis require a team approach, and the addition of anti-inflammatory agents such as corticosteroids. Typically, this might include an infectious disease specialist, a neurologist, a neuroradiologist, an ophthalmologist and a neurosurgeon.[60]

Albendazole has the drug of choice for neurocysticercosis with better efficacy than praziquantel and less drug interactions with steroids and seizure medications.[61, 62] Often albendazole is combined with praziquantel due to evidence demonstrating improved effect with combination therapy but in this context interactions with corticosteroids and seizures medications need be managed.[63] It is the inflammatory response in the brain that is largely responsible for seizures, encephalitis, and elevated intracranial pressure. The results of two double-blind, placebo-controlled trials in patients with a solitary enhancing lesion, and a third double-blind, placebo-controlled trial comparing the evolution of brain parenchymal lesions on CT after three months of treatment was summarized by Garcia.[6] Only one of these trials showed benefit from albendazole in terms of resolution of images and seizures. The current recommendation is that therapeutic decisions on using albendazole (15 mg/kg daily for 10-14 days) with or without praziquantel (50mg/kg for 10 days) need to be tailored to the individual patient, based on the number, location, and viability of the cysticerci.[6, 63] All patients selected for treatment with anthelminthic drugs should undergo a prior ophthalmologic exam in order to rule out intraocular cysts and be counseled about the risk of treatment-induced seizures.

Guidelines on the use of anthelminthic chemotherapy have been published.[64] Since patients with single ring-enhancing lesions on CT scans often improve spontaneously without any therapy, they can be followed and not given albendazole or steroids.[65, 66] In the case of multiple viable cysticerci, most clinicians suggest treatment with albendazole and prednisone, with monitoring for elevations in intracranial pressure and seizures.[4, 6]

Because both albendazole and praziquantel kill cysticerci and exacerbate brain inflammation and edema, patients being treated for neurocysticercosis also require steroids, usually dexamethasone, to reduce swelling. Dexamethasone affects the blood levels of both praziquantel and albendazole, so drug doses of both may need to be adjusted.[67] Additional medical management with anticonvulsants is also a critical component of the long-term management of *T. solium*-induced seizures.

Neurosurgical management with placement of ventricular shunts is often required for complicated neurocysticercosis involving cerebrospinal obstruction and hydrocephalus. Surgical management may also be required for spinal lesions and eye lesions.

Prevention and Control

Taenia solium is a significant public health problem, even outside the endemic areas, due to the association of cysticercosis with the adult infections.[68] For example, an outbreak of cysticercosis was reported among an orthodox Jewish community in New York City resulting from the ingestion of *T. solium* eggs passed from domestic employees who were recent emigrants from Latin America.[69]

It has been suggested that recent emigrants from countries in which *T. solium* infection is endemic should be screened for tapeworm infection before they are employed as housekeepers or food handlers.[69]

In many impoverished regions in developing countries, pigs are more affordable than cows, since pigs behave like omnivores. That is why owners allow them to roam free and eat garbage and human feces.[6] The infection in pigs is preventable by protecting their feed from contamination with human feces. Individual infection is prevented by thoroughly cooking pork, or by freezing it at -10 °C for a minimum of 5 days. Cysticerci can survive in meat refrigerated at 4°C for up to 30 days.[70]

In 2003, the World Health Assembly identified several measures to control *T. solium* infection including; 1. identification and treatment of individuals who carry the adult tapeworm, 2. universal or selected treatment with praziquantel to reduce the prevalence in areas where *T. solium* infection is endemic, 3. veterinary sanitary measures, such as enforced meat inspection and control, 4. improvement of pig husbandry, and treatment of infected animals with single-dose therapy, and 5. case management, reporting and surveillance of people with cysticercosis. Community-based interventions comprised of sanitation and pig management highly effective in disease control.[71] Ring-screening strategies have been proposed to control *T. solium* infection.[72] Anthelminthic chemotherapy programs need to be linked with other health programs using a wider integrated approach.[10] In 2012, *T. solium* was added by the WHO to their list of neglected zoonotic diseases that they felt could be targeted for effective control.[16, 17]

Inoculation of pigs with recombinant antigens cloned from parasite oncosphere mRNA appears to be an effective vaccine, and could be used to reduce the incidence of adult tapeworm in a few countries, such as Mexico, where public health programs can be integrated with prevention on the farm.[37, 73-75] In one experimental study, treating all pigs eliminated 100% of viable cysticerci.[76] Serological testing in the abattoir is now also possible.[77] Any of these three approaches, or in combination, could significantly reduce transmission of *T. solium* to humans, if applied rigorously to commercial pig farms in endemic areas.

Some black bears in California have acquired cysticercosis, most likely as the result of feeding at garbage dumps near campgrounds.[78] Hunting bears is a popular sport in the United States, and distributing meat from kills to neighbors is common practice among hunters. Hunter organizations should issue warnings, advising hunters that any meat obtained from carnivores or omnivores should be cooked well before eating.

References

1. Bush, A. O.; Lafferty, K. D.; Lotz, J. M.; Shostak, A. W., Parasitology meets ecology on its own terms: Margolis et al. revisited. *J Parasitol* **1997**, *83* (4), 575-83.
2. Pojmanska, T., [A review of ecologic terms used in current parasitology]. *Wiad Parazytol* **1993**, *39* (3), 285-97.
3. Pawlowski, Z.; Allan, J.; Sarti, E., Control of Taenia solium taeniasis/cysticercosis: from research towards implementation. *Int J Parasitol* **2005**, *35* (11-12), 1221-32.
4. Coyle, C. M., Neurocysticercosis: an update. *Curr Infect Dis Rep* **2014**, *16* (11), 437.
5. Coyle, C. M.; Mahanty, S.; Zunt, J. R.; Wallin, M. T.; Cantey, P. T.; White, A. C., Jr.; O'Neal, S. E.; Serpa, J. A.; Southern, P. M.; Wilkins, P.; McCarthy, A. E.; Higgs, E. S.; Nash, T. E., Neurocysticercosis: neglected but not forgotten. *PLoS Negl Trop Dis* **2012**, *6* (5), e1500.
6. Garcia, H. H.; Gonzalez, A. E.; Eveans, C. A. W.; Gilman, R. H., The Cysticercosis Working Group in Peru. *Lancet* **2003**, *361*, 547-56.

7.   Nsengiyumva, G.; Druet-Cabanac, M.; Ramanankandrasana, B.; Bouteille, B.; Nsizabira, L.; Preux, P. M., Cysticercosis as a major risk factor for epilepsy in Burundi, east Africa. *Epilepsia* **2003**, *44* (7), 950-5.

8.   Mwidunda, S. A.; Carabin, H.; Matuja, W. B.; Winkler, A. S.; Ngowi, H. A., A school based cluster randomised health education intervention trial for improving knowledge and attitudes related to Taenia solium cysticercosis and taeniasis in Mbulu district, northern Tanzania. *PLoS One* **2015**, *10* (2), e0118541.

9.   Zammarchi, L.; Strohmeyer, M.; Bartalesi, F.; Bruno, E.; Munoz, J.; Buonfrate, D.; Nicoletti, A.; Garcia, H. H.; Pozio, E.; Bartoloni, A.; Group, C. P. S., Epidemiology and management of cysticercosis and Taenia solium taeniasis in Europe, systematic review 1990-2011. *PLoS One* **2013**, *8* (7), e69537.

10.   Fifty Sixth World Health Organization, Control of neurocysticercosis, Report by the Health Assembly. http://www.who.int **2003**.

11.   Despommier, D. D., Tapeworm infection--the long and the short of it. *N Engl J Med* **1992**, *327* (10), 727-8.

12.   Richards, F. O.; Schantz, P. M.; Ruiz-Tiben, E.; Sorvillo, F. J., Cysticercosis in Los Angeles County. *JAMA* **1985**, *254* (24), 3444-8.

13.   DeGiorgio, C.; Pietsch-Escueta, S.; Tsang, V.; Corral-Leyva, G.; Ng, L.; Medina, M. T.; Astudillo, S.; Padilla, N.; Leyva, P.; Martinez, L.; Noh, J.; Levine, M.; del Villasenor, R.; Sorvillo, F., Sero-prevalence of Taenia solium cysticercosis and Taenia solium taeniasis in California, USA. *Acta neurologica Scandinavica* **2005**, *111* (2), 84-8.

14.   Cantey, P. T.; Coyle, C. M.; Sorvillo, F. J.; Wilkins, P. P.; Starr, M. C.; Nash, T. E., Neglected parasitic infections in the United States: cysticercosis. *Am J Trop Med Hyg* **2014**, *90* (5), 805-9.

15.   Hotez, P. J., Neglected infections of poverty in the United States of America. *PLoS Negl Trop Dis* **2008**, *2* (6), e256.

16.   Fleury, A.; Trejo, A.; Cisneros, H.; Garcia-Navarrete, R.; Villalobos, N.; Hernandez, M.; Villeda Hernandez, J.; Hernandez, B.; Rosas, G.; Bobes, R. J.; de Aluja, A. S.; Sciutto, E.; Fragoso, G., Taenia solium: Development of an Experimental Model of Porcine Neurocysticercosis. *PLoS Negl Trop Dis* **2015**, *9* (8), e0003980.

17.   WHO, Accelerating work to overcome the global impact of neglected tropical diseases A roadmap for implementation. *Geneva, 2012. Available from: whqlibdocwhoint/hq/2012/WHO_HTM_NTD_20121_ engpdf* **2012**.

18.   Cox, F. E., History of human parasitology. *Clin Microbiol Rev* **2002**, *15* (4), 595-612.

19.   Tyson, E., Lumbricus latus, or a discourse read before the Royal Society, of the joynted worm, wherein great many mistakes of former writers concerning it, are remarked; its natural history from more exact information is attempted; and the whole urged, as a difficulty against doctrine of univocal generation. *Philos Trans* **1683**, *13*, 113-144.

20.   Plater, F., Praxeos Medicae Opus. *Basel* **1656**.

21.   Goeze, J. A. E.; Blankenburg, P. A., Versuch ciner Naturgeschichte der Eingeweiderwumer Thierischer Korper. *Pape* **1782**.

22.   Hartmann, P. J., Miscellanea curiosa sive ephemeridium medicophysicarum Germanicarum Academiae Imperialis Leopoldineae naturae curiosorum decuriae II. *Observatio 34 Literis Joonnis Ernesti Adelbuneri Nurnberg pp 1688*, 58-59.

23.   Kuchenmeister, F., The Cysticercus cellulosus transformed within the organism of man into Taenia solium. *Lancet* **1861**, *i*, 39.

24.   Kuchenmeister, F., Experimenteller nachweis, dass Cysticercus cellulosae innerhalb des menschlichen darmkanales sichlil in Taenia solium umwandelt. *Wiener Medizinische Wochenschrift* **1855**, *5*, 1-4.

25.   Merchant, M. T.; Aguilar, L.; Avila, G.; Robert, L.; Flisser, A.; Willms, K., Taenia solium: description of the intestinal implantation sites in experimental hamster infections. *J Parasitol* **1998**, *84* (4), 681-5.

26.   Camacho, S. D.; Ruiz, A. C.; Uribe Beltran M; K., W., Serology as an indicator of Taenia solium tapeworm infections in a rural community in Mexico. *Trans Trop Med Hyg* **1990**, *84*, 563-566.

27.   de Aluja, A. S.; Villalobos, A. N.; Plancarte, A.; Rodarte, L. F.; Hernandez, M.; Sciutto, E., Experimental Taenia solium cysticercosis in pigs: characteristics of the infection and antibody response. *Vet Parasitol* **1996**, *61* (1-2), 49-59.

28.   Rodriguez-Contreras, D.; Skelly, P. J., Molecular and functional characterization and tissue localization of 2 glucose transporter homologues (TGTP1 and TGTP2) from the tapeworm Taenia solium. *Parasitology*

1998, *117*, 579-88.

29. Sciutto, E.; Fragoso, G.; Hernandez, M.; Rosas, G.; Martinez, J. J.; Fleury, A.; Cervantes, J.; Aluja, A.; Larralde, C., Development of the S3Pvac vaccine against porcine Taenia solium cysticercosis: a historical review. *J Parasitol* **2013,** *99* (4), 686-92.

30. Gauci, C.; Jayashi, C.; Lightowlers, M. W., Vaccine development against the Taenia solium parasite: the role of recombinant protein expression in Escherichia coli. *Bioengineered* **2013,** *4* (5), 343-7.

31. Silver, S. A.; Erozan, Y. S.; Hruban, R. H., Cerebral cysticercosis mimicking malignant glioma: a case report. *Acta cytologica* **1996,** *40* (2), 351-7.

32. White, A. C., Jr.; Robinson, P.; Kuhn, R., Taenia solium cysticercosis: host-parasite interactions and the immune response. *Chem Immunol* **1997,** *66*, 209-30.

33. Leid, R. W.; Suquet, C. M.; Tanigoshi, L., Parasite defense mechanisms for evasion of host attack; a review. *Vet Parasitol* **1987,** *25* (2), 147-62.

34. Laclette, J. P.; Landa, A.; Arcos, L.; Willms, K.; Davis, A. E.; Shoemaker, C. B., Paramyosin is the Schistosoma mansoni (Trematoda) homologue of antigen B from Taenia solium (Cestoda). *Molecular and biochemical parasitology* **1991,** *44* (2), 287-95.

35. Laclette, J. P.; Shoemaker, C. B.; Richter, D.; Arcos, L.; Pante, N.; Cohen, C.; Bing, D.; Nicholson-Weller, A., Paramyosin inhibits complement C1. *J Immunol* **1992,** *148* (1), 124-8.

36. Restrepo, B. I.; Llaguno, P.; Sandoval, M. A.; Enciso, J. A.; Teale, J. M., Analysis of immune lesions in neurocysticercosis patients: central nervous system response to helminth appears Th1-like instead of Th2. *Journal of neuroimmunology* **1998,** *89* (1-2), 64-72.

37. Lightowlers, M. W., Eradication of Taenia solium cysticercosis: a role for vaccination of pigs. *International journal for parasitology* **1999,** *29* (6), 811-7.

38. Song, E. K.; Kim, I. H.; Lee, S. O., Unusual manifestations of Taenia solium infestation. *Journal of gastroenterology* **2004,** *39* (3), 288-91.

39. Del Giudice, P.; Bernard, E.; Perrin, C.; Marty, P.; Le Fichoux, Y.; Ortonne, J. P.; Michiels, J. F.; Dellamonica, P., Subcutaneous cysticercosis. *Annales de dermatologie et de venereologie* **1996,** *123* (8), 474-7.

40. Salgado, P.; Rojas, R.; Sotelo, J., Cysticercosis. Clinical classification based on imaging studies. *Archives of internal medicine* **1997,** *157* (17), 1991-7.

41. Fleury, A.; Cardenas, G.; Adalid-Peralta, L.; Fragoso, G.; Sciutto, E., Immunopathology in Taenia solium neurocysticercosis. *Parasite Immunol* **2016,** *38* (3), 147-57.

42. Mitchell, W. G.; Crawford, T. O., Intraparenchymal cerebral cysticercosis in children: diagnosis and treatment. *Pediatrics* **1988,** *82* (1), 76-82.

43. Nash, T. E.; Patronas, N. J., Edema associated with calcified lesions in neurocysticercosis. *Neurology* **1999,** *53* (4), 777-81.

44. Dorny, P.; Brandt, J.; Zoli, A.; Geerts, S., Immunodiagnostic tools for human and porcine cysticercosis. *Acta tropica* **2003,** *87* (1), 79-86.

45. Chapman, A.; Vallejo, V.; Mossie, K. G.; Ortiz, D.; Agabian, N.; Flisser, A., Isolation and characterization of species-specific DNA probes from Taenia solium and Taenia saginata and their use in an egg detection assay. *Journal of clinical microbiology* **1995,** *33* (5), 1283-8.

46. Praet, N.; Verweij, J. J.; Mwape, K. E.; Phiri, I. K.; Muma, J. B.; Zulu, G.; van Lieshout, L.; Rodriguez-Hidalgo, R.; Benitez-Ortiz, W.; Dorny, P.; Gabriel, S., Bayesian modelling to estimate the test characteristics of coprology, coproantigen ELISA and a novel real-time PCR for the diagnosis of taeniasis. *Trop Med Int Health* **2013,** *18* (5), 608-14.

47. Yamasaki, H.; Allan, J. C.; Sato, M. O.; Nakao, M.; Sako, Y.; Nakaya, K.; Qiu, D.; Mamuti, W.; Craig, P. S.; Ito, A., DNA differential diagnosis of taeniasis and cysticercosis by multiplex PCR. *J Clin Microbiol* **2004,** *42* (2), 548-53.

48. Yamasaki, H.; Allan, J. C.; Sato, M. O.; Nakao, M.; Sako, Y.; Nakaya, K.; Qiu, D.; Mamuti, W.; Craig, P. S.; Ito, A., DNA differential diagnosis of taeniasis and cysticercosis by multiplex PCR. *Journal of clinical microbiology* **2004,** *42* (2), 548-53.

49. Jeri, C.; Gilman, R. H.; Lescano, A. G.; Mayta, H.; Ramirez, M. E.; Gonzalez, A. E.; Nazerali, R.; Garcia, H. H., Species identification after treatment for human taeniasis. *Lancet* **2004,** *363* (9413), 949-50.

50. Allan, J. C.; Avila, G.; Garcia Noval, J.; Flisser, A.; Craig, P. S., Immunodiagnosis of taeniasis by

coproantigen detection. *Parasitology* **1990,** *101,* 473-7.

51. Wilkins, P. P.; Allan, J. C.; Verastegui, M.; Acosta, M.; Eason, A. G.; Garcia, H. H.; Gonzalez, A. E.; Gilman, R. H.; Tsang, V. C., Development of a serologic assay to detect Taenia solium taeniasis. *Am J Trop Med Hyg* **1999,** *60* (2), 199-204.

52. Leite, C. C.; Jinkins, J. R.; Escobar, B. E.; Magalhães, A. C.; Gomes, G. C.; Dib, G.; Vargas, S. A.; Zee, C.; Watanabe, A. T., MR imaging of intramedullary and intradural-extramedullary spinal cysticercosis. *AJR Am J Roentgenol* **1997,** *169* (6), 1713-7.

53. Tsang, V. C.; Brand, J. A.; Boyer, A. E., An enzyme-linked immunoelectrotransfer blot assay and glycoprotein antigens for diagnosing human cysticercosis (Taenia solium). *J Infect Dis* **1989,** *159* (1), 50-9.

54. Proano-Narvaez, J. V.; Meza-Lucas, A.; J., Laboratory diagnosis of human neurocysticercosis: double-blind comparison of enzyme-linked immunosorbent assay and electroimmunotransfer blot assay. *Microbiol* **2002,** *40* 2115-18.

55. Gekeler, F.; Eichenlaub, S.; Mendoza, E. G.; Sotelo, J.; Hoelscher, M.; Löscher, T., Sensitivity and specificity of ELISA and immunoblot for diagnosing neurocysticercosis. *Eur J Clin Microbiol Infect Dis* **2002,** *21* (3), 227-9.

56. The Medical Letter. **2000.**

57. Richards, F.; Schantz, P. M., Treatment of Taenia solium infections. *Lancet* **1985,** *1* (8440), 1264-5.

58. Keeling, J. E. D., The chemotherapy of cestode infections. *Adv Chemother* **1978,** *3,* 109-152.

59. Del Brutto, O. H., Neurocysticercosis. *Continuum (Minneap Minn)* **2012,** *18* (6 Infectious Disease), 1392-416.

60. Wilson, M.; Bryan, R. T.; Fried, J. A.; Ware, D. A.; Schantz, P. M.; Pilcher, J. B.; Tsang, V. C., Clinical evaluation of the cysticercosis enzyme-linked immunoelectrotransfer blot in patients with neurocysticercosis. *J Infect Dis* **1991,** *164* (5), 1007-9.

61. Sotelo, J.; Del Brutto, O. H.; Roman, G. C., Cysticercosis. *Current clinical topics in infectious diseases* **1996,** *16,* 240-59.

62. Bittencourt, P. R.; Gracia, C. M.; Martins, R.; Fernandes, A. G.; Diekmann, H. W.; Jung, W., Phenytoin and carbamazepine decreased oral bioavailability of praziquantel. *Neurology* **1992,** *42* (3 Pt 1), 492-6.

63. Garcia, H. H.; Lescano, A. G.; Gonzales, I.; Bustos, J. A.; Pretell, E. J.; Horton, J.; Saavedra, H.; Gonzalez, A. E.; Gilman, R. H.; Cysticercosis Working Group in, P., Cysticidal Efficacy of Combined Treatment With Praziquantel and Albendazole for Parenchymal Brain Cysticercosis. *Clin Infect Dis* **2016,** *62* (11), 1375-9.

64. Garcia, H. H.; Evans, C. A. W.; Nash, T. E., Current consensus guidelines for treatment of neurocysticercosis. *Clin Microbiol Rev* **2002,** *15,* 747-56.

65. Carpio, A.; Escobar, A.; Hauser, W. A., Cysticercosis and epilepsy: a critical review. *Epilepsia* **1998,** *39* (10), 1025-40.

66. Sotelo, J.; del Brutto, O. H.; Penagos, P.; Escobedo, F.; Torres, B.; Rodriguez-Carbajal, J.; Rubio-Donnadieu, F., Comparison of therapeutic regimen of anticysticercal drugs for parenchymal brain cysticercosis. *Journal of neurology* **1990,** *237* (2), 69-72.

67. Sotelo, J.; Jung, H., Pharmacokinetic optimisation of the treatment of neurocysticercosis. *Clinical pharmacokinetics* **1998,** *34* (6), 503-15.

68. Lara-Aguilera, R.; Mendoza-Cruz, J. F.; Martinez-Toledo, J. L.; Macias-Sanchez, R.; Willms, K.; Altamirano-Rojas, L.; Santamaria-Llano, A., Taenia solium taeniasis and neurocysticercosis in a Mexican rural family. *Am J Trop Med Hyg* **1992,** *46* (1), 85-8.

69. Schantz, P. M.; Moore, A. C.; Muñoz, J. L.; Hartman, B. J.; Schaefer, J. A.; Aron, A. M.; Persaud, D.; Sarti, E.; Wilson, M.; Flisser, A., Neurocysticercosis in an Orthodox Jewish community in New York City. *N Engl J Med* **1992,** *327* (10), 692-5.

70. Fan, P. C.; Ma, Y. X.; Kuo, C. H.; Chung, W. C., Survival of Taenia solium cysticerci in carcasses of pigs kept at 4 C. *J Parasitol* **1998,** *84* (1), 174-5.

71. Carabin, H.; Traore, A. A., taeniasis and cysticercosis control and elimination through community-based interventions. *Curr Trop Med Rep* **2014,** *1* (4), 181-193.

72. O'Neal, S. E.; Moyano, L. M.; Ayvar, V.; Rodriguez, S.; Gavidia, C.; Wilkins, P. P.; Gilman, R. H.; Garcia, H. H.; Gonzalez, A. E.; Cysticercosis Working Group in, P., Ring-screening to control endemic

transmission of Taenia solium. *PLoS Negl Trop Dis* **2014,** *8* (9), e3125.

73.   Manoutcharian, K.; Rosas, G.; Hernandez, M.; Fragoso, G.; Aluja, A.; Villalobos, N.; Rodarte, L. F.; Sciutto, E., Cysticercosis: identification and cloning of protective recombinant antigens. *J Parasitol* **1996,** *82* (2), 250-4.

74.   Lightowlers, M. W.; Gauci, C. G., Vaccines against cysticercosis and hydatidosis. *Vet Parasitol* **2001,** *101* (3-4), 337-52.

75.   Molinari, J. L.; Rodríguez, D.; Tato, P.; Soto, R.; Arechavaleta, F.; Solano, S., Field trial for reducing porcine Taenia solium cysticercosis in Mexico by systematic vaccination of pigs. *Vet Parasitol* **1997,** *69* (1-2), 55-63.

76.   Gonzales, A. E.; Garcia, H. H.; Gilman, R. H.; Gavidia, C. M.; Tsang, V. C.; Bernal, T.; Falcon, N.; Romero, M.; Lopez-Urbina, M. T., Effective, single-dose treatment or porcine cysticercosis with oxfendazole. *Am J Trop Med Hyg* **1996,** *54* (4), 391-4.

77.   D'Souza, P. E.; Hafeez, M., Detection of Taenia solium cysticercosis in pigs by ELISA with an excretory-secretory antigen. *Vet Res Commun* **1999,** *23* (5), 293-8.

78.   Theis, J. H.; Cleary, M.; Syvanen, M.; Gilson, A.; Swift, P.; Banks, J.; Johnson, E., DNA-confirmed Taenia solium cysticercosis in black bears (Ursus americanus) from California. *Am J Trop Med Hyg* **1996,** *55* (4), 456-8.

30. *Diphyllobothrium latum*
(Linnaeus 1758)

Introduction

Diphyllobothrium latum belongs to the order Pseudophyllidea and usually achieves a length of 2-15 meters, but has achieved a length of 25 meters, making it the longest parasite to infect humans.[1] It is estimated that as many as 20 million people may be infected worldwide by fish tapeworms.; mainly *Diphyllobothrium latum,* but also *Diphyllobothrium pacificum, D. nihonkaiense, D. cordatum, D. ursi, D. dendriticum, D. lanceolatum, D. dalliae,* and *D. yonagoensis.*[23] The fish tapeworm can grow at a rate of 22 cm/day, releasing 1,000,000 eggs per day, and live for up to 25 years.[4-6] It is acquired by eating raw or under-cooked fish and for that reason it is commonly referred to as the fish or broad tapeworm. As with all other

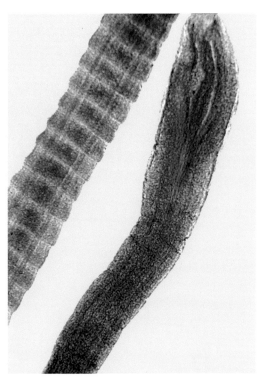

Figure 30.2. The scolex and mature proglottids of *D. latum.* Courtesy H. Zaiman.

adult tapeworms, it lives in the lumen of the small intestine and usually does little harm to its host. It has a unique affinity for absorbing vitamin B12, and as a result the infection can have pathological consequences for some infected individuals.

All species in this group of tapeworms have similar complex life cycles. In most cases they use invertebrates (e.g., copepods) and freshwater fish as intermediate hosts.

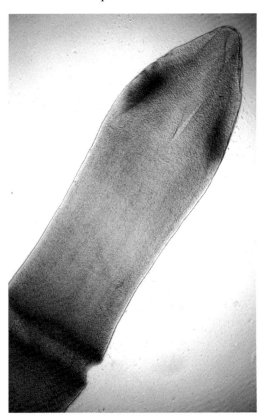

Figure 30.1. The plerocercoid stage of *D. latum.* This is the infective stage for the definitve host.

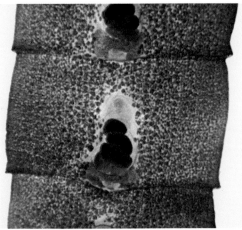

Figure 30.3. Mature proglottids of *D. latum.*

Diphyllobothrium latum

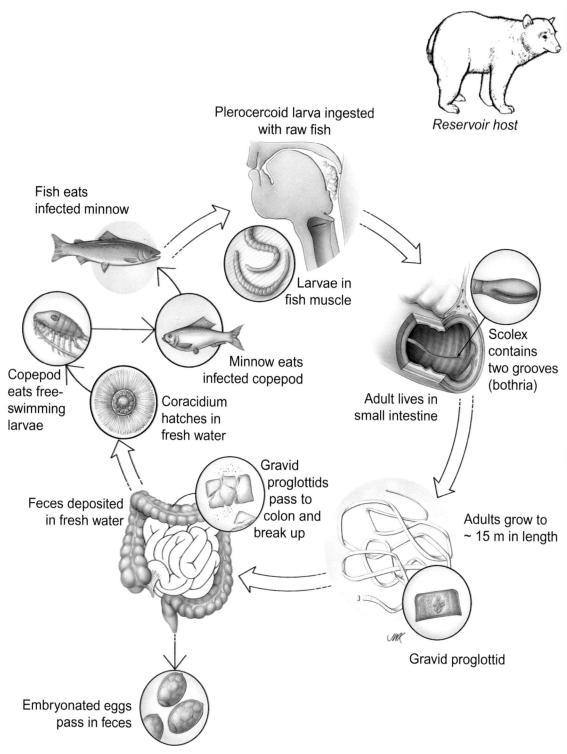

Reservoir host

Plerocercoid larva ingested
with raw fish

Fish eats
infected minnow

Larvae in
fish muscle

Scolex
contains
two grooves
(bothria)

Copepod
eats free-
swimming
larvae

Minnow eats
infected copepod

Coracidium
hatches in
fresh water

Adult lives in
small intestine

Gravid
proglottids
pass to
colon and
break up

Feces deposited
in fresh water

Adults grow to
~ 15 m in length

Gravid proglottid

Embryonated eggs
pass in feces

Parasitic Diseases 6th Ed. Parasites Without Borders www.parasiteswithoutborders.com

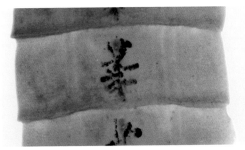

Figure 30.4. Gravid proglottids of *D. latum*.

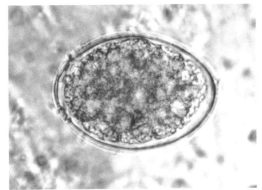

Figure 30.5. Unembryonated egg of *D. latum*. 65 x 45 μm

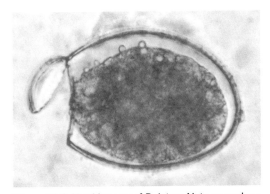

Figure 30.6. Hatching egg of *D. latum*. Note operculum.

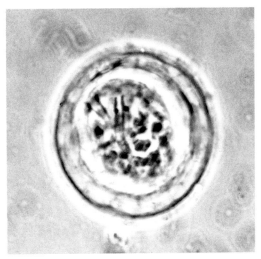

Figure 30.7. Ciliated coracidium. 60 μm in diameter.

Most carnivores are susceptible to infection with *D. latum*, including dog, bear, cat, fox, martin, mink, and other wild mammals. Some of these hosts are important reservoirs for the human infection.

D. latum, the major fish tapeworm of humans, will be the model in this chapter for all the others. It is still common throughout Scandinavia, though prevalence in that region has decreased in recent years due in large part, to vastly improved sanitation.[7, 8] The infection was probably introduced to North America (especially in the Great Lakes region and in Lake Winnipeg, Manitoba) by northern European immigrants.[9] Today, new infections are reported commonly in Russia, Brazil, and Japan,[9] although infections have also been reported in Asia, Europe and the Americas. Overall, it is believed that the number of new cases of *D. latum* infection are declining in North America but human *D. nihonkaiense* infection has been reported recently from Washington state in the United States.[10, 11] A related sub-species, *D. latum* var. *parvum* infects humans in Korea and China.[12] In circumpolar regions, infection due to *D. dendriticum* (a more benign variant) is common in both people and animals.[13] A related species, *Adenocephalus pacificus* (syn. *Diphyllobothrium pacificum*), has been reported from the Pacific Coast of South America - Peru, Chile, and Ecuador – and may be an important species in the region (possibly linked to ceviche consumption).[14]

Historical Information

Descriptions of what appears to have been infection due to the broad or fish tapeworm go back thousands of years, with evidence of human infection in Peru from 10,000-4,000

BCE from archaelogical evidence.[15] In 1609, the Swiss physician Félix Plater observed and reported that *Diphyllobothrium latum* infected humans.[16] In 1751, Carl Linnaeus classified *Diphyllobothrium latum*.[17] In 1917, Constantine Janicki and Felix Rosen, in a series of elegant epidemiological observations and experiments, described and illustrated its complex life cycle, including copepods, fish, and then the human host.[18]

Life Cycle

Infection begins when undercooked or raw fish, infected with the plerocercoid metacestode of the parasite, is eaten (Fig. 30.1). In the northern hemisphere, pike and percids are the most common source of infection in many regions of the world.[9] After ingestion, the parasite is released from the fish's flesh in the stomach. The plerocercoid larvae, now free of fish muscle, pass to the small intestine and attach to the intestinal wall by applying their two bothria (grooves) to the epithelial surface. They grow and develop into the adult worms (Fig. 30.2), becoming fully-formed strobilae within three months. In human infection, eggs begin to pass into the stool 15-45 days after ingestion of the infected fish.[6] Usually, only one tapeworm of *D. latum* infects a given individual, but patients can harbor multiple infections. The adult fish tapeworm usually has a life span of 4.5 years can live for

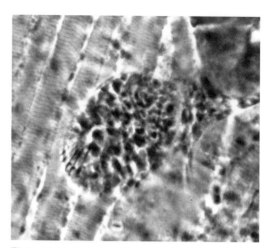

Figure 30.9. Procercoid stage of *D. latum* in tissues of *Diaptomus* spp. Note hooklets. (Phase-contrast)

as long as 25 years.[9]

Proglottids (segments) are greater in width than length (Figs. 30.3, 30.4), and contain both sets of sex organs. Proglottids fertilize eggs in nearby segments. As fertilized proglottids become gravid, eggs (Fig. 30.5) exit from the centrally located uterine pore, entering into the lumen of the small intestine. Gravid segments can also break off from the strobila and disintegrate in the small intestine. The fertilized, unembryonated eggs pass out of the host with the feces and must be deposited in freshwater if the life cycle is to continue.

The eggs measure 70 µm and embryonate over a 9-12 day period before hatching (Fig. 30.6). The motile coracidium (Fig. 30.7) (ciliated oncosphere) emerges from the egg and immediately begins to swim. Free-living coracidia can live for 3-4 days before exhausting their food reserves. Motile coracidia attract the attention of zooplankton crustacean predators (e.g., *Cyclops* spp. and *Diaptomus* spp.) (Fig. 30.8) and become ingested. Instead of being digested by the crustacean intermediate host, the coracidium burrows into the body cavity and develops into an immature metacestode, referred to as a procercoid (Fig. 30.9).

When infected crustacea are consumed by small freshwater fish, particularly various species of minnows, the procercoid is freed

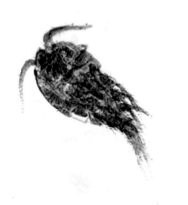

Figure 30.8. *Diaptomus* spp. infected with *D. latum.*

from the crustacean and penetrates the wall of the small intestine of the fish, eventually lodging in the muscles, or various viscera, such as the liver and gonads. It then differentiates and grows into a plerocercoid metacestode, the infective stage for humans. Upon death of this second intermediate host, the plerocercoids in viscera are triggered to migrate to the muscles.[6]

When infected minnows are eaten by large predator fish species such as members of the perch, pike, and salmonid families, plerocercoids can be transferred to the body muscles of these larger fish. Carnivores, including humans, often consume these larger fish and a resulting intestinal tapeworm infection can then develop.

Cellular and Molecular Pathogenesis

Pseudophyllidean tapeworms absorb large quantities of vitamin B12 and their analogues. They employ a tegumental cyanocobalamin receptor that has a high affinity for several analogues of this compound, including cobalamin, and mediate dissociation of the vitamin B12-intrinsic factor complex.[19] Cobalamin is converted to adenosyl-cobalamin, a coenzyme for methyl-malonyl-CoA mutase. Anaerobic energy metabolism relies on the production of propionate and these two enzymes are integral to that metabolic pathway.[20] These tapeworms have the ability to absorb B12 at an absorption rate of 100:1 relative to that of the infected host.[6] Almost half of all patients infected with *D. latum* develop decreased B12 levels, but only a minority develop clinically apparent anemia. It appears that host factors, the number of infecting worms, and the specific tapeworm involved determines the risk of developing B12 deficiency and macrocytic hypochromic anemia.[3]

Clinical Disease

In most individuals, infection with the fish tapeworm results in no obvious symptoms. Infections with multiple worms may cause nonspecific symptoms such as watery diarrhea, fatigue, and rarely mechanical obstruction of the small bowel.[21-23] Exhaustion of vitamin B12 is a slow process, taking many months to years.[24] The full picture of megaloblastic anemia due to B12 deficiency is indistinguishable from that due to other causes. While up to 40% of infected individuals will have B12 deficiency, less than 2% of infected individuals develop megaloblastic anemia.[25] The reason for the relative infrequency of megaloblastic anemia among most of those infected with of *D. latum* is not well understood. There may be host genetic factors that predispose certain infected individuals to suffer the effects of this deficiency. One study indicated that patients with megaloblastic anemia due to infection with *D. latum* had less intrinsic factor than those who were free of anemia, but who also harbored the worm. This observation has not been confirmed by other studies.[25] Eosinophilia has been reported in a number of cases.[23, 26]

Diagnosis

Segments of worm in stool (Figs. 30.3, 30.4) sometimes alert patients to the fact that they harbor a tapeworm but most proglottids break up in the intestinal tract before exiting the host. Diagnosis is typically made by microscopic identification of non-embryonated eggs (Figs. 30.5, C.58.) in stool. Molecular tests are available for diagnosis that also allow for species determination, but most diagnosis is done using visual microscopy.[6]

Treatment

The drug of choice is praziquantel (5-10 mg/kg once).[27] Niclosamide is an alternative therapy that appears to be effective.[6]

Prevention and Control

In sylvatic settings, numerous reservoir hosts are potentially important for maintaining the life cycle. Interference with this phase of its ecology would be very difficult, if not impossible. On an individual basis, the best way to avoid infection with *D. latum* is to avoid eating freshwater fish unless it is well cooked or once frozen. Sushi is predominantly made from saltwater fish species that do not acquire *D. latum* or related tapeworm species. A few cases have been reported from eating sushi prepared from Pacific coast salmon, which spend a portion of their life in freshwater.[28] The culinary habit among many Jewish mothers or grandmothers of teaching their daughters to prepare gefilte fish by tasting the raw mixture led many a female to acquire this infection in the United States, and was popularized in a medical anthropological description by Desowitz.[29] Today, proper disposal of human feces in the Great Lakes region of the United States has greatly reduced prevalence of *D. latum*. In Scandinavian countries, gravlax and a wide variety of other marinated raw fish dishes, remain sources of infection for this tapeworm.

References

1. von Bonsdorff, B., Diphyllobothriasis in man. *Academic Press, New York, NY.* **1977**.
2. Chai, J. Y.; Darwin Murrell, K.; Lymbery, A. J., Fish-borne parasitic zoonoses: status and issues. *Int J Parasitol* **2005**, *35* (11-12), 1233-54.
3. Jimenez, J. A.; Rodriguez, S.; Gamboa, R.; Rodriguez, L.; Garcia, H. H.; Cysticercosis Working Group in, P., Diphyllobothrium pacificum infection is seldom associated with megaloblastic anemia. *Am J Trop Med Hyg* **2012**, *87* (5), 897-901.
4. Kuhlow, F., [Studies on the development of Diphyllobothrium latum]. *Z Tropenmed Parasitol* **1955**, *6* (2), 213-25.
5. Dogiel, V. A., Allgemeine Parasitologie. *Parasitol. Schriftenr.* **1963**, *16*, 1-523.
6. Scholz, T.; Garcia, H. H.; Kuchta, R.; Wicht, B., Update on the human broad tapeworm (genus diphyllobothrium), including clinical relevance. *Clin Microbiol Rev* **2009**, *22* (1), 146-60, Table of Contents.
7. Kyronseppa, H., The occurrence of human intestinal parasites in Finland. *Scand Dis* **1993**, *25* (5), 671-3.
8. Dick, T. A.; Nelson, P. A.; Choudhury, A., Diphyllobothriasis: update on human cases, foci, patterns and sources of human infections and future considerations. *Southeast Asian J Trop Med Public Health* **2001**, *32 Suppl 2*, 59-76.
9. Dick, T. A.; Nelson, P. A.; Choudhury, A., Diphyllobothriasis: update on human cases, foci, patterns and sources of human infections and future considerations. *The Southeast Asian journal of tropical medicine and public health* **2001**, *32 Suppl 2*, 59-76.
10. Torres, P.; Franjola, R.; Weitz, J. C.; Peña, G.; Morales, E., [New records of human diphyllobothriasis in Chile (1981-1992), with a case of multiple Diphyllobothrium latum infection]. *Boletin chileno de parasitologia* **1993**, *48* (3-4), 39-43.
11. Fang, F. C.; Billman, Z. P.; Wallis, C. K.; Abbott, A. N.; Olson, J. C.; Dhanireddy, S.; Murphy, S. C., Human Diphyllobothrium nihonkaiense infection in Washington State. *J Clin Microbiol* **2015**, *53* (4), 1355-7.
12. Lee, S. H.; Chai, J. Y.; Seo, M.; Kook, J.; Huh, S.; Ryang, Y. S.; Ahn, Y. K., Two rare cases of Diphyllobothrium latum parvum type infection in Korea. *The Korean journal of parasitology* **1994**, *32* (2), 117-20.
13. Curtis, M. A.; Bylund, G., Diphyllobothriasis: fish tapeworm disease in the circumpolar north.

Arctic medical research **1991,** *50* (1), 18-24.

14. Kuchta, R.; Serrano-Martinez, M. E.; Scholz, T., Pacific Broad Tapeworm Adenocephalus pacificus as a Causative Agent of Globally Reemerging Diphyllobothriosis. *Emerg Infect Dis* **2015,** *21* (10), 1697-703.

15. Reinhard, K. J.; Barnum, S. V., Parasitology as an interpretative tool in archaeology. *Am. Antiq* **1991,** *57,* 231–245.

16. Plater, F., Praxeos seu de cognoscendis, praedicendis praecudensis curandiso affectibus homini incommodantibus tractatus tertius et ultimus. *De vitiis libris duobus agens quorum primum corpis secundus Exretorum vitia continet Typis Conradi Waldkirchii* **1609.**

17. Linnaeus, C., Taenia osculis lateralibus solitaris. *Amoenitates Academicae Holmiae Laurentium Salvium 2,* 80-81.

18. Janicki, C., Le cycle evolutif du Dibothriocephalus latus L. *Soc Neuchateloise Sci Natur Bull* **1917,** *42,* 19-53.

19. Friedman, P. A.; Weinstein, P. P.; Mueller, J. F.; Allen, R. H., Characterization of cobalamin receptor sites in brush-border plasma membranes of the tapeworm Spirometra mansonoides. *The Journal of biological chemistry* **1983,** *258* (7), 4261-5.

20. Smyth, J. D.; McManus, D. P., The Physiology and Biochemistry of Tapeworms. 1989.

21. Shimizu, T.; Kinoshita, K.; Tokuda, Y., Diphyllobothrium nihonkaiense infection linked to chilled salmon consumption. *BMJ Case Rep* **2012,** *2012.*

22. Lee, S. H.; Park, H.; Yu, S. T., Diphyllobothrium latum infection in a child with recurrent abdominal pain. *Korean J Pediatr* **2015,** *58* (11), 451-3.

23. Nawa, Y.; Hatz, C.; Blum, J., Sushi delights and parasites: the risk of fishborne and foodborne parasitic zoonoses in Asia. *Clin Infect Dis* **2005,** *41* (9), 1297-303.

24. Goodman, K. I.; Salt, W. B., Vitamin B12 deficiency. Important new concepts in recognition. *Postgraduate medicine* **1990,** *88* (3), 147-50, 153.

25. Saarni, M.; Nyberg, W.; al., e., Symptoms in carriers of Diphyllobothrium latum and in uninfected controls. *Acta Med Scand* **1963,** *173* 147-154.

26. Arizono, N.; Yamada, M.; Nakamura-Uchiyama, F.; Ohnishi, K., Diphyllobothriasis associated with eating raw pacific salmon. *Emerg Infect Dis* **2009,** *15* (6), 866-70.

27. Groll, E., Praziquantel for cestode infections in man. *Acta Trop* **1980,** *37* (3), 293-6.

28. Hutchinson, J. W.; Bass, J. W.; Demers, D. M.; Myers, G. B., Diphyllobothriasis after eating raw salmon. *Hawaii medical journal* **1997,** *56* (7), 176-7.

29. Desowitz, R. S., New Guinea Tapeworms and Jewish Grandmothers: of Parasites and People. *W W Norton Co Pubs* **1981.**

31. Tapeworms of Minor Medical Importance

Hymenolepis nana
(Siebold 1852)

Introduction

Hymenolepis nana, in the order Cyclophyllidea, has a worldwide distribution, and infects mostly children, with prevalence in children as high as 25% in certain areas.[1-3] In Asia and elsewhere, *H. nana* infection is a common infection among children living in poor neighborhoods and in institutional settings.[4, 5] As its species name implies, this is a small tapeworm, measuring 34-45 mm in length. The adult consists of 150-200 proglottids, and lives in the lumen of the small intestine, loosely attached to the epithelial cells of the villi. Its scolex has four suckers and a single row of hooks. Rodents are significant reservoir hosts for this tapeworm. Like *Strongyloides stercoralis*, *Hymenolepis nana* is able to complete its entire life cycle within the human host. Autoinfection results in a high worm burden, particularly in immunosuppressed patients.[6, 7] In 2015, malignant transformation and metastasis of cells from *Hymenolepsis nana* in an HIV-1 infected

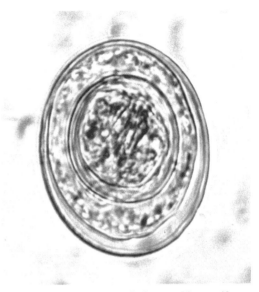

Figure 31.2. Egg of *Hymenolepis nana*. 35 μm x 40 μm.

individual was described.[8]

A second related species, *Hymenolepis microstoma*, has been described in *H. nana*-infected patients from remote communities in Western Australia.[9]

Historical Information

In 1852, Theodore Bilharz identified *Hymenolepis nana* when he discovered it on autopsy of a six-year-old boy who died of meningitis, and whose small intestine harbored numerous adult parasites.[10] In 1887, Giovanni Grassi demonstrated that *H. nana* could have a direct transmission cycle in rats without an intermediate host.[11] In 1911, Charles Nicholl and Edward A. Minchin demonstrated that *H. nana* can also have an indirect transmission cycle involving fleas or beetles as intermediate hosts.[12] In 1921, Y. Saeki determined that *H. nana* could have a direct transmission cycle in humans.

Life Cycle

Infection can begin in one of two ways; by ingesting the cysticercoid metacestode (Fig. 31.1) along with an infected insect, or by ingesting embronated eggs. Infective

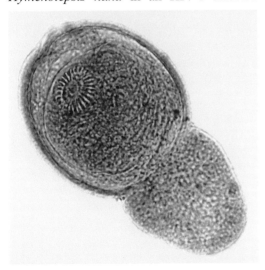

Figure 31.1. The cysticercoid of *Hymenolepis nana*. 350 μm x 200 μm.

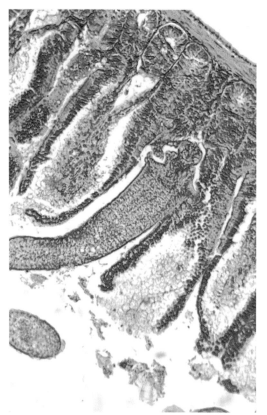

Figure 31.3. Histological section of *H. nana, in situ.*

stages of *H. nana* are sometimes present in tenebrio larvae (i.e., meal worms often found contaminating cereals and grains) or in rat feces. If eggs are ingested (Fig 31.2), the oncospheres hatch in the small intestine and penetrate the lamina propria of a villus. There, each larva differentiates into the cysticercoid (juvenile stage). This stage reenters the intestinal lumen, and attaches to the surface of the villous tissue (Fig. 31.3), where it rapidly differentiates into an immature adult parasite with four suckers and a single row of hooklets (Fig. 31.4). *H. nana* grows to full maturity within a three to four-week period. If the cysticercoid is ingested, then it attaches to the wall of the small intestine and differentiates and matures to the adult worm, usually within a two-week period. Although the lifespan of an adult worm is only 4-6 weeks, internal autoinfection can allow an infection to last for years.[13]

Mating between nearby proglottids (Fig. 31.5) produces hundreds of fertilized eggs. Gravid segments break off from the strobila and disintegrate in the small intestine, releasing the fertilized, embryonated eggs. Autoinfection, with released eggs hatching directly within the intestine, is a possibility, but rarely occurs, as immunity to reinfection develops in most instances.[14] Eggs deposited in the feces may be ingested by the larvae of beetles, or by rodents, or by humans. In the invertebrate host, the oncospheres hatch and penetrate the gut and enter the hemocele where they differentiate into cysticercoid metacestodes.

Cellular and Molecular Pathogenesis

Infection is usually self-limited in adult patients, but not in very young children, probably reflecting the age-specificity of development of protective immunity, and is most likely a consequence of children ingest-

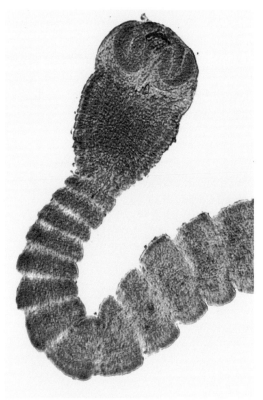

Figure 31.4. Scolex of *Hymenolepis nana.* It has four suckers as well as hooks.

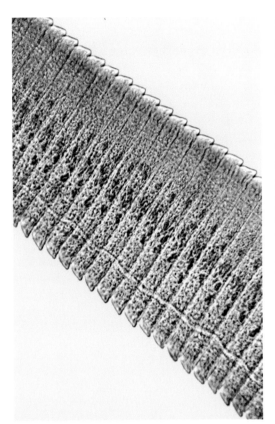

Figure 31.5. Mature proglottids of *Hymenolepis nana*. 400 μm wide.

ing infected insects. The cysticercoid stage is relatively non-immunogenic, allowing for autoinfection to develop. In contrast, infection initiated by ingestion of the egg stage triggers a rapid and robust protective immune response.[15, 16] A low but detectable protective humoral immune response occurs as the result of exposure to the entire life cycle, and is transferable to a naive host.[1, 17] In experimental infections of mice, the cysticercoid attracts eosinophils by secreting factors into the local area of infection, especially during reinfection, and these host cells may play a role in preventing establishment of new infections with *Hymenolepis nana*.[18, 19] In addition, regardless of the immunological background of the mouse strain, INF-γ is always a dominant feature of their response to infection, and expulsion of worms may be due directly to the upregulation of this peptide. Antibodies of the IgE class may also play a role in protec-

tion.[20, 21] It appears that immunity to this parasite is multifactorial, involving both Th1 and Th2 responses.[17]

Clinical Disease

Most infections are not clinically apparent. Heavy infections are accompanied by diarrhea.[5] It is not clear whether *Hymenolepis nana* causes symptoms such as abdominal pain, headache, and itching around the anus, or if these complaints are due to co-infection with other pathogens.

Diagnosis

Microscopic identification of embryonated eggs (Fig. 32.2) in the stool is the definitive diagnosis. When whole pieces of strobila are passed, they can be identified directly, or the eggs can be expressed from gravid proglottids and then identified.

Treatment

Praziquantel is the drug of choice because it affects both the cysticercoid in the villus tissue and the adult.[22-25] A higher dose (25 mg/kg once) is required for other tapeworms. In contrast, niclosamide kills the adult, but it is not effective against the metacestode.[26] If niclosamide is the only drug available, treatment for several days or re-examining the patient's stool after therapy is required, because an additional course of therapy may be necessary. Nitazoxanide has been investigated as a broad-spectrum antiparasitic for children with multiple intestinal protozoa and helminths, including *H. nana* and may be an alternative therapy.[27-29]

Prevention and Control

Preventing contamination of food and water supplies with human feces and infected fleas and beetles is the best approach to controlling *H. nana* infection. In treating individuals, especially small children, it is sometimes difficult to achieve a cure, due to autoinfection. Rodent reservoir hosts contaminate the environment and, in many situations, controlling their populations has reduced the incidence of infection, but more often than not, rodent populations cannot be reduced. Reinfection in endemic areas is the norm.

Hymenolepis diminuta
(Rudolphi 1819)

Introduction

Hymenolepis dimunuta is found throughout the world and has many reservoir hosts, including dogs, cats, and many species of rodents. As with *H. nana*, it is primarily an infection of children.[12]

Historical Information

In 1819, Karl Rudolphi described the morphology of *Hymenolepis diminuta*.[30] In 1858, David Weinland described the infection in humans.[31]

Life Cycle

Infection begins when the cysticercoid is ingested with the infected insect. The immature worm attaches to the intestinal wall with the aid of four suckers on its scolex. The adult worm matures within 18 days, and grows to 50 cm in length. The strobila contains about 1,000 proglottids at any one time.

Gravid proglottids detach from the strobila and disintegrate in the small intestine. Eggs (Fig. 31.6) pass with the feces, and must be ingested by an appropriate intermediate host, either the larva of fleas or flour beetles (*Tenebrio* spp.), to continue the life cycle. In contrast to eggs of *H. nana*, *H. diminuta* ova are not infectious for humans. When eggs were experimentally fed to *Tenebrio molitor*

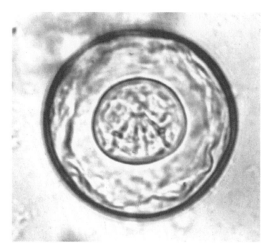

Figure 31.6. Egg of *H. diminuta*. 75 μm in diameter.

larvae, some eggs passed through their gut tract, and were incorporated within the fecal pellets. There, they remained infective for 48 hours, allowing infection to spread among the remaining insect larvae.[32]

The egg hatches within the lumen of the insect gut, and the oncosphere penetrates into the hemocele and develops into the cysticercoid, the infective stage for humans. The life cycle is completed when a human eats an infected insect. Other vertebrates (e.g., rats, mice, and dogs) also serve as definitive hosts. Beetle to beetle transmission may be even more significant than cycles involving vertebrate intermediates, and may serve to free this parasite from reliance on the presence of an additional host to complete its life cycle.[32]

Cellular and Molecular Pathogenesis

Hymenolepis diminuta is a well-studied tapeworm, and continues to serve as a model for all adult tapeworms infecting warm-blooded mammals.[33, 34] Despite the wealth of knowledge accumulated on this cestode, little is known of its pathophysiology in humans owing to the rarity with which it infects humans.[35, 36]

Clinical Disease

H. diminuta appears to induce no tissue

damage. Usually there are no clinical symptoms attributable to this infection, although infections with more than ten worms have been associated with abdominal pain, anorexia, and irritability [37-39] In experimental infection in rats, *H. diminuta* has subtle effects on gut transit time and the myoelectric potential, but whether this is the case in human infection has yet to be demonstrated.[40]

Diagnosis

Identification of eggs (Fig. 31.6, C.61) in the stool is the definitive method of diagnosis. Occasionally, whole segments of adult worms, which can be identified directly, are also passed in the feces. It is possible to extract eggs from such gravid segments and identify them.

Treatment

A single dose of Praziquantel is the drug of choice. Niclosamide given for several days is an effective alternative drug.[35] Adaptation of *H. diminuta* to the golden hamster has created a model laboratory infection for the *in vivo* testing of new anti-cestode drugs.[41]

Prevention and Control

H. diminuta, like *H. nana*, must be controlled both in the infected individual and in the reservoir host, but the latter is an unrealistic goal in most rural and suburban situations, particularly in less developed countries. Community efforts are aimed at curtailing contamination of food, especially whole grains and processed flour, by insects that could harbor the intermediate stage of the worm.

Dipylidium caninum
(Linnaeus 1758)

Introduction

Dipylidium caninum lives in the lumen of the small intestine of the dog, cat, fox, hyena, and occasionally human. The name of the genus is of Greek origin, and means "double pore" or "double opening."

Life Cycle

The infection is acquired by ingesting an infected adult flea, usually *Ctenocephalides canis* or *C. felis* (Fig. 38.23). The cysticercoid is released from the flea by the digestive enzymes of the host. The scolex (Fig. 32.7) attaches to the villous surface of the small intestine, and within 25 days, the adult worm begins passing gravid proglottids (Fig. 31.8). These segments disintegrate and release eggs (Fig. 31.9), which pass in feces to the external environment. Flea larvae ingest eggs. As with *H. diminuta*, the oncosphere penetrates the hemocele of the immature insect host and develops into the cysticercoid. This stage is infective for humans. Children can be infected by coming in close contact with dogs or cats, and inadvertently swallowing an infected adult flea.

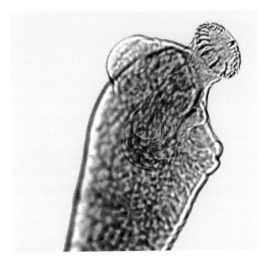

Figure 31.7. Scolex of *Dipylidium caninum*. Note the four suckers and hooks.

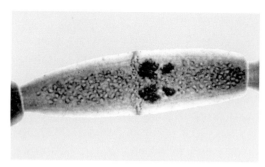

Figure 31.8. Double-pored gravid proglottid of *Dipylidium caninum*. 200 μm in width.

Clinical Disease

D. caninum does not usually cause any recognized clinical disease, but a few case reports have suggested a number of symptoms, such as mild abdominal pain, diarrhea, pruritus ani, failure to thrive, and irritability, may be association with infection.[42-45] Most *D. caninum* infections occur in children less than 8 years of age.[46]

Diagnosis

The diagnosis is made by microscopically identifying the characteristic egg clusters (Fig. 31.9) in the patient's stool. If proglottids are available, they, too, are readily identifiable.

Treatment

Praziquantel or niclosamide are the drugs of choice.[47, 48]

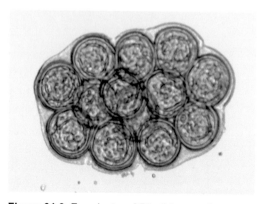

Figure 31.9. Egg cluster of *Dipylidium caninum*.

Prevention and Control

Eradication of fleas in pets and treating infected animals with niclosamide greatly reduce the chances of human infection.

Mesocestoides spp.
(Valliant 1863)

Introduction

Cestodes, in the genus *Mesocestoides*, infect numerous species of mammals and birds. Human infections have been reported.[49] Most of the cases reported from the U.S. were caused by *Mesocestoides variabilis*.[50] The life cycle of mesocestoides is complex, involving a coprophagous arthropod as the first intermediate host, and birds, snakes, lizards, amphibians, rodents, or other mammalian carnivores as the second intermediate host. The infective stage, known as a tetrathyridium, develops in the second intermediate host. Tetrathyridia are usually about 1 cm long and contain an invaginated scolex with four suckers. Humans acquire the parasite by eating the tetrathyridia, which can develop to an adult worm in the gut, or migrate to the peritoneal cavity. Cases of mesocestoides infection have been described in the United States, but the mode of acquisition is not known.[49] A case of mesocestoides infection from a 19 month-old boy in Alexandria, Louisiana, has led to the suggestion that the infection is food-borne, possibly in association with the culinary customs of the Acadian and Creole communities in this region. Treatment of the adult tapeworm with praziquantel or niclosamide is effective.[50]

Spirometra spp.

Spirometra mansonoides and other related *Spirometra* spp. are pseudophyllidian tapeworms that cause a closely related series of metacestode infections in humans (some are life-threatening), collectively referred to as sparganosis. Cases of sparganosis have been reported from Southeast Asia, Japan, China, especially on the island of Hainan, Africa, Italy, and the United States.[51, 52] The definitive hosts for the many species of spirometra are cats, birds, canines, and a number of other carnivores.[51, 53]

The life cycles of *Spirometra spp.* are complex and similar to that of *Diphyllobothrium latum* (see Chapter 30). The definitive hosts harbor the adult tapeworm in their small intestinal tract. When they defecate into freshwater, the unembryonated eggs hatch and the released free-swimming coracidia are eaten by copepods. The parasites then develop into the procercoid stage that is infectious for second intermediate hosts; amphibians, fish, reptiles, and birds. These animals ingest the infected copepods, releasing the procercoids that penetrate the intestinal tract and develop to the plerocercoid stage in muscle tissue. This stage is infective for definitive hosts; warm-blooded predator species that prey on these infected cold-blooded animals.[54]

Human infection results from ingestion of raw or undercooked flesh of any of the numerous intermediate hosts, and from application of such flesh as poultices. This practice is very common in some areas of the world, particularly on the island of Hainan, where over 30% of the frogs harbor the juvenile stage of spirometra.[55, 56] The skin of numerous cold-blooded vertebrates contains a variety of closely related peptides, referred to as megainins.[57] These amphipathic peptides are related to gramicidin, and have potent anti-microbial activities.[58] Employing frog and fish skins for medical use has a chemotherapeutic basis. As with any other therapy, the use of cold-blooded vertebrate skin as a poultice can have unwanted "side effects." In this case, the user may develop a parasitic infection. The plerocercoid stage can migrate out of the poultice and into the subcutaneous tissues, stimulated by the rise in temperature from the human host. If the poultice is placed over an open wound, or the eye, the immature parasite may enter the site. In the eye, the inner surface of the lid is the initial site of infection.[59, 60] The surrounding tissues proliferate, becoming edematous and painful (unilateral periorbital edema), because the larva secretes a version of growth hormone (GH) similar in activity to mammalian GH.[61] The pleurocercoid may migrate beyond the eye lid into the brain, where it continues to grow. Neurological symptoms follow.[62] Occasionally, patients die of neurological complications of infection with *Spirometra* spp..

Diagnosis is either based on identification of the worm after removal or biopsy. There is an ELISA test for sparganosis with high levels of sensitivity and specificity that can be useful in making the diagnosis.[63, 64] In the case of early eye involvement, removal of the larva from the space between the lower lid and the eyeball results in complete remission. Larvae often migrate behind the eye, and even into the brain via the optic nerve, making easy removal of the parasite impossible.[65] In these instances, surgery is necessary. Subcutaneous lesions are often removed by surgery, as treatment with antihelminthic therapy such as with praziquantil is associated with limited success.[65] Prevention is difficult, because of the effectiveness and popularity of poultice use for a variety of medical problems, including photophobia due to chickenpox.[66]

Taenia spp. (other than *T. saginata* and *T.solium*)

Taenia spp. (e.g., *T. multiceps, T. brauni, T. serialis*) is a group of cyclophyllidian tapeworms that, as adults, infect dogs and other canidae. Intermediate hosts include domestic cattle, horses, goats, and some wild herbivorous animals of Africa. Humans become infected with the metacestode (juvenile stage), known as coenurus, which resembles cysts found in the intermediate hosts. Human infections have been largely confined to the

African continent, but a few cases have been described from France, England, and North and South America.

The larva routinely invades the central nervous system (brain, eyes, spinal cord). Other space-occupying lesions resemble this infection, such as those caused by cysticerci and hydatid cysts.

Diagnosis is based on clinical, epidemiologic, and laboratory findings. No serologic tests are currently available.

Treatment involves surgery if the lesion is accessible. Although albendazole, praziquantel and other antihelminthic therapies have been used, it is unclear how efficacious these are.[67] Recommendations for prevention are limited, because reservoir hosts include such a large number of species of wild animals.

References

1. Gomez-Priego, A.; Godinez-Hana, A. L.; Gutierrez-Quiroz, M.; R., Detection of serum antibodies in human Hymenolepis infection by enzyme immunoassay. *Trans Trop Med Hyg* **1991**, *85*, 645-647.

2. Crompton, D. W., How much human helminthiasis is there in the world? *J Parasitol* **1999**, *85* (3), 397-403.

3. Thompson, R. C., Neglected zoonotic helminths: Hymenolepis nana, Echinococcus canadensis and Ancylostoma ceylanicum. *Clin Microbiol Infect* **2015**, *21* (5), 426-32.

4. Mirdha, B. R.; Samantray, J. C., Hymenolepis nana: a common cause of paediatric diarrhoea in urban slum dwellers in India. *Journal of tropical pediatrics* **2002**, *48* (6), 331-4.

5. Sirivichayakul, C.; Radomyos, P.; Praevanit, R.; Pojjaroen-Anant, C.; Wisetsing, P., Hymenolepis nana infection in Thai children. *Journal of the Medical Association of Thailand = Chotmaihet thangphaet* **2000**, *83* (9), 1035-8.

6. Heyneman, D., Studies on helminth immunity. III. Experimental verification of autoinfection from cysticercoids of Hymenolepis nana in the white mouse. *J Infect Dis* **1961**, *109*, 10-8.

7. Ito, A., Hymenolepis nana: immunogenicity of a lumen phase of the direct cycle and failure of autoinfection in BALB/c mice. *Exp Parasitol* **1982**, *54* (1), 113-20.

8. Muehlenbachs, A.; Bhatnagar, J.; Agudelo, C. A.; Hidron, A.; Eberhard, M. L.; Mathison, B. A.; Frace, M. A.; Ito, A.; Metcalfe, M. G.; Rollin, D. C.; Visvesvara, G. S.; Pham, C. D.; Jones, T. L.; Greer, P. W.; Velez Hoyos, A.; Olson, P. D.; Diazgranados, L. R.; Zaki, S. R., Malignant Transformation of Hymenolepis nana in a Human Host. *N Engl J Med* **2015**, *373* (19), 1845-52.

9. Macnish, M. G.; Ryan, U. M.; Behnke, J. M.; Thompson, R. C. A., Detection of the rodent tapeworm Rodentolepis (=Hymenolepis) microstoma in humans. A new zoonosis? *International journal for parasitology* **2003**, *33* (10), 1079-85.

10. Bilharz, T.; von Siebold, C. T., Ein Beitrag zur Helminhographia humana, aus brieflichen Mitteilungen des Dr. Bilharz in Cairo, nenst Bermerkungen von Prof. C. Th. von Siebold in Breslau. *Z. Wiss. Zool.* **1852**, *4*, 53-76.

11. Grassi, B., Entwicklungscyclus der Taenia nanna. Dritte Praliminarnote. *Centralblatt für Bakteriologie und Parasitenkunde* **1887**, *2*, 305-312.

12. Riley, W. A.; Shannin, W. R., The Rat Tapeworm, Hymenolepos diminuta. In Man. *The Journal of Parasitology* **1922**, *8* (3), 109-117.

13. Fan, P. C., Infectivity and development of the human strain of Hymenolepis nana in ICR mice. *Southeast Asian J Trop Med Public Health* **2005**, *36* (1), 97-102.

14. Andreassen, J.; Collier, L.; Balows, A.; Sussman, M.; Cox, F. E. G.; Kreier, J. P.; Wakelin, D., Intestinal Tapeworms. 1998; p 520-537.

15. Menan, E. I.; Nebavi, N. G.; Adjetey, T. A.; Assavo, N. N.; Kiki-Barro, P. C.; Kone, M., [Profile of intestinal helminthiases in school aged children in the city of Abidjan]. *Bull Soc Pathol Exot* **1997**, *90* (1), 51-4.

16. Ito, A.; Onitake, K.; Sasaki, J.; Takami, T., Hymenolepis nana: immunity against oncosphere challenge in mice previously given viable or non-viable oncospheres of H. nana, H. diminuta, H.

microstoma and Taenia taeniaeformis. *Int J Parasitol* **1991,** *21* (2), 241-5.

17. Palmas, C.; Wakelin, D.; Gabriele, F., Transfer of immunity against Hymenolepis nana in mice with lymphoid cells or serum from infected donors. *Parasitology* **1984,** *89 (Pt 2),* 287-93.

18. Niwa, A.; Miyazato, T., Reactive oxygen intermediates from eosinophils in mice infected with Hymenolepis nana. *Parasite immunology* **1996,** *18* (6), 285-95.

19. Conchedda, M.; Bortoletti, G.; Gabriele, F.; Wakelin, D.; Palmas, C., Immune response to the cestode Hymenolepis nana: cytokine production during infection with eggs or cysts. *International journal for parasitology* **1997,** *27* (3), 321-7.

20. Asano, K.; Muramatsu, K., Importance of interferon-gamma in protective immunity against Hymenolepis nana cysticercoids derived from challenge infection with eggs in BALB/c mice. *International journal for parasitology* **1997,** *27* (11), 1437-43.

21. Watanabe, N.; Nawa, Y.; Okamoto, K.; Kobayashi, A., Expulsion of Hymenolepis nana from mice with congenital deficiencies of IgE production or of mast cell development. *Parasite immunology* **1994,** *16* (3), 137-44.

22. Bouree, P., [Efficacy of a single dose of praziquantel as treatment for Taenia saginata and Hymenolepis nana]. *Pathol Biol (Paris)* **1988,** *36* (5 Pt 2), 759-61.

23. Bouree, P., Successful treatment of Taenia saginata and Hymenolepis nana by single oral dose of praziquantel. *J Egypt Soc Parasitol* **1991,** *21* (2), 303-7.

24. Pedro Rde, J.; Deberaldini, E. R.; de Souza Dias, L. C.; Goto, M. M., [Treatment of school children with Hymenolepis nana with praziquantel]. *AMB Rev Assoc Med Bras* **1982,** *28* (9-10), 216-7.

25. Schenone, H., Praziquantel in the treatment of Hymenolepis nana infections in children. *Am J Trop Med Hyg* **1980,** *29* (2), 320-1.

26. Maggi, P.; Brandonisio, O.; Carito, V.; Bellacosa, C.; Epifani, G.; Pastore, G., Hymenolepis nana parasites in adopted children. *Clin Infect Dis* **2005,** *41* (4), 571-2.

27. Diaz, E.; Mondragon, J.; Ramirez, E.; Bernal, R., Epidemiology and control of intestinal parasites with nitazoxanide in children in Mexico. *The American journal of tropical medicine and hygiene* **2003,** *68* (4), 384-5.

28. Rossignol, J. F.; Maisonneuve, H., Nitazoxanide in the treatment of Taenia saginata and Hymenolepis nana infections. *Am J Trop Med Hyg* **1984,** *33* (3), 511-2.

29. Chero, J. C.; Saito, M.; Bustos, J. A.; Blanco, E. M.; Gonzalvez, G.; Garcia, H. H.; Cysticercosis Working Group in, P., Hymenolepis nana infection: symptoms and response to nitazoxanide in field conditions. *Trans R Soc Trop Med Hyg* **2007,** *101* (2), 203-5.

30. Rudolphi, C. A., Entozoorum Synopsis cui Accedunt Mantissa Duplex et Indeces Locuplet. *Issimi Berolini* **1819**.

31. Weinland, D. F., Human Cestodes. An Essay on the Tapeworms of Man. 1858.

32. Pappas, P. W.; Barley, A. J., Beetle-to-beetle transmission and dispersal of Hymenolepis diminuta (Cestoda) eggs via the feces of Tenebrio molitor. *The Journal of parasitology* **1999,** *85* (2), 384-5.

33. Arai, H. P., Biology of the Tapeworm Hymenolepis diminuta. 1980.

34. Andreassen, J.; Bennet-Jenkins, E. M.; Bryant, C., Immunology and biochemistry of Hymenolepis diminuta. *Advances in parasitology* **1999,** *42,* 223-75.

35. Kalaivani, R.; Nandhini, L.; Seetha, K. S., Hymenolepis diminuta infection in a school-going child: A rare case report. *Australas Med J* **2014,** *7* (9), 379-81.

36. Kilincel, O.; Ozturk, C. E.; Gun, E.; Oksuz, S.; Uzun, H.; Sahin, I.; Kilic, N., [A rare case of Hymenolepis diminuta infection in a small child]. *Mikrobiyol Bul* **2015,** *49* (1), 135-8.

37. Wiwanitkit, V., Overview of hymenolepis diminuta infection among Thai patients. *MedGenMed : Medscape general medicine* **2004,** *6* (2), 7.

38. Hamrick, H. J.; Bowdre, J. H.; Church, S. M., Rat tapeworm (Hymenolepis diminuta) infection in a child. *The Pediatric infectious disease journal* **1990,** *9* (3), 216-9.

39. Tena, D.; Pérez Simón, M.; Gimeno, C.; Pérez Pomata, M. T.; Illescas, S.; Amondarain, I.; González, A.; Domínguez, J.; Bisquert, J., Human infection with Hymenolepis diminuta: case report from Spain. *Journal of clinical microbiology* **1998,** *36* (8), 2375-6.

40. Dwinell, M. B.; Bass, P.; Schaefer, D. M.; Oaks, J. A., Tapeworm infection decreases intestinal

transit and enteric aerobic bacterial populations. *The American journal of physiology* **1997**, *273* (2 Pt 1), G480-5.

41.   Ostlind, D. A.; Mickle, W. G.; Smith, S. K.; Cifelli, S.; Ewanciw, D. V., The Hymenolepis diminuta-golden hamster (Mesocricetus auratus) model for the evaluation of gastrointestinal anticestode activity. *The Journal of parasitology* **2004**, *90* (4), 898-9.

42.   Hamrick, H. J.; Drake, W. R.; Jones, H. M.; Askew, A. P.; Weatherly, N. F., Two cases of dipylidiasis (dog tapeworm infection) in children: update on an old problem. *Pediatrics* **1983**, *72* (1), 114-7.

43.   Manyam, K. S.; Stump, K.; Picut, C., Observations in a case of Dipylidium caninum infection. *Vet Med Small Anim Clin* **1980**, *75* (1), 66.

44.   Narasimham, M. V.; Panda, P.; Mohanty, I.; Sahu, S.; Padhi, S.; Dash, M., Dipylidium caninum infection in a child: a rare case report. *Indian J Med Microbiol* **2013**, *31* (1), 82-4.

45.   Szwaja, B.; Romanski, L.; Zabczyk, M., A case of Dipylidium caninum infection in a child from the southeastern Poland. *Wiad Parazytol* **2011**, *57* (3), 175-8.

46.   Molina, C. P.; Ogburn, J.; Adegboyega, P., Infection by Dipylidium caninum in an infant. *Archives of pathology & laboratory medicine* **2003**, *127* (3), e157-9.

47.   Jones, W. E., Niclosamide as a treatment for Hymenolepis diminuta and Dipylidium caninum infection in man. *Am J Trop Med Hyg* **1979**, *28* (2), 300-2.

48.   Schenone, H.; Thompson, L.; Quero, M. S., [Infection by Dipylidium caninum in a young girl treated with praziquantel]. *Bol Chil Parasitol* **1987**, *42* (3-4), 74-5.

49.   Schultz, L. V.; Roberto, R. R.; Rutherford, G. W.; Hummert, B.; Lubell, I., Mesocestoides (Cestoda) infection in a California child. *The Pediatric infectious disease journal* **1992**, *11* (4), 332-4.

50.   Fuentes, M. V.; Galán-Puchades, M. T.; Malone, J. B., Short report: a new case report of human Mesocestoides infection in the United States. *The American journal of tropical medicine and hygiene* **2003**, *68* (5), 566-7.

51.   Walker, M. D.; Zunt, J. R., Neuroparasitic infections: cestodes, trematodes, and protozoans. *Semin Neurol* **2005**, *25* (3), 262-77.

52.   Pampiglione, S.; Fioravanti, M. L.; Rivasi, F., Human sparganosis in Italy. Case report and review of the European cases. *APMIS* **2003**, *111* (2), 349-54.

53.   Hughes, A. J.; Biggs, B. A., Parasitic worms of the central nervous system: an Australian perspective. *Intern Med J* **2002**, *32* (11), 541-53.

54.   Lescano, A. G.; Zunt, J., Other cestodes: sparganosis, coenurosis and Taenia crassiceps cysticercosis. *Handb Clin Neurol* **2013**, *114*, 335-45.

55.   Kean, B. H.; Ellsworth, R. M.; Sun, T., Color Atlas / Text of Ophthalmic Parasitology. 1991; p 195-200.

56.   Despommier, D., People, Parasites, and Plowshares. 2014.

57.   Oren, Z.; Shai, Y., Mode of action of linear amphipathic alpha-helical antimicrobial peptides. *Biopolymers* **1998**, *47* (6), 451-63.

58.   Bechinger, B., Structure and functions of channel-forming peptides: magainins, cecropins, melittin and alamethicin. *The Journal of membrane biology* **1997**, *156* (3), 197-211.

59.   Otranto, D.; Eberhard, M. L., Zoonotic helminths affecting the human eye. *Parasit Vectors* **2011**, *4*, 41.

60.   Wiwanitkit, V., Ocular sparganosis. *Orbit* **2014**, *33* (6), 474.

61.   Phares, K., An unusual host-parasite relationship: the growth hormone-like factor from plerocercoids of spirometrid tapeworms. *International journal for parasitology* **1996**, *26* (6), 575-88.

62.   Song, T.; Wang, W. S.; Zhou, B. R.; Mai, W. W.; Li, Z. Z.; Guo, H. C.; Zhou, F., CT and MR characteristics of cerebral sparganosis. *AJNR Am J Neuroradiol* **2007**, *28* (9), 1700-5.

63.   Cui, J.; Li, N.; Wang, Z. Q.; Jiang, P.; Lin, X. M., Serodiagnosis of experimental sparganum infections of mice and human sparganosis by ELISA using ES antigens of Spirometra mansoni spargana. *Parasitol Res* **2011**, *108* (6), 1551-6.

64.   Liu, L. N.; Zhang, X.; Jiang, P.; Liu, R. D.; Zhou, J.; He, R. Z.; Cui, J.; Wang, Z. Q., Serodiagnosis

of sparganosis by ELISA using recombinant cysteine protease of Spirometra erinaceieuropaei spargana. *Parasitol Res* **2015,** *114* (2), 753-7.

65.   Tan, T. Y.; Lui, C. C.; Chen, H. J.; Liou, C. W., Cerebral sparganosis: case report. *Changgeng yi xue za zhi / Changgeng ji nian yi yuan = Chang Gung medical journal / Chang Gung Memorial Hospital* **1999,** *22* (2), 287-92.

66.   Chang, J. H.; Lin, O. S.; Yeh, K. T., Subcutaneous sparganosis--a case report and a review of human sparganosis in Taiwan. *The Kaohsiung journal of medical sciences* **1999,** *15* (9), 567-71.

67.   El-On, J.; Shelef, I.; Cagnano, E.; Benifla, M., Taenia multiceps: a rare human cestode infection in Israel. *Vet Ital* **2008,** *44* (4), 621-31.

32. Juvenile Tapeworm Infections of Humans

Echinococcus granulosus
(Batsch 1786)

Echinococcus multilocularis
(Leuckart 1863)

Introduction

Echinococcus granulosus lives as an adult parasite in the small intestine of its definitive host – domestic dogs and other canidae. It is one of the smallest cestodes, measuring 5 mm in length. The strobila consists of a scolex and three segments (Fig. 32.1). Sheep and other herbivores serve as intermediate hosts, acquiring infection by eating embryonated eggs that contaminate grazing pastures. Humans are also susceptible to the juvenile stage of the parasite, which may develop to a large, fluid-filled cyst, often exceeding 40 cm in diameter. The condition is referred to as hydatid disease. Although both *Echinococcus granulosus and Echinococcus multilocularis* cause infection in humans, 95% of the cases of human disease are due to *Echinococcus granulosus*.[1] It is estimated that an annual loss of US $194,000,000 or 285,000 disability-adjusted life years is due to echinococcosis worldwide.[2]

Distribution of *E. granulosus* coincides with sheep husbandry. Eurasia, especially the Russian Federation and Central Asia and China (including Tibet), Mediterranean countries (especially, Turkey, Lebanon and Syria), North and East Africa (especially, Egypt, Sudan, and Kenya), and Australia have the highest prevalence.[3-5] Mongolia is also an important source of hydatid disease.[6] Infection has been totally eradicated from Iceland, Ireland, and Greenland but not from other island communities, such as Cyprus and New Zealand.[2, 7]

Small, endemic areas of infection exist

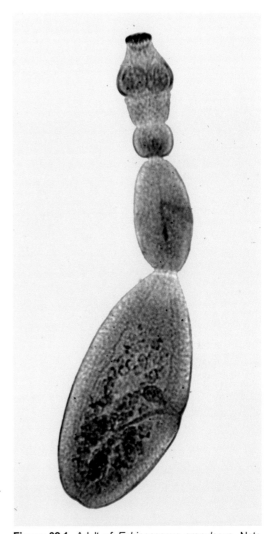

Figure 32.1. Adult of *Echinococcus granulosus*. Note suckers and hooks on scolex. The worm is 5.5 mm long.

in the United States, primarily in California, Utah, New Mexico, Alaska and Arizona, where local transmission to humans has been documented.[8-10] A number of cases have also been described in the lower Mississippi River Valley.[11]

Indigenous peoples of the Canadian Arctic, especially the Inuit, are infected with a northern variant, *E. granulosus var. canadensis*, acquired in a sylvatic cycle involving moose and caribou (cervids), wolves, and sled dogs.[3, 12, 13] Two cases reported from Alaska were unusually severe.[13] In Lapland (i.e., northern Scandinavian countries), herd-

Echinococcus granulosus

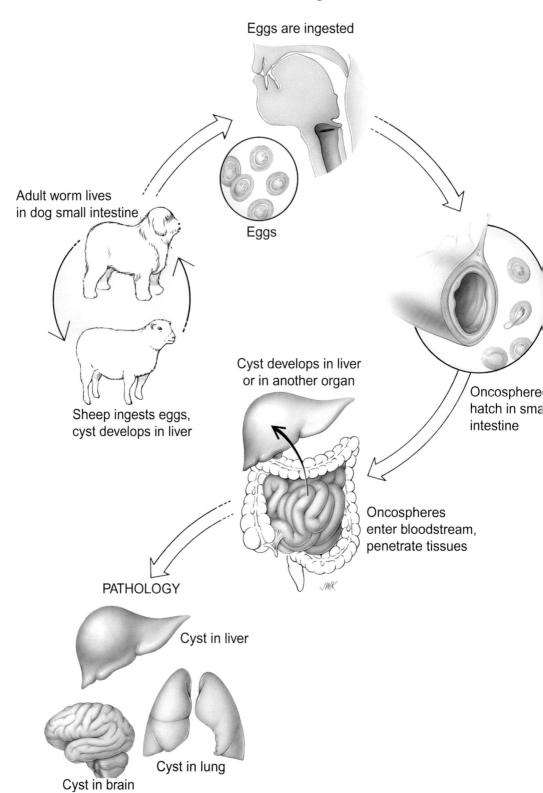

Eggs are ingested

Eggs

Adult worm lives
in dog small intestine

Sheep ingests eggs,
cyst develops in liver

Cyst develops in liver
or in another organ

Oncosphere
hatch in sma
intestine

Oncospheres
enter bloodstream,
penetrate tissues

PATHOLOGY

Cyst in liver

Cyst in lung

Cyst in brain

Parasitic Diseases 6th Ed. Parasites Without Borders www.parasiteswithoutborders.com

ing of reindeer as well as artificial introduction of reindeer is associated with this infection.[14]

Historical Information

Descriptions of the massive cysts seen in slaughtered animals can be found in multiple ancient texts from Babylon, Greece, and Rome.[15] In 1766, Pierre Pallas described the hydatid cyst of *Echinococcus granulosus*, in which he sketched cysts that he removed from the viscera of mice, and compared them with those recovered by others from human infections.[16] In 1782, Johann Goeze, in his classic monograph, depicted the juveniles (i.e., protoscolices).[17] In 1853, Carl Von Siebold described the adult worms in the dog and demonstrated that echinococcus cysts from sheep gave rise to adult tapeworms when fed to dogs.[18] In 1863, Bernhard Naunyn fed the contents of hydatid cysts from a human infection to dogs, and recovered adult tapeworms in them.[19] These experiments provided the essential link between the animal and human infection cycles.

Life Cycle

Echinococcus granulosus adults live in the canine small intestine. Multiple infection is the rule, with hundreds to thousands of adult worms occupying the greater portion of the upper half of the small intestine. The gravid segment (one per adult tapeworm) breaks off and disintegrates in the large bowel, releasing hundreds of infective eggs (Figs. 28.5, 29.5), which then pass out with the feces. Sheep, as well as other domestic animals (e.g., cattle, pigs, and horses), and humans acquire the juvenile stage by ingesting embryonated eggs. Each intermediate host species (sheep, cattle, pig, and horse) seems to have evolved a separate, genetically definable strain of parasite.[20] The oncosphere hatches in the small intestine, enters

the bloodstream, and in the vast majority of cases, reaches the liver via the portal circulation (Fig. 32.2).[21-23] Other organs can also be invaded, including brain, lung, heart, bones, eyes and kidney.[24-30] Once in the tissue, the larva synthesizes a hyaline membrane, and becomes surrounded by it. This membrane differentiates into an outer, acellular laminate structure, and an inner, cellular germinal layer (Fig. 32.3, 32.11). The inner surface of the germinal layer gives rise to protoscolices (Fig. 32.5) (i.e., the infectious stage for the definitive host), and more outer membrane material.

The hydatid cyst requires several months to years in order to develop, mature and fill with fluid (Fig. 32.6). The fluid is under pressure, and the wall, while substantial, can rupture if severely traumatized. The entire cyst can contain millions of protoscolices. The diameter of the mature outer cyst varies from 2 to 20 cm, and sometimes is even larger. The fluid portion of the cyst contains both host and parasite proteins. A canine host must ingest the hydatid cyst and its contents (i.e., the protoscolices) to complete the life cycle. This commonly occurs when infected sheep are slaughtered (Fig. 32.11), and organs containing hydatid cysts are discarded or fed to dogs.

The protoscolex, released from the hydatid cyst, attaches itself to the wall of the small intestine aided by its four suckers and a row of hooklets (Fig. 32.6). New gravid proglottids are produced within about 2 months. Dogs do not seem to become ill from the effects of even heavy intestinal infections, which may exceed a million adult worms.

Cellular and Molecular Pathogenesis

There is minimal host reaction to a living hydatid cyst, but little is known regarding the nature of the immune responses directed at the parasite, and the antigens it secretes into the cyst fluid. Evidence suggests that the production of immunosuppressive substances by the parasite suppress host responses for the life of the cyst.[31-34] Studies indicate a potential role for IL-21 in echinococcosis.[35] Cysts can remain alive for months to years. In contrast to the cysts, the eggs and the oncospheres of *E. granulosus* are immunogenic, and elicit protective immunity. This feature might provide a mechanism by which intermediate hosts, including humans, control the number of oncospheres that ultimately develop into hydatid cysts.[3]

Clinical Disease

The primary exposure and initial infection are thought to always be asymptomatic with symptoms only occurring coincident with cyst development. Hydatid disease develops as the result of rapid growth of the cyst (or cysts), and subsequent expansion of the cyst wall. The liver is the most common site of hydatid cyst development (Fig. 32.9), followed by the lungs. More than 90 percent of cysts develop in these two organs. Cysts have been reported to infect almost all of the

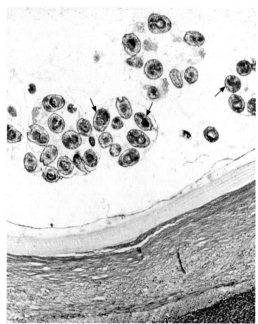

Figure 32.3. Histological section of an hydatid cyst with capsules filled with protoscolices (arrows) of *Echinococcus granulosus*. Each protoscolex measures approx. 13-14 µm in length.

visceral organs, including the bone marrow (Fig. 32.10) or brain, the latter usually with fatal results. If a cyst ruptures, the entire contents (fluid and protoscolices) spill into the surrounding tissues or body cavity (e.g., peritoneum, pleural cavity). When such an event occurs, an immediate anaphylactic reaction may ensue.[36, 37] Moreover, cyst contents can seed the area, and invade new tissues to produce second-generation hydatid cysts (Fig. 32.10). Even a few cells from the germinal membrane can re-establish an entire hydatid cyst, as each cell of the germinal membrane has a stem cell-like ability to reproduce a full hydatid cyst. Avoiding contact with hydatid cyst contents and is sterilizing the germinal layer is essential as the mortality rate of 2-4% usually seen in cases of cystic echinococcus may be increased if patients are improperly treated.

Approximately 60 percent of hydatid cysts are asymptomatic. Symptoms, when present, are those of a large space-occupying lesion. If the liver is involved, it becomes

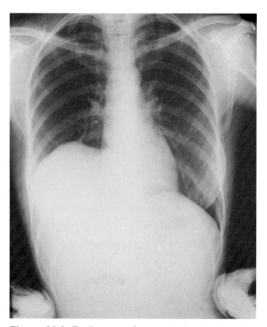

Figure 32.2. Radiogram of upper body showing elevation in right lobe of liver due to a large hydatid cyst.

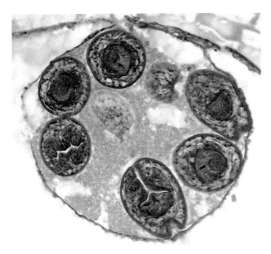

Figure 32.4. Brood capsule with protoscolices of *Echinococcus granulosus*.

enlarged (Fig. 32.3). The cyst presents as a palpable, soft, non-tender, intrahepatic mass. The uninvolved bulk of the liver remains normal. Involvement of the lung is usually identified by chance on a radiograph, or by the presence of bloody sputum, in which protoscolices or hooklets (Fig. 32.7) can be found. Patients may describe the sputum they produce as salty if it is due to a leaking hydatid cyst in the lungs.[38] Expansion and rupture of liver hydatid cysts into the biliary tree can result in secondary cholangitis, biliary obstruction, and intraperitoneal rupture.[39] Lung cysts can rupture into the bronchial tree and cause the development of a bronchobiliary fistula. Rupture of a cyst, wherever it is lodged, may occur even after relatively minor blunt trauma, and often leads to an allergic reaction. It may be mild and limited to urticaria, or may take the form of anaphylactic shock, requiring immediate intervention. Most patients with the northern variant of echinococcosis have asymptomatic lung cysts that are usually detected on chest radiographs obtained for other reasons (e.g., tuberculosis screening).

Diagnosis

An accurate case history is essential to the diagnosis of hydatid disease. Ownership

of dogs, life on a sheep farm – even during childhood, and especially in endemic areas – and/or a history of travel to endemic areas are important factors in ruling in this disease.

Within the last decade, the diagnostic algorithms for hydatid disease have been modified based on increasing experience with radiologic imaging modalities, including ultrasound, CT, and MRI. Currently ultrasound is the recommended modality with a reported 90% sensitivity for hepatic hydatidosis but this is still controversial as some investigations suggest CT might be superior.[40] Despite this recommendation, in many resource-rich countries both CT and MRI are widely used.[1] The major radiological criteria have been standardized and management is now guided by an expert consensus generated under the aegis of the World Health Organization Informal Working Group on Echinococcosis (WHO-IWGE).[41]

Imaging by MRI frequently reveals a mixture of hyperdensities and hypodensities, with scattered calcifications (Fig. 32.8).[42] Internal septae and daughter cysts are often demonstrable, and such evidence is strongly suggestive of the diagnosis.

Serodiagnosis is also useful both for pri-

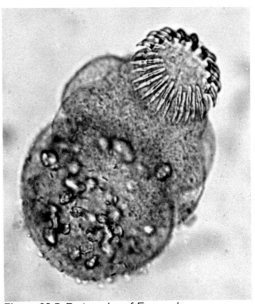

Figure 32.5. Protoscolex of *E. granulosus*.

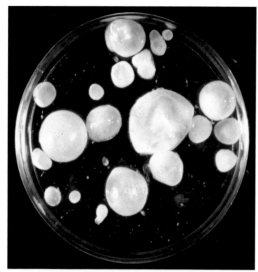

Figure 32.6. Petri dish filled with daughter cysts of *Echinococcus granulosus*.

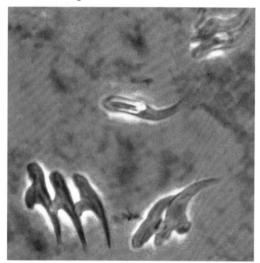

Figure 32.7. Hooklets of a protoscolex. Each hooklet measures approx. 2 μm in length.

mary diagnosis and following patients during and after their medical or surgical management.[43] ELISA, for the detection of echinococcus antibodies, is the test of choice, and employs hydatid fluid antigen. In addition, efforts are underway to refine the ELISA using specific antigens, including two known as antigen 5 and lipoprotein antigen B.[44] Of patients with hepatic cystic echinococcosis, 30-40% have negative serologies, possibly due to the ability of *E. granulosus* antigens to inhibit B cell activity and proliferation.[45] Patients with intact cysts have a high false-

negative rate; presumably because these patients do not experience sufficient antigen challenge to induce a detectable antibody response. Efforts are underway to develop tests that detect circulating echinococcus antigens. Eosinophilia is an uncommon finding in patients with hydatid disease.[46]

A definitive diagnosis of echinococcosis can be made by microscopically identifying hooklets (Fig. 32.7) in any sample, sputum being the most common. This is usually the case in long-term infections, in which all cells within the cyst have died, and the only remaining evidence of infection are the hooklets and portions of the acellular, laminate outer membrane of the cyst wall. Biopsy of cysts is absolutely contra-indicated, due to their metastatic nature.

Treatment

Treatment of hydatid disease is driven by cyst size, location, and stage.[47] Hydatid cysts

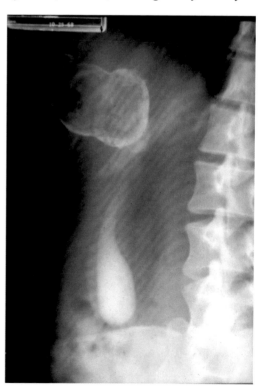

Figure 32.8. Radiogram of a calcified hydatid cyst of *Echinococcus granulosus*.

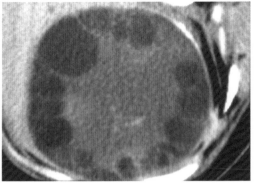

Figure 32.9. Radiogram of a liver infected with multiple hydatid cysts of *Echinococcus granulosus*.

undergo an increase in size of 1-5 cm per year with calcification occurring 5-10 years post infection, but this development varies depending on host as well as parasite factors.[48, 49] These hydatid cysts develop, enlarge, fill with protoscolices and daughter cysts and undergoe a defined evolution over years with predictable features.[47] As the hydatid cyst

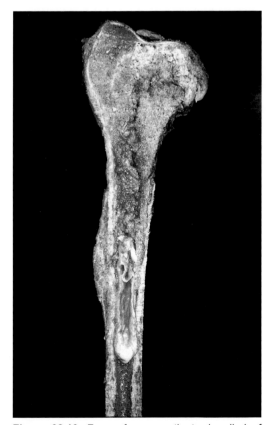

Figure 32.10. Femur from a patient who died of hydatid disease of the bone. Courtesy W. Johnson.

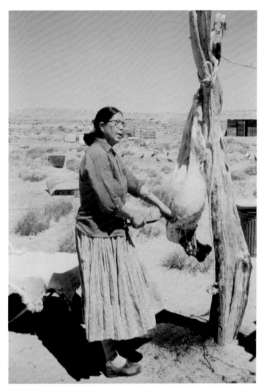

Figure 32.11. Navajo butchering a sheep. The organs containing hydatid cysts are occasionally fed to their dogs, thus completing the life cycle. Courtesy P.M.Schantz.

develops, it goes through a series of defined stages that guide the choice of optimum therapy from stage cystic echinococcosis (CE) stage 1 to CE5.

Treatment of patients with hydatid cysts often requires both surgical and medical interventions.[41] Surgical intervention is the usual approach to cure for patients with large cysts and complex cysts. Care must be taken to prevent inadvertent rupture of the cysts. Successful removal depends on the location of the cyst. Historically, a variety of strategies have been devised to prevent or minimize spillage of cyst contents. This includes preoperative use of anthelminthic drugs and the use of protoscolicidal compounds such as 95% ethanol, hypertonic saline and cetrimide.

Introduced in the mid-1980s, the PAIR technique (Puncture, Aspiration, Injection, Re-aspiration) with ultrasound guidance has

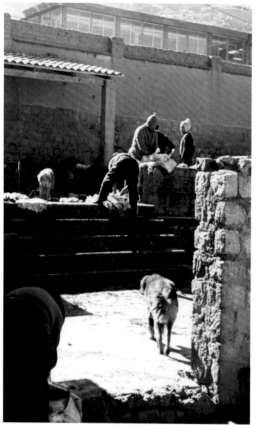

Figure 32.12. Peruvian slaughter house. Organs from sheep containing hydatid cysts are routinely fed to the numerous dogs that frequent these unsanitary, unsupervised rural establishments.

replaced the need for laparotomy and surgery for some patients.[50, 51] The risk of complications from PAIR appear to be greatly improved through the use of adjuvant anthelminthic chemotherapy started one month prior to performing this procedure. More recently laproscopic surgery has emerged as a viable alternative for surgical treatment.[52] For pulmonary cysts antihelminthic therapy is usually started after cyst removal with concerns that treatment may weaken the cyst wall leading to cyst rupture.

Albendazole 400 mg bid x 1-6 months or, for children, 15 mg/kg/d (max. 800 mg) x 1-6 months has been used successfully to treat hydatid disease, particularly when surgical removal was impossible. Chemotherapy can result in cyst regression or collapse, although prolonged courses of therapy are usually required.[46, 50, 51] It has been estimated that treatment can result in the disappearance of up to 48 percent of cysts and a substantial reduction in size of an additional 24 percent.[51] Albendazole is preferable to mebendazole because the former is metabolized to a sulfoxide derivative, which exhibits antiparasitic activity and is widely distributed in the tissues. In many areas of the world praziquantel is added and patients are given both albendazole and praziquantel in response to evidence of praziquantel's protoscolicidal activity.[53-56] Therapeutic responses can be monitored radiographically and serologically. Reversible liver toxicity has been reported with prolonged therapy with albendazole.[57, 58] As outlined in the section on trichuriasis, the benzimidazole antihelminthics, including albendazole, are teratogenic and embryotoxic in laboratory animals. Both drugs are considered category C agents in the United States. Before use in pregnancy the risks versus benefits must be weighed.

Prevention and Control

Infection of domestic dogs with *E. granulosus* can be prevented. Control is best achieved by avoiding feeding dogs (Figs.

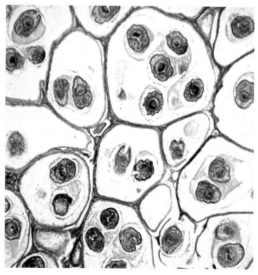

Figure 32.13. *Echinococcus multilocularis* alveolar cyst from an infected vole.

32.11, 32.12) any infected organs of slaughtered sheep, or other animals, and by periodically treating dogs prophylactically with niclosamide, arecoline hydrobromide, or praziquantel.[51] An arecoline control program in dogs has resulted in the near-elimination of *E. granulosus* infection in New Zealand and Tasmania. In Iceland, mass slaughter of infected sheep and dogs led to the total eradication of the disease. Attempts to duplicate that effort in Cyprus were not as successful.[59] Strict regulations regarding the importation of animal products that might carry *E. granulosus* eggs (e.g., animal hides of various carnivores, fishing flies, etc.) is a requirement for this control strategy to be effective. A recombinant peptide vaccine, EG95, induces high levels of protection in sheep, and may prove useful in situations where cost of production and ease of distribution are not important factors (i.e., the developed world).[60] Canine vaccination, which is currently being tested, may be critical in many areas of the world.[61, 62]

Echinococcus multilocularis

Echinococcus multilocularis infects wild Caenidae, such as fox, and can also infect domestic dogs. The intermediate hosts are usually rodents (e.g., voles, field mice, ground squirrels).[63] The biology of the infection in humans resembles the situation found in the intermediate hosts. *E. multilocularis* results in discrete cysts (alveolar echinococcosis) (Fig. 32.13) that metastasize from a single location, except for the fact that *E. multilocularis* does not produce protoscolices in human infection, only membranes that grow and bisect whatever organ they happen to be in, confounding the diagnosis of this unusual parasitic disease. In rodents, protoscolices are found in each daughter cyst.

This infection is prevalent among fur trappers and others whose occupations bring them in close contact with wild foxes and populations with close contact with dogs that regularly feed on infected rodents.[64] This includes urban areas where reservoir hosts could expand from foxes to domesticated dogs and cats. Alveolar echinococcosis has emerged to the point where it is endemic in the northern hemisphere including western Europe, where it is considered a re-emerging disease due, in part, to the banning of fox hunting in a number of Common Market countries.[65] It is also prevalent in the Russian Federation and Central Asia, China (especially in western and central regions), and northern Japan (Hokkaido). In North America, human infections have been reported from Alaska and in the upper Midwest and Northern Plains along the Canadian border.

Infection begins when the intermediate host ingests the egg. The oncosphere hatches in the small intestine and invades the liver by the hematogenous route. It transforms, and then grows into an alveolar type of cyst, characterized by numerous daughter cysts, as compared to hydatid cysts, that grow as a single membrane-bounded unit. Foxes and dogs ingest infected liver containing numerous protoscolices, which leads to infection with the adult worm, thereby completing the life cycle.

In humans, the incubation period of larval infection with *E. multilocularis* is long, with incubation periods of 5-15 years. The initial exposure often occurs during childhood, but the disease has been recognized mainly in older adults.[66] Alveolar disease can be highly aggressive disease specifically affecting the liver as the primary target organ. The membrane proliferates indefinitely and causes progressive destruction of the liver parenchyma, which can lead to hepatic failure. In some cases this may lead to direct extension to the lungs and rarely metastasis to the CNS.[67] Although initially asymptomatic as the disease progresses infected individuals may develop hepatomegaly, jaundice, multiple palpable abdominal masses, epigastric pain, and weight loss. If untreated, the mortality of clinically apparent disease can be as high as 50-75%.[64]

HLA type may play a role in a given individual's risk of developing further disease after chemotherapy. Re-growth of the parasite was significantly more prevalent in patients with haplotype HLA-DQB1 *02 than those with haplotype HLA-DRB1 *1157.[68] IL-10 production was also higher in infected individuals, and may relate to the lack of development of protective immunity.[69] Other investigators have noted an important role of Interleukin-5 and a robust Th2 response to infection with *E. multilocularis*.[70]

Diagnosis is based on radiographic imaging findings which show tumor like lesions with areas of calcification.[71] Serologic testing by ELISA is both highly sensitive and specific and allows distinction between *E. multilocularis* and *E. granulosus*.[72, 73] Directed biopsy of the lesion can often establish the diagnosis.[63]

Surgical resection is the preferred approach to treatment with the entire larval mass being removed as part of a hepatic wedge or pulmonary lobe resection.[64] Long-term adjuvant chemotherapy with albendazole or mebendazole improves the 10-year survival rate.[74, 75] Nitazoxanide has some demonstrated *in vitro* activity against *E. multilocularis* and may prove to be a useful alternative therapy.[76]

Prevention relates to the handling of animal furs, subsequent oral contamination with eggs, and transmission from infected dogs or cats to humans. Trappers and those involved in animal husbandry in the fur industry should be educated to exercise caution when handling carcasses and processing furs. Use of oral baits laced with therapeutic doses of praziquantel for control of *E. multilocularis* infections in foxes has been effective in certain areas.[77] Monthly treatment of dogs at high risk with praziquantel may be an effective approach.

References

1. Griffin, D. O.; Donaghy, H. J.; Edwards, B., Management of serology negative human hepatic hydatidosis (caused by Echinococcus granulosus) in a young woman from Bangladesh in a resource-rich setting: A case report. *IDCases* **2014**, *1* (2), 17-21.
2. Budke, C. M.; Deplazes, P.; Torgerson, P. R., Global socioeconomic impact of cystic echinococcosis. *Emerging infectious diseases* **2006**, *12* (2), 296-303.
3. Garcia, H. H.; Gonzalez, A. E.; Eveans, C. A. W.; Gilman, R. H., The Cysticercosis Working Group in Peru. *Lancet* **2003**, *361*, 547-56.
4. Moro, P. L.; Schantz, P. M., Echinococcosis: historical landmarks and progress in research and control. *Ann Trop Med Parasitol* **2006**, *100* (8), 703-14.
5. Abdybekova, A.; Sultanov, A.; Karatayev, B.; Zhumabayeva, A.; Shapiyeva, Z.; Yeshmuratov, T.; Toksanbayev, D.; Shalkeev, R.; Torgerson, P. R., Epidemiology of echinococcosis in Kazakhstan: an update. *J Helminthol* **2015**, *89* (6), 647-50.
6. Ito, A.; Budke, C. M., The present situation of echinococcoses in Mongolia. *J Helminthol* **2015**, *89* (6), 680-8.
7. Economides, P.; Christofi, G.; Gemmell, M. A., Control of Echinococcus granulosus in Cyprus and comparison with other island models. *Veterinary parasitology* **1998**, *79* (2), 151-63.
8. Stojkovic, M.; Rosenberger, K.; Kauczor, H. U.; Junghanss, T.; Hosch, W., Diagnosing and staging of cystic echinococcosis: how do CT and MRI perform in comparison to ultrasound? *PLoS neglected tropical diseases* **2012**, *6* (10), e1880.
9. Moro, P.; Schantz, P. M., Cystic echinococcosis in the Americas. *Parasitology international* **2006**, *55 Suppl*, S181-6.
10. Schantz, P. M., Echinococcosis in American Indians living in Arizona and New Mexico: a review of recent studies. *American journal of epidemiology* **1977**, *106* (5), 370-9.
11. Daly, J. J.; McDaniel, R. C.; Husted, G. S.; Harmon, H., Unilocular hydatid cyst disease in the

mid-South. *JAMA* **1984,** *251* (7), 932-3.

12.   Finlay, J. C.; Speert, D. P., Sylvatic hydatid disease in children: case reports and review of endemic Echinococcus granulosus infection in Canada and Alaska. *The Pediatric infectious disease journal* **1992,** *11* (4), 322-6.

13.   McManus, D. P.; Zhang, L.; Castrodale, L. J.; Le, T. H.; Pearson, M.; Blair, D., Short report: molecular genetic characterization of an unusually severe case of hydatid disease in Alaska caused by the cervid strain of Echinococcus granulosus. *The American journal of tropical medicine and hygiene* **2002,** *67* (3), 296-8.

14.   Sweatman, G. K., The Significance of the Artificial Introduction of Reindeer (Rangifer Tarandus) and Moose (Alces Alces) in the Spread of Hydatid Disease (Echinococcus Granulosus). *Ann Trop Med Parasitol* **1964,** *58*, 307-14.

15.   Cox, F. E., History of human parasitology. *Clin Microbiol Rev* **2002,** *15* (4), 595-612.

16.   Pallas, P. S., Miscellanea Zoologica: Quibus Novae Imprimis Atque Obscure Animalium Species Describuntur Et Observationibus Iconibusque Illustrantur. 1766.

17.   Goeze, J. A. E.; Blankenburg, P. A., Versuch ciner Naturgeschichte der Eingeweiderwumer Thierischer Korper. *Pape* **1782.**

18.   Seibold, C. T.; Z., Von Uber die Verwandlung der Echinococcus-brut in Taenia. *Zool* **1853,** *4* 409-424.

19.   Naunyn, B., Uber die zu Echinococcus hominis gehorige Taenia. *Arch Anat Physiol Wissenschr Med* **1863**, 412-416.

20.   Haag, K. L.; Araújo, A. M.; Gottstein, B.; Siles-Lucas, M.; Thompson, R. C.; Zaha, A., Breeding systems in Echinococcus granulosus (Cestoda; Taeniidae): selfing or outcrossing? *Parasitology* **1999,** *118 (Pt 1)*, 63-71.

21.   Heath, D. D.; Holcman, B.; Shaw, R. J., Echinococcus granulosus: the mechanism of oncosphere lysis by sheep complement and antibody. *International journal for parasitology* **1994,** *24* (7), 929-35.

22.   Holcman, B.; Heath, D. D.; Shaw, R. J., Ultrastructure of oncosphere and early stages of metacestode development of Echinococcus granulosus. *International journal for parasitology* **1994,** *24* (5), 623-35.

23.   Harris, A.; Heath, D. D.; Lawrence, S. B.; Shaw, R. J., Echinococcus granulosus: ultrastructure of epithelial changes during the first 8 days of metacestode development in vitro. *International journal for parasitology* **1989,** *19* (6), 621-9.

24.   Diaz-Menendez, M.; Perez-Molina, J. A.; Norman, F. F.; Perez-Ayala, A.; Monge-Maillo, B.; Fuertes, P. Z.; Lopez-Velez, R., Management and outcome of cardiac and endovascular cystic echinococcosis. *PLoS Negl Trop Dis* **2012,** *6* (1), e1437.

25.   Nourbakhsh, A.; Vannemreddy, P.; Minagar, A.; Toledo, E. G.; Palacios, E.; Nanda, A., Hydatid disease of the central nervous system: a review of literature with an emphasis on Latin American countries. *Neurol Res* **2010,** *32* (3), 245-51.

26.   Rexiati, M.; Mutalifu, A.; Azhati, B.; Wang, W.; Yang, H.; Sheyhedin, I.; Wang, Y., Diagnosis and surgical treatment of renal hydatid disease: a retrospective analysis of 30 cases. *PLoS One* **2014,** *9* (5), e96602.

27.   Sen, S.; Venkatesh, P.; Chand, M., Primary intraocular hydatid cyst with glaucoma. *J Pediatr Ophthalmol Strabismus* **2003,** *40* (5), 312-3.

28.   Sinav, S.; Demirci, A.; Sinav, B.; Oge, F.; Sullu, Y.; Kandemir, B., A primary intraocular hydatid cyst. *Acta Ophthalmol (Copenh)* **1991,** *69* (6), 802-4.

29.   Babitha, F.; Priya, P. V.; Poothiode, U., Hydatid cyst of bone. *Indian J Med Microbiol* **2015,** *33* (3), 442-4.

30.   Pazarci, O.; Oztemur, Z.; Bulut, O., Treatment of Bifocal Cyst Hydatid Involvement in Right Femur with Teicoplanin Added Bone Cement and Albendazole. *Case Rep Orthop* **2015,** *2015*, 824824.

31.   Dixon, J. B., Echinococcosis. *Comparative immunology, microbiology and infectious diseases* **1997,** *20* (1), 87-94.

32.   Gottstein, B.; Hemphill, A., Immunopathology of echinococcosis. *Chemical immunology* **1997,** *66*,

177-208.

33. Wang, Y.; Zhou, H.; Shen, Y.; Wang, Y.; Wu, W.; Liu, H.; Yuan, Z.; Xu, Y.; Hu, Y.; Cao, J., Impairment of dendritic cell function and induction of CD4(+)CD25(+)Foxp3(+) T cells by excretory-secretory products: a potential mechanism of immune evasion adopted by Echinococcus granulosus. *BMC Immunol* **2015,** *16*, 44.

34. Zheng, Y., Strategies of Echinococcus species responses to immune attacks: implications for therapeutic tool development. *Int Immunopharmacol* **2013,** *17* (3), 495-501.

35. Zhang, F.; Pang, N.; Zhu, Y.; Zhou, D.; Zhao, H.; Hu, J.; Ma, X.; Li, J.; Wen, H.; Samten, B.; Fan, H.; Ding, J., CCR7(lo)PD-1(hi) CXCR5(+) CD4(+) T cells are positively correlated with levels of IL-21 in active and transitional cystic echinococcosis patients. *BMC Infect Dis* **2015,** *15*, 457.

36. Nunnari, G.; Pinzone, M. R.; Gruttadauria, S.; Celesia, B. M.; Madeddu, G.; Malaguarnera, G.; Pavone, P.; Cappellani, A.; Cacopardo, B., Hepatic echinococcosis: clinical and therapeutic aspects. *World journal of gastroenterology : WJG* **2012,** *18* (13), 1448-58.

37. Minciullo, P. L.; Cascio, A.; David, A.; Pernice, L. M.; Calapai, G.; Gangemi, S., Anaphylaxis caused by helminths: review of the literature. *European review for medical and pharmacological sciences* **2012,** *16* (11), 1513-8.

38. Nakamura, K.; Ito, A.; Yara, S.; Haranaga, S.; Hibiya, K.; Hirayasu, T.; Sako, Y.; Fujita, J., A case of pulmonary and hepatic cystic Echinococcosis of CE1 stage in a healthy Japanese female that was suspected to have been acquired during her stay in the United Kingdom. *Am J Trop Med Hyg* **2011,** *85* (3), 456-9.

39. Irkoruucu, O.; Reyhan, E.; Erdem, H., The detection of cysto-biliary communications during surgery for liver hydatid cysts: let's speak the unspoken. *Clinics (Sao Paulo)* **2012,** *67* (2), 179.

40. Dhar, P.; Chaudhary, A.; Desai, R.; Agarwal, A.; Sachdev, A., Current trends in the diagnosis and management of cystic hydatid disease of the liver. *The Journal of communicable diseases* **1996,** *28* (4), 221-30.

41. Brunetti, E.; Kern, P.; Vuitton, D. A.; Writing Panel for the, W.-I., Expert consensus for the diagnosis and treatment of cystic and alveolar echinococcosis in humans. *Acta tropica* **2010,** *114* (1), 1-16.

42. Agildere, A. M.; Aytekin, C.; J., MRI of hydatid disease of the liver: a variety of sequences. *Assist Tomogr* **1998,** *22*, 718-24.

43. Gottstein, B., Molecular and immunological diagnosis of echinococcosis. *Clinical microbiology reviews* **1992,** *5* (3), 248-61.

44. Chemale, G.; Ferreira, H. B.; Barrett, J.; Brophy, P. M.; Zaha, A., Echinococcus granulosus antigen B hydrophobic ligand binding properties. *Biochimica et biophysica acta* **2005,** *1747* (2), 189-94.

45. Zhang, W.; McManus, D. P., Recent advances in the immunology and diagnosis of echinococcosis. *FEMS immunology and medical microbiology* **2006,** *47* (1), 24-41.

46. Schaefer, J. W.; Khan, M. Y., Echinococcosis (Hydatid disease): lessons from experience with 59 patients. *Reviews of infectious diseases* **1991,** *13* (2), 243-7.

47. Gharbi, H. A.; Hassine, W.; Brauner, M. W.; Dupuch, K., Ultrasound examination of the hydatic liver. *Radiology* **1981,** *139* (2), 459-63.

48. Moro, P. L.; Gilman, R. H.; Verastegui, M.; Bern, C.; Silva, B.; Bonilla, J. J., Human hydatidosis in the central Andes of Peru: evolution of the disease over 3 years. *Clinical infectious diseases : an official publication of the Infectious Diseases Society of America* **1999,** *29* (4), 807-12.

49. Frider, B.; Larrieu, E.; Odriozola, M., Long-term outcome of asymptomatic liver hydatidosis. *Journal of hepatology* **1999,** *30* (2), 228-31.

50. Filice, C.; Brunetti, E., Use of PAIR in human cystic echinococcosis. *Acta tropica* **1997,** *64* (1-2), 95-107.

51. Pelaez, V.; Kugler, C., PAIR as percutaneous treatment of hydatid liver cysts. *Acta Tropica* **2000,** *75*, 197-202.

52. Chen, X.; Cen, C.; Xie, H.; Zhou, L.; Wen, H.; Zheng, S., The Comparison of 2 New Promising Weapons for the Treatment of Hydatid Cyst Disease: PAIR and Laparoscopic Therapy. *Surg Laparosc Endosc Percutan Tech* **2015,** *25* (4), 358-62.

53. Alvela-Suarez, L.; Velasco-Tirado, V.; Belhassen-Garcia, M.; Novo-Veleiro, I.; Pardo-Lledias, J.;

Romero-Alegria, A.; Perez del Villar, L.; Valverde-Merino, M. P.; Cordero-Sanchez, M., Safety of the combined use of praziquantel and albendazole in the treatment of human hydatid disease. *Am J Trop Med Hyg* **2014,** *90* (5), 819-22.

54.   Bygott, J. M.; Chiodini, P. L., Praziquantel: neglected drug? Ineffective treatment? Or therapeutic choice in cystic hydatid disease? *Acta Trop* **2009,** *111* (2), 95-101.

55.   De, S.; Pan, D.; Bera, A. K.; Sreevatsava, V.; Bandyopadhyay, S.; Chaudhuri, D.; Kumar, S.; Rana, T.; Das, S.; Das, S. K.; Suryanaryana, V. V.; Singh, M. N.; Bhattacharya, D., In vitro assessment of praziquantel and a novel nanomaterial against protoscoleces of Echinococcus granulosus. *J Helminthol* **2012,** *86* (1), 26-9.

56.   Moreno, M. J.; Urrea-Paris, M. A.; Casado, N.; Rodriguez-Caabeiro, F., Praziquantel and albendazole in the combined treatment of experimental hydatid disease. *Parasitol Res* **2001,** *87* (3), 235-8.

57.   Horton, R. J., Albendazole in treatment of human cystic echinococcosis: 12 years of experience. *Acta tropica* **1997,** *64* (1-2), 79-93.

58.   Rowley, A. H.; Shulman, S. T.; Donaldson, J. S.; Schantz, P. M., Albendazole treatment of recurrent echinococcosis. *The Pediatric infectious disease journal* **1988,** *7* (9), 666-7.

59.   Beard, T. C., The elimination of echinococcosis from Iceland. *Bulletin of the World Health Organization* **1973,** *48* (6), 653-60.

60.   Woollard, D. J.; Gauci, C. G.; Heath, D. D.; Lightowlers, M. W., Epitope specificities and antibody responses to the EG95 hydatid vaccine. *Parasite immunology* **1998,** *20* (11), 535-40.

61.   Petavy, A. F.; Hormaeche, C.; Lahmar, S.; Ouhelli, H.; Chabalgoity, A.; Marchal, T.; Azzouz, S.; Schreiber, F.; Alvite, G.; Sarciron, M. E.; Maskell, D.; Esteves, A.; Bosquet, G., An oral recombinant vaccine in dogs against Echinococcus granulosus, the causative agent of human hydatid disease: a pilot study. *PLoS neglected tropical diseases* **2008,** *2* (1), e125.

62.   Zhang, W.; McManus, D. P., Vaccination of dogs against Echinococcus granulosus: a means to control hydatid disease? *Trends in parasitology* **2008,** *24* (9), 419-24.

63.   Moro, P.; Schantz, P. M., Echinococcosis: a review. *Int J Infect Dis* **2009,** *13* (2), 125-33.

64.   Wilson, J. F.; Rausch, R. L., Alveolar hydatid disease. A review of clinical features of 33 indigenous cases of Echinococcus multilocularis infection in Alaskan Eskimos. *Am J Trop Med Hyg* **1980,** *29* (6), 1340-55.

65.   Schweiger, A.; Ammann, R. W.; Candinas, D.; Clavien, P. A.; Eckert, J.; Gottstein, B.; Halkic, N.; Muellhaupt, B.; Prinz, B. M.; Reichen, J.; Tarr, P. E.; Torgerson, P. R.; Deplazes, P., Human alveolar echinococcosis after fox population increase, Switzerland. *Emerg Infect Dis* **2007,** *13* (6), 878-82.

66.   Lukaschenko, N. P.; J., Problems of epidemiology and prophylaxix of alveolar (multilocular echinococcosis): a general review-with particular reference to the USSR. *Int* **1971,** *1*, 125-134.

67.   Kammerer, W. S.; Schantz, P. M., Echinococcal disease. *Infect Dis Clin North Am* **1993,** *7* (3), 605-18.

68.   Eiermann, T. H.; Bettens, F.; Tiberghien, P.; Schmitz, K.; Beurton, I.; Bresson-Hadni, S.; Ammann, R. W.; Goldmann, S. F.; Vuitton, D. A.; Gottstein, B.; Kern, P., HLA and alveolar echinococcosis. *Tissue antigens* **1998,** *52* (2), 124-9.

69.   Godot, V.; Harraga, S.; Deschaseaux, M.; Bresson-Hadni, S.; Gottstein, B.; Emilie, D.; Vuitton, D. A., Increased basal production of interleukin-10 by peripheral blood mononuclear cells in human alveolar echinococcosis. *European cytokine network* **1997,** *8* (4), 401-8.

70.   Sturm, D.; Menzel, J.; Gottstein, B.; Kern, P., Interleukin-5 is the predominant cytokine produced by peripheral blood mononuclear cells in alveolar echinococcosis. *Infect Immun* **1995,** *63* (5), 1688-97.

71.   Didier, D.; Weiler, S.; Rohmer, P.; Lassegue, A.; Deschamps, J. P.; Vuitton, D.; Miguet, J. P.; Weill, F., Hepatic alveolar echinococcosis: correlative US and CT study. *Radiology* **1985,** *154* (1), 179-86.

72.   Gottstein, B.; Jacquier, P.; Bresson-Hadni, S.; Eckert, J., Improved primary immunodiagnosis of alveolar echinococcosis in humans by an enzyme-linked immunosorbent assay using the Em2plus antigen. *Journal of clinical microbiology* **1993,** *31* (2), 373-6.

73.   Carmena, D.; Benito, A.; Eraso, E., The immunodiagnosis of Echinococcus multilocularis infection. *Clin Microbiol Infect* **2007,** *13* (5), 460-75.

74.   Schantz, P. M.; Brandt, F. H.; Dickinson, C. M.; Allen, C. R.; Roberts, J. M.; Eberhard, M. L., Effects of albendazole on Echinococcus multilocularis infection in the Mongolian jird. *The Journal of infectious diseases* **1990,** *162* (6), 1403-7.

75.   Eckert, J.; Deplazes, P., Biological, epidemiological, and clinical aspects of echinococcosis, a zoonosis of increasing concern. *Clin Microbiol Rev* **2004,** *17* (1), 107-35.

76.   Reuter, S.; Manfras, B.; Merkle, M.; Harter, G.; Kern, P., In vitro activities of itraconazole, methiazole, and nitazoxanide versus Echinococcus multilocularis larvae. *Antimicrob Agents Chemother* **2006,** *50* (9), 2966-70.

77.   Takahashi, K.; Uraguchi, K.; Hatakeyama, H.; Giraudoux, P.; Romig, T., Efficacy of anthelmintic baiting of foxes against Echinococcus multilocularis in northern Japan. *Vet Parasitol* **2013,** *198* (1-2), 122-6.

VII. The Trematodes

The class Trematoda, in the phylum Platyhelminthes, consists of two orders, Monogenea and Digenea. All are obligate parasites. Trematodes of medical importance only occur in the order Digenea, and include the blood flukes, the intestinal flukes, and the tissue flukes. They are mainly found throughout the tropics and subtropics, while a few species are encountered in temperate zones, as well.

Trematodes undergo complex developmental cycles in their intermediate and definitive hosts. But, as complex as trematode biology is, offering seemingly numerous opportunities for interrupting their life cycles, eradication of any medically important species has occurred to only a limited extent in specific geographic areas such as *Schistosoma mansoni* in China and *S. japonicum* in Japan.

Trematodes maintain their site location within the host using their two suckers, one anterior and one ventral. The anterior sucker also serves as the opening to the oral cavity, into which host tissues are ingested. The outer surface of the adult is covered with a tegument similar in design and function to the tegument of cestodes. It serves as an absorbing surface for both large and small molecular-weight molecules. The tegument is covered by membrane-bound microvilli, underneath which are mitochondria, pinocytes, and other structures facilitating nutrient acquisition.

In addition, trematodes have a functional blind gut into which they ingest tissues of the host. Ingested material is pumped down into the bifurcated intestinal tract, where digestion occurs, aided by enzymes (e.g., proteases, lipases, aminopeptidases, esterases). Since the gut has no exit, wastes are regurgitated into the host. These worms obtain a wide variety of nutrients in several different ways, making it difficult to develop drugs or immune-based therapies to interrupt metabolic processes.

Several layers of muscle lie just below the tegument, allowing trematodes to move about freely within the host. This activity can result in severe pathological consequences for the host, particularly in the case of *Fasciola. hepatica, Paragonimus. westermani* and the schistosomes.

A pair of dorsal ganglia gives rise to lateral peripheral nerves running the length of the body, and they innervate the muscle layers. Commissures from the lateral nerves also innervate various organs, including the gut, and reproductive organs. The flukes have no body cavity; rather, organs are embedded in the parenchyma.

In addition to solid wastes, trematodes excrete small molecular-compounds using a network of tubules that connect to collecting organelles known as flame cells. These, in turn, connect to the excretory pore at the tegumental surface of the parasite.

The digeneic trematodes employ one of three reproductive strategies; 1. self-fertilization, in which the same worm possesses both sets of reproductive organs (e.g., *Fasciola hepatica*), 2. cross-fertilization between two worms possessing both sets of reproductive organs (e.g., *Paragonimus westermani*), or 3. fertilization between worms of the opposite sex, as is the case among the schistosomes.

Egg production is complex, involving a series of specialized organs. The ovum, supplied with yolk from the vitelline glands, is fertilized within the uterus and becomes surrounded by a shell within the Mehlis' gland. It exits from the parasite through the genital pore, usually situated in between the anterior and ventral suckers.

Once the eggs reach freshwater, or, for some species, a suitable terrestrial niche, they are either stimulated to hatch in the external environment, or they hatch after being ingested by the next host. There, they undergo asexual reproduction, eventually increasing in numbers many-fold, compared to the single entering miracidium. Intermediate hosts include snail species that live in freshwater or terrestrial habitats. In addition, other invertebrates, including ants and other insects, and a variety of cold-blooded vertebrates, including fish and crabs, function as intermediate hosts for medically important species of trematodes. Plants (e.g., watercress and water chestnuts), are sites on which some species of metacercariae encyst.

Many species of adult trematodes are acquired by ingesting the intermediate stage (i.e., the metacercaria), but a few (notably the schistosomes) can actively penetrate unbroken skin.

Site selection by trematodes within the human host is poorly understood. It is determined by a complex interplay between chemical and physical niches, which represent environmental cues for the parasite, and the receiving and translation of those cues by the nervous system of the parasite. Some drugs interfere with trematode nervous system functions (e.g., praziquantel), resulting in profound changes in worm behavior. Under those conditions, elimination of the parasite is possible.

33. The Schistosomes

Schistosoma mansoni
(Sambon 1907)

Schistosoma japonicum
(Katsurada 1904)

Schistosoma haematobium
(Bilharz 1852)

Schistosoma mekongi
(Bilharz 1852)

Schistosoma intercalatum
(Fischer 1934)

Introduction

Five trematode species in the genus *Schistosoma*; *Schistosoma mansoni, S. haematobium, S. japonicum, S. mekongi,* and *S. intercalatum* cause a series of related diseases in humans referred to as schistosomiasis, with sporadic reports of other cases being caused by less common species. *S. intercalatum*, a parasite of cattle in West Africa, is a less common cause of disease in humans than the other schistosomes. Except for *S. haematobium* that produces urinary tract disease and female genital schistosomiasis,

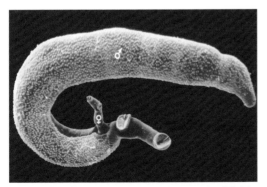

Figure 33.1. Scanning electron micrograph of *Schistosoma mansoni* adults. (From Kessel and Shih: Scanning Electron Microscopy in Biology. Springer-Verlag, 1976. Reproduced with permission).

the human schistosomes primarily affect the intestine and liver. Chronic schistosomiasis also causes physical growth and cognitive delays in children.[1] The Global Burden of Disease Study in 2013 estimates that almost 300 million people suffer with some form of schistosomiasis, with approximately 90 percent of the cases found in Africa.[2] Additional estimates indicate that schistosomiasis causes up to 200,000 deaths each year.[3] In addition to those infected, a total of almost 800 million people are at risk worldwide.[4, 5] Schistosomes that infect humans are largely tropical in distribution, reflecting the geographical distribution of their intermediate host snail species. Poverty is a second critical factor, as it is for many human parasitic diseases.[6] Forced migration of people due to armed conflict throughout many parts of the world, including Africa, and encroachment into natural systems (e.g., constructing irrigation canals and dams), have resulted in regional increases in schistosomiasis.

Schistosoma mansoni is found throughout most of sub-Saharan Africa, Egypt and the Sudan, parts of the Middle East, some parts of South America (including Brazil, Venezuela and the Guyanas), and some islands in the Caribbean. It is the only form of schistosomiasis found in the New World and is believed to have been introduced over hundreds of years through the middle passage of the Atlantic slave trade.[7] Its intermediate hosts are aquatic snails in the genus *Biomphalaria*. Reservoir hosts for *S. mansoni* include baboons and monkeys in Africa. They play no significant role in the epidemiology of human disease.

Schistosoma haematobium is prevalent in most parts of Africa, and in some parts of the Middle East. An outbreak of *Schistosoma haematobium* was also reported in Corsica, France that was most likely initiated by an infected individual from Africa who had migrated there.[8, 9] Its aquatic intermediate host snails are in the genus *Bulinus*. There are no important reservoir hosts for this trematode

Schistosoma mansoni

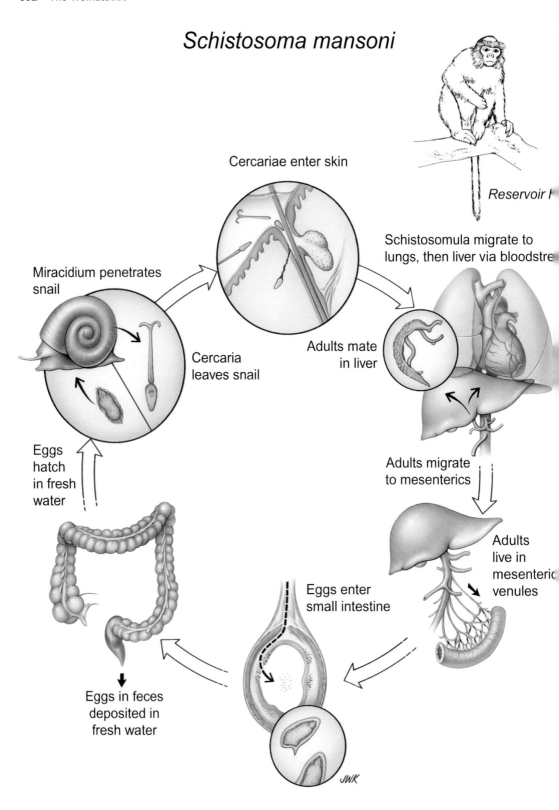

Cercariae enter skin

Reservoir H

Schistosomula migrate to lungs, then liver via bloodstre

Miracidium penetrates snail

Cercaria leaves snail

Adults mate in liver

Eggs hatch in fresh water

Adults migrate to mesenterics

Adults live in mesenteric venules

Eggs enter small intestine

Eggs in feces deposited in fresh water

JWK

species, although during an isolated outbreak in the Omo River Valley of Ethiopia among white-water rafters, the origin of the outbreak was traced back to monkeys.[10] *S. haematobium* causes urinary tract and female genital schistosomiasis (urogenital schistosomiasis) – in East and South African countries such as Tanzania, Zimbabwe, Malawi, Mozambique, and KwaZulu-Natal South Africa, urogenital schistosomiasis is a major co-factor in their HIV/AIDS epidemic.[11]

Schistosoma intercalatum occasionally infects people in Cameroon, Gabon, and Democratic Republic of Congo.[12-14]

Schistosoma japonicum occurs in China, Malaysia, the Philippines, and, to a small extent, Indonesia. It was eradicated from Japan as of 1977.[15] Its amphibious intermediate host snails are in the genus *Oncomelania*. In contrast to the other schistosomes, zoonotic transmission occurs on a regular basis. There are important reservoir hosts for *S. japonicum*, including water buffalo, cattle and pigs.[16] *S. mekongi,* a closely related species, is found in the Mekong River in Southeast Asia. Although similar in morphology and life cycle to *S. japonicum, S. mekongi* is genetically distinct.[17] There are no autochthonous infections in the United States with any of the above species of schistosomes because there are no appropriate species of intermediate host snails, and, most importantly, sanitary disposal of feces and urine is the general rule. Thousands of Caribbean, African and Southeast Asian immigrants and refugees may be infected, so clinicians who practice only in the United States must still be knowledgeable regarding this potentially life-threatening parasitic infection.

Historical Information

Paleoparasitologists have found *S. haematobium* eggs in mummies dating as far back as 1250 BCE.[18] It has been suggested that ancient Egyptians believed the advent of manhood was heralded by the appearance of blood in the urine, analogous to the onset of menstruation in women, but there remains controversy about this and possible references to schistosoma-induced hematuria in early Egyptian papyri.[19] Hematuria in males, in fact, represents a late manifestation of *S. haematobium* infection.

In 1798, A. J. Renoult, a French army surgeon put forth the first modern description of what is believed to have been hematuria due to *S. haematobium*. Renoult described the epidemic of haematuria seen in Napoleon's soldiers who invaded Egypt.[20] Cases were subsequently described among troops involved in the Second Anglo-Boer War (1899-1902).[21] In 1851 and 1852, Theodor Bilharz and Ernst von Siebold reported human cases of *Schistosoma haematobium*, described the adult worm and made the connection with the appearance of blood in the urine (hematuria).[22-24] They identified this as

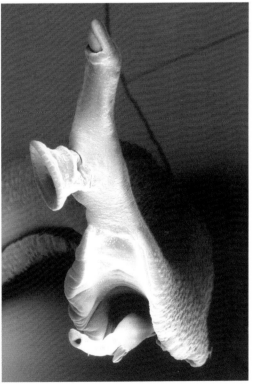

Figure 33.2. Scanning electron micrograph of adult schistosomes. Notice gynecophoral canal with female inside. Photo D. Scharf.

Schistosoma japonicum

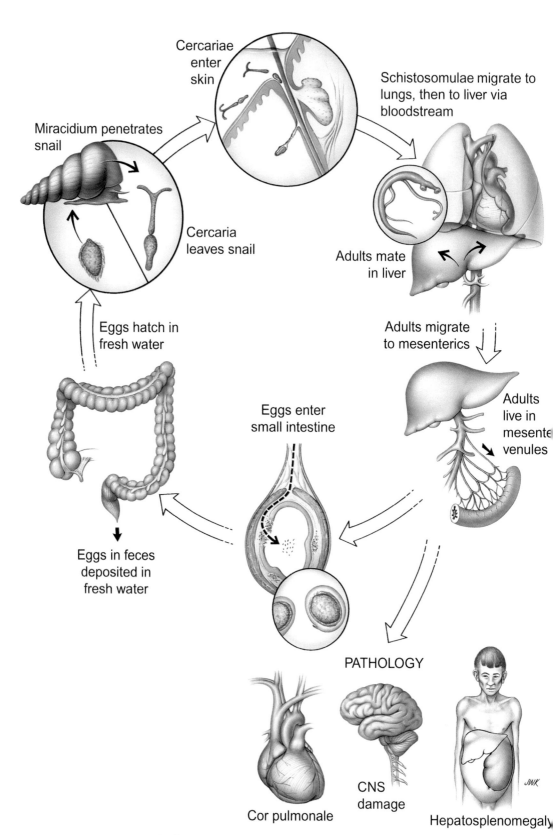

Cercariae enter skin

Schistosomulae migrate to lungs, then to liver via bloodstream

Miracidium penetrates snail

Cercaria leaves snail

Adults mate in liver

Eggs hatch in fresh water

Adults migrate to mesenterics

Eggs enter small intestine

Adults live in mesente venules

Eggs in feces deposited in fresh water

PATHOLOGY

Cor pulmonale

CNS damage

Hepatosplenomegaly

JWK

a parasite that occupied the venous plexus of the bladder and whose eggs possessed a terminal spine. In 1854, Wilhelm Griesinger described in detail the clinical disease and its pathology.[25] Griesinger noted the relation of the infection to the involvement of the bladder and ureters. In 1918, Robert Leiper described the life cycle of *S. haematobium*, its intermediate host, and its morphology.[26] He also carried out experimental infections with *S. haematobium* in various indigenous animals of northern Egypt, and proved that rats and mice were susceptible.

Although the symptoms associated with *Schistosoma haematobium* are perhaps easier to recognize in early writings, other forms of schistosomiasis came to be recognized and understood. In 1902, Patrick Manson described a case of schistosomiasis in an Englishman who had traveled extensively throughout the Caribbean, and in whose stool, but not his urine, he found many eggs with lateral spines.[27] In 1907, Louis Sambon recognized two blood flukes, on the basis of morphology and origin of the eggs in stool and urine.[28] In tribute to Manson, Sambon named this new organism after him, *Schistosoma mansoni*.[24] In 1908, Piraja de Silva also discovered *S. mansoni* in South America.[29] By 1918, Leiper had conducted extensive investigations on schistosomiasis, and reported the life cycle of *S. mansoni*, in which he described its snail intermediate host, and morphology of the adult worms.[26]

Giving credit for the discovery of *Schistosoma japonicum* is less straightforward. In 1888, Tokuho Majima described a case of cirrhosis and linked the presence of *Schistosoma japonicum* with this disease.[30] In 1904, Fujiro Katsurada described *S. japonicum* adult worms from infected cats.[31] At the same time, John Catto, working in Singapore, described an identical adult worm in a patient who died of cholera.[32] Catto named it *S. cattoi*, but his publication was delayed, and the name *S. japonicum* was accepted instead.

In 1904, Kenji Kawanishi made the correlation between the clinical condition, Katayama fever (acute schistosomiasis), and the presence of *S. japonicum* adults, after finding eggs of this parasite in the stools of patients suffering from the acute phase of the infection.[33] Kan Fujinami and Hatchitaro Nakamura in 1909, and Yoenji Miyagawa in 1912, independently reported on the details of the life cycle.[34, 35] In 1914, Keinosuke Miyairi and Masatsugu Suzuki, identified *Oncomelania* spp. snails as the intermediate hosts.[36]

S. japonicum infection has had a major impact on the history of modern China. It is believed that Mao's troops were unable to launch an amphibious assault on Taiwan in the late 1940s because they developed Katayama fever while encamped along the Yangtze River.[37] Later on during the Great Leap Forward, Mao mobilized tens of thousands of workers to either bury *Oncomelania* snails along the clay banks of rice paddy irrigation canals, or remove them by hand, one by one.[38]

In the 1900s, a number of additional species of schistosomes, including *S. mekongi,* and *S. intercalatum*, were discovered and their life cycles, specific snail intermediates, and disease manifestations were described.[39]

Life Cycle

Schistosomes have separate sexes (Fig. 33.1); the female measures 15 mm in length, and the male is 10 mm long. Schistosome adults remain *in copula* (Fig. 33.2) for most of their life span, living attached by their oral and ventral sucker disks to the endothelium of the veins (Figs. 33.3a, 33.3b). *S. mansoni* lives in the inferior mesenteric veins that drain the intestine, while *S. japonicum* and *S. mekongi* live in the superior mesenteric veins. *S. japonicum* adult worms can also find their way to the choroid plexus, the venules around the spinal column, and other ectopic locations. *S. haematobium* is found almost exclusively in the venus plexus that drains the urinary

Schistosoma haematobium

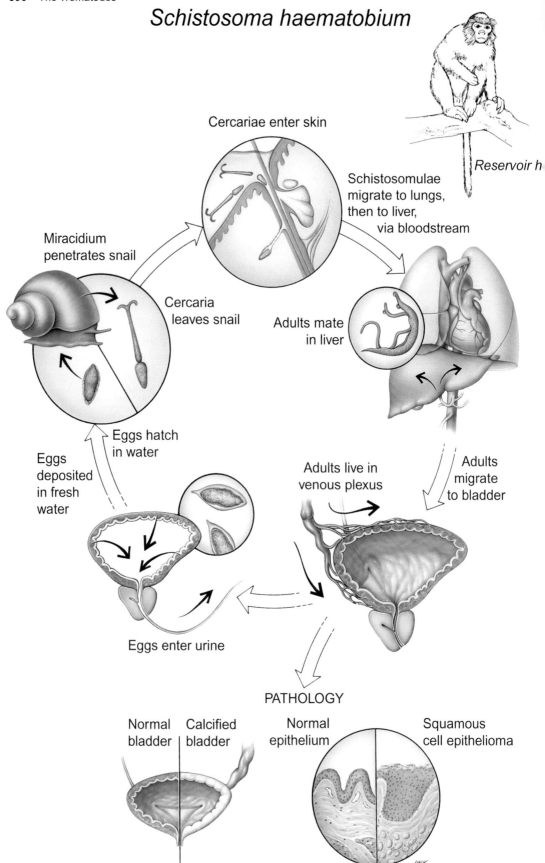

Cercariae enter skin

Reservoir h

Schistosomulae
migrate to lungs,
then to liver,
via bloodstream

Miracidium
penetrates snail

Cercaria
leaves snail

Adults mate
in liver

Eggs hatch
in water

Eggs
deposited
in fresh
water

Adults live in
venous plexus

Adults
migrate
to bladder

Eggs enter urine

PATHOLOGY

| Normal bladder | Calcified bladder | Normal epithelium | Squamous cell epithelioma |

JWK

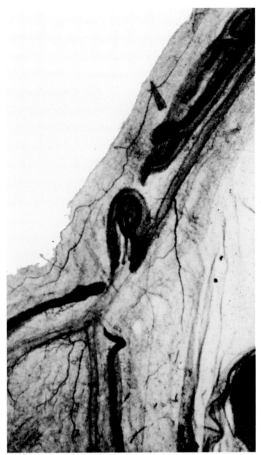

Figure 33.3a. Adult schistosomes *in situ*. The elongated worms appear dark due to the ingestion of hemoglobin.

bladder. The routes by which adult schistosomes arrive at these sites has been studied for various species using a number of different animal models, and is known to involve migration through various capillary beds.[40] Worms live 5-8 years, on average, although some live as long as 37 years.[41] Schistosomes are facultative anaerobes, deriving energy primarily through the degradation of glucose and glycogen, and utilizing sophisticated transport mechanisms for glucose uptake and utilization.[42]

Adult schistosomes utilize hemoglobin as a primary source of amino acids, which is ingested into their blind, bifurcated gut.[25] They employ a hemoglobinase, digesting the globin portion of the molecule, and detoxifying the heme moiety into a pigment before it

is regurgitated back into the bloodstream.[43] The female lies within the gynecophoral canal of the male (Fig. 33.2). This muscular, tegumental fold extends down both sides of the male, and may enable the female to feed on blood, by assisting in pumping blood into their esophagus. Single sex infections with females, or females experimentally separated from males, then re-introduced into the same host, do not produce eggs, presumably due to their inability to obtain a blood meal.

Free amino acids and glucose are transported across the tegument by active transport mechanisms. They store excess glucose as glycogen. The tegumental surface of male *S. mansoni* is covered with finger-like projections, termed "papillae", while male *S. haematobium* have more widely spaced, shorter, finger-like projections, termed "tubercles". Evidence suggests that these projections have a sensory function.[44]

Females *in copula* lay eggs throughout their lives. The eggs of *S. mansoni* are oval, and possess a lateral spine (Fig. 33.4); those of *S. japonicum* and *S. mekongi* are globu-

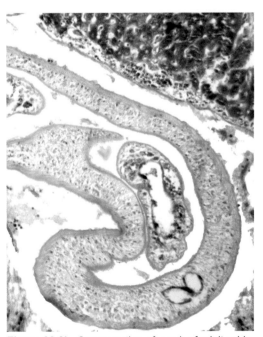

Figure 33.3b. Cross section of a pair of adult schistosomes *in situ* in a mesenteric venule.

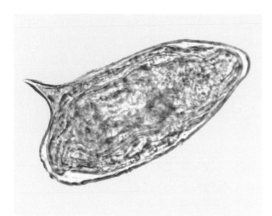

Figure 33.4. Egg of *Schistosoma mansoni*. Note lateral spine. 150 μm x 60 μm.

lar and lack a large easily identifiable spine (Fig. 33.5a, 33.5b); those of *S. haematobium* are oval, with a terminal spine (Fig. 33.6). *S. mansoni* females produce, on average, 300 eggs per day, while *S. japonicum* and *S. mekongi* shed some 1500-3000 eggs daily. *S. haematobium* produce hundreds of eggs per day.[45] When the female worm applies her ventral sucker to the endothelial surface, eggs pass through the birth pore located above the ventral sucker, encounter endothelial cells and penetrate into the surrounding connective tissue. The larvae, in the eggs, secrete lytic enzymes facilitating this process. Eggs collect in the sub-mucosa (Fig. 33.7) before lysing their way into the lumen of the small intestine, or, in the case of *S. haematobium*, the lumen of the bladder.

When adult females raise their ventral

suckers, eggs inadvertently escape into the circulation, which carries them to the liver via the portal circulation. Nearly 50% of all *S. mansoni* eggs produced end up in the liver, a dead end for the life cycle. Eggs that reach the lumen of the small intestine are included in the fecal mass. Eggs of *S. haematobium* must traverse the wall of the bladder (Fig. 33.8) before exiting the host in the urine. In both cases, the egg's penchant for penetrating tissues causes the infected individual significant pathological consequences.

For the life cycle to continue, eggs in feces or urine must be deposited in freshwater. There, environmental cues trigger the larva stage, termed the miracidium, to hatch (Fig. 33.9). This ciliated, free-swimming stage (Fig. 33.10) seeks out its appropriate snail intermediate host, relying on a gradient of appropriate low molecular weight signal(s) emanating from the proper snail host to do so. In essence, the snail becomes a chemical homing device for the parasite.

Upon finding the right snail (Figs. 33.11,

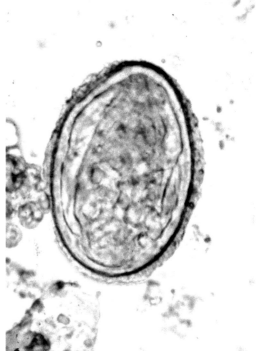

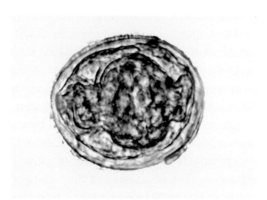

Figure 33.5a. Egg of *Schistosoma japonicum*. No spine can be seen. 85 μm x 60 μm.

Figure 33.5b. Egg of *Schistosoma mekongi*. No spine can be seen. 65 μm x 50 μm.

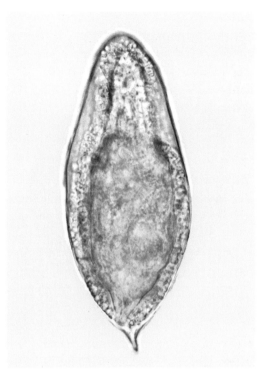

Figure 33.6. Egg of *Schistosoma haematobium.* Note terminal spine. 155 μm x 55 μm.

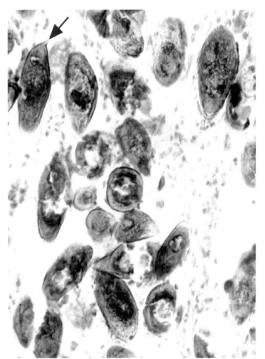

Figure 33.8. *S. haematobium* eggs in bladder wall. Note terminal spine (arrow).

33.12), the miracidium penetrates the soft, fleshy foot, facilitated by a different set of proteolytic enzymes than it used to exit from the mammalian host. The miracidium invades the snail's lymph spaces, and then takes up

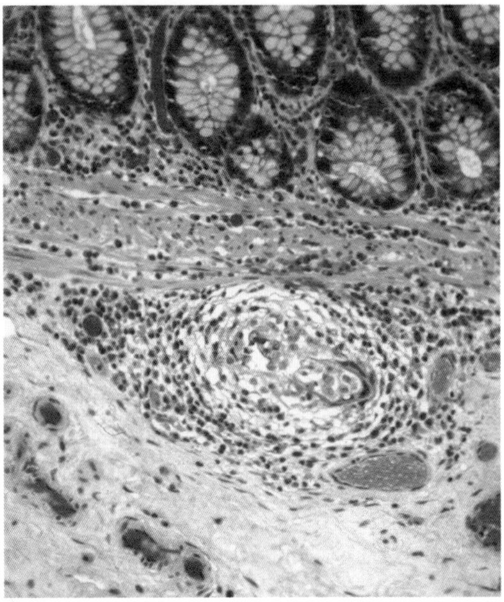

Figure 33.7. Schistosome egg in tissue of the small intestine. Note intense granuloma.

residence in its hepatopancreas.

A series of remarkable transformations then ensue, beginning with production of the sporocyst. This stage gives rise to daughter sporocysts, which, in turn, produce cercariae, the infectious stage for humans. During each stage of development, there is an increase in the number of individuals. A single miracidium of *S. mansoni* produces some 4,000 genetically identical cercariae (Fig. 33.13). Throughout the process, the snail somehow manages to remain alive, even when it becomes infected with numerous miracidia. An infection that results in the production of more than 40,000 cercariae overwhelms the snail, and it dies. Each miracidium is either male or female, as are the resulting cercariae.

Cercariae exit from the snail aided by yet another set of proteolytic enzymes. Cercariae are positively phototropic and negatively geotropic. They accumulate at the surface of water, and swim about seeking their definitive host by following gradients of chemical cues,

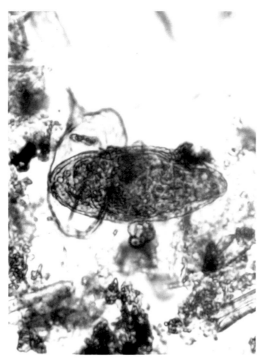

Figure 33.9. Miracidium of *S. mansoni* caught in the act of hatching.

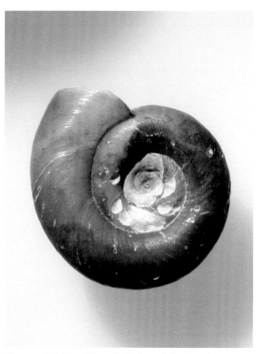

Figure 33.11. *Biomphalaria glabrata*, the most common intermediate snail host for *S. mansoni*.

including linoleic acid, that emanate from human skin. Cercariae must infect within 8 hours after emerging from its snail host; oth-

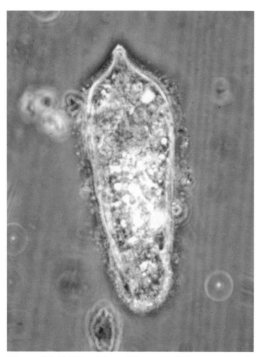

Figure 33.10. Miracidium of *S. mansoni*. Phase contrast.

erwise they exhaust their glycogen reserves and die.

Infection in the human host is initiated when the cercariae penetrate unbroken skin. With regards to *S. mansoni*, this step requires about 0.5 hour, but occurs much more rapidly with *S. japonicum*.[46] Skin penetration is usually through a hair follicle, and is facilitated by release of another set of proteases and eicosanoids.[47] Cercariae shed their tails, and rapidly transform within the dermal layer

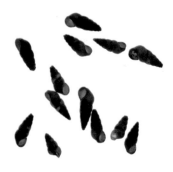

Figure 33.12. *Oncomelania nosophora*, a snail intermediate host for *S. japonicum*.

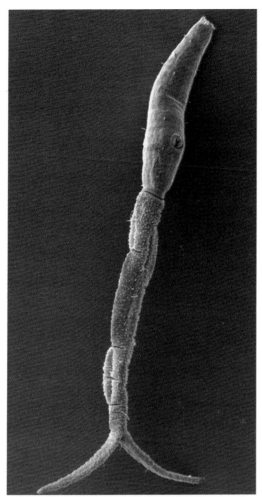

Figure 33.13. Scanning electron micrograph of a cercaria of *S. mansoni*. Photo D. Scharf.

of skin into the schistosomula stage. After approximately 2 days, the schistosomulae migrate through the bloodstream to the capillaries of the lung, where they remain for another several days. It is here that the immature worms acquire their ability to incorporate host serum proteins onto their tegumental surface. This "camouflage" has the profound effect of convincing the leukocytes that the worm is "self," enabling the parasite to live out a long, and prosperous life inside its new host. In addition, the worm possesses a β-2-microglobulin-like molecule that aids in confusing immune defense cells, particularly macrophages, in their attempt to recognize parasite antigens. Schistosomulae migrate

from the lungs via the blood stream to the liver, where they mature to adult worms. Both sexes produce pheromones that are mutually attractive, and eventually worms of opposite sex find each other in the vastness of the parenchymal tissue. They mate there, and migrate out into the mesenteric circulation *in copula*. *S. mansoni* and *S. japonicum* worm pairs live in the small mesenteric veins that drain the intestines, while *S. haematobium* worm pairs live in the bladder venous plexus and possibly small veins that drain the female genital tract. Egg production begins shortly thereafter. Other mammalian species, including baboons, rhesus monkeys, chimpanzees, mice, and rats, can be experimentally infected with the cercariae of *S. mansoni*. Few viable eggs are produced in the rat, however.

Cellular and Molecular Pathogenesis

Adult schistosomes and the larval form usually do not cause significant pathological damage in the host through an active modulation of the host immune system.[48, 49] Evidence indicates that the adult worm pair elicits remarkably little in the way of host immunopathologic responses as a consequence of a unique cloaking strategy of antigen-masking its surface with host serum proteins that prevents the host from recognizing tegumental antigens.[50] They also shed tegumental components regularly, avoiding long-term exposure of that biologically active layer to its host immune surveillance system.[51] Adult schistosomes living in the venous circulation have the capacity to harbor enteric bacteria affixed to their surface. This relationship can result in the introduction of enteric bacteria, such as *Salmonella*, directly into the bloodstream. As a result there is a well-described association between chronic schistosomiasis and so-called enteric fevers from non-typhoidal salmonellosis.[52]

In contrast to adults, the eggs produced by the worm pairs result in profound immunopathologic responses. This phenomenon accounts for almost all of the pathology and clinical manifestations of schistosomiasis. For *S. japonicum* and *S. mansoni,* egg deposition occurs in the circulation of the small intestine and liver (Fig. 33.14) to produce intestinal and hepatic fibrosis, whereas *S. haematobium* egg deposition occurs in the circulation of the bladder to produce fibrosis leading in many cases to an obstructive uropathy. Heavy egg deposition occurs predominantly in individuals with large numbers of adult worms. Clinical illness caused by schistosomiasis generally occurs only in people who suffer from recurrent heavy worm burdens. Increasing evidence suggests that a component of this phenomenon depends on host genetic factors.[53] In this regard, the same genes specific for susceptibility to *Schistosoma mansoni* have been identified in people living in Africa and South America.[54] In a study in the Sudan, a specific gene locus was associated with advanced liver disease confirming epidemiologic observations of fibrosis occurring in families.[55] Furthermore, immunocompromised individuals with HIV shed fewer eggs in stool exams than similar individuals without HIV.[56] The soluble secretions from schistosome eggs, termed soluble egg antigens (SEAs), trigger host inflammatory and immune responses that result in granuloma formation, and are T cell-dependent, and include prominent Th2 components.[57, 58] Th2 bias downregulates other Th1 responses, and result in altered patterns of host susceptibility to other infectious pathogens, possibly including the human immunodeficiency virus.[59, 60] The pathogenesis of granuloma formation also requires host-derived production of TNF.[61] The diameters of the granulomas vary with the age of the infection. In newly acquired infections, granulomas are large, causing displacement of normal tissue with fibrotic, epithelioid reactions. Over time, eggs elicit less and less volume of granulomatous tissue. This reaction appears to be under the regulation of IL-12.[62]

Granulomas form around eggs that collect in the intestinal wall and results in fibrosis. Erosion of the submucosa and villous tissue also occurs, presumably by the action of secreted proteolytic enzymes from the miracidiae within the eggs. In heavy infection, gastrointestinal hemorrhage results from damage to the submucosa.

Eggs swept back into the liver block presinusoidal capillaries, and induce granulomas there, as well. The presence of granulomas causes tissue fibrosis, and eventually leads to obstruction of the hepatic vasculature. Fibrosis of most of the portal areas incorporating the blood vessels leads to pipe stem fibrosis (Symmer's Fibrosis) (Fig. 33.15), and, ultimately, to portal hypertension. Clinically, this manifests as hepatosplenomegaly, the extent of which is dependent partially on host major histocompatibility class II alleles.[63] Development of collateral circulation follows, including esophageal varices. Parenchymal liver

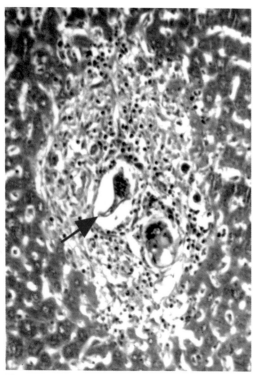

Figure 33.14. Granuloma in liver surrounding eggs of *S. mansoni.* Note the lateral spine (arrow).

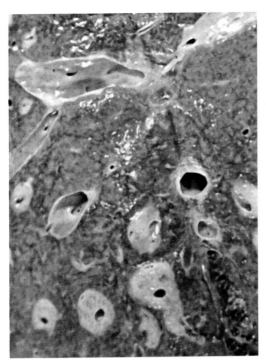

Figure 33.15. Pipe stem fibrosis in liver due to heavy infection with *S. mansoni*. Note normal liver tissue next to fibrotic vessels.

cells remain unaffected by granulomas, and, hence, liver function remains normal.

Portal hypertension forces eggs to bypass the liver, and many are carried to the spleen, which becomes enlarged, further contributing to increased pressure in portal circulation. Infection with *S. japonicum* results in a greater number of granulomas, and consequently greater morbidity because this species produces, on average, five to ten times more eggs than *S. mansoni*. Collateral circulation may also wash eggs into the lung capillary beds, occasionally leading to pulmonary fibrosis and *cor pulmonale*.

Accumulation of *S. haematobium* eggs around the bladder and ureters leads to granuloma formation and fibrosis. Calcification of dead eggs in the bladder wall (Fig. 33.16) results in rigidity of the bladder, and subsequent increased hydrostatic pressure in the ureters and kidneys. The bladder epithelium develops pseudopolyps (Fig. 33.17), which can transform into transitional squamous cell carcinoma in untreated patients (Fig. 33.18).

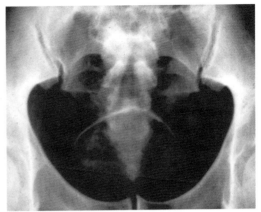

Figure 33.16. X-ray showing calcified dome of the bladder due to chronic infection with *S. haematobium*.

In some patients with long-standing disease (in all major types of schistosomiasis), deposition of immune complexes in kidneys can lead to basement membrane disease.[62]

Emerging evidence over the last decade confirms that *S. haematobium* eggs also gain access to the female genital tract to cause female genital schistosomiasis. Granulomas in the uterus, cervix, and vagina produce ulcerative lesions, which are rich in inflammatory cells. These lesions presumably provide conduits for the entry of HIV/AIDS during intercourse.[11] Through such mechanisms, *S. haematobium* infection is linked to a 3-4 fold increase in acquiring HIV/AIDS.

Penetration of the skin by cercariae is dependent on the release of parasite-derived

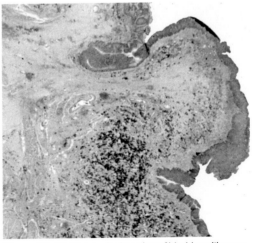

Figure 33.17. Histological section of bladder with pseudopolyp due to chronic infection with *S. haematobium*.

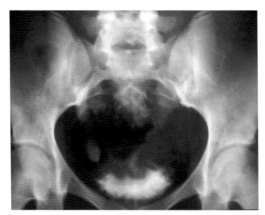

Figure 33.18. X-ray of bladder with a squamous cell tumor induced by *S. haematobium* eggs.

proteases and eicosanoids. The process of host entry typically causes no major reaction, but repeated exposure can lead to sensitization, and the development of a maculopapular rash (Fig. 33.19), characterized by IgE or IgG antibodies and an eosinophilic infiltrate. This is particularly true of accidental skin penetration by avian or bovine schistosomes. Many schistosomes specifically parasitic for animals can cause aberrant infections in humans. Avian schistosomes of the genera *Austro-*

bilharzia, *Trichobilharzia*, and *Ornithobilharzia*, and other mammalian schistosomes (*Schistosoma matthei* and *Schistosomatium douthitti*) are included in this group. The cercariae of these species cause a hypersensitivity skin reaction (cercarial dermatitis), known as "clam digger's itch" or "swimmer's itch" (Fig. 33.20).

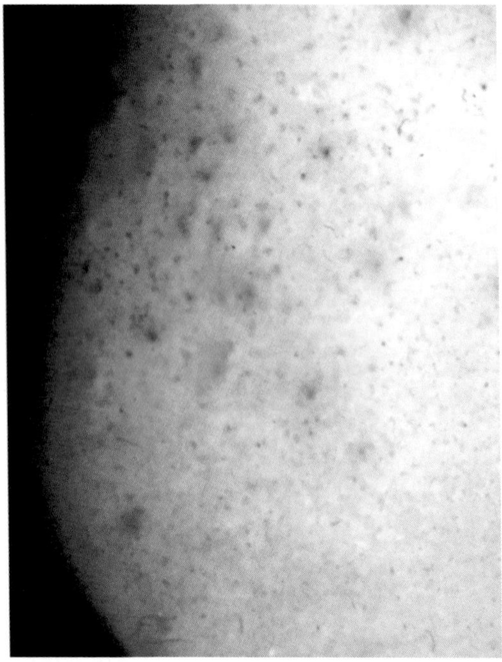

Cellular and humoral responses to both penetrating cercariae and migrating schistosomulae are a critical component of naturally acquired immunity to human schistosomiasis. This hypothesis derives from experimental evidence showing that cercariae attenuated by exposure to ionizing radiation (e.g., x-rays, gamma-rays or ultraviolet light), can penetrate skin and migrate through the tissues without being able to transform into schistosomulae. In so doing they elicit protective immune responses, including IL-13.[64-66] These observations are the basis for an experimental vaccine in non-human

Figure 33.19. Thigh of a child suffering from a maculopapular rash ("swimmer's itch") due to the cercariae of a schistosome species that normally infects birds.

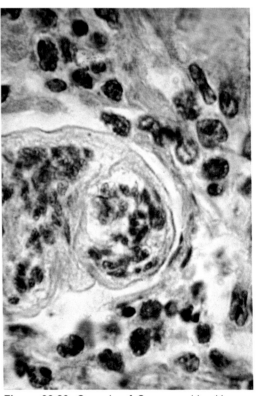

Figure 33.20. Cercaria of *S. mansoni* in skin surrounded by eosinophils.

primates. The cercariae must remain alive in order to secrete the antigens associated with vaccine protection. In humans living in endemic regions, this process may take years of exposure to cercariae. Until then, young children have a particular problem mounting an effective immune response to invading schistosomulae. The mechanism by which children during their early years of exposure to cercariae and invading schistosomulae are susceptible to the parasite but then become resistant over time is unclear, but appears to be due to age related aspects of the innate immune response.[45, 67] One hypothesis is that young children respond initially to the parasite by producing IgG_4 blocking antibodies.[68] It has been suggested that blocking antibodies delay the development of protective IgE that is needed for the resistance to infection that older people have developed in endemic areas.

Current understanding of Th1 and Th2 immune mechanisms encourages the use of recombinant schistosome proteins to produce a practical vaccine.[69, 70] Animal protection studies have used several naturally purified or recombinant proteins such as paramyosin, calpain, tetraspanin, and others with good results in a mouse model, although the mechanism of protection is still under investigation.[71, 72] Studies in the Philippines in a population with risk of exposure to S. japonicum demonstrated that individuals with predominantly Th1 cellular immune responses appeared resistant to initial infection.[73, 74]

Clinical Disease

As in other helminth infections, clinical disease resulting from schistosomes usually occurs only in heavily-infected individuals. The clinical manifestations of acute schistosomiasis occur predominantly in S. japonicum and S. mansoni infections. This condition is sometimes known as "Katayama fever". The classical disease attributed to schistosomia-

sis occurs during chronic infections. Chronic infection with S. haematobium can also lead to squamous cell carcinoma of the bladder.

Acute schistosomiasis (Katayama fever)

The dramatic clinical manifestations of Katayama fever occur most commonly in new immigrants who experience intense levels of exposure to either S. japonicum or S. mansoni cercariae. The name reflects the early descriptions of this syndrome in the Katayama District of Japan.[75] The symptoms are often dramatic and appear approximately 4-8 weeks after initial exposure, when adult worm pairs begin releasing their eggs in the tissues. Some investigators believe that Katayama fever resembles some of the manifestations of serum sickness. There is also a clinical resemblance to typhoid fever. Patients experience hepatosplenomegaly and lymphadenopathy as well as an impressive eosinophilia. The affected individual is frequently febrile and has flu-like symptoms, including cough and headache. At this stage of the illness, schistosome eggs may not yet have appeared in the feces.

Chronic schistosomiasis

This manifestation of infection occurs as a consequence of many years of progressive injury resulting from chronic egg deposition in the tissues and the resulting granuloma formation (Fig. 33.21). The injury has an immunopathological basis. In the case of S. japonicum and S. mansoni infection, the injury occurs when eggs are deposited in the wall of the intestine and in the liver parenchyma. With S. haematobium, injury occurs in the bladder. The extent of injury depends on chronic worm burden, so chronic schistosomiasis occurs predominantly in individuals who are predisposed to repeated heavy infections.[68] In a population with repeated high exposures to cercariae, less than a quar-

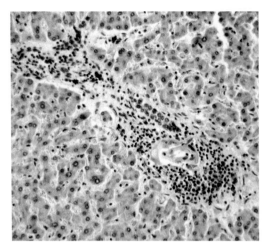

Figure 33.21. Granuloma surrounding an egg of *S. mansoni* in liver tissue.

ter develop heavy infection and only 10% of these individuals with heavy infection develop periportal fibrosis.

S. japonicum and *S. mansoni* infections result in chronic intestinal. Children with intestinal schistosomiasis develop intermittent abdominal pain, sometimes accompanied with bloody diarrhea. The blood loss and ulceration of intestinal schistosomiasis may result in iron deficiency and anemia. This may explain why chronic schistosomiasis during childhood can result in physical growth retardation similar to that described for intestinal nematode infections. Stunting becomes most prominent at the age of peak intensity (usually between 8 and 20-years of age).[76] It is partly reversible by specific anti-helmintic therapy.[77]

Hepatomegaly results from portal fibrosis. Splenomegaly follows, and in advanced cases, the spleen may fill much of the left side of the abdomen. Patients may also develop symptoms of hypersplenism. Portal obstructive disease due to schistosomiasis is similar to other causes in that it leads to hematemesis from ruptured esophageal varices. As a result of portal hypertension, and the consequent development of a collateral circulation, schistosome eggs are washed into the lungs, where they induce granulomatous inflammation, leading to obstructive disease culminating in

cor pulmonale. As noted above, long standing infections can cause nephrotic syndrome, resulting from the deposition of immune complexes onto the glomerular membrane.

S. haematobium, unlike the other three major schistosomes, causes involvement of the urinary tract, which is characterized by an inflammatory response induced by the secretions of the miracidia inside the eggs as they are deposited in the wall of the bladder. Patients with chronic *S. haematobium* infection develop hematuria as well as symptoms that mimic urinary tract infections such as dysuria and increased urinary frequency. Over time the inflammatory changes in the bladder may result in fibrosis that can lead to an obstructive uropathy. This sometimes results in hydronephrosis or hydroureter. The resulting urinary stasis can sometimes lead to secondary bacterial urinary tract infections that may exacerbate the scarring and fibrosis.

Bladder carcinoma

A characteristic type of bladder carcinoma occurs in regions where *S. haematobium* is endemic. In contrast to adenocarcinoma, the most common type of bladder cancer in industrialized countries, some patients with chronic *S. haematobium* go on to develop squamous cell carcinoma. Evidence suggests that the eggs of *S. haematobium* are able to induce this through a number of mechanisms including the action of estrogen metabolites.[78] Squamous cell carcinoma is the most common type of bladder cancer in parts of Egypt, as well as elsewhere in Africa. Over time, it is possible that *S. haematobium* eggs may function as a human carcinogen that elicits metaplastic changes in the bladder.[79]

Female genital schistosomiasis

Egg deposition in the uterus, cervix, and lower genital tract produces a painful and stigmatizing condition known as female genital schistosomiasis (FGS). FGS is associated with bleeding, vaginal itching, and pain on sexual intercourse. On colposcopic exam FGS presents as "sandy patches" that correspond to the presence of schistosome granulomas. These patches bleed easily on contact. FGS also has important psychosocial consequences and has been linked to stigma, marital discord, and depression. There is also a strong association between FGS and acquiring HIV/AIDS during sex, with some estimates indicating that FGS is a major co-factor in Africa's AIDS epidemic.[11]

CNS schistosomiasis

Rarely, schistosomes induce focal inflammatory reactions within the central nervous system, caused by deposition of eggs in the spinal cord and the brain.[80] S. mansoni and S. haematobium are more likely to do so in the spinal cord, and S. japonicum in the brain. Inflammation due to eggs may result in focal transverse myelitis and encephalopathy.

Diagnosis

Diagnosing schistosomiasis can be done through detection of the parasite or the host immune response. Definitive diagnosis is made by microscopically identifying schistosome eggs in stool or urine (Figs. 33.4, 33.5a, 33.5b, 33.6). If a single stool examination is negative, concentration of a specimen collected over a 24-hour period is required, because the number of eggs in stool can be few. Quantitative egg counts are sometimes useful for epidemiologic studies attempting to determine infection intensities. For light infections, or in patients from whom egg excretion is intermittent, and from whom eggs cannot be found in stool, a rectal biopsy can be carried out (Fig. 33.22). The tissue is squashed between two microscope slides and examined under the low-power lens of a microscope. If eggs are detected, they can

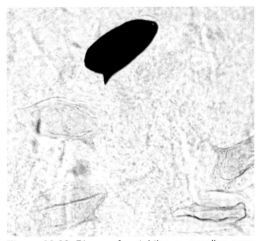

Figure 33.22. Biopsy of rectal tissue revealing eggs of *S. mansoni*. Note calcified egg, indicating that the infection was chronic.

then be observed under higher power and examined for the presence of "flame" cells (excretory cells). If they are flickering (as in a flame), then the miracidium in the egg is alive, and the patient has an active infection. Treatment must then be entertained. If no live eggs are seen, or if they are calicified, then it is likely that the infection is no longer active, and treatment is not necessary. It is helpful to refer to the specimen as a "rectal snip", rather than a biopsy, to preclude its fixation and subsequent sectioning, which would make the identification of live miracidia in eggs impossible.

While most schistosome eggs appear in feces, urine should examined for the presence of eggs of *S. haematobium* if this species is suspected. The urine sample should generally be collected close to noon, when egg excretion is usually maximal. Urine may have to be concentrated by sedimentation to reveal the few eggs present. *S. haematobium* eggs may also be seen in stool and rectal snip specimens, but their numbers are typically small in these samples. Diagnosis of female genital schistosomiasis requires training to identify the characteristic sandy patches associated with this condition. Confirmatory microscopy is a useful aid but not always available in resource-poor settings.

A number of additional tests have become available for the diagnosis of schistosomiasis. Two schistosome glycoprotein antigens known as CCA and CAA that circulate in the bloodstream of acutely-infected patients have been identified and can now be tested for using both qualitative and quantitative assays that are currently available.[81-83] These assays can be easily applied to urine samples.[84, 85] A number of nucleic acid amplification tests (NAATS) have been developed that allow for detection as well as schistosome speciation.[86-88]

Antibodies develop 6 to 12 weeks after exposure and tend to become positive before eggs are evident in urine or stool.[89] There are a number of serological tests available with western blot confirmatory testing, as well.[90] Since serologies remain positive for long periods after treatment of infection, they can not be used for follow-up and are difficult to use to monitor repeat infections in endemic areas.[91]

Portable ultrasound imaging has been shown to be clinically useful in the diagnosis of schistosomiasis. Ultrasound can define the extent of Symmer's fibrosis in patients with *S. mansoni* or *S. japonicum* infections, while the chronic obstructive changes associated with *S. haematobium* infection can also be detected.[92]

Treatment

Optimal treatment depends on whether one is treating acute schistosomiasis syndrome (Katayama fever) or the chronic phase of the disease. Since the acute schistosomiasis syndrome is a hypersensitivity reaction to the parasitic antigens, antihelminthic therapy results in exacerbation of symptoms in about half of those treated.[93] Short course treatment with corticosteroids and delay of antihelminthic therapy improves symptoms, leads to decreased morbidity and avoids the clinical deterioration seen with acute use of antihel-minthic treatment.[93, 94] Acute treatment with antihelminthic therapy is also not required to prevent the chronic manifestations of schistosomiasis.[95] How long to wait after the acute syndrome subsides before initiating antihelminthic therapy is unknown, but it seems prudent to wait for a period (6 weeks according to some) after resolution of the acute symptoms to start treatment when the worms have fully matured, as praziquantel, the drug of choice for schistosomiasis, is not active against the larval stage.[95] Treatment can then be repeated once 4-6 weeks after this first treatment course.

For treatment of chronic schistosomiasis, praziquantel is the drug of choice for most species of schistosomes. This drug is well-tolerated, is associated with few side effects (nausea, epigastric pain, dizziness, and general malaise), has a very high therapeutic index, and a single dose is usually sufficient to greatly reduce the worm burden in individuals in endemic areas with high worm burdens, and to cure those with low worm burdens.[96-98] Praziquantel interferes with calcium ion influx across the tegument, resulting in spastic paralysis of the worm. At higher doses, the tegument develops blebs and is unmasked, making it susceptible to immune attack.[99] In younger patients, praziquantel may also reverse some of the pathology associated with Symmer's fibrosis.[100] There is evidence that part of its effectiveness is due to synergism with the host's humoral immune response.[101] Because it is effective in a single dose, it has been used in control programs (see below). For patients no longer in endemic areas, test of cure is recommended with repeat testing for eggs in urine or stool no sooner than 3 to 6 months after treatment.[102] When treatment is initiated patients should be monitored for evidence of CNS disease, as treatment can cause an acute inflammatory response in patients who have eggs in the CNS. If this develops, prompt and prolonged therapy with corticosteroids is critical to prevent worsening of neurological symptoms and irreversible damage.[103, 104]

Praziquantel is now inexpensive and the World Health assembly has endorsed community treatment of school-age children in endemic areas. The Schistosomaisis Control Initiative (SCI) based at Imperial College, London, is leading global efforts to provide mass drug administration of praziquantel. Currently, praziquantel is being provided in a "rapid impact" of interventions, which includes mass-drug treatment for intestinal helminth infections, lymphatic filariasis, and onchocerciasis.[105] Unfortunately, political obstacles have so far failed to link this approach with antiretroviral drug therapy for HIV/AIDS. Millions of girls and women living in poverty in Africa have been denied access to an inexpensive backdoor approach to HIV/AIDS prevention.[106] Resistance has occurred and a number of treatment failures have been reported.[107-109]

Alternatives to praziquantel are limited in use due to a higher frequency of adverse reactions and differences in spectrum of activity. Oxamniquine is an alternate drug with good anti-parasitic activity. In some regions, oxamniquine is as effective as praziquantel for the treatment of infections with *S. mansoni*, and metrifonate is effective for the treatment of *S. haematobium* infections.[110] The anti-malarial drug artemether has been studied in China as a chemprophylactic agent in patients who anticipate high levels of exposure to *S. japonicum* and *S. mansoni* cercariae during seasonal floods. Chemoprophylactic activity of artemether was present but lower against *S. haematobium.[111]* The efficacy of praziquantel is enhanced when combined with artemether, and the combination might prevent the emergence of resistance to praziquantel when used in widespread and repeated community treatment.[112]

Treatment should be carried out only in patients with active schistosome infections. Portocaval or splenorenal shunts should be avoided in untreated schistosomiasis, because they increase the probability of eggs reaching the lungs. If such a shunt is mandated by the intensity of portal hypertension, it should be carried out only after treating with any of the above-mentioned drugs.

Prevention and Control

Schistosomes' success in carrying out their life cycles is dependent upon complex ecological interactions with a wide variety of invertebrate and vertebrate host species. They appear to have numerous weak points in their quest to complete their life cycles. Numerous control programs have attempted to take advantage of these "weak points." Control programs in the Middle East and North Africa have nearly succeeded in schistosome elimination, while programs in China and Brazil have also achieved remarkable success.[113-116] Although more challenging for less-developed countries, a number of programs including mass treatment to reduce worm burden have improved the situation for many.[117, 118]

Prevention of schistosomiasis by individuals requires that they never come in contact with infested freshwater. This suggestion is impossible to carry out in much of the world because of many complex economic, cultural, and behavioral patterns. In addition, it may be necessary for many people to be in contact with freshwater for agricultural or other food-gathering purposes. Temporary visitors to endemic areas can heed the advice to avoid potential sources of infection. Dam building in Africa has helped increase the spread of schistosomiasis (Fig. 33.23).

Control of schistosomiasis at the community level has been directed at; 1. eradication of snail intermediate hosts with molluscacides, and biologic agents, 2. public health education, 3. sanitation, or other engineering interventions concerning fresh water supplies, and 4. chemotherapy with praziquantel and oxamniquine.[119, 120] Control of *S. japoni-*

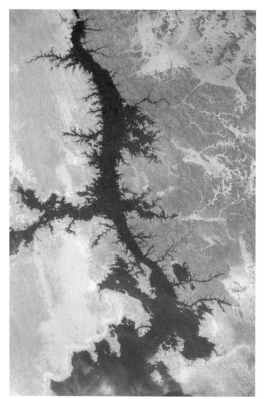

Figure 33.23. Lake Nasser and the Aswan High Dam in Egypt. Photo S. Musgrave, astronaut *extraordinaire*.

farming and using horses (a non-susceptable host) as draft animals instead.[15]

The gold standard of control for schistosomiasis has been mass-drug administration of praziquantel, with the London-based Schistosomiasis Control Initiative leading the way to providing tens of millions of people access to this essential medicine. Support for such programs of mass-drug administration comes through overseas development agencies such as USAID, DFID (United Kingdom), and some private donations, including an innovative New York-based END Fund, and a Washington DC based END7 campaign based at the Sabin Vaccine Institute. Studies in endemic areas have shown that while praziquantel is effective at treating large populations, there is a high rate of post-treatment reinfection. This necessitates frequent administration of the drug, although this tactic is frequently not possible in poor, developing rural areas without the support of the international community.[121] Control of the infection with anthelminthic drugs alone is difficult. There is also concern about the emergence of praziquantel drug resistance.[122]

Investigations into vaccinations and new therapeutics are currently underway and offer hope for improved methods to help address this neglected tropical disease.[45, 62, 69, 71, 72, 123-129]

cum is complicated by the occurrence of reservoir hosts, such as water buffalo and cattle, in many regions of Asia, particularly in China. In Japan, this problem was overcome mainly by eliminating the use of water buffalo in rice

References

1. Gurarie, D.; Wang, X.; Bustinduy, A. L.; King, C. H., Modeling the effect of chronic schistosomiasis on childhood development and the potential for catch-up growth with different drug treatment strategies promoted for control of endemic schistosomiasis. *Am J Trop Med Hyg* **2011,** *84* (5), 773-81.

2. Global Burden of Disease Study, C., Global, regional, and national incidence, prevalence, and years lived with disability for 301 acute and chronic diseases and injuries in 188 countries, 1990-2013: a systematic analysis for the Global Burden of Disease Study 2013. *Lancet* **2015,** *386* (9995), 743-800.

3. Rollinson, D.; Knopp, S.; Levitz, S.; Stothard, J. R.; Tchuem Tchuente, L. A.; Garba, A.; Mohammed, K. A.; Schur, N.; Person, B.; Colley, D. G.; Utzinger, J., Time to set the agenda for schistosomiasis elimination. *Acta Trop* **2013,** *128* (2), 423-40.

4. Utzinger, J.; Raso, G.; Brooker, S.; De Savigny, D.; Tanner, M.; Ornbjerg, N.; Singer, B. H.; N'Goran E, K., Schistosomiasis and neglected tropical diseases: towards integrated and sustainable control and a word of caution. *Parasitology* **2009,** *136* (13), 1859-74.

5.   Steinmann, P.; Keiser, J.; Bos, R.; Tanner, M.; Utzinger, J., Schistosomiasis and water resources development: systematic review, meta-analysis, and estimates of people at risk. *Lancet Infect Dis* **2006,** *6* (7), 411-25.

6.   King, C. H., Parasites and poverty: the case of schistosomiasis. *Acta Trop* **2010,** *113* (2), 95-104.

7.   Lammie, P. J.; Lindo, J. F.; Secor, W. E.; Vasquez, J.; Ault, S. K.; Eberhard, M. L., Eliminating lymphatic filariasis, onchocerciasis, and schistosomiasis from the americas: breaking a historical legacy of slavery. *PLoS Negl Trop Dis* **2007,** *1* (2), e71.

8.   Douard, A.; Cornelis, F.; Malvy, D., Urinary schistosomiasis in France. *Int J Infect Dis* **2011,** *15* (7), e506-7.

9.   Berry, A.; Mone, H.; Iriart, X.; Mouahid, G.; Aboo, O.; Boissier, J.; Fillaux, J.; Cassaing, S.; Debuisson, C.; Valentin, A.; Mitta, G.; Theron, A.; Magnaval, J. F., Schistosomiasis haematobium, Corsica, France. *Emerg Infect Dis* **2014,** *20* (9), 1595-7.

10. Fuller, G. K.; Lemma, A.; Haile, T., Schistosomiasis in Omo National Park of southwest Ethiopia. *The American journal of tropical medicine and hygiene* **1979,** *28* (3), 526-30.

11. Kjetland, E. F.; Hegertun, I. E.; Baay, M. F.; Onsrud, M.; Ndhlovu, P. D.; Taylor, M., Genital schistosomiasis and its unacknowledged role on HIV transmission in the STD intervention studies. *Int J STD AIDS* **2014,** *25* (10), 705-15.

12. Chu, T.; Liao, C.; Huang, Y.; Chang, Y.; Costa, A.; Ji, D.; Nara, T.; Tsubouchi, A.; Chang, P. W.; Chiu, W.; Fan, C., Prevalence of Schistosoma intercalatum and S. haematobium Infection among Primary Schoolchildren in Capital Areas of Democratic Republic Of Sao Tome and Principe, West Africa. *Iran J Parasitol* **2012,** *7* (1), 67-72.

13. Dufillot, D.; Duong, T. H.; Koko, J.; Eko Eni, L.; Kombila, M., [Prevalence of Schistosoma intercalatum intestinal bilharziasis in children hospitalized the urban area of Gabon]. *Arch Pediatr* **1995,** *2* (10), 1023-4.

14. World Health Organization. *Weekly Epidemiol Rec 171* **1989,** *64*.

15. Minai, M.; Hosaka, Y.; Ohta, N., Historical view of schistosomiasis japonica in Japan: implementation and evaluation of disease-control strategies in Yamanashi Prefecture. *Parasitology international* **2003,** *52* (4), 321-6.

16. Hotez, P. J.; Zheng, F.; Long-qi, X.; Ming-gang, C.; Shu-hua, X.; Shu-xian, L.; Blair, D.; McManus, D. P.; Davis, G. M., Emerging and reemerging helminthiases and the public health of China. *Emerging infectious diseases* **1997,** *3* (3), 303-10.

17. Kongklieng, A.; Kaewkong, W.; Intapan, P. M.; Sanpool, O.; Janwan, P.; Thanchomnang, T.; Lulitanond, V.; Sri-Aroon, P.; Limpanont, Y.; Maleewong, W., Molecular differentiation of Schistosoma japonicum and Schistosoma mekongi by real-time PCR with high resolution melting analysis. *Korean J Parasitol* **2013,** *51* (6), 651-6.

18. Ruffer, M. A., Note on the Presence of "Bilharzia Haematobia" in Egyptian Mummies of the Twentieth Dynasty [1250-1000 B.C.]. *Br Med J* **1910,** *1* (2557), 16.

19. Nunn, J. F.; Tapp, E., Tropical diseases in ancient Egypt. *Trans R Soc Trop Med Hyg* **2000,** *94* (2), 147-53.

20. Renoult, A. J., Notice sur l'he´maturie qu'e´prouvent les Europe´ens dans la haute Egypte et la Nubie. *J. Gen. Med. Chir. Pharm* **1808,** *17*, 366-370.

21. Cox, F. E., History of human parasitology. *Clin Microbiol Rev* **2002,** *15* (4), 595-612.

22. Bilharz, T.; von Siebold, C. T., Ein Beitrag zur Helminhographia humana, aus brieflichen Mitteilungen des Dr. Bilharz in Cairo, nenst Bermerkungen von Prof. C. Th. von Siebold in Breslau. *Z. Wiss. Zool.* **1852,** *4*, 53-76.

23. Bilharz, T., Fernere mittheilungen u¨ber Distomun haematobium. *Z. Wiss. Zool.* **1853,** *4*, 454-456.

24. Kean, B. H.; Mott, K. E.; Russell, A. J., Tropical medicine and parasitology: classic investigations. *Cornell University Press, Ithaca, NY* **1978**.

25. Griesinger, W., Klinische und anatomische Beobachtungen uber die Krankheiten von Aegypten. *Arch Physiol Heilk* **1854,** *13*, 528-575.

26. Leiper, R. T., Researches on Egyptian Bilharziosis. 1918.

27. Manson, P., Report of a Case of Bilharzia from the West Indies. *British medical journal* **1902,** *2* (2190), 1894-5.

28. Sambon, L. W.; J., New or little known African entozoa. *Med Hyg 117* **1907**, *10*.

29. Piraja de Silva, M. A., Contribucao para o estudo da schistosomiasena Bahia. *Brazil Med* **1908**, *2* 281-283.

30. Majima, T., A strange case of liver cirrhosis caused by parasitic ova. *Tokyo Igakkai Zasshi* **1888**, *2*, 898-901.

31. Katsurada, F., The etiology of a parasitic disease. *Iji Shimbun* **1904**, *669*, 1325-1332.

32. Catto, J., SCHISTOSOMA CATTOI, A NEW BLOOD FLUKE OF MAN. *British medical journal* **1905**, *1* (2297), 11-26.2.

33. Kawanishi, K., A report on a study of the "Katayama disease" in Higo-No-Kuni. *Tokyo Ig Za* **1904**, *18*, 31-48.

34. Fujinami, K.; Nakamura, H., Katayama disease in Hiroshima prefecture: route of infection, development of the worm in the host and animals in Katayama disease in Hiroshima prefecture (Japanese blood sucking worm disease-schistosomiasis japonica). . *Kyoto Ig Za* **1909**, *6*, 224-252.

35. Miyagawa, Y., Uber den Wanderungsweg des Schistosomum japonicum von der Haut bis zum Pfortadersystem und uber die Korperkonstitution der jungsten Wurmer zur Zeit der Hautinvasion. *Zentralbl Bakteriol Parasit Lnfekt* **1912**, *66*, 406-417.

36. Miyairi, K.; Suzuki, M., Der Zwischenwirt der Schistosoma japonicum Katsurada. *Mitt Med Fakultat Kaiserlichen Univ Kyushu* **1914**, *1* 187-197.

37. Kierman, F. A., The blood fluke that saved Formosa. *Harper Magazine* **1959**, 45-47.

38. Hotez, P., Forgotten People, Forgotten Diseases: The Neglected Tropical Diseases and their Impact on Global Health and Development. **2013**.

39. Foster, W. D., A history of parasitology. *Livingstone, Edinburgh, United Kingdom.* **1965**.

40. Wilson, R. A., The saga of schistosome migration and attrition. *Parasitology* **2009**, *136* (12), 1581-92.

41. Vermund, S. H.; Bradley, D. J.; Ruiz-Tiben, E., Survival of Schistosoma mansoni in the human host: estimates from a community-based prospective study in Puerto Rico. *The American journal of tropical medicine and hygiene* **1983**, *32* (5), 1040-8.

42. You, H.; Stephenson, R. J.; Gobert, G. N.; McManus, D. P., Revisiting glucose uptake and metabolism in schistosomes: new molecular insights for improved schistosomiasis therapies. *Front Genet* **2014**, *5*, 176.

43. Chappell, C. L.; Kalter, D. C.; Dresden, M. H., The hypersensitivity response to the adult worm proteinase, SMw32, in Schistosoma mansoni infected mice. *The American journal of tropical medicine and hygiene* **1988**, *39* (5), 463-8.

44. Kruger, F. J.; Hamilton-Attwell, V. L., The morphology of a sensory receptor in the nippled tubercles of Schistosoma mattheei. *Onderstepoort J Vet Res* **1985**, *52* (2), 111-2.

45. McManus, D. P.; Loukas, A., Current status of vaccines for schistosomiasis. *Clin Microbiol Rev* **2008**, *21* (1), 225-42.

46. Ruppel, A.; Chlichlia, K.; Bahgat, M., Invasion by schistosome cercariae: neglected aspects in Schistosoma japonicum. *Trends in parasitology* **2004**, *20* (9), 397-400.

47. Cohen, F. E.; Gregoret, L. M.; Amiri, P.; Aldape, K.; Railey, J.; McKerrow, J. H., Arresting tissue invasion of a parasite by protease inhibitors chosen with the aid of computer modeling. *Biochemistry* **1991**, *30* (47), 11221-9.

48. Jenkins, S. J.; Hewitson, J. P.; Jenkins, G. R.; Mountford, A. P., Modulation of the host's immune response by schistosome larvae. *Parasite Immunol* **2005**, *27* (10-11), 385-93.

49. Cai, P.; Gobert, G. N.; You, H.; McManus, D. P., The Tao survivorship of schistosomes: implications for schistosomiasis control. *Int J Parasitol* **2016**.

50. Sepulveda, J.; Tremblay, J. M.; DeGnore, J. P.; Skelly, P. J.; Shoemaker, C. B., Schistosoma mansoni host-exposed surface antigens characterized by sera and recombinant antibodies from schistosomiasis-resistant rats. *Int J Parasitol* **2010**, *40* (12), 1407-17.

51. Collins, J. J.; Wendt, G. R.; Iyer, H.; Newmark, P. A., Stem cell progeny contribute to the schistosome host-parasite interface. *Elife* **2016**, *5*.

52. Gendrel, D.; Kombila, M.; Beaudoin-Leblevec, G.; Richard-Lenoble, D., Nontyphoidal salmonellal septicemia in Gabonese children infected with Schistosoma intercalatum. *Clinical infectious*

diseases : an official publication of the Infectious Diseases Society of America **1994,** *18* (1), 103-5.

53. Webster, J. P.; Gower, C. M.; Blair, L., Do hosts and parasites coevolve? Empirical support from the Schistosoma system. *Am Nat* **2004,** *164 Suppl 5,* S33-51.

54. Chiarella, J. M.; Goldberg, A. C.; Abel, L.; Carvalho, E. M.; Kalil, J.; Dessein, A., Absence of linkage between MHC and a gene involved in susceptibility to human schistosomiasis. *Brazilian journal of medical and biological research = Revista brasileira de pesquisas medicas e biologicas / Sociedade Brasileira de Biofisica ... [et al.]* **1998,** *31* (5), 665-70.

55. Dessein, A. J.; Hillaire, D.; Elwali, N. E.; Marquet, S.; Mohamed-Ali, Q.; Mirghani, A.; Henri, S.; Abdelhameed, A. A.; Saeed, O. K.; Magzoub, M. M.; Abel, L., Severe hepatic fibrosis in Schistosoma mansoni infection is controlled by a major locus that is closely linked to the interferon-gamma receptor gene. *American journal of human genetics* **1999,** *65* (3), 709-21.

56. Karanja, D. M.; Boyer, A. E.; Strand, M.; Colley, D. G.; Nahlen, B. L.; Ouma, J. H.; Secor, W. E., Studies on schistosomiasis in western Kenya: II. Efficacy of praziquantel for treatment of schistosomiasis in persons coinfected with human immunodeficiency virus-1. *The American journal of tropical medicine and hygiene* **1998,** *59* (2), 307-11.

57. Warren, K. S.; Ser, A., The pathology of schistosome infections. *Helminth Abstr* **1973,** *42* 591-633.

58. King, C. L.; Xianli, J.; Malhotra, I.; Liu, S.; Mahmoud, A. A.; Oettgen, H. C., Mice with a targeted deletion of the IgE gene have increased worm burdens and reduced granulomatous inflammation following primary infection with Schistosoma mansoni. *Journal of immunology (Baltimore, Md. : 1950)* **1997,** *158* (1), 294-300.

59. Pearce, E. J.; Caspar, P.; Grzych, J. M.; Lewis, F. A.; Sher, A., Downregulation of Th1 cytokine production accompanies induction of Th2 responses by a parasitic helminth, Schistosoma mansoni. *The Journal of experimental medicine* **1991,** *173* (1), 159-66.

60. Curry, A. J.; Else, K. J.; Jones, F.; Bancroft, A.; Grencis, R. K.; Dunne, D. W., Evidence that cytokine-mediated immune interactions induced by Schistosoma mansoni alter disease outcome in mice concurrently infected with Trichuris muris. *The Journal of experimental medicine* **1995,** *181* (2), 769-74.

61. Haseeb, M. A.; Shirazian, D. J.; Preis, J., Elevated serum levels of TNF-alpha, sTNF-RI and sTNF-RII in murine schistosomiasis correlate with schistosome oviposition and circumoval granuloma formation. *Cytokine* **2001,** *15* (5), 266-9.

62. Wynn, T. A., Development of an antipathology vaccine for schistosomiasis. *Annals of the New York Academy of Sciences* **1996,** *797,* 191-5.

63. Secor, W. E.; del Corral, H.; dos Reis, M. G.; Ramos, E. A.; Zimon, A. E.; Matos, E. P.; Reis, E. A.; do Carmo, T. M.; Hirayama, K.; David, R. A.; David, J. R.; Harn, D. A., Association of hepatosplenic schistosomiasis with HLA-DQB1*0201. *The Journal of infectious diseases* **1996,** *174* (5), 1131-5.

64. Bickle, Q. D.; Andrews, B. J.; Doenhoff, M. J.; Ford, M. J.; Taylor, M. G., Resistance against Schistosoma mansoni induced by highly irradiated infections: studies on species specificity of immunization and attempts to transfer resistance. *Parasitology* **1985,** *90 (Pt 2),* 301-12.

65. Mangold, B. L.; Dean, D. A., The role of IgG antibodies from irradiated cercaria-immunized rabbits in the passive transfer of immunity to Schistosoma mansoni-infected mice. *The American journal of tropical medicine and hygiene* **1992,** *47* (6), 821-9.

66. Dessein, A.; Kouriba, B.; Eboumbou, C.; Dessein, H.; Argiro, L.; Marquet, S.; Elwali, N.-E. M. A.; Rodrigues, V.; Li, Y.; Doumbo, O.; Chevillard, C., Interleukin-13 in the skin and interferon-gamma in the liver are key players in immune protection in human schistosomiasis. *Immunological reviews* **2004,** *201,* 180-90.

67. Gryseels, B.; Polman, K.; Clerinx, J.; Kestens, L., Human schistosomiasis. *Lancet* **2006,** *368* (9541), 1106-18.

68. Acosta, L. P.; McManus, D. P.; Aligui, G. D. L.; Olveda, R. M.; Tiu, W. U., Antigen-specific antibody isotype patterns to schistosoma japonicum recombinant and native antigens in a defined population in Leyte, the Philippines. *The American journal of tropical medicine and hygiene* **2004,** *70* (5), 549-55.

69. Siddiqui, A. A.; Siddiqui, B. A.; Ganley-Leal, L., Schistosomiasis vaccines. *Hum Vaccin* **2011,** *7*

(11), 1192-7.

70. El Ridi, R.; Tallima, H.; Selim, S.; Donnelly, S.; Cotton, S.; Gonzales Santana, B.; Dalton, J. P., Cysteine peptidases as schistosomiasis vaccines with inbuilt adjuvanticity. *PLoS One* **2014,** *9* (1), e85401.

71. Kojima, S.; Nara, T.; Tada, S.; Tsuji, M., A vaccine trial for controlling reservoir livestock against schistosomiasis japonica. *Proceedings of the 9th International Congress of Parasitology Bologna* **1998,** 489-494.

72. Hotez, P. J.; Bethony, J. M.; Diemert, D. J.; Pearson, M.; Loukas, A., Developing vaccines to combat hookworm infection and intestinal schistosomiasis. *Nat Rev Microbiol* **2010,** *8* (11), 814-26.

73. Acosta, L. P.; Aligui, G. D. L.; Tiu, W. U.; McManus, D. P.; Olveda, R. M., Immune correlate study on human Schistosoma japonicum in a well-defined population in Leyte, Philippines: I. Assessment of 'resistance' versus 'susceptibility' to S. japonicum infection. *Acta tropica* **2002,** *84* (2), 127-36.

74. Acosta, L. P.; Waine, G.; Aligui, G. D. L.; Tiu, W. U.; Olveda, R. M.; McManus, D. P., Immune correlate study on human Schistosoma japonicum in a well-defined population in Leyte, Philippines: II. Cellular immune responses to S. japonicum recombinant and native antigens. *Acta tropica* **2002,** *84* (2), 137-49.

75. Kajihara, N.; Hirayama, K., The War against a Regional Disease in Japan A History of the Eradication of Schistosomiasis japonica. *Trop Med Health* **2011,** *39* (1 Suppl 1), 3-44.

76. McGarvey, S. T.; Aligui, G.; Daniel, B. L.; Peters, P.; Olveda, R.; Olds, G. R., Child growth and schistosomiasis japonica in northeastern Leyte, the Philippines: cross-sectional results. *The American journal of tropical medicine and hygiene* **1992,** *46* (5), 571-81.

77. Stephenson, L. S.; Latham, M. C.; Kurz, K. M.; Kinoti, S. N., Single dose metrifonate or praziquantel treatment in Kenyan children. II. Effects on growth in relation to Schistosoma haematobium and hookworm egg counts. *The American journal of tropical medicine and hygiene* **1989,** *41* (4), 445-53.

78. Santos, J.; Gouveia, M. J.; Vale, N.; Delgado Mde, L.; Goncalves, A.; da Silva, J. M.; Oliveira, C.; Xavier, P.; Gomes, P.; Santos, L. L.; Lopes, C.; Barros, A.; Rinaldi, G.; Brindley, P. J.; da Costa, J. M.; Sousa, M.; Botelho, M. C., Urinary estrogen metabolites and self-reported infertility in women infected with Schistosoma haematobium. *PLoS One* **2014,** *9* (5), e96774.

79. Hodder, S. L.; Mahmoud, A. A.; Sorenson, K.; Weinert, D. M.; Stein, R. L.; Ouma, J. H.; Koech, D.; King, C. H., Predisposition to urinary tract epithelial metaplasia in Schistosoma haematobium infection. *The American journal of tropical medicine and hygiene* **2000,** *63* (3-4), 133-8.

80. Scrimgeour, E. M.; Gajdusek, D. C., Involvement of the central nervous system in Schistosoma mansoni and S. haematobium infection. A review. *Brain : a journal of neurology* **1985,** *108 (Pt 4),* 1023-38.

81. van Dam, G. J.; Wichers, J. H.; Ferreira, T. M. F.; Ghati, D.; van Amerongen, A.; Deelder, A. M., Diagnosis of schistosomiasis by reagent strip test for detection of circulating cathodic antigen. *Journal of clinical microbiology* **2004,** *42* (12), 5458-61.

82. van Dam, G. J.; de Dood, C. J.; Lewis, M.; Deelder, A. M.; van Lieshout, L.; Tanke, H. J.; van Rooyen, L. H.; Corstjens, P. L., A robust dry reagent lateral flow assay for diagnosis of active schistosomiasis by detection of Schistosoma circulating anodic antigen. *Exp Parasitol* **2013,** *135* (2), 274-82.

83. Gundersen, S. G.; Ravn, J.; Haagensen, I., Early detection of circulating anodic antigen (CAA) in a case of acute schistosomiasis mansoni with Katayama fever. *Scand J Infect Dis* **1992,** *24* (4), 549-52.

84. Coulibaly, J. T.; N'Gbesso, Y. K.; Knopp, S.; N'Guessan, N. A.; Silue, K. D.; van Dam, G. J.; N'Goran, E. K.; Utzinger, J., Accuracy of urine circulating cathodic antigen test for the diagnosis of Schistosoma mansoni in preschool-aged children before and after treatment. *PLoS Negl Trop Dis* **2013,** *7* (3), e2109.

85. Coulibaly, J. T.; Knopp, S.; N'Guessan, N. A.; Silue, K. D.; Furst, T.; Lohourignon, L. K.; Brou, J. K.; N'Gbesso, Y. K.; Vounatsou, P.; N'Goran, E. K.; Utzinger, J., Accuracy of urine circulating cathodic antigen (CCA) test for Schistosoma mansoni diagnosis in different settings of Cote

d'Ivoire. *PLoS Negl Trop Dis* **2011,** *5* (11), e1384.

86. Schunk, M.; Kebede Mekonnen, S.; Wondafrash, B.; Mengele, C.; Fleischmann, E.; Herbinger, K. H.; Verweij, J. J.; Geldmacher, C.; Bretzel, G.; Loscher, T.; Zeynudin, A., Use of Occult Blood Detection Cards for Real-Time PCR-Based Diagnosis of Schistosoma Mansoni Infection. *PLoS One* **2015,** *10* (9), e0137730.

87. Sady, H.; Al-Mekhlafi, H. M.; Ngui, R.; Atroosh, W. M.; Al-Delaimy, A. K.; Nasr, N. A.; Dawaki, S.; Abdulsalam, A. M.; Ithoi, I.; Lim, Y. A.; Chua, K. H.; Surin, J., Detection of Schistosoma mansoni and Schistosoma haematobium by Real-Time PCR with High Resolution Melting Analysis. *Int J Mol Sci* **2015,** *16* (7), 16085-103.

88. Meurs, L.; Brienen, E.; Mbow, M.; Ochola, E. A.; Mboup, S.; Karanja, D. M.; Secor, W. E.; Polman, K.; van Lieshout, L., Is PCR the Next Reference Standard for the Diagnosis of Schistosoma in Stool? A Comparison with Microscopy in Senegal and Kenya. *PLoS Negl Trop Dis* **2015,** *9* (7), e0003959.

89. Jones, M. E.; Mitchell, R. G.; Leen, C. L., Long seronegative window in schistosoma infection. *Lancet* **1992,** *340* (8834-8835), 1549-50.

90. Kinkel, H. F.; Dittrich, S.; Baumer, B.; Weitzel, T., Evaluation of eight serological tests for diagnosis of imported schistosomiasis. *Clin Vaccine Immunol* **2012,** *19* (6), 948-53.

91. Rabello, A. L.; Garcia, M. M.; Pinto da Silva, R. A.; Rocha, R. S.; Katz, N., Humoral immune responses in patients with acute Schistosoma mansoni infection who were followed up for two years after treatment. *Clin Infect Dis* **1997,** *24* (3), 304-8.

92. Hatz, C.; Jenkins, J. M.; Morrow, R. H.; Tanner, M., Ultrasound in schistosomiasis--a critical look at methodological issues and potential applications. *Acta tropica* **1992,** *51* (1), 89-97.

93. Jaureguiberry, S.; Paris, L.; Caumes, E., Acute schistosomiasis, a diagnostic and therapeutic challenge. *Clin Microbiol Infect* **2010,** *16* (3), 225-31.

94. Harries, A. D.; Cook, G. C., Acute schistosomiasis (Katayama fever): clinical deterioration after chemotherapy. *J Infect* **1987,** *14* (2), 159-61.

95. Grandiere-Perez, L.; Ansart, S.; Paris, L.; Faussart, A.; Jaureguiberry, S.; Grivois, J. P.; Klement, E.; Bricaire, F.; Danis, M.; Caumes, E., Efficacy of praziquantel during the incubation and invasive phase of Schistosoma haematobium schistosomiasis in 18 travelers. *Am J Trop Med Hyg* **2006,** *74* (5), 814-8.

96. Utzinger, J.; N'Goran, E. K.; N'Dri, A.; Lengeler, C.; Tanner, M., Efficacy of praziquantel against Schistosoma mansoni with particular consideration for intensity of infection. *Trop Med Int Health* **2000,** *5* (11), 771-8.

97. Kramer, C. V.; Zhang, F.; Sinclair, D.; Olliaro, P. L., Drugs for treating urinary schistosomiasis. *Cochrane Database Syst Rev* **2014,** *8,* CD000053.

98. Danso-Appiah, A.; Utzinger, J.; Liu, J.; Olliaro, P., Drugs for treating urinary schistosomiasis. *Cochrane Database Syst Rev* **2008,** (3), CD000053.

99. Greenberg, R. M., Are Ca2+ channels targets of praziquantel action? *International journal for parasitology* **2005,** *35* (1), 1-9.

100. Homeida, M. A.; el Tom, I.; Nash, T.; Bennett, J. L., Association of the therapeutic activity of praziquantel with the reversal of Symmers' fibrosis induced by Schistosoma mansoni. *The American journal of tropical medicine and hygiene* **1991,** *45* (3), 360-5.

101. Brindley, P. J.; Sher, A., The chemotherapeutic effect of praziquantel against Schistosoma mansoni is dependent on host antibody response. *Journal of immunology (Baltimore, Md. : 1950)* **1987,** *139* (1), 215-20.

102. Lucey, D. R.; Maguire, J. H., Schistosomiasis. *Infect Dis Clin North Am* **1993,** *7* (3), 635-53.

103. Silva, L. C.; Maciel, P. E.; Ribas, J. G.; Souza-Pereira, S. R.; Antunes, C. M.; Lambertucci, J. R., Treatment of schistosomal myeloradiculopathy with praziquantel and corticosteroids and evaluation by magnetic resonance imaging: a longitudinal study. *Clin Infect Dis* **2004,** *39* (11), 1618-24.

104. Ferrari, T. C.; Moreira, P. R.; Cunha, A. S., Clinical characterization of neuroschistosomiasis due to Schistosoma mansoni and its treatment. *Acta Trop* **2008,** *108* (2-3), 89-97.

105. Molyneux, D. H.; Hotez, P. J.; Fenwick, A., "Rapid-impact interventions": how a policy of

integrated control for Africa's neglected tropical diseases could benefit the poor. *PLoS Med* **2005**, *2* (11), e336.

106. Hotez, P. J.; Molyneux, D. H.; Fenwick, A.; Ottesen, E.; Ehrlich Sachs, S.; Sachs, J. D., Incorporating a rapid-impact package for neglected tropical diseases with programs for HIV/ AIDS, tuberculosis, and malaria. *PLoS Med* **2006**, *3* (5), e102.

107. Silva, I. M.; Thiengo, R.; Conceicao, M. J.; Rey, L.; Lenzi, H. L.; Pereira Filho, E.; Ribeiro, P. C., Therapeutic failure of praziquantel in the treatment of Schistosoma haematobium infection in Brazilians returning from Africa. *Mem Inst Oswaldo Cruz* **2005**, *100* (4), 445-9.

108. Wang, W.; Dai, J. R.; Li, H. J.; Shen, X. H.; Liang, Y. S., Is there reduced susceptibility to praziquantel in Schistosoma japonicum? Evidence from China. *Parasitology* **2010**, *137* (13), 1905-12.

109. Melman, S. D.; Steinauer, M. L.; Cunningham, C.; Kubatko, L. S.; Mwangi, I. N.; Wynn, N. B.; Mutuku, M. W.; Karanja, D. M.; Colley, D. G.; Black, C. L.; Secor, W. E.; Mkoji, G. M.; Loker, E. S., Reduced susceptibility to praziquantel among naturally occurring Kenyan isolates of Schistosoma mansoni. *PLoS Negl Trop Dis* **2009**, *3* (8), e504.

110. King, C. H.; Lombardi, G.; Lombardi, C.; Greenblatt, R.; Hodder, S.; Kinyanjui, H.; Ouma, J.; Odiambo, O.; Bryan, P. J.; Muruka, J., Chemotherapy-based control of schistosomiasis haematobia. II. Metrifonate vs. praziquantel in control of infection-associated morbidity. *The American journal of tropical medicine and hygiene* **1990**, *42* (6), 587-95.

111. Utzinger, J.; Chollet, J.; You, J.; Mei, J.; Tanner, M.; Xiao, S., Effect of combined treatment with praziquantel and artemether on Schistosoma japonicum and Schistosoma mansoni in experimentally infected animals. *Acta tropica* **2001**, *80* (1), 9-18.

112. Ngoran, E. K.; Utzinger, J., Randomized, double blind placebo controlled trial of oral artemether for the prevention of patent S hematobium infections *AmJ Trop Med Hyg* **2003**, 24-32.

113. Engels, D.; Chitsulo, L.; Montresor, A.; Savioli, L., The global epidemiological situation of schistosomiasis and new approaches to control and research. *Acta tropica* **2002**, *82* (2), 139-46.

114. Jordan, P., Schistosomiasis--research to control. *The American journal of tropical medicine and hygiene* **1977**, *26* (5 Pt 1), 877-86.

115. Liu, R.; Dong, H. F.; Jiang, M. S., What is the role of health education in the integrated strategy to control transmission of Schistosoma japonicum in China? *Parasitol Res* **2012**, *110* (5), 2081-2.

116. Wang, L. D.; Chen, H. G.; Guo, J. G.; Zeng, X. J.; Hong, X. L.; Xiong, J. J.; Wu, X. H.; Wang, X. H.; Wang, L. Y.; Xia, G.; Hao, Y.; Chin, D. P.; Zhou, X. N., A strategy to control transmission of Schistosoma japonicum in China. *N Engl J Med* **2009**, *360* (2), 121-8.

117. Cleland, C. R.; Tukahebwa, E. M.; Fenwick, A.; Blair, L., Mass drug administration with praziquantel reduces the prevalence of Schistosoma mansoni and improves liver morbidity in untreated preschool children. *Trans R Soc Trop Med Hyg* **2014**, *108* (9), 575-81.

118. Chaula, S. A.; Tarimo, D. S., Impact of praziquantel mass drug administration campaign on prevalence and intensity of Schistosoma haemamtobium among school children in Bahi district, Tanzania. *Tanzan J Health Res* **2014**, *16* (1), 1-8.

119. Unrau, G. O., Individual household water supplies as a control measure against Schistosoma mansoni. A study in rural St Lucia. *Bulletin of the World Health Organization* **1975**, *52* (1), 1-8.

120. Jobin, W. R.; Brown, R. A.; Vélez, S. P.; Ferguson, F. F., Biological control of Biomphalaria glabrata in major reservoirs of Puerto Rico. *The American journal of tropical medicine and hygiene* **1977**, *26* (5 Pt 1), 1018-24.

121. Olveda, R. M.; Daniel, B. L.; Ramirez, B. D.; Aligui, G. D.; Acosta, L. P.; Fevidal, P.; Tiu, E.; de Veyra, F.; Peters, P. A.; Romulo, R.; Domingo, E.; Wiest, P. M.; Olds, G. R., Schistosomiasis japonica in the Philippines: the long-term impact of population-based chemotherapy on infection, transmission, and morbidity. *The Journal of infectious diseases* **1996**, *174* (1), 163-72.

122. Herwaldt, B. L.; Tao, L. F.; van Pelt, W.; Tsang, V. C.; Bruce, J. I., Persistence of Schistosoma haematobium infection despite multiple courses of therapy with praziquantel. *Clinical infectious diseases : an official publication of the Infectious Diseases Society of America* **1995**, *20* (2), 309-15.

123. Pearce, E. J., Progress towards a vaccine for schistosomiasis. *Acta tropica* **2003**, *86* (2-3), 309-13.

124.   Bergquist, R.; Al-Sherbiny, M.; Barakat, R.; Olds, R., Blueprint for schistosomiasis vaccine development. *Acta tropica* **2002,** *82* (2), 183-92.

125.   Capron, A.; Capron, M.; Dombrowicz, D.; Riveau, G., Vaccine strategies against schistosomiasis: from concepts to clinical trials. *International archives of allergy and immunology* **2001,** *124* (1-3), 9-15.

126.   Onkanga, I. O.; Mwinzi, P. N.; Muchiri, G.; Andiego, K.; Omedo, M.; Karanja, D. M.; Wiegand, R. E.; Secor, W. E.; Montgomery, S. P., Impact of two rounds of praziquantel mass drug administration on Schistosoma mansoni infection prevalence and intensity: a comparison between community wide treatment and school based treatment in western Kenya. *Int J Parasitol* **2016**.

127.   Almeida, G. T.; Lage, R. C.; Anderson, L.; Venancio, T. M.; Nakaya, H. I.; Miyasato, P. A.; Rofatto, H. K.; Zerlotini, A.; Nakano, E.; Oliveira, G.; Verjovski-Almeida, S., Synergy of Omeprazole and Praziquantel In Vitro Treatment against Schistosoma mansoni Adult Worms. *PLoS Negl Trop Dis* **2015,** *9* (9), e0004086.

128.   Buro, C.; Beckmann, S.; Oliveira, K. C.; Dissous, C.; Cailliau, K.; Marhofer, R. J.; Selzer, P. M.; Verjovski-Almeida, S.; Grevelding, C. G., Imatinib treatment causes substantial transcriptional changes in adult Schistosoma mansoni in vitro exhibiting pleiotropic effects. *PLoS Negl Trop Dis* **2014,** *8* (6), e2923.

129.   Basra, A.; Mombo-Ngoma, G.; Melser, M. C.; Diop, D. A.; Wurbel, H.; Mackanga, J. R.; Furstenau, M.; Zoleko, R. M.; Adegnika, A. A.; Gonzalez, R.; Menendez, C.; Kremsner, P. G.; Ramharter, M., Efficacy of mefloquine intermittent preventive treatment in pregnancy against Schistosoma haematobium infection in Gabon: a nested randomized controlled assessor-blinded clinical trial. *Clin Infect Dis* **2013,** *56* (6), e68-75.

34. *Clonorchis sinensis* (Looss 1907)

Opisthorchis viverrini

Opisthorchis felineus

Introduction

There are three major fish-borne liver flukes of major significance for human health; *Clonorchis sinensis, Opisthorchis viverrini,* and *Opisthorchis felineus.*[1] *Clonor-chis sinensis* is endemic mostly in China and Korea (North and South), but it is found elsewhere in Southeast Asia and is acquired by eating raw or undercooked freshwater fish.[2] *Opisthorchis viverrini* is endemic to northern Thailand, Vietnam, Cambodia, and Laos where it is also a major liver fluke species, *O. felineus,* can be found in Siberia, but a new focus recently emerged in Italy.[1, 3-6] The biology, pathogenesis, and clinical disease of all three species are similar, so in most of this chapter *C. sinensis* will be presented as the model organism for fish-borne liver flukes affecting humans, and on occasion the unique differences of *Opisthorchis viverrini,* and *O. felineus* will be mentioned.

C. sinensis has numerous reservoir hosts, including dogs and cats. More than 25 million people in the Far East are infected with these fish-borne liver flukes, and some estimate that up to one fourth of Chinese immigrants to the United States harbor these flukes.[2, 7] Approximately 10 million people in northern Thailand are infected with *O. viverini,* and 16 million in the former USSR with *O. felineus.*[8, 9] These liver flukes have been identified as potent inducers of carcinogenesis and major causes of bile duct cancer (cholangiocarcinoma).[10, 11]

Historical information

In 1875, James McConnell described the adult fluke in a patient who died at a hospital in Calcutta, India, and Arthur Looss renamed it *C. sinensis* in 1907.[7, 12] In 1887, Isao Ijima demonstrated that *C. sinensis* infects animals, establishing the concept of reservoir hosts for this parasite.[13] In 1910, Haraujiro Kobayashi identified freshwater fish as the intermediate vertebrate hosts.[14] In 1918, Masatomo Muto extended these studies in Japan by identifying snails in the genus *Bulimus* as the first intermediate host.[15] It is now known that the genus of snail responsible for harboring the intermediate stages of these trematodes varies from

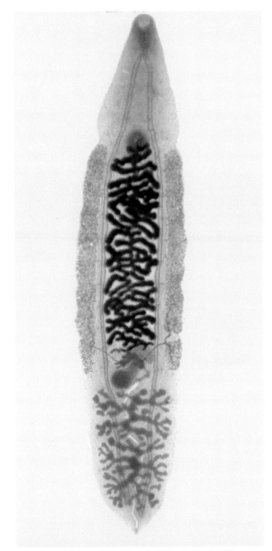

Figure 34.1. An adult *Clonorchis sinensis*. 19 mm x 3.5 mm.

Clonorchis sinensis

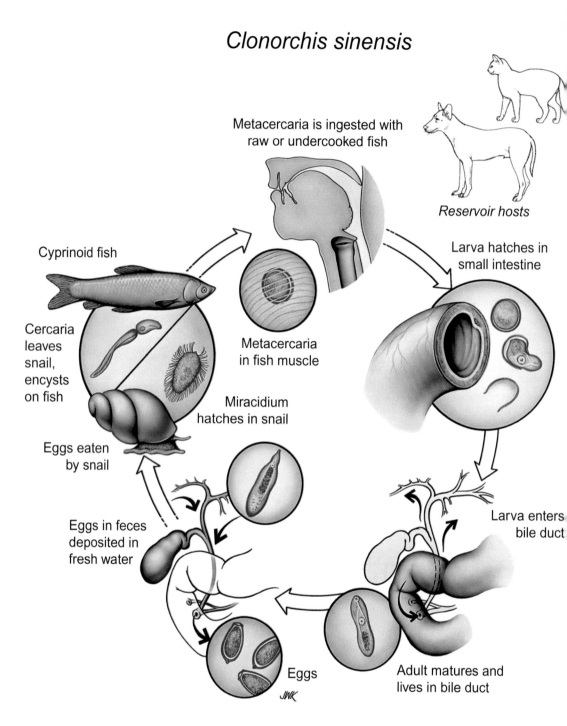

Metacercaria is ingested with
raw or undercooked fish

Reservoir hosts

Cyprinoid fish

Larva hatches in
small intestine

Cercaria
leaves
snail,
encysts
on fish

Metacercaria
in fish muscle

Miracidium
hatches in snail

Eggs eaten
by snail

Larva enters
bile duct

Eggs in feces
deposited in
fresh water

Eggs

Adult matures and
lives in bile duct

JWK

Parasitic Diseases 6th Ed. Parasites Without Borders www.parasiteswithoutborders.com

region to region, with at least eight different species already described for *C. sinensis*.[16]

Life Cycle

Infection begins when the definitive host ingests a raw, pickled, salted, smoked, frozen or undercooked fish or crustacean harboring the metacercaria (Fig. 34.2).[17, 18] There are multiple species of freshwater fish that may harbor this parasite and, despite referring to these as fish-borne liver flukes, it has been discovered that freshwater crustaceans, such as shrimp, may also act as an intermediate host.[17] The ingested larval stage excysts in the small intestine and transforms into the immature fluke. The flukes then enter the biliary system through the ampulla of Vater, migrate up the bile duct (Fig. 34.3), remaining there, growing to adulthood within several weeks.[19] The method of travel up the bile ducts to reach intrahepatic sites in the biliary system is in contrast to the migration of *Fasciola hepatica,* which penetrates Glisson's capsule, and then migrates through the liver parenchyma before ending up in the extrahepatic biliary ducts.[19] The mature parasite (Fig. 34.1) measures 20 mm by 3.5 mm, and lives in the lumen of the bile duct, feeding on epithelium. Each parasite may live for up to 26 years in the biliary system.[20] Since each worm has both male and female reproductive organs, self-fertilization is the norm. Single worms

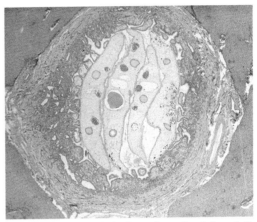

Figure 34.3. Histological section of adults of *C. sinensis* in bile duct.

are capable of producing eggs without the requirement of finding a mate. Egg production follows self-fertilization. Embryonated eggs (Fig. 34.4) pass from the common bile duct into the small intestine and are excreted with the feces. These eggs must reach freshwater in order to continue the life cycle. In experimental infections, adult worms produce 1000-4000 eggs per day, and in human infection egg production is about 4000 eggs per day per worm.[21]

Eggs are eaten by the intermediate host snail, (in most of Asia, *Parafossarulus* spp.), stimulating the miracidium to hatch. The miracidia then penetrate the intestinal wall. Flukes undergo a process of asexual maturation with development to the sporocyst, then the redia stage, then cercariae. Cercariae emerge from the snail approximately 95 days later.[18] The

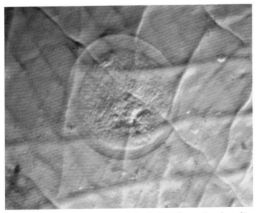

Figure 34.2. Metacercaria of *C. sinensis, in situ,* under the scales of a grass carp. 165 μm.

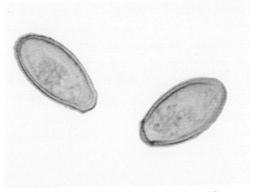

Figure 34.4. Eggs of *C. sinensis*. 30 μm x 15 μm.

cercarial stage is highly motile, and when it encounters an appropriate host such as a cyprinid fish, it encysts under the scales, transforming to the metacercaria. Encystment can also occur under the exoskeleton of various fresh-water crustacea (e.g., crabs, crayfish, and shrimp), completing the life cycle.[17]

Cellular and Molecular Pathogenesis

Adult worms induce eosinophilic inflammatory reactions after they attach to the bile duct and begin feeding.[22, 23] In heavy infection, these changes may lead to desquamation of the biliary epithelium, formation of crypts, and metaplasia.[24, 25] *C. sinensis* elicits the production of specific IgE antibodies in serum and bile.[26] Chronic clonorchis and opisthorchis infections elicit reactions resulting in intermittent obstruction of the biliary tree, as well the introduction of pyogenic bacteria into the infection sites.[27] Through this process, chronic liver fluke infection can result in recurrent ascending cholangitis and pancreatitis.[16, 28-31] Over time, the presence of these fish-borne trematodes in the biliary tree may result in squamous metaplastic changes that lead to cholangiocarcinoma.[32] This is particularly true of heavy *O. viverini* infections in Thailand that can be associated with a 15-fold increase in risk of developing this unusual form of cancer. A much higher percentage of patients who died of cholangiocarcinoma had coexistent opisthorchiasis than did those who died of other causes.[25] The molecular basis of helminth induced carcinogenesis has been reviewed.[33]

Clinical Disease

The symptoms seen in patients both acutely and chronically infected by these fish-borne trematodes are mostly determined by inoculum of metacercariae and worm burden. In acute infections with few metacercariae, patients are often asymptomatic, while patients infected with large numbers of metacercariae may present with right upper quadrant abdominal discomfort and tenderness, nausea, diarrhea, and headache.[34] Heavy chronic infections can result in hepatomegaly, right upper quadrant tenderness, and eosinophilia.[16] Heavy infections can facilitate the sequestration of pyogenic bacteria behind areas of intrahepatic biliary narrowing, causing recurrent ascending cholangitis and pancreatitis.[16, 28-31] Very heavy infections can lead to anorexia, cachexia and weight loss with elevated alkaline phosphatase but normal hepatic transaminase levels. There does seem to be an anatomical preference for the left lobe of the liver that has been explained by small differences in the anatomy that cause these parasites to favor this portion of the liver.[7] Cholangiocarcinoma (bile duct carcinoma) is a long-standing sequelae due to chronic fibrosis and infection. It has a high mortality in Asia.

Diagnosis

Four weeks after initial infection, eggs of these fish-borne trematodes start to be released into human feces, so a microscopic examination of a concentrated sample of feces is the definitive gold standard test.[7] In light infection eggs may be detectable in concentrated specimens. During periods of biliary obstruction, when patients may present for care, eggs may not be detected in the stool.[35] Flukes may be detected by endoscopic retrograde cholangiopancreatography (ERCP). The presence of flukes in the biliary tract may also be observed using ultrasound, CT, MRI and cholangiography.[36-40] A variety of serological tests, including Western blot and ELISA, are available, but can not distinguish between current and past infection, and may cross react with other parasitic infections.[41, 42] Nucleic acid amplification tests (NAAT) such as polymerase chain reaction (PCR) tests and loop-mediated isothermal amplification (LAMP) have been developed to improve the sensitivity of egg detection in stool, but are not used routinely in the clinics where most of these cases are seen.[43-46]

Treatment

Praziquantel is the drug of choice for treating *Clonorchis sinensis*, *Opisthorchis viverini,* and *O. felineus*.[47] Albendazole is also effective for *Clonorchis sinensis* but shows only modest efficacy for the treatment of *Opisthorchis viverini* and *O. felineus*.[48, 49]

Prevention and Control

Ingestion of contaminated raw, under-cooked, pickled, frozen, salted, smoked or dried freshwater fish or crustaceans is the source of infection with *Clonorchis sinensis* and its close relatives. In many parts of Asia it is a common practice to grind fish containing metacercariae into a paste together with spices and condiments to produce a dish roughly equivalent to ceviche. This concoction is a prime source of liver fluke infection. Thoroughly cooking contaminated fish and crustaceans is the most effective way of eliminating the parasite on an individual basis.[16] At least one form of biliary carcinoma is preventable by changes in eating habits. Centuries-old culinary preferences in most endemic areas do not allow for this possibility, and in some areas the ingestion of raw fish has important roles in traditional cultural, and religious contexts.[7] There is also a long held myth that hot spices and the consumption of alcohol along with the raw fish will be protective, but there is no evidence to support this belief.[7]

The advent of large-scale aquaculture of grass carp, and related fishes in areas where fecal contamination of the ponds from infected hosts occurs on a regular basis, results in the establishment of infection in the fish population.[16, 31] Animal reservoirs make control of this parasite difficult at best. Ammonium sulfate kills the eggs of clonorchis, and so it is recommended as a treatment for human feces destined to be used as fertilizer.

Molluscicides, alone, have not been used successfully for eradicating the intermediate snail hosts are there concerns about the impact of their use on the environment.[50] In combination with regular draining of ponds, they have been moderately effective in controlling infection in fish. While human vaccines are being tested and studied, a vaccination strategy targeting the freshwater fish is being studied and tested as well.[51]

References

1.   Petney, T. N.; Andrews, R. H.; Saijuntha, W.; Wenz-Mucke, A.; Sithithaworn, P., The zoonotic, fish-borne liver flukes Clonorchis sinensis, Opisthorchis felineus and Opisthorchis viverrini. *Int J Parasitol* **2013,** *43* (12-13), 1031-46.

2.   Stauffer, W. M.; Sellman, J. S.; Walker, P. F., Biliary liver flukes (Opisthorchiasis and Clonorchiasis) in immigrants in the United States: often subtle and diagnosed years after arrival. *Journal of travel medicine* **2004,** *11* (3), 157-9.

3.   Sripa, B.; Kaewkes, S.; Intapan, P. M.; Maleewong, W.; Brindley, P. J., Food-borne trematodiases in Southeast Asia epidemiology, pathology, clinical manifestation and control. *Adv Parasitol* **2010,** *72*, 305-50.

4.   Kruthong, S.; Lerdverasirikul, P.; R., Opisthorchis viverini infection in rural communities in northeast Thailand. *Trans Med Hyg* **1987,** *81*, 1-414.

5.   Giboda, M.; Ditrich, O.; Scholz, T.; Viengsay, T.; Bouaphanh, S., Human Opisthorchis and Haplorchis infections in Laos. *Transactions of the Royal Society of Tropical Medicine and Hygiene* **1991,** *85* (4), 538-40.

6. Wunderink, H. F.; Rozemeijer, W.; Wever, P. C.; Verweij, J. J.; van Lieshout, L., Foodborne trematodiasis and Opisthorchis felineus acquired in Italy. *Emerg Infect Dis* **2014**, *20* (1), 154-5.

7. Qian, M. B.; Utzinger, J.; Keiser, J.; Zhou, X. N., Clonorchiasis. *Lancet* **2015**.

8. Schwartz, D. A., Cholangiocarcinoma associated with liver fluke infection: a preventable source of morbidity in Asian immigrants. *The American journal of gastroenterology* **1986**, *81* (1), 76-9.

9. WHO, Control of food-borne trematode infections: Report of a WHO study group. *Report Series No 849 Organization* **1995**.

10. Sithithaworn, P.; Yongvanit, P.; Duenngai, K.; Kiatsopit, N.; Pairojkul, C., Roles of liver fluke infection as risk factor for cholangiocarcinoma. *J Hepatobiliary Pancreat Sci* **2014**, *21* (5), 301-8.

11. Sripa, B.; Brindley, P. J.; Mulvenna, J.; Laha, T.; Smout, M. J.; Mairiang, E.; Bethony, J. M.; Loukas, A., The tumorigenic liver fluke Opisthorchis viverrini--multiple pathways to cancer. *Trends Parasitol* **2012**, *28* (10), 395-407.

12. McConnell, J. F. P., Anatomy and pathological relations of a new species of liver fluke. *Lancet* **1875**, *2* 271-274.

13. Ijima, I.; J., Notes on Diastoma endemicum. *Baelz Sci Imperial Univ Jpn* **1887**, *1*, 47-50.

14. Kobayashi, H., On the life cycle and morphology of Clonorchis sinensis. *Centr BakterParasit InfectKrank* **1914**, *75*, 299-317.

15. Muto, S., On the primary intermediate host of Clonorchis sinensis. *Chuo Igakakai Zasshi* **1918**, *25*, 49-52.

16. Lun, Z.-R.; Gasser, R. B.; Lai, D.-H.; Li, A.-X.; Zhu, X.-Q.; Yu, X.-B.; Fang, Y.-Y., Clonorchiasis: a key foodborne zoonosis in China. *The Lancet. Infectious diseases* **2005**, *5* (1), 31-41.

17. Yang, L. D.; Hu, M.; Gui, A. F., [An epidemiological study on clonorchiasis sinensis in Hubei Province]. *Zhonghua Yu Fang Yi Xue Za Zhi* **1994**, *28* (4), 225-7.

18. Liang, C.; Hu, X. C.; Lv, Z. Y.; Wu, Z. D.; Yu, X. B.; Xu, J.; Zheng, H. Q., [Experimental establishment of life cycle of Clonorchis sinensis]. *Zhongguo Ji Sheng Chong Xue Yu Ji Sheng Chong Bing Za Zhi* **2009**, *27* (2), 148-50.

19. Kim, T. I.; Yoo, W. G.; Kwak, B. K.; Seok, J. W.; Hong, S. J., Tracing of the Bile-chemotactic migration of juvenile Clonorchis sinensis in rabbits by PET-CT. *PLoS Negl Trop Dis* **2011**, *5* (12), e1414.

20. Attwood, H. D.; Chou, S. T., The longevity of Clonorchis sinensis. *Pathology* **1978**, *10* (2), 153-6.

21. Kim, J. H.; Choi, M. H.; Bae, Y. M.; Oh, J. K.; Lim, M. K.; Hong, S. T., Correlation between discharged worms and fecal egg counts in human clonorchiasis. *PLoS Negl Trop Dis* **2011**, *5* (10), e1339.

22. Sun, T., Pathology and immunology of Clonorchis sinensis infection of the liver. *Annals of clinical and laboratory science* **1984**, *14* (3), 208-15.

23. Yen, C. M.; Chen, E. R.; Hou, M. F.; Chang, J. H., Antibodies of different immunoglobulin isotypes in serum and bile of patients with clonorchiasis. *Annals of tropical medicine and parasitology* **1992**, *86* (3), 263-9.

24. Pungpak, S.; Akai, P. S.; Longenecker, B. M.; Ho, M.; Befus, A. D.; Bunnag, D., Tumour markers in the detection of opisthorchiasis-associated cholangiocarcinoma. *Transactions of the Royal Society of Tropical Medicine and Hygiene* **1991**, *85* (2), 277-9.

25. Srivatanakul, P.; Sriplung, H.; Deerasamee, S., Epidemiology of liver cancer: an overview. *Asian Pacific journal of cancer prevention : APJCP* **2004**, *5* (2), 118-25.

26. Yong, T. S.; Park, S. J.; Lee, D. H.; Yang, H. J.; Lee, J., Identification of IgE-reacting Clonorchis sinensis antigens. *Yonsei medical journal* **1999**, *40* (2), 178-83.

27. Ho, C. S.; Wesson, D. E., Recurrent pyogenic cholangitis in Chinese immigrants. *The American journal of roentgenology, radium therapy, and nuclear medicine* **1974**, *122* (2), 368-74.

28. McFadzen, A. J. S.; Yeung, R. T. T.; R., Acute pancreatitis due to Clonorchis sinensis. *Trans Trop Med Hyg 466* **1966**, *60*.

29. Haswell-Elkins, M. R.; Mairiang, E.; Mairiang, P.; Chaiyakum, J.; Chamadol, N.; Loapaiboon, V.; Sithithaworn, P.; Elkins, D. B., Cross-sectional study of Opisthorchis viverrini infection and cholangiocarcinoma in communities within a high-risk area in northeast Thailand. *International journal of cancer. Journal international du cancer* **1994**, *59* (4), 505-9.

30. Thamavit, W.; Bhamarapravati, N.; Sahaphong, S.; Vajrasthira, S.; Angsubhakorn, S., Effects of dimethylnitrosamine on induction of cholangiocarcinoma in Opisthorchis viverrini-infected Syrian golden hamsters. *Cancer research* **1978,** *38* (12), 4634-9.
31. Wang, K. X.; Zhang, R. B.; Cui, Y. B.; Tian, Y.; Cai, R.; Li, C. P., Clinical and epidemiological features of patients with clonorchiasis. *World J Gastroenterol* **2004,** *10* (3), 446-8.
32. Okuda, K.; Kubo, Y.; Okazaki, N.; Arishima, T.; Hashimoto, M., Clinical aspects of intrahepatic bile duct carcinoma including hilar carcinoma: a study of 57 autopsy-proven cases. *Cancer* **1977,** *39* (1), 232-46.
33. Brindley, P. J.; da Costa, J. M.; Sripa, B., Why does infection with some helminths cause cancer? *Trends Cancer* **2015,** *1* (3), 174-182.
34. Liang, S. D.; Wu, Y. R.; Pan, Y. L., [Analysis on 2175 admitted cases of clonorchiasis sinensis in Guigang City]. *Zhongguo Ji Sheng Chong Xue Yu Ji Sheng Chong Bing Za Zhi* **2008,** *26* (5), 374-5.
35. Joo, K. R.; Bang, S. J., A bile based study of Clonorchis sinensis infections in patients with biliary tract diseases in Ulsan, Korea. *Yonsei Med J* **2005,** *46* (6), 794-8.
36. Choi, D.; Hong, S. T., Imaging diagnosis of clonorchiasis. *Korean J Parasitol* **2007,** *45* (2), 77-85.
37. Jeong, Y. Y.; Kang, H. K.; Kim, J. W.; Yoon, W.; Chung, T. W.; Ko, S. W., MR imaging findings of clonorchiasis. *Korean J Radiol* **2004,** *5* (1), 25-30.
38. Lim, J. H., Radiologic findings of clonorchiasis. *AJR Am J Roentgenol* **1990,** *155* (5), 1001-8.
39. Choi, B. I.; Kim, H. J.; Han, M. C.; Do, Y. S.; Han, M. H.; Lee, S. H., CT findings of clonorchiasis. *AJR Am J Roentgenol* **1989,** *152* (2), 281-4.
40. Lim, J. H.; Ko, Y. T.; Lee, D. H.; Kim, S. Y., Clonorchiasis: sonographic findings in 59 proved cases. *AJR Am J Roentgenol* **1989,** *152* (4), 761-4.
41. Kim, S. I., A Clonorchis sinensis-specific antigen that detects active human clonorchiasis. *The Korean journal of parasitology* **1998,** *36* (1), 37-45.
42. Kim, C. S.; Min, D. Y.; J., Immunodiagnosis of clonorchiasis using a recombinant antigen. *Korean* **1998,** *36,* 183-90.
43. Kim, E. M.; Verweij, J. J.; Jalili, A.; van Lieshout, L.; Choi, M. H.; Bae, Y. M.; Lim, M. K.; Hong, S. T., Detection of Clonorchis sinensis in stool samples using real-time PCR. *Ann Trop Med Parasitol* **2009,** *103* (6), 513-8.
44. Parvathi, A.; Umesha, K. R.; Kumar, S.; Sithithaworn, P.; Karunasagar, I.; Karunasagar, I., Development and evaluation of a polymerase chain reaction (PCR) assay for the detection of Opisthorchis viverrini in fish. *Acta Trop* **2008,** *107* (1), 13-6.
45. Umesha, K. R.; Kumar, S.; Parvathi, A.; Duenngai, K.; Sithithaworn, P.; Karunasagar, I.; Karunasagar, I., Opisthorchis viverrini: detection by polymerase chain reaction (PCR) in human stool samples. *Exp Parasitol* **2008,** *120* (4), 353-6.
46. Arimatsu, Y.; Kaewkes, S.; Laha, T.; Hong, S. J.; Sripa, B., Rapid detection of Opisthorchis viverrini copro-DNA using loop-mediated isothermal amplification (LAMP). *Parasitol Int* **2012,** *61* (1), 178-82.
47. Hsu, C. C.; Kron, M. A., Clonorchiasis and praziquantel. *Archives of internal medicine* **1985,** *145* (6), 1002-3.
48. Liu, Y. H.; Wang, X. G.; Gao, P.; Qian, M. X., Experimental and clinical trial of albendazole in the treatment of Clonorchiasis sinensis. *Chin Med J (Engl)* **1991,** *104* (1), 27-31.
49. Pungpark, S.; Bunnag, D.; Harinasuta, T., Albendazole in the treatment of opisthorchiasis and concomitant intestinal helminthic infections. *Southeast Asian J Trop Med Public Health* **1984,** *15* (1), 44-50.
50. Sithithaworn, P.; Andrews, R. H.; Nguyen, V. D.; Wongsaroj, T.; Sinuon, M.; Odermatt, P.; Nawa, Y.; Liang, S.; Brindley, P. J.; Sripa, B., The current status of opisthorchiasis and clonorchiasis in the Mekong Basin. *Parasitol Int* **2012,** *61* (1), 10-6.
51. Wang, X.; Chen, W.; Tian, Y.; Mao, Q.; Lv, X.; Shang, M.; Li, X.; Yu, X.; Huang, Y., Surface display of Clonorchis sinensis enolase on Bacillus subtilis spores potentializes an oral vaccine candidate. *Vaccine* **2014,** *32* (12), 1338-45.

35. *Fasciola hepatica*
(Linnaeus 1758)

Introduction

Fasciola hepatica, the sheep liver fluke, is acquired by eating contaminated leafy wild plants (e.g., watercress) that grow at the littoral zone of standing bodies of freshwater. Facioliasis is a zoonosis, infecting wild animals and livestock of all kinds, and is endemic throughout Central America, the British Isles, southeastern United States, Africa, Europe (especially Turkey), Asia, the Middle East, and South America.[1,2] Although less frequent in other parts of the world, cases have been reported in the United States and Australia.[3,4] New Zealand also used to have *F. hepatica,* but aggressive eradication programs in the 1960s and '70s have eradicated it from that island country.[5] *F. hepatica* infects millions of

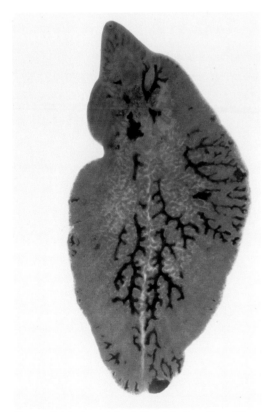

Figure 35.1. An adult of *Fasciola hepatica*. 30mm x 14 mm.

people worldwide and has been reported in more than 50 countries.[6-9]

Intensity of infection in humans is always associated with animal husbandry.[10] In areas of South America, such as Peru and Bolivia, there is a high prevalence, particularly in the northwestern altiplano of Bolivia, near Lake Titicaca.[11] *Fasciola gigantica* is a closely related species infecting cattle and wild herbivores in Africa and Asia, and can on rare occasions also infect humans.[12-15]

Historical Information

The writings of Jean de Brie in 1379 indicate that shepherds not only knew of the infection, but also strongly suspected that contaminated watercress was a source of the parasite.[16] In 1684, Francesco Redi described the adult parasite he obtained from a rabbit.[17] In 1758, Carl Linnaeus named this parasite *Fasciola hepatica*.[18,19] In 1881, Friedrich Leuckart and Algernon Thomas independenly described most of the biological aspects of its life cycle.[20,21] In 1892, Adolfo Lutz conducted experiments in guinea pigs proving that the adult parasite was acquired by swallowing the infective stage.[22]

Life Cycle

Infection is initiated by ingestion of encysted metacercariae that are firmly attached to littoral vegetation, particularly watercress, in standing bodies of freshwater (e.g., farm ponds).[23] They excyst in the small intestine, penetrate the intestinal wall, and migrate in the peritoneal cavity to the surface of the liver. Metacercariae penetrate Glisson's capsule and enter the parenchymal tissue of the liver. Migrating metacercariae track through the liver causing necrosis and fibrosis. Only a small number reach the biliary tree to develop to sexual maturity. Maturation to reproductive adults takes up to 4 months. The adult fluke is large, measuring 35 mm by 15

Fasciola hepatica

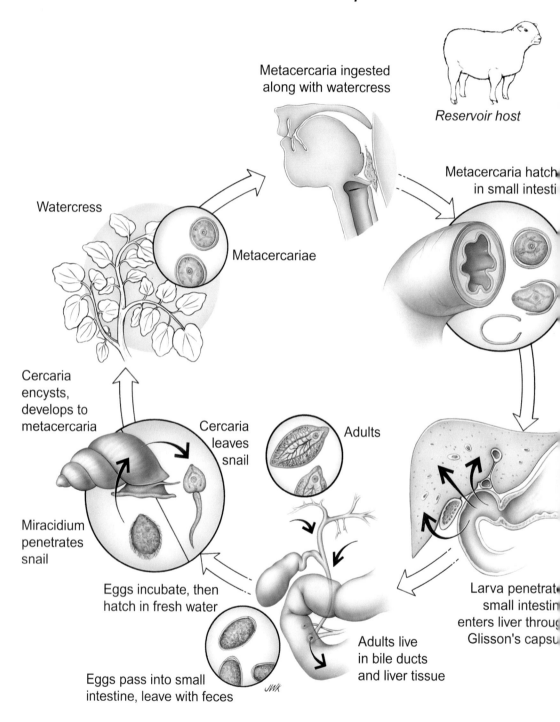

Metacercaria ingested
along with watercress

Reservoir host

Metacercaria hatch
in small intesti

Watercress

Metacercariae

Cercaria
encysts,
develops to
metacercaria

Cercaria
leaves
snail

Adults

Miracidium
penetrates
snail

Eggs incubate, then
hatch in fresh water

Larva penetrat
small intestin
enters liver throug
Glisson's capsu

Adults live
in bile ducts
and liver tissue

Eggs pass into small
intestine, leave with feces

mm (Fig. 35.1) and can live in the biliary tree for over a decade.

Both the immature worms and adults feed on liver parenchymal tissue (*foie gras d'homme*) and epithelial cells lining the bile ducts (Fig. 35.2). Self-fertilization leads to egg production. These large worms spend their lives burrowing through the liver, aided by their muscular oral suckers, creating tunnels into which are deposited eggs and waste products.

Fertilized, unembryonated eggs (Fig. 35.3) pass out of the liver through the common duct, enter the small intestine, and become included into the fecal mass.

Eggs must be deposited in freshwater in order to embryonate, which may take as long as 9-15 days. The miracidium is stimulated to hatch by exposure to direct sunlight, and after emerging from the egg, it is a free-swim-

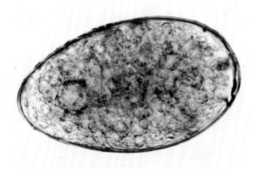

Figure 35.3. Egg of *F. hepatica.* 140 μm x 85 μm.

ming organism until it finds its snail host. The most common snail species for *F. hepatica* is *Lymnea truncatula* but many other species of Lymneid snails (e.g., *Fossaria modicella*) support the growth and development of this fluke throughout the world. The miracidium penetrates the snail's body wall, and finds its way to the hepatopancreas. After sequential development, first into sporocysts, then into rediae, the cercariae (Fig. 35.4) emerge from the snail. They then attach to the surfaces of littoral vegetation, where they become encysted. Within the cyst they transform into the environmentally resistant, infective stage, the metacercaria. This stage can live and remain infective for several months.

Ingested metacercariae sometimes find their way to tissues other than the liver (e.g., brain, kidney).[24, 25] In this case, they become aberrant infections and pass eggs that cannot find their way out of the body.

Cellular and Molecular Pathogenesis

Adult *Fasciola hepatica* secrete large quantities of proline which stimulates bile epithelial cells to divide and hypertrophy, creating the "lawn" of cells on which the fluke periodically grazes, presumably with the aid of its muscular oral sucker and secreted proteases.[26, 27] While moving through liver tissue this fluke creates trauma. Tunnels and abscesses form that are filled with necrotic

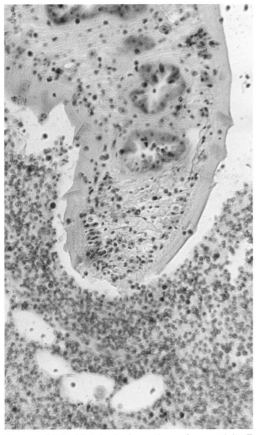

Figure 35.2. Histological section of an adult *F. hepatica* in liver.

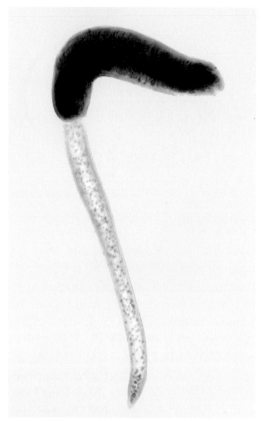

Figure 35.4. Cercaria of *F. hepatica*. 100 μm.

cell debris, worm excreta, and fertilized eggs. Fascioliasis induces high levels of circulating eosinophils throughout the infection period.[28, 29]

Halzoun (pharyngitis and laryngeal edema) is a condition specific to the Middle East associated with consumption of raw sheep liver that, although previously attributed to *Fasciola hepatica,* may in most cases be due to other parasitic infections.[30, 31]

Clinical Disease

Individuals may develop symptoms related to the migration of the immature worms within a month after becoming infected.[29] Many infected persons are asymptomatic during this early phase, while symptomatic patients may report fever, pain in the right upper quadrant of the abdomen, headache, generalized malaise, myalgia, weight loss, and urticaria.[32] Eosinophilia is

a prominent feature. Prominent radiographic findings on contrast CT have been reported as "hypoattenuating tracts" that follow the path of helminth invasion from the liver capsule.[33] Symptoms usually develop 6-12 weeks after exposure, and generally last for about 6 weeks. In heavy infections, the liver can be enlarged and tender. A right-sided pleural effusion with eosinophilia has been described.[34, 35]

Acute disease tends to be proportional to the number of ingested metacercariae. Chronic disease is usually proportional to the number of adult worms in the biliary system. During the chronic stage of the disease, dull pain and obstruction of bile ducts can occur. There are usually no changes in liver function tests, and jaundice is not a usual finding, but has been reported.[32] The gallbladder may become severely damaged in heavy infection. Fasciola in sites other than liver may cause no symptoms, or it may be present as a small tumor mass. If the parasite invades the brain, it can induce focal neurological abnormalities.

Diagnosis

Diagnosis begins with a clinical suspicion of exposure to *F. hepatica* from a carefully obtained history. It is only after enough time has gone by (up to 4 months) that mature adults, present in the biliary tree, release eggs into the stool. During acute infection, serology usually becomes positive while the metacercariae are migrating through the liver parenchyma. Most patients will present at this stage with high levels of circulating eosinophils.[29] Serological tests can be useful in ruling in the diagnosis at this stage of the infection and have excellent sensitivity and specificity.[36-38] *Fasciola hepatica* circulating antigen tests, also with excellent sensitivity and specificity, are available and correlate with burden of infection.[39, 40]

When mature flukes are present in the biliary system, microscopic identification of eggs in the stool is a definitive method of diagnosis. Eggs may be detected in the feces, in bile aspirates, or in duodenal aspirates. These unembryonated eggs (Fig. 35.3) are yellow-brown and measure 130-150 micrometers by 60-90 micrometers wide.

Imaging techniques such as ultrasonography, computed tomography (CT), cholangiography, endoscopic cholangiopancreatography (ERCP) and MRI may be helpful in making the diagnosis of fascioliasis.[41-44] During acute disease, linear tracts can be seen in the liver, while filling defects and adult flukes can be visualized in the biliary system during chronic disease.

Treatment

Triclabendazole is the drug of choice for treatment of infection with *Fasciola hepatica*.[29, 45-48] Although triclabendazole is not FDA approved or generally available in the United States, it can be obtained from the CDC under an investigational protocol. Praziquantel, which is excellent for treating infections with other flukes, is not effective against fasciola, nor are mebendazole, albendazole, or artesunate.[49-51] Nitazoxanide appears to be an inferior but alternate therapy with some demonstrated efficacy.[52, 53] Successfully treated patients will develop negative serologies 6-12 months after clearing their parasites.

Prevention and Control

Periodic draining of ponds can best control fasciola, reducing littoral plant growth to a minimum. Protecting freshwater supplies and regularly surveying herds and herders for the presence of the parasites can achieve further control of the spread of fascioliasis in domestic animals. In this regard, an ELISA test detected experimentally and naturally-infected calves with a high degree of sensitivity and specificity.[37] When infections are detected, appropriate treatment in both groups is warranted. Snail elimination with molluscicides has not been successful. Education of farm personnel regarding the mode of acquisition of the infection is essential to eliminating transmission due to human fecal contamination of freshwater aquatic habitats. Vaccines have been developed for animal use that have demonstrated some degree of efficacy in terms of reduction in egg production and worm burdens.[54] Despite significant advances in vaccine development, no human or animal vaccine is in current use.[55]

References

1. Mas-Coma, M. S.; Esteban, J. G.; Bargues, M. D., Epidemiology of human fascioliasis: a review and proposed new classification. *Bull World Health Organ* **1999,** *77* (4), 340-6.
2. Bosnak, V. K.; Karaoglan, I.; Sahin, H. H.; Namiduru, M.; Pehlivan, M.; Okan, V.; Mete, A. O., Evaluation of patients diagnosed with fascioliasis: A six-year experience at a university hospital in Turkey. *J Infect Dev Ctries* **2016,** *10* (4), 389-94.
3. Weisenberg, S. A.; Perlada, D. E., Domestically acquired fascioliasis in northern California. *Am J Trop Med Hyg* **2013,** *89* (3), 588-91.
4. Sivagnanam, S.; van der Poorten, D.; Douglas, M. W., Hepatic lesions and eosinophilia in an urban dweller. *Liver Int* **2014,** *34* (4), 643.
5. Charleston, W. A.; McKenna, P. B., Nematodes and liver fluke in New Zealand. *N Z Vet J* **2002,** *50* (3 Suppl), 41-7.
6. Lukambagire, A. H.; McHaile, D. N.; Nyindo, M., Diagnosis of human fascioliasis in Arusha region, northern Tanzania by microscopy and clinical manifestations in patients. *BMC Infect Dis* **2015,** *15* (1), 578.
7. Nyindo, M.; Lukambagire, A. H., Fascioliasis: An Ongoing Zoonotic Trematode Infection. *Biomed*

Res Int **2015,** *2015,* 786195.

8.   Keiser, J.; Utzinger, J., Food-borne trematodiases. *Clin Microbiol Rev* **2009,** *22* (3), 466-83.

9.   Mas-Coma, S., Epidemiology of fascioliasis in human endemic areas. *J Helminthol* **2005,** *79* (3), 207-16.

10.   Esteban, J.-G.; Gonzalez, C.; Curtale, F.; Muñoz-Antoli, C.; Valero, M. A.; Bargues, M. D.; el-Sayed, M.; el-Wakeel, A. A. W.; Abdel-Wahab, Y.; Montresor, A.; Engels, D.; Savioli, L.; Mas-Coma, S., Hyperendemic fascioliasis associated with schistosomiasis in villages in the Nile Delta of Egypt. *The American journal of tropical medicine and hygiene* **2003,** *69* (4), 429-37.

11.   Hillyer, G. V.; Soler de Galanes, M.; Rodriguez-Perez, J.; Bjorland, J.; Silva de Lagrava, M.; Ramirez Guzman, S.; Bryan, R. T., Use of the Falcon assay screening test--enzyme-linked immunosorbent assay (FAST-ELISA) and the enzyme-linked immunoelectrotransfer blot (EITB) to determine the prevalence of human fascioliasis in the Bolivian Altiplano. *The American journal of tropical medicine and hygiene* **1992,** *46* (5), 603-9.

12.   Menon, P.; Sinha, A. K.; Rao, K. L.; Khurana, S.; Lal, S.; Thapa, B. R., Biliary Fasciola gigantica infestation in a nonendemic area - An intraoperative surprise. *J Pediatr Surg* **2015,** *50* (11), 1983-6.

13.   Fang, W.; Chen, F.; Yang, Q., [Case report: Fasciola gigantica infection treated by triclabendazole]. *Zhongguo Ji Sheng Chong Xue Yu Ji Sheng Chong Bing Za Zhi* **2013,** *31* (2), Inside front page.

14.   Bestas, R.; Yalcin, K.; Cicek, M., Cholestasis caused by Fasciola gigantica. *Turkiye Parazitol Derg* **2014,** *38* (3), 201-4.

15.   Chen, J. X.; Chen, M. X.; Ai, L.; Xu, X. N.; Jiao, J. M.; Zhu, T. J.; Su, H. Y.; Zang, W.; Luo, J. J.; Guo, Y. H.; Lv, S.; Zhou, X. N., An Outbreak of Human Fascioliasis gigantica in Southwest China. *PLoS One* **2013,** *8* (8), e71520.

16.   de Brie, J., Le Bon Berger ou le Vray Regime et Gouvenement de Bergers et Bergeres: Compose par le Rustique Jehan de Brie le Bon Berger (1379). Isidor Liseux, Paris. **1879.**

17.   Redi, F., Osservazioni di Francesco Redi. *Intorno Agli Animali Viventi che si Trovano Negli Animali Viventi Piero Matini Florence* **1684.**

18.   Lima Wdos, S.; Soares, L. R.; Barcante, T. A.; Guimaraes, M. P.; Barcante, J. M., Occurrence of Fasciola hepatica (Linnaeus, 1758) infection in Brazilian cattle of Minas Gerais, Brazil. *Rev Bras Parasitol Vet* **2009,** *18* (2), 27-30.

19.   Cox, F. E., History of human parasitology. *Clin Microbiol Rev* **2002,** *15* (4), 595-612.

20.   Leuckart, F. R., Zur Entwicklungsgeschichte des Lerberegels. *Zool Anz* **1881,** *4,* 641-646.

21.   Thomas, A. P. W.; R., J., Report of experiments on the development of the liver fluke, Fasciola hepatica. *Soc Engi* **1881,** *17* 1-28.

22.   Lutz, A., Zur Lebensgeschichte des Distoma hepaticum. *Zentralbi Bakteriol Parasit* **1892,** *11,* 783-796.

23.   Mas-Coma, S.; Bargues, M. D.; Valero, M. A., Fascioliasis and other plant-borne trematode zoonoses. *Int J Parasitol* **2005,** *35* (11-12), 1255-78.

24.   Catchpole, B. N.; Snow, D., Human ectopic fascioliasis. *Lancet* **1952,** *2* 711-712.

25.   Arjona, R.; Riancho, J. A.; Aguado, J. M.; Salesa, R.; González-Macías, J., Fascioliasis in developed countries: a review of classic and aberrant forms of the disease. *Medicine* **1995,** *74* (1), 13-23.

26.   Modavi, S.; Isseroff, H., Fasciola hepatica: collagen deposition and other histopathology in the rat host's bile duct caused by the parasite and by proline infusion. *Experimental parasitology* **1984,** *58* (3), 239-44.

27.   Wijffels, G. L.; Panaccio, M.; Salvatore, L.; Wilson, L.; Walker, I. D.; Spithill, T. W., The secreted cathepsin L-like proteinases of the trematode, Fasciola hepatica, contain 3-hydroxyproline residues. *The Biochemical journal* **1994,** *299 (Pt 3),* 781-90.

28.   Demirci, M.; Korkmaz, M.; Sakru, N.; Kaya, S.; Kuman, A., Diagnostic importance of serological methods and eosinophilia in tissue parasites. *Journal of health, population, and nutrition* **2002,** *20* (4), 352-5.

29.   Saba, R.; Korkmaz, M.; Inan, D.; Mamikoğlu, L.; Turhan, O.; Günseren, F.; Cevikol, C.; Kabaalioğlu, A., Human fascioliasis. *Clinical microbiology and infection : the official publication*

of the European Society of Clinical Microbiology and Infectious Diseases **2004,** *10* (5), 385-7.

30. Khalil, G.; Haddad, C.; Otrock, Z. K.; Jaber, F.; Farra, A., Halzoun, an allergic pharyngitis syndrome in Lebanon: the trematode Dicrocoelium dendriticum as an additional cause. *Acta Trop* **2013,** *125* (1), 115-8.

31. Saleha, A. A., Liver fluke disease (fascioliasis): epidemiology, economic impact and public health significance. *The Southeast Asian journal of tropical medicine and public health* **1991,** *22 Suppl,* 361-4.

32. Arjona, R.; Riancho, J. A.; Aguado, J. M.; Salesa, R.; Gonzalez-Macias, J., Fascioliasis in developed countries: a review of classic and aberrant forms of the disease. *Medicine (Baltimore)* **1995,** *74* (1), 13-23.

33. Patel, N. U.; Bang, T. J.; Dodd, G. D., 3rd, CT findings of human Fasciola hepatica infection: case reports and review of the literature. *Clin Imaging* **2016,** *40* (2), 251-5.

34. Corredoira, J. C.; Perez, R.; Casariego, E.; Varela, J.; Lopez, M. J.; Torres, J., [Eosinophilic pleural effusion caused by Fasciola hepatica]. *Enferm Infecc Microbiol Clin* **1990,** *8* (4), 258-9.

35. Moretti, G.; Broustet, A.; Beylot, J.; Amouretti, M., [Pleural effusion revealing and a recapitulating Fasciola hepatica distomatosis]. *Bord Med* **1971,** *4* (4), 1181-2 passim.

36. O'Neill, J., On the presence of a filaria in "crawcraw." *Lancet* **1875,** *1*, 265-266.

37. Rokni, M. B.; Massoud, J.; O'Neill, S. M.; Parkinson, M.; Dalton, J. P., Diagnosis of human fasciolosis in the Gilan province of Northern Iran: application of cathepsin L-ELISA. *Diagnostic microbiology and infectious disease* **2002,** *44* (2), 175-9.

38. Gonzales Santana, B.; Dalton, J. P.; Vasquez Camargo, F.; Parkinson, M.; Ndao, M., The diagnosis of human fascioliasis by enzyme-linked immunosorbent assay (ELISA) using recombinant cathepsin L protease. *PLoS Negl Trop Dis* **2013,** *7* (9), e2414.

39. Hassan, M. M.; Saad, M.; Hegab, M. H.; Metwally, S., Evaluation of circulating Fasciola antigens in specific diagnosis of fascioliasis. *J Egypt Soc Parasitol* **2001,** *31* (1), 271-9.

40. Almazan, C.; Avila, G.; Quiroz, H.; Ibarra, F.; Ochoa, P., Effect of parasite burden on the detection of Fasciola hepatica antigens in sera and feces of experimentally infected sheep. *Vet Parasitol* **2001,** *97* (2), 101-12.

41. Zali, M. R.; Ghaziani, T.; Shahraz, S.; Hekmatdoost, A.; Radmehr, A., Liver, spleen, pancreas and kidney involvement by human fascioliasis: imaging findings. *BMC gastroenterology* **2004,** *4*, 15.

42. Cevikol, C.; Karaali, K.; Senol, U.; Kabaalioglu, A.; Apaydin, A.; Saba, R.; Luleci, E., Human fascioliasis: MR imaging findings of hepatic lesions. *Eur Radiol* **2003,** *13* (1), 141-8.

43. Van Beers, B.; Pringot, J.; Geubel, A.; Trigaux, J. P.; Bigaignon, G.; Dooms, G., Hepatobiliary fascioliasis: noninvasive imaging findings. *Radiology* **1990,** *174* (3 Pt 1), 809-10.

44. Dias, L. M.; Silva, R.; Viana, H. L.; Palhinhas, M.; Viana, R. L., Biliary fascioliasis: diagnosis, treatment and follow-up by ERCP. *Gastrointest Endosc* **1996,** *43* (6), 616-20.

45. el-Karaksy, H.; Hassanein, B.; Okasha, S.; Behairy, B.; Gadallah, I., Human fascioliasis in Egyptian children: successful treatment with triclabendazole. *Journal of tropical pediatrics* **1999,** *45* (3), 135-8.

46. Marcos, L. A.; Terashima, A.; Gotuzzo, E., Update on hepatobiliary flukes: fascioliasis, opisthorchiasis and clonorchiasis. *Curr Opin Infect Dis* **2008,** *21* (5), 523-30.

47. Marcos, L. A.; Tagle, M.; Terashima, A.; Bussalleu, A.; Ramirez, C.; Carrasco, C.; Valdez, L.; Huerta-Mercado, J.; Freedman, D. O.; Vinetz, J. M.; Gotuzzo, E., Natural history, clinicoradiologic correlates, and response to triclabendazole in acute massive fascioliasis. *Am J Trop Med Hyg* **2008,** *78* (2), 222-7.

48. Villegas, F.; Angles, R.; Barrientos, R.; Barrios, G.; Valero, M. A.; Hamed, K.; Grueninger, H.; Ault, S. K.; Montresor, A.; Engels, D.; Mas-Coma, S.; Gabrielli, A. F., Administration of triclabendazole is safe and effective in controlling fascioliasis in an endemic community of the Bolivian Altiplano. *PLoS Negl Trop Dis* **2012,** *6* (8), e1720.

49. Fand, Z.; Kamal, M.; Mansour, N.; R., Praziquantel and Fasciola hepatica infection. *Trans Trop Med Hyg 813* **1989,** *83*.

50. Hien, T. T.; Truong, N. T.; Minh, N. H.; Dat, H. D.; Dung, N. T.; Hue, N. T.; Dung, T. K.; Tuan, P. Q.; Campbell, J. I.; Farrar, J. J.; Day, J. N., A randomized controlled pilot study of artesunate

versus triclabendazole for human fascioliasis in central Vietnam. *Am J Trop Med Hyg* **2008**, *78* (3), 388-92.

51.   Cabada, M. M.; White, A. C., Jr., New developments in epidemiology, diagnosis, and treatment of fascioliasis. *Curr Opin Infect Dis* **2012**, *25* (5), 518-22.

52.   Rossignol, J. F.; Abaza, H.; Friedman, H., Successful treatment of human fascioliasis with nitazoxanide. *Trans R Soc Trop Med Hyg* **1998**, *92* (1), 103-4.

53.   Favennec, L.; Jave Ortiz, J.; Gargala, G.; Lopez Chegne, N.; Ayoub, A.; Rossignol, J. F., Double-blind, randomized, placebo-controlled study of nitazoxanide in the treatment of fascioliasis in adults and children from northern Peru. *Aliment Pharmacol Ther* **2003**, *17* (2), 265-70.

54.   Espino, A. M.; Hillyer, G. V., A novel Fasciola hepatica saposinlike recombinant protein with immunoprophylactic potential. *The Journal of parasitology* **2004**, *90* (4), 876-9.

55.   Molina-Hernandez, V.; Mulcahy, G.; Perez, J.; Martinez-Moreno, A.; Donnelly, S.; O'Neill, S. M.; Dalton, J. P.; Cwiklinski, K., Fasciola hepatica vaccine: we may not be there yet but we're on the right road. *Vet Parasitol* **2015**, *208* (1-2), 101-11.

36. *Paragonimus westermani*
(Kerbert 1878)

Paragonimus kellicotti
(Ward 1908)

Introduction

There are more than 40 species in the genus *Paragonimus,* but only nine are responsible for the majority of cases in humans; *P. westermani, P. africanus, P. heterotremus, P. kellicotti, P. mexicanus, P. siamensis, P. skrjabini, P. miyazakii, and P. uterobilateralis.*[1-10] An estimated 20 million people are infected with *Paragonimus* spp. worldwide.[11] The most commonly reported trematode in this genus to cause human disease is *Paragonimus westermani.* While most members of this genus are relatively restricted in distribution, *Paragonimus westermani* is widely found throughout the world.[11] *P. westermani* will be presented as the model organism for

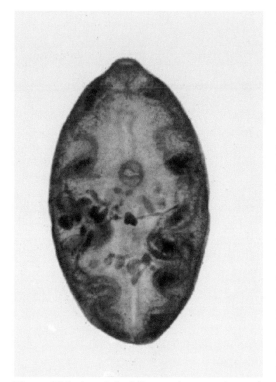

Figure 36.1. An adult of *Paragonimus westermani.* 10mm x 5 mm.

food-borne lung flukes affecting humans, but *P. kellicotti*, which is indigenous to the United States, and certain other paragonimus species will be mentioned.[12-14]

Although hermaphroditic, most *Paragonimus* spp. do not self-fertilize. Instead they live typically as 2 or more worms in cysts or cavities, usually in lung tissue.[13] Paragonimiasis occurs throughout Japan, China, Korea, Vietnam, Thailand, Cambodia, India, Micronesia, Indonesia, Papua New Guinea, and the Philippines.[15-17] *P. westermani* infects a wide range of reservoir hosts, including fox, civet, tiger, leopard, panther, mongoose, wolf, pig, dog, and cat. It employs numerous crustaceans as intermediate hosts and that is what accounts for its global distribution.[11]

The genus *Paragonimus* is diverse.[5, 18] Several other species routinely infect humans: *P. skrjabini* and *P. miyazakii* in Japan, *P. africanus* in Cameroon, *P. uterobilateralis* in Liberia and Nigeria, and *P. mexicanus* and *P. ecuadoriensis* in Latin America.[5] *P. kellicoti*, a lung fluke of mink and opossums in the United States, has also caused infection in humans.[12]

Historical Information

In 1878, Coenraad Kerbert described the adult worm that he isolated at autopsy from a Bengal tiger.[19] In 1916, Koan Nakagawa implicated the freshwater crab as the intermediate host in the transmission of *P. westermani.*[20] In 1915, Sadamu Yokagawa deciphered the correct route of migration of the immature adult fluke in the mammalian host.[21] In 1880, one year after the first human case was described in an individual living in Taiwan, Erwin Von Baelz and Patrick Manson reported on most of the clinical features of the disease, and also identified eggs of *P. westermani* in the sputum of patients with hemoptysis. [22, 23] In 1899, Max Braun established the genus *Paragonimus,* with the name derived from the Greek words "para" (on the side of)

Paragonimus westermani

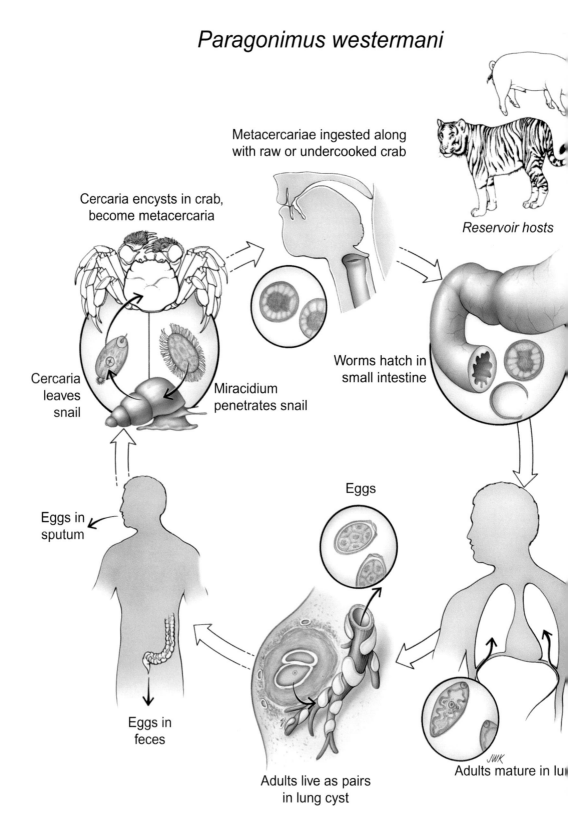

Metacercariae ingested along with raw or undercooked crab

Cercaria encysts in crab, become metacercaria

Reservoir hosts

Worms hatch in small intestine

Cercaria leaves snail

Miracidium penetrates snail

Eggs in sputum

Eggs

Eggs in feces

Adults live as pairs in lung cyst

Adults mature in lu

JWK

and gonimos" (genitalia).[24]

Life Cycle

The adult of *P. westermani* is large, measuring 10-12 mm in length and 5-7 mm in width (Fig. 36.1). It induces a fibrotic capsule of tissue at the periphery of the lung and lives there, usually as 2 or more worms. More than 50 species of crustaceans are able to support the next stage of the life cycle with freshwater crabs (e.g., *Eriocheir* spp., *Potamon* spp., *Potamiscus* spp.) as the most common intermediate hosts throughout most of the Far East.[13] In many Asian countries, crabs are eaten raw or undercooked. In the U.S., *P. kelicotti* infection results from eating uncooked crayfish.[25]

Infection begins by ingesting the metacercariae (Fig. 36.2), that excyst in the small intestine.[13] Metacercariae penetrate into the abdominal cavity, and within several days, develop to immature flukes. The worms migrate to the lungs by penetrating the diaphragm, and mature to reproductive adults within 8-12 weeks (Fig. 36.3). Worms also locate to aberrant sites, including brain, liver, intestines, muscle, skin, and testes. In these sites, passage of eggs to the external environment is not possible.

The pair of adults usually cross-fertilize

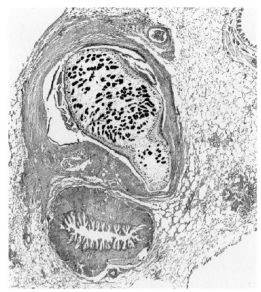

Figure 36.3. Histological section of an adult *P. westermani* in lung.

each other. Both diploid and triploid forms of the adult *P. westermani* exist.[18] The triploid form produces eggs via parthenogenesis. Egg production begins about 30 days after ingestion of the metacercariae. Eggs (Fig. 36.4) pass fertilized, but unembryonated, into the surrounding tissue. Eventually, they reach the bronchioles and are included into the sputum that also contains blood and debris from the necrotic lesions created by the adults. Because some of the sputum is swallowed, eggs can be recovered from feces as well as sputum. The eggs must reach freshwater to

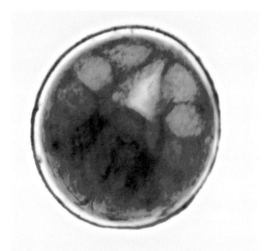

Figure 36.2. Metacercaria of *P. westermani*. 34 μm.

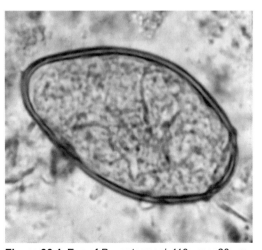

Figure 36.4. Egg of *P. westermani*. 110 μm x 60 μm.

embryonate. The miracidium develops over a 3-week period, after which it hatches and seeks out its intermediate snail host (e.g., *Melania* spp., *Semisulcospira* spp., and *Thiara* spp.). In contrast to other trematodes such as *Schistosoma* spp., *Paragonimus* spp. are able to mature in a large variety of snail species.[13] *Paragonimus* spp. develop through the sporocyst and redia stages into cercariae, which then exit from the snail and encyst on and within crustacean intermediate hosts. In the case of the crab, the metacercariae infect all organs.

Cellular and Molecular Pathogenesis

Immature worms of *P. westermani* do not cause clinical disease, either on their way from the small intestine to the abdominal cavity, or during the last leg of their journey to the lung tissue, except in the case of heavy infection.[26-29] In contrast, mature adult worms in the lung form cysts that eventually communicate with the bronchioles.[24] Triploid forms of the parasite are considered more pathogenic than diploid forms. The diploid forms are smaller and will form cysts only if sexual partners are found.[24] The inflammatory responses to paragonimus cysts are characterized by a variety of cells, but eosinophils usually predominate. Charcot-Leyden crystals can frequently be found in the sputum of infected individuals. Specific IgG and IgE antibodies are produced throughout the infection, but appear to have no protective function.[30] Several stages of *P. westermani* secrete cysteine proteases that cleave IgG molecules, and the worm may employ this strategy to avoid immune damage by the host.[31] Infections last somewhat longer than a year, after which adult worms die and become calcified.

Larval stages of several zoonotic species of paragonimus such as *P. skrjabini* and *P. miyazakii* can cause extensive damage to the tissues as they migrate throughout the viscera.[24]

Clinical Disease

The clinical manifestations of paragonimiasis include acute early infection and late or chronic disease. Early infection occurs between the time of ingestion of infective metacercariae, and lasts up until flukes mature into egg producing adults. During this stage of infection some patients may remain asymptomatic, while others present with diarrhea, fever, chest pain, fatigue, urticaria, epigastric pain, and eosinophilia.[26-29] Patients may go on to develop cough with blood-tinged sputum, dyspnea, increasing leukocytosis and eosinophilia, and transient pulmonary infiltrates. In some situations patients may present with cutaneous manifestations, noting painless subcutaneous swellings that are migratory.[32] These subcutaneous nodules contain juvenile flukes.[24]

Mature lung flukes trigger late stage infection. Cough and recurrent hemoptysis are the most common clinical features.[33, 34] Patients may also present with chest pain, dyspnea, fever, or chills.[13] Depending on the severity of the infection and the frequency of bacterial superinfections, there may be pneumothorax and pleural effusion, with consequent pleural adhesions.

An often fatal clinical outcome results from extrapulmonary paragonimiasis. Immature flukes may migrate to a number of tissues, including the brain. Cerebral paragonimiasis is thought to be rare, estimated to occur in less than 1 percent of symptomatic individuals infected with *P. westermani,* but is associated with a significantly higher mortality rate than pulmonary disease.[35] Cerebral paragonimiasis may be more common with other *Paragonimiasis* spp. such as *P. kellicotti.*[36, 37]

Diagnosis

Diagnostic modality is based on the stage of the disease. Late-stage disease is diagnosed by microscopic identification of eggs in the sputum, bronchoalveolar lavage fluid, and more rarely in stool.[38, 39] A number of cases of acid-fast bacilli-negative pulmonary infections are due to paragonimiasis. One distinguishing feature is the presence of Charcot-Leyden crystals on histopathology.[40] Eggs can be visualized microscopically using using wet preps. For many years, acid-fast staining of sputum specimens destroyed paragonimus eggs. This issue has been overcome using modern Ziehl-Neelsen staining and use of a 10x rather than the standard 100x objective employed in the diagnosis of mycobacterial infections.[38, 39]

If sputum or other body fluids, such as CSF or pleural fluid, is negative for eggs on repeated sampling, indirect evidence of infection can be obtained by use of serological tests, such as ELISA and Western blot.[41-43] These tests are particularly helpful in early stage disease as well as extrapulmonary disease. Immunoblot testing is available from the CDC and ELISA tests are available from commercial laboratories.[13, 27] Serology is also used in the diagnosis of *P. kellicotti* infection in the US.[25] Antigen detection tests have been developed, but are not routinely used in clinical practice.[44] Molecular tests using nucleic acid amplification testing (NAAT) are being developed that allow for species identification.[45] There is also a simple and rapid intradermal test, performed by injecting diluted paragonimus antigen into the skin.[24] Over 2 million people have been skin tested in China, with an overall positivity rate of 20%.[24] Both the serologic and intradermal assays indicate either current or past exposure to the infection.

Imaging tests such as computed tomography (CT) and fluorodeoxyglucose-positron emission tomography (FDG-PET) can help with the diagnosis but are not definitive.[46-48] In many cases migratory tracks through and between the pleura and lung parenchyma as a result of helminth invasion can be visual-ized.[49] Clinical diagnosis depends on suspicion of paragonimiasis in any patient from an endemic area who has the characteristic pulmonary disease. Pulmonary paragonimiasis must be distinguished from chronic bronchiectasis, lung abscess due to other causes, and tuberculosis.[16, 50] Cerebral paragonimiasis must be distinguished from brain tumors, and lesions caused by other helminths (i.e., juvenile tapeworms and *Fasciola hepatica*). The subcutaneous nodules of *P. skrjabini* must be differentiated from other forms of cutaneous larva migrans and gnathostomiasis.[24]

Treatment

The drug of choice against *Paragonimus* spp. is praziquantel, while triclabendazole is an alternative drug with similar efficacy.[24, 50-54] Another regimen that has been used is multiple rounds of praziquantel alternating with albendazole.[55] The complications of pleural effusions and subsequent fibrosis may sometimes require surgical management, including decortication.[13]

Prevention and Control

Because of its numerous reservoir hosts and its worldwide distribution, many consider control of this parasite in animals to be impractical in most parts of the world.[13] Due to cultural eating habits favoring the acquisition of this parasite, control of paragonimus infection is difficult, and would require a comprehensive approach.[56] For example, "drunken hairy crab" is traditionally eaten live, and in the modern city of Shanghai, its considered *haute cuisine*. Treatment of infected individuals, sanitation changes, and behavioral changes in handling and cooking intermediate crustacean hosts all have a role to play in the control of paragonimiasis. In certain endemic regions of the world, mass chemotherapy has been attempted to reduce prevalence rates.[57-60] Boiling the invertebrate host for several minutes until the meat has congealed and turned opaque can kill the metacercariae. Marinat- ing and salting of crabs or other crustaceans does not reliably kill these infective stages.[24]

References

1.   Iwagami, M.; Rajapakse, R. P.; Paranagama, W.; Okada, T.; Kano, S.; Agatsuma, T., Ancient divergence of Paragonimus westermani in Sri Lanka. *Parasitol Res* **2008,** *102* (5), 845-52.
2.   Iwagami, M.; Rajapakse, R. P.; Yatawara, L.; Kano, S.; Agatsuma, T., The first intermediate host of Paragonimus westermani in Sri Lanka. *Acta Trop* **2009,** *109* (1), 27-9.
3.   Iwagami, M.; Rajapakse, R. P.; Paranagama, W.; Agatsuma, T., Identities of two Paragonimus species from Sri Lanka inferred from molecular sequences. *J Helminthol* **2003,** *77* (3), 239-45.
4.   Iwagami, M.; Ho, L. Y.; Su, K.; Lai, P. F.; Fukushima, M.; Nakano, M.; Blair, D.; Kawashima, K.; Agatsuma, T., Molecular phylogeographic studies on Paragonimus westermani in Asia. *J Helminthol* **2000,** *74* (4), 315-22.
5.   Iwagami, M.; Monroy, C.; Rosas, M. A.; Pinto, M. R.; Guevara, A. G.; Vieira, J. C.; Agatsuma, Y.; Agatsuma, T., A molecular phylogeographic study based on DNA sequences from individual metacercariae of Paragonimus mexicanus from Guatemala and Ecuador. *Journal of helminthology* **2003,** *77* (1), 33-8.
6.   Iwagami, M.; Monroy, C.; Rosas, M. A.; Pinto, M. R.; Guevara, A. G.; Vieira, J. C.; Agatsuma, Y.; Agatsuma, T., A molecular phylogeographic study based on DNA sequences from individual metacercariae of Paragonimus mexicanus from Guatemala and Ecuador. *J Helminthol* **2003,** *77* (1), 33-8.
7.   Agatsuma, T.; Iwagami, M.; Sato, Y.; Iwashita, J.; Hong, S. J.; Kang, S. Y.; Ho, L. Y.; Su, K. E.; Kawashima, K.; Abe, T., The origin of the triploid in Paragonimus westermani on the basis of variable regions in the mitochondrial DNA. *J Helminthol* **2003,** *77* (4), 279-85.
8.   Blair, D.; Chang, Z.; Chen, M.; Cui, A.; Wu, B.; Agatsuma, T.; Iwagami, M.; Corlis, D.; Fu, C.; Zhan, X., Paragonimus skrjabini Chen, 1959 (Digenea: Paragonimidae) and related species in eastern Asia: a combined molecular and morphological approach to identification and taxonomy. *Syst Parasitol* **2005,** *60* (1), 1-21.
9.   Doanh, P. N.; Horii, Y.; Nawa, Y., Paragonimus and paragonimiasis in Vietnam: an update. *Korean J Parasitol* **2013,** *51* (6), 621-7.
10.   Chai, J. Y., Paragonimiasis. *Handb Clin Neurol* **2013,** *114*, 283-96.
11.   Furst, T.; Keiser, J.; Utzinger, J., Global burden of human food-borne trematodiasis: a systematic review and meta-analysis. *Lancet Infect Dis* **2012,** *12* (3), 210-21.
12.   Mariano, E. G.; Borja, S. R.; Vruno, M. J., A human infection with Paragonimus kellicotti (lung fluke) in the United States. *American journal of clinical pathology* **1986,** *86* (5), 685-7.
13.   Procop, G. W., North American paragonimiasis (Caused by Paragonimus kellicotti) in the context of global paragonimiasis. *Clin Microbiol Rev* **2009,** *22* (3), 415-46.
14.   Diaz, J. H., Paragonimiasis acquired in the United States: native and nonnative species. *Clin Microbiol Rev* **2013,** *26* (3), 493-504.
15.   Kim, E.-A.; Juhng, S.-K.; Kim, H. W.; Kim, G. D.; Lee, Y. W.; Cho, H. J.; Won, J. J., Imaging findings of hepatic paragonimiasis : a case report. *Journal of Korean medical science* **2004,** *19* (5), 759-62.
16.   Singh, T. N.; Singh, H. R.; Devi, K. S.; Singh, N. B.; Singh, Y. I., Pulmonary paragonimiasis. *The Indian journal of chest diseases & allied sciences* **2004,** *46* (3), 225-7.
17.   Owen, I. L., Parasitic zoonoses in Papua New Guinea. *Journal of helminthology* **2005,** *79* (1), 1-14.
18.   Blair, D., Genomes of Paragonimus westermani and related species: current state of knowledge. *International journal for parasitology* **2000,** *30* (4), 421-6.
19.   Kerbert, C., Zur Trematodenkenntnis. *Zool Anz* **1878,** *1*, 271-273.
20.   Nakagawa, K.; J., The mode of infection in pulmonary distomiasis: certain fresh water crabs as intermediate hosts of Paragonimus westermani. *Dis* **1916,** *18*, 131-142.
21.   Yokogawa, S., On the route of migration of Paragonimus westermani in the definitive host. *aiwan Igakkai Zasshi* **1915,** *152*, 685-700.

22. Von Baelz, E. O. E., Uber Parasitare Haemoptoe (gregarinosis pulmonum). Zentralbl Med Wissenschr. **1880,** *18* 721-722.
23. Manson, P., Distoma ringeri: Medical Report for the Half Year Ended 30 September. 1880; Vol. 2, p 10-12.
24. Blair, D.; Xu, Z. B.; Agatsuma, T., Paragonimiasis and the genus Paragonimus. *Advances in parasitology* **1999,** *42,* 113-222.
25. Fischer, P. U.; Weil, G. J., North American paragonimiasis: epidemiology and diagnostic strategies. *Expert Rev Anti Infect Ther* **2015,** *13* (6), 779-86.
26. Zhong, H. L.; He, L. Y.; Xu, Z. B.; Cao, W. J., Recent progress in studies of paragonimus and paragonimiasis control in China. *Chin Med J (Engl)* **1981,** *94* (8), 483-94.
27. Kagawa, F. T., Pulmonary paragonimiasis. *Semin Respir Infect* **1997,** *12* (2), 149-58.
28. DeFrain, M.; Hooker, R., North American paragonimiasis: case report of a severe clinical infection. *Chest* **2002,** *121* (4), 1368-72.
29. Uchiyama, F.; Morimoto, Y.; Nawa, Y., Re-emergence of paragonimiasis in Kyushu, Japan. *Southeast Asian J Trop Med Public Health* **1999,** *30* (4), 686-91.
30. Kong, Y.; Ito, A.; Yang, H. J.; Chung, Y. B.; Kasuya, S.; Kobayashi, M.; Liu, Y. H.; Cho, S. Y., Immunoglobulin G (IgG) subclass and IgE responses in human paragonimiases caused by three different species. *Clinical and diagnostic laboratory immunology* **1998,** *5* (4), 474-8.
31. Chung, Y. B.; Yang, H. J.; Kang, S. Y.; Kong, Y.; Cho, S. Y., Activities of different cysteine proteases of Paragonimus westermani in cleaving human IgG. *The Korean journal of parasitology* **1997,** *35* (2), 139-42.
32. Hatano, Y.; Katagiri, K.; Ise, T.; Yamaguchi, T.; Itami, S.; Nawa, Y.; Takayasu, S., Expression of Th1 and Th2 cytokine mRNAs in freshly isolated peripheral blood mononuclear cells of a patient with cutaneous paragonimiasis. *J Dermatol Sci* **1999,** *19* (2), 144-7.
33. Singh, T. S.; Mutum, S. S.; Razaque, M. A., Pulmonary paragonimiasis: clinical features, diagnosis and treatment of 39 cases in Manipur. *Trans R Soc Trop Med Hyg* **1986,** *80* (6), 967-71.
34. Im, J. G.; Whang, H. Y.; Kim, W. S.; Han, M. C.; Shim, Y. S.; Cho, S. Y., Pleuropulmonary paragonimiasis: radiologic findings in 71 patients. *AJR Am J Roentgenol* **1992,** *159* (1), 39-43.
35. Singh, T. S.; Khamo, V.; Sugiyama, H., Cerebral paragonimiasis mimicking tuberculoma: First case report in India. *Trop Parasitol* **2011,** *1* (1), 39-41.
36. Centers for Disease, C.; Prevention, Human paragonimiasis after eating raw or undercooked crayfish --- Missouri, July 2006-September 2010. *MMWR Morb Mortal Wkly Rep* **2010,** *59* (48), 1573-6.
37. Lane, M. A.; Barsanti, M. C.; Santos, C. A.; Yeung, M.; Lubner, S. J.; Weil, G. J., Human paragonimiasis in North America following ingestion of raw crayfish. *Clin Infect Dis* **2009,** *49* (6), e55-61.
38. Barennes, H.; Slesak, G.; Buisson, Y.; Odermatt, P., Paragonimiasis as an important alternative misdiagnosed disease for suspected acid-fast bacilli sputum smear-negative tuberculosis. *Am J Trop Med Hyg* **2014,** *90* (2), 384-5.
39. Slesak, G.; Inthalad, S.; Basy, P.; Keomanivong, D.; Phoutsavath, O.; Khampoui, S.; Grosrenaud, A.; Amstutz, V.; Barennes, H.; Buisson, Y.; Odermatt, P., Ziehl-Neelsen staining technique can diagnose paragonimiasis. *PLoS Negl Trop Dis* **2011,** *5* (5), e1048.
40. Luo, J.; Wang, M. Y.; Liu, D.; Zhu, H.; Yang, S.; Liang, B. M.; Liang, Z. A., Pulmonary Paragonimiasis Mimicking Tuberculous Pleuritis: A Case Report. *Medicine (Baltimore)* **2016,** *95* (15), e3436.
41. Ikeda, T., Cystatin capture enzyme-linked immunosorbent assay for immunodiagnosis of human paragonimiasis and fascioliasis. *The American journal of tropical medicine and hygiene* **1998,** *59* (2), 286-90.
42. Slemenda, S. B.; Maddison, S. E.; Jong, E. C.; Moore, D. D., Diagnosis of paragonimiasis by immunoblot. *The American journal of tropical medicine and hygiene* **1988,** *39* (5), 469-71.
43. Dekumyoy, P.; Waikagul, J.; Eom, K. S., Human lung fluke Paragonimus heterotremus: differential diagnosis between Paragonimus heterotremus and Paragonimus westermani infections by EITB. *Tropical medicine & international health : TM & IH* **1998,** *3* (1), 52-6.

44. Zhang, Z.; Zhang, Y.; Liu, L.; Dong, C.; Zhang, Y.; Wu, Z.; Piessens, W. F., Antigen detection assay to monitor the efficacy of praziquantel for treatment of Paragonimus westermani infections. *Trans R Soc Trop Med Hyg* **1996,** *90* (1), 43.

45. Intapan, P. M.; Kosuwan, T.; Wongkham, C.; Maleewong, W., Genomic characterization of lung flukes, Paragonimus heterotremus, P. siamensis, P. harinasutai, P. westermani and P. bangkokensis by RAPD markers. *Vet Parasitol* **2004,** *124* (1-2), 55-64.

46. Lee, I. J.; Seo, J.; Kim, D. G., Organizing pneumonia by paragonimiasis and coexistent aspergilloma manifested as a pulmonary irregular nodule. *Case Rep Radiol* **2011,** *2011*, 692405.

47. Kim, K. U.; Lee, K.; Park, H. K.; Jeong, Y. J.; Yu, H. S.; Lee, M. K., A pulmonary paragonimiasis case mimicking metastatic pulmonary tumor. *Korean J Parasitol* **2011,** *49* (1), 69-72.

48. Song, J. U.; Um, S. W.; Koh, W. J.; Suh, G. Y.; Chung, M. P.; Kim, H.; Kwon, O. J.; Jeon, K., Pulmonary paragonimiasis mimicking lung cancer in a tertiary referral centre in Korea. *Int J Tuberc Lung Dis* **2011,** *15* (5), 674-9.

49. Akaba, T.; Takeyama, K.; Toriyama, M.; Kubo, A.; Mizobuchi, R.; Yamada, T.; Tagaya, E.; Kondo, M.; Sakai, S.; Tamaoki, J., Pulmonary Paragonimiasis: The Detection of a Worm Migration Track as a Diagnostic Clue for Uncertain Eosinophilic Pleural Effusion. *Intern Med* **2016,** *55* (5), 503-6.

50. Johnson, R. J.; Johnson, J. R., Paragonimiasis in Indochinese refugees. Roentgenographic findings with clinical correlations. *The American review of respiratory disease* **1983,** *128* (3), 534-8.

51. Johnson, R. J.; Jong, E. C.; Dunning, S. B.; Carberry, W. L.; Minshew, B. H., Paragonimiasis: diagnosis and the use of praziquantel in treatment. *Reviews of infectious diseases* **1985,** *7* (2), 200-6.

52. Udonsi, J. K., Clinical field trials of praziquantel in pulmonary paragonimiasis due to Paragonimus uterobilateralis in endemic populations of the Igwun Basin, Nigeria. *Trop Med Parasitol* **1989,** *40* (1), 65-8.

53. Ripert, C.; Couprie, B.; Moyou, R.; Gaillard, F.; Appriou, M.; Tribouley-Duret, J., Therapeutic effect of triclabendazole in patients with paragonimiasis in Cameroon: a pilot study. *Transactions of the Royal Society of Tropical Medicine and Hygiene* **1992,** *86* (4), 417.

54. Keiser, J.; Utzinger, J., Chemotherapy for major food-borne trematodes: a review. *Expert opinion on pharmacotherapy* **2004,** *5* (8), 1711-26.

55. Hu, Y.; Qian, J.; Yang, D.; Zheng, X., Pleuropulmonary paragonimiasis with migrated lesions cured by multiple therapies. *Indian J Pathol Microbiol* **2016,** *59* (1), 56-8.

56. Sharma, O. P., The man who loved drunken crabs. A case of pulmonary paragonimiasis. *Chest* **1989,** *95* (3), 670-2.

57. Kim, J. S.; Bang, F. B., [A Follow-Up Study To Evaluate The Efficacy Of Mass Chemotherapy For Control Of Paragonimiasis]. *Kisaengchunghak Chapchi* **1974,** *12* (1), 8-13.

58. Kim, J. S., Mass Chemotherapy In The Control Of Paragonimiasis. *Kisaengchunghak Chapchi* **1969,** *7* (1), 6-14.

59. Xu, Z. B., Studies on clinical manifestations, diagnosis and control of paragonimiasis in China. *Southeast Asian J Trop Med Public Health* **1991,** *22 Suppl,* 345-8.

60. Choi, D. W., Paragonimus and paragonimiasis in Korea. *Kisaengchunghak Chapchi* **1990,** *28 Suppl,* 79-102.

37. Trematodes of Minor Medical Importance

Besides the trematode infections already identified as major causes of human disease throughout the world, other trematode species continue to have a negative impact on the human condition, but not quite to the extent of schistosomiasis, for example. A few of these "rare" infections are actually not so rare in some geographic regions, and deserve more than a mention, since cases of exotic infections are becoming more common in western clinics due to increased immigration from those regions. Many of them are zoonotic and classify as emerging infections in some locales.[1] They include at least 59 different species of intestinal flukes found in Southeast Asia.[2]

Fasciolopsis buski
(Lankaster 1857)

The three trematodes composing the family Fasciolidae are; *Fasciola hepatica, Fasciola gigantica,* and *Fasciolopsis buski.*[3] *Fasciola hepatica* is considered a trematode of major human importance. (see Chapter 35) *Fasciola gigantica* is very similar in biology and geography to *F. hepatica* and will not be discussed further in this section. *Fasciolopsis buski*, the giant intestinal fluke, is a large trematode (Fig. 37.1), similar in morphology to *F. hepatica. F. buski* is the most common intestinal trematode infection in humans, and lives attached to the columnar epithelium of the small intestine. Infection occurs in China, Taiwan, Vietnam, Thailand, Bangladesh, and India (including the Bihar State).[4-7] Reservoir hosts include dogs and rabbits.

Life Cycle

The infectious stage for mammals is the metacercaria, which is found on the husks of the seeds of littoral freshwater plants (e.g., lotus, water chestnut, water caltrop and other commercial crops in which human feces is used as fertilizer). Once eaten, the metacercaria excysts in the small intestine and attaches to the luminal surface. The adult matures within 2-4 months, and measures 20-30 mm by 10 mm. In contrast to the longer life spans of other trematodes, *Fasciolopsis buski* only lives for about one year. After self-fertilization, egg-laying begins. The large, ovoid, unembryonated eggs (Fig. 37.2) are passed out with the fecal mass. If they reach warm (i.e., 25°–30°C) freshwater, they immediately undergo embryogenesis, and hatch within 5-8 weeks. The miracidium that emerges penetrates a snail (e.g., *Segmentina* spp. and *Heppentis* spp.), and develops sequentially first into sporocysts, then rediae, and finally into cercariae. After leaving the

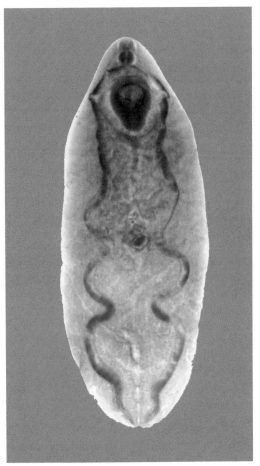

Figure 37.1. An adult of *Fasciolopsis buski*. 25 mm x 10mm.

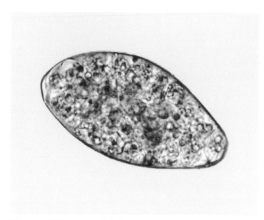

Figure 37.2. Egg of *F. buski*. 140 μm x 80 μm.

snail, the cercariae swim about and come to rest on littoral vegetation. The metaceracaria develops and then encysts there, awaiting ingestion by an unsuspecting host.

Clinical Disease

The worm feeds on columnar epithelial cells, injuring the tissue. Light infection does not cause clinical disease, although intermittent diarrhea may result. Heavy infection (i.e., hundreds of worms) produces continuous diarrhea, nausea, vomiting, fever, intestinal hemorrhage, obstruction of the ampula of Vater, blockage of the common bile duct, and in extreme cases, blockage of the small intestine. Abdominal pain is a common complaint, simulating the signs and symptoms of peptic ulcer. Allergic-type reactions with swelling of the legs and face have been reported. Hypoproteinemia, vomiting, anemia, and weight loss have been described in heavily-infected children.[8] An elevated level of circulating eosinophils is a common feature of even light infection with *F. buski*.

Diagnosis

Definitive diagnosis is by microscopic identification of the egg or flukes in stool or vomit.[9, 10]

Treatment

The drug of choice is praziquantel.[11, 12]

Prevention and control

Proper disposal of human feces is the primary method of control. For travellers to endemic areas one should make sure that all aquatic plants are well-cooked prior to ingestion. Reservoir hosts apparently play a role in the maintenance of this parasite in endemic regions, and consequently it is recommended that raw aquatic plants are not fed to pigs.[13] The habit of shucking water chestnuts by placing the seed pod in one's mouth and biting through the tough, outer husk, exposes one to the infection. This activity is still common in some areas, but public health education programs have helped reduce infection.[6]

Echinostoma spp.

The genus *Echinostoma* has at least 24 species with 15 capable of infecting humans.[1, 14] These trematodes are found throughout Southeast Asia with endemic foci in Korea, China, India, Indonesia, Thailand, the Philippines, and Malaysia.[14-16] Their life cycles are similar to that of fasciola, except that the metacercariae encyst in various species of snails, tadpoles, or freshwater fish.[17] Adults live in the small intestine, and the symptoms they induce depend on the degree of infection. Diarrhea, nausea, vomiting, and abdominal pain are commonly experienced, usually accompanied by fever.

Heterophyes heterophyes
(Siebold 1852)

Metagonimus yokogawai
(Katsurada 1912)

Heterophyes heterophyes (Fig. 37.3) and *Metagonimus yokogawai* (Fig. 37.4) are small flukes that live primarily in the small intestine. They cause little damage there. *H. heterophyes* is found throughout Asia, the Middle East, and Africa. *M. yokogawai* is also common in Asia, but foci of infections have been reported in Spain and Russia. A few human infections with *H. nocens*, a related species, have been reported from Korea.[18]

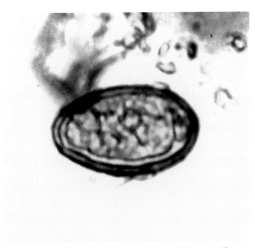

Figure 37.4. Egg of *H. heterophyes*. 25 μm x 13 μm.

Life Cycles

Infection begins with the ingestion of encysted metacercariae that live just under the skin of certain freshwater fishes (e.g., grass carp).[19] The metacercariae excyst in the small intestine and develop into adult worms.

Although a rare event, instead of remaining in the small intestine, adult worms can migrate to other organs, such as the heart or brain, where they cause focal granulomas, with variable clinical consequences. Both species of trematodes self-fertilize, and egg production ensues shortly thereafter. The fully-embryonated eggs pass out with the fecal mass into brackish or freshwater.

H. heterophyes primarily infects snails of the genus *Cerithidia*, while those of *M. yokogawai* infect snails in the genera *Semisulcospira* and *Thiara*. The embryonated eggs are ingested by their respective snail hosts, and hatch inside, releasing the miracidia. This stage undergoes sequential development in the snail, first to sporocysts, then to rediae, and finally to cercariae. The cercariae penetrate out of the snail, and like those of *Clonorchis sinensis*, encyst under the skin of freshwater fish, or in frogs, tadpoles, or even another snail.[14] The species of intermediate hosts for both of these parasites varies widely with the geographic locale. In Asia, the intermediate hosts are cyprinoid and salmonid fishes, and in the Middle East, mullet and tilapia are primarily involved with the life cycle.

Clinical Disease

Like other trematode infections, the clinical presentation is thought to be determined

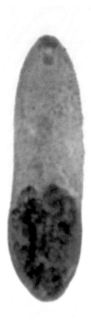

Figure 37.3. An adult of *Heterophyes heterophyes*. 2 mm x 0.5 mm.

in large part by the worm burden.[20] Epigastric distress, fatigue, diarrhea, weight loss and malaise have been reported for heavy infection, along with belching, headache, nausea, vomiting, and even urinary incontinence.[18, 21]

Diagnosis

Diagnosis is usually based on recovery and identification of eggs in feces. The eggs (Figs. 37.5, 37.6) of *H. heterophyes* and *M. yokogawai* closely resemble those of *C. sinensis*. They must be carefully differentiated by their absence of a terminal knob and a collar at the

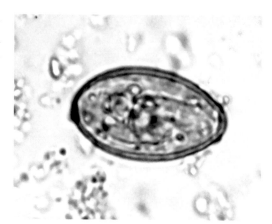

Figure 37.6. Egg of *M. yokogawai*. 25 μm x 15 μm.

operculum. Eggs and even adult flukes have been recovered on endoscopy.[22-24]

Treatment

The drug of choice is praziquantel. Mebendazole may be an alternative, but less efficacious option.[25]

Prevention and control

Echinostomiasis can be prevented by eating only cooked fish, and by controlling the indiscriminate use of untreated human feces as fertilizer.[1, 17, 19] Protection of fish ponds from contamination with human feces and control of snail populations are potentially helpful.[14]

Nanophyetus salmincola
(Chapin 1927)

Although *Nanophyetus salmincola* may be the most common trematode in the United States, it tends to mostly infect animals, and only rarely infects humans.[26] *Nanophyetus salmincola* infects dogs, foxes, and coyotes in eastern Siberia and in the Pacific Northwest of the United States, where it produces "salmon poisoning" or "elokomin fluke fever" as a result of a rickettsia, *Neorickettsia helmintheca*, which is co-transmitted with the parasite.[27] Human infection has also been

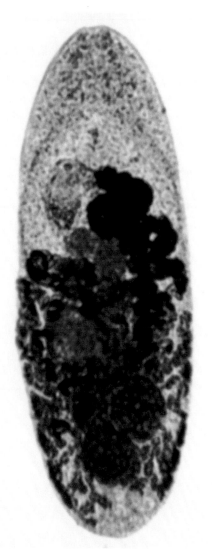

Figure 37.5. An adult of *Metagonimus yokogawai*. 2.5 mm x 0.6 mm.

described, resulting in diarrhea, nausea, vomiting, cachexia, anorexia, and elevated levels of circulating eosinophils.[28] *N. salmincola* infection is diagnosed by the presence of characteristic eggs in the stools, along with a history of ingestion of raw or poorly cooked salmon.[28]

References

1. Fried, B.; Graczyk, T. K.; Tamang, L., Food-borne intestinal trematodiases in humans. *Parasitology research* **2004**, *93* (2), 159-70.
2. Chai, J. Y.; Shin, E. H.; Lee, S. H.; Rim, H. J., Foodborne intestinal flukes in Southeast Asia. *Korean J Parasitol* **2009**, *47 Suppl*, S69-102.
3. Keiser, J.; Utzinger, J., Food-borne trematodiases. *Clin Microbiol Rev* **2009**, *22* (3), 466-83.
4. Wiwanitkit, V.; Suyaphan, A., High prevalence of HBsAg seropositivity in Hilltribers in the Mae Jam district in northern Thailand. *MedGenMed : Medscape general medicine* **2002**, *4* (3), 26.
5. Bhatti, H. S.; Malla, N.; Mahajan, R. C.; Sehgal, R., Fasciolopslasis--a re-emerging infection in Azamgarh (Uttar Pradesh). *Indian journal of pathology & microbiology* **2000**, *43* (1), 73-6.
6. Graczyk, T. K.; Gilman, R. H.; Fried, B., Fasciolopsiasis: is it a controllable food-borne disease? *Parasitology research* **2001**, *87* (1), 80-3.
7. Achra, A.; Prakash, P.; Shankar, R., Fasciolopsiasis: Endemic focus of a neglected parasitic disease in Bihar. *Indian J Med Microbiol* **2015**, *33* (3), 364-8.
8. Gupta, A.; Xess, A.; Sharma, H. P.; Dayal, V. M.; Prasad, K. M.; Shahi, S. K., Fasciolopsis buski (giant intestinal fluke)--a case report. *Indian journal of pathology & microbiology* **1999**, *42* (3), 359-60.
9. Naher, B. S.; Shahid, A. T.; Khan, K. A.; Nargis, S.; Hoque, M. M., Fasciolopsiasis in a five year old girl. *Mymensingh Med J* **2013**, *22* (2), 397-9.
10. Le, T. H.; Nguyen, V. D.; Phan, B. U.; Blair, D.; McManus, D. P., Case report: unusual presentation of Fasciolopsis buski in a Vietnamese child. *Trans R Soc Trop Med Hyg* **2004**, *98* (3), 193-4.
11. Taraschewski, H.; Mehlhorn, H.; Bunnag, D.; Andrews, P.; Thomas, H., Effects of praziquantel on human intestinal flukes (Fasciolopsis buski and Heterophyes heterophyes). *Zentralblatt fur Bakteriologie, Mikrobiologie, und Hygiene. Series A, Medical microbiology, infectious diseases, virology, parasitology* **1986**, *262* (4), 542-50.
12. Chai, J. Y., Praziquantel treatment in trematode and cestode infections: an update. *Infect Chemother* **2013**, *45* (1), 32-43.
13. Inpankaew, T.; Murrell, K. D.; Pinyopanuwat, N.; Chhoun, C.; Khov, K.; Sem, T.; Sorn, S.; Muth, S.; Dalsgaard, A., A survey for potentially zoonotic gastrointestinal parasites of dogs and pigs in Cambodia. *Acta Parasitol* **2015**, *60* (4), 601-4.
14. Toledo, R.; Esteban, J. G., An update on human echinostomiasis. *Trans R Soc Trop Med Hyg* **2016**, *110* (1), 37-45.
15. Park, S. K.; Kim, D.-H.; Deung, Y.-K.; Kim, H.-J.; Yang, E.-J.; Lim, S.-J.; Ryang, Y.-S.; Jin, D.; Lee, K.-J., Status of intestinal parasite infections among children in Bat Dambang, Cambodia. *The Korean journal of parasitology* **2004**, *42* (4), 201-3.
16. Huffman, J. E.; Fried, B., Echinostoma and echinostomiasis. *Advances in parasitology* **1990**, *29*, 215-69.
17. Anantaphruti, M. T., Parasitic contaminants in food. *The Southeast Asian journal of tropical medicine and public health* **2001**, *32 Suppl 2*, 218-28.
18. Chai, J.-Y.; Park, J.-H.; Han, E.-T.; Shin, E.-H.; Kim, J.-L.; Guk, S.-M.; Hong, K.-S.; Lee, S.-H.; Rim, H.-J., Prevalence of Heterophyes nocens and Pygydiopsis summa infections among residents of the western and southern coastal islands of the Republic of Korea. *The American journal of tropical medicine and hygiene* **2004**, *71* (5), 617-22.
19. Chai, J.-Y.; Lee, S.-H., Food-borne intestinal trematode infections in the Republic of Korea. *Parasitology international* **2002**, *51* (2), 129-54.
20. Graczyk, T. K.; Fried, B., Echinostomiasis: a common but forgotten food-borne disease. *Am J Trop*

Med Hyg **1998,** *58* (4), 501-4.

21. Chang, Y. D.; Sohn, W. M.; Ryu, J. H.; Kang, S. Y.; Hong, S. J., A human infection of Echinostoma hortense in duodenal bulb diagnosed by endoscopy. *Korean J Parasitol* **2005,** *43* (2), 57-60.

22. Jung, W. T.; Lee, K. J.; Kim, H. J.; Kim, T. H.; Na, B. K.; Sohn, W. M., A case of Echinostoma cinetorchis (Trematoda: Echinostomatidae) infection diagnosed by colonoscopy. *Korean J Parasitol* **2014,** *52* (3), 287-90.

23. Toledo, R.; Munoz-Antoli, C.; Esteban, J. G., Intestinal trematode infections. *Adv Exp Med Biol* **2014,** *766*, 201-40.

24. Esteban, J. G.; Munoz-Antoli, C.; Toledo, R.; Ash, L. R., Diagnosis of human trematode infections. *Adv Exp Med Biol* **2014,** *766*, 293-327.

25. Chen, Y.; Xu, G.; Feng, Z.; Guo, Z.; Lin, J.; Fang, Y., Studies on efficacy of praziquantel and mebendazole-medicated salt in treatment of Echinochasmus fujianensis infection. *Southeast Asian J Trop Med Public Health* **1997,** *28* (2), 344-6.

26. Eastburn, R. L.; Fritsche, T. R.; Terhune, C. A., Jr., Human intestinal infection with Nanophyetus salmincola from salmonid fishes. *Am J Trop Med Hyg* **1987,** *36* (3), 586-91.

27. Headley, S. A.; Scorpio, D. G.; Vidotto, O.; Dumler, J. S., Neorickettsia helminthoeca and salmon poisoning disease: a review. *Vet J* **2011,** *187* (2), 165-73.

28. Eastburn, R. L.; Fritsche, T. R.; Terhune, C. A., Human intestinal infection with Nanophyetus salmincola from salmonid fishes. *The American journal of tropical medicine and hygiene* **1987,** *36* (3), 586-91.

VIII. The Arthropods

Arthropods directly influence humans' well-being, not only because they are hosts of parasitic organisms and vectors of a wide variety of pathogens, but also by causing tissue damage and disease. They also affect human health by reducing the availability of food. Insects destroy an estimated 20% of all food crops, and this destruction continues despite the increasing use of pesticides in fields and storage areas. Livestock are also affected by arthropod-borne infections. Vast areas of Africa are short of protein foods because cattle suffer a number of vector-borne diseases, including trypanosomiasis transmitted by tsetse flies and a variety of tick-transmitted diseases.

Although the pathogenic effects of arthropods are most pronounced in the tropics, they are by no means negligible in the United States and other temperate areas. Lyme disease and anaplasmosis, which are transmitted by ticks, have spread rapidly throughout the United States. *Aedes albopictus*, the Asian tiger mosquito, has been introduced in shipments of used automobile tires into the southern United States and has spread as far north as central Ohio, Indiana, and Illinois; moreover, the introduced strain of the mosquito is apparently able to survive the winter in the egg stage in temperate climates. The same species has been introduced into Europe and South America. *Ae. albopictus* can be an efficient vector of dengue, chikungunya and Zika virus. In 1999, reports surfaced about the introduction and rapid spread across the Eastern United States of another pest mosquito, *Ochlerotatus japonicus*. Introductions of new species should not be unexpected and point to the ease with which such introductions can occur. The unexpected appearance in New York City in 1999 of mosquito-transmitted human infections of the West Nile virus, and its subsequent spread throughout the United States, should reinforce our awareness of vulnerability to invasion by both pathogens and vectors.

Although fear has been expressed that blood-feeding arthropods, especially mosquitoes, could transmit the AIDS virus, a large body of epidemiological and experimental evidence fails to support this hypothesis.

Even though arthropods cause problems for humans and livestock, they are also beneficial as pollinators, producers of honey, natural regulators of harmful insects, and essential members of food chains.

The phylum Arthropoda contains an enormous diversity of members, with the number of species exceeding that of all other phyla combined. The arthropods share a number of characteristics that distinguish them from all other animal groups, although some of these features are absent in a particular species or group at some period of development. Nevertheless, all species in the phylum are identifiable.

Among the morphologic characteristics are bilateral symmetry, a hard exoskeleton, a segmented body, and paired, jointed appendages. The term arthropod, derived from Greek, means "jointed foot."

Growth by metamorphosis is another characteristic of the arthropods. In some groups, growth is gradual; each change from one stage to the next is known as a molt, and gives rise to a stage somewhat larger but morphologically similar to its predecessor (incomplete metamorphosis). Among the spiders, eight or nine immature stages may precede the final molt to the sexually mature adult. Another developmental strategy involves the egg, the larva, the pupa and the adult. In this case, each stage is morphologically distinct (complete metamorphosis). Examples include the flies and the fleas.

The application of the tools of molecular biology to the study of arthropods is pervasive. Most dramatic are the various genome projects. The genome of *Anopheles gambiae*, the most important of the African malaria vectors, is complete, and work on *An. funestus* is nearing completion. The genomes of *Aedes aegypti*, the Yellow Fever mosquito, *Culex pipiens* the vector of West Nile Virus and *Ixodes scapularis,* the primary vector or Lyme Disease in the U.S. have been completed. Mitochondrial genomes for the sand flies *Phlebotomus papatasi* and *P.* chinesis have been reported. The value of these programs and their use in eventual control of the diseases these vectors transmit remains to be determined.

38. Insects

Introduction

The insects have two distinct types of development. The more primitive insect orders pass through a series of stages by incomplete metamorphosis (Fig. 38.1). A typical life cycle involves the egg, a (usually) fixed number of immature nymph stages, and the mature adult stage. The insect molts between stages, sheds its old exoskeleton, and reveals a new skin within. Nymphs are similar to the adult, but lack wings and are sexually immature.

In contrast, complete metamorphosis is characteristic of some of the more advanced insect orders, including the flies (Diptera) (Fig. 38.2) and the fleas, Siphonaptera (Fig 38.3). The life cycle of an insect exhibiting complete metamorphosis includes the egg, larval stages, a pupa stage, and the adult stage.

Table 38.1 lists arthropods of importance to human health, the pathogens they harbor and transmit, and the diseases they cause. The methods by which the arthropod vectors transmit pathogens vary. Some pathogens, unchanged by any interaction with the vector, are transmitted mechanically from one host to another on contaminated legs or mouthparts of the arthropod or in its feces. Other pathogens require passage through the arthropod as part of their life cycle. In such cases, the pathogens undergo specific developmental changes, which usually include multiplication, within the arthropod.

Arthropods can also be pathogens themselves. They can infest the host, migrating through the body or developing *in situ* while feeding on host tissue. Other arthropods cause mechanical injury through bites, chemical injury through injection of toxins, or allergic reactions to the materials they transmit via the bite or sting. Moreover, entomophobia and arachnophobia (i.e., fear of insects and arachnids, particularly spiders) are not uncommon psychological conditions.[1,2]

The salivary secretions of arthropods in general, and insects in particular, have proven to be extraordinarily complex. These secretions serve as potent immunogens and stimulate the bothersome allergic reactions to the insect's bite. They also serve, in many cases, to carry the viral, bacterial, protozoal or nematode pathogens for which so many arthropods serve as vectors. These salivary secretions evolved not to cause allergic responses or convey pathogens, but for a much more basic reason. They facilitate the capacity of the arthropod to take blood from a host whose physiology and defense mechanisms are designed to prevent the loss of blood.

In almost all blood-sucking arthropods studied to date, the saliva of each species has at least one anticlotting, one vasodilator and one antiplatelet compound. The molecular diversity of these compounds is great, even among closely related genera of blood feeders.[3,4]

Diptera: The Flies

No single group of insects has so affected human evolution, development, or history as the Diptera, the order of insects comprised of flies and mosquitoes. Malaria, yellow fever, elephantiasis, sleeping sickness, dengue, and river blindness are among the more serious diseases carried by members of this large order. Notorious as vectors of pathogenic organisms of humans and animals, dipterans are also important for the mechanical damage (i.e., myiasis) caused by their larvae and the allergic responses caused by the bites of some adults.

Flies develop by complete metamorphosis and have distinct larval, pupal, and adult forms. Larvae are usually vermiform, often living in water or damp places or developing in living or dead tissue. Pupae represent a non-feeding transitional stage. Adult dipter-

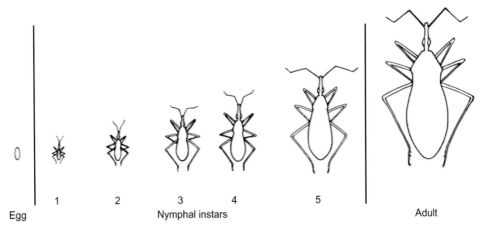

Figure 38.1. Incomplete metamorphosis in insects. Typical example of incomplete metamorphosis is the kissing bug, *Rhodnius prolixus*. Immature stages are wingless, smaller versions of the winged adult. All stages, except the egg, have three pairs of legs. The number of nymphal stages varies with the species.

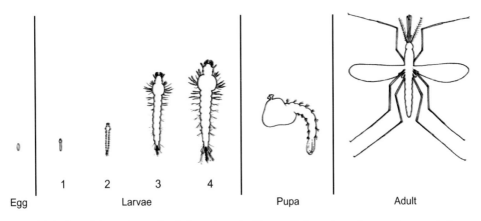

Figure 38.2. Complete metamorphosis in an insect with aquatic immature stages. The anopheles mosquito begins as an egg laid on the surface of water and develops through four larval stages and a single pupal stage to a sexually mature, winged adult.

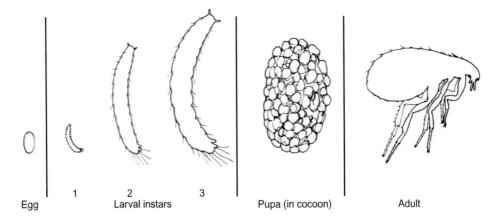

Figure 38.3. Complete metamorphosis in an insect with terrestrial immature stages. The flea begins as an egg laid on the fur of the host or in the nest area. Several maggot-like larval stages are followed by a single pupal stage, encased in a sand-covered cocoon, from which a wingless, sexually mature adult flea emerges.

Table 38.1. Arthropods of medical importance.

Order and representative species	Common name	Geographic distribution	Effects on humans
Insecta			
Anoplura (sucking lice)			
Pediculus humanus humanus	Body louse	Worldwide	Skin reactions to bites, vectors of rickettsiae and spirochetes
P. humanus capitis	Head louse	Worldwide	Skin reaction to bites
Phthirus pubis	Crab louse	Worldwide	Skin reaction to bites
Heteroptera (true bugs)			
Cimex lectularius	Bed bug	Worldwide	Skin reaction to bites
C. hemipterus	Tropical bed bug	Tropical and subtropical	
Triatoma infestans	Kissing bug, cone-nosed bug	Tropical and subtropical regions of the New World	Skin reaction to bites, vectors of *Trypanosoma cruzi*, the cause of Chagas disease
Rhodnius prolixus			
Panstrongylus megistus			
Hymenoptera (bees, wasps, ants)			
Apis mellifera	Honey bee	Worldwide	Painful sting, potential anaphylaxis
Bombus spp.	Bumble bee	Worldwide	Painful sting, potential anaphylaxis
Various genera and species of the family Vespidae	Wasp, hornet, yellow jacket	Worldwide	Painful sting, potential anaphylaxis
Solenopsis spp.	Fire ant	Tropical America, southeastern United States	Painful bite and multiple stings, potential anaphylaxis
Diptera (flies, mosquitoes, and their relatives)			
Ceratopogonidae *Culicoides* spp. *Leptoconops* spp.	No-see-um, sand fly	Worldwide	Serious biting pest, skin reaction to bites, vectors of several filariid nematodes
Psychodidae *Phlebotomus* spp. *Lutzomyia* spp.	sand fly	Worldwide	Skin reaction to bites, vectors of *Leishmania*, Pappataci fever, and Carrion's disease
Simuliidae *Simulium* spp.	Blackfly, buffalo gnat	Worldwide	Serious biting pests, skin reaction to bites, vectors of *Onchocerca* and *Mansonella*
Culicidae *Aedes* spp. *Anopheles* spp. *Culex* spp. *Culiseta* spp. *Mansonia* spp.	Mosquito	Worldwide	Serious biting pests, skin reaction to bites, vectors of viruses, protozoa, and filaria
Tabanidae *Tabanus* spp.	Horsefly	Worldwide	Biting pests, painful bite followed by skin reaction
Chrysops spp.	Deerfly	Worldwide	Biting pests, vectors of tularemia and *Loa loa*.
Muscidae *Musca domestica*	Housefly	Worldwide	Mechanical disseminator of pathogens
Stomoxys calcitrans	Stablefly	Worldwide	Serious biting pest
Glossina spp.	Tsetse fly	Africa	Vector of trypanosomes of humans and animals
Calliphoridae Cuterebridae Sarcophagidae Larvae of various genera and species	Maggots	Worldwide	Myiasis, accidental or obligate development of larval flies in human tissue
Siphonaptera (fleas)			
Xenopsylla cheopis	Oriental rat flea	Worldwide	Vector of bubonic plague
Ctenocephalides felis	Cat flea	Worldwide	Biting pest
C. canis	Dog flea		
Pulex irritans	Human flea	Worldwide	Biting pest, plague vector
Tunga penetrans	Chigoe flea	Africa and South America	Infestation of toes, feet and legs, causing severe pain and secondary infection

ans, which usually possess wings, have only one pair (*diptera* means "two wings"). The mouthparts of the adults may be adapted for biting, piercing flesh, and sucking blood, or only for sucking fluids.

Diptera is a large order, divided into three suborders containing over 100 families. Only nine families are of medical concern. The most primitive suborder, the Nematocera, contains four medically important families: Ceratopogonidae, Psychodidae, Simuliidae, and Culicidae. In the suborder Brachycera, only the Tabanidae are of any medical significance; in the third suborder, Cyclorrhapha, the Muscidae, Gasterophilidae, Cuterebridae, and Oestridae are of major concern.

Ceratopogonidae: The Biting Midges

Ceratopogonids, commonly called punkies, no-see-ums, sand flies, or midges, are minute (0.4-5.0 mm long), slender, blood-sucking dipterans. They constitute a serious pest problem in many areas of the tropics, the temperate zones, and in the Arctic. Most of the species that affect humans belong to two genera, *Culicoides* and *Leptoconops*, which act as vectors of several filariids that infect humans in Africa and the New World. Species of culicoides may also serve as vectors of filariids and viruses that infect animals including humans.

Life Cycle

Ceratopogonid larvae develop in aquatic or semi-aquatic habitats, often in freshwater, but usually in brackish water or tidal flats. Some important species are associated with the highly polluted runoff from livestock holding areas. Larval stages are long, slender, and maggot-like; in some species they undergo diapause, a state of arrested development, for as long as three years while awaiting optimal environmental conditions. Adult female ceratopogonids require blood for the production of their eggs. They typically feed at dusk and may attack in large numbers.

Pathogenesis

The mouthparts of ceratopogonids are short and lancet-like, producing a painful bite. Because of their large numbers, they can be important pests, particularly in beach and resort areas near salt marshes. Bites can produce local lesions that persist for hours or days. Sensitized individuals develop allergic reactions.

Midges of the genus *Culicoides* are the main vectors of the filariid nematodes: *Mansonella perstans* and *M. streptocerca* in Africa, and *M. ozzardi* in the New World tropics.

Control

Ceratopogonids develop in a wide range of habitats, and each species presents its own special problems with respect to control. Salt marsh habitats can be drained or channeled and other breeding sites modified, but treatment of breeding sites with insecticides remains the most effective short-term control measure. Window screens are ineffective unless they are treated with insecticides, because they allow these minute insects easy entry. Commercial mosquito repellents containing diethyltoluamide (DEET) may be useful against some of the common species of these pests.

Psychodidae: Mothflies or Sand flies

A single subfamily of the Psychodidae, the Phlebotominae, of tropical, subtropical, and temperate regions – contains members that suck blood. Phlebotomine sand flies are small (1-3 mm), hairy, delicate, weak-flying insects that feed on a wide range of cold- and warm-blooded animals, and transmit a number of viral, bacterial, and protozoan infections. Flies of the genera *Phlebotomus* and *Lutzomyia* are important as vectors of the leishmaniae.

Historical Information

In 1921, Edouard and Etienne Sergent demonstrated the role of phlebotomine flies in the transmission of leishmaniasis.[5]

Life Cycle

Phlebotomine larvae develop in non-aquatic habitats such as moist soil, animal burrows, termite nests, loose masonry, stone-walls, or rubbish heaps. The four larval stages are completed within 2-6 weeks; the pupa stage may last 8-14 days. The adults (Fig. 38.4) are weak fliers, exhibiting a hopping movement rather than sustained flight. Only female phlebotomines require blood, feeding usually at night. Some species prefer to feed on humans, but none are exclusively anthropophilic; they feed on dogs and rodents as well.

Pathogenesis

The mouthparts of the female phlebotomine are short and adapted for piercing and sucking. The bite may be painful, producing

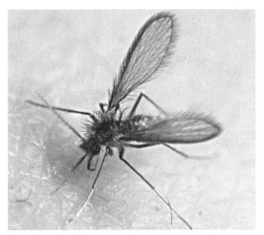

Fig. 38.4. Adult female phlebotomine sand fly, *Lutzomyia anthophora*. Courtesy J. Ribeiro

an itchy local lesion. Sensitized individuals may show severe allergic reactions. The saliva of the sand fly is particularly complex and contains a number of potent compounds that can influence the susceptibility of human macrophages to invasion by promastigotes of leishmania introduced by the feeding vector. The use of components of sand fly saliva as a vaccine to prevent infection is being actively pursued and has received encouraging preliminary results.

Although phlebotomines cause problems in some areas as pests, they are of particular concern as vectors of a number of diseases. Bartonellosis (also called Carrion's disease, Oroya fever, or verruga peruana) is a South American disease transmitted from human to human by *Lutzomyia verrucarum* and related species. It is caused by the bacterium *Bartonella bacilliformis*, which invades erythrocytes and reticuloendothelial cells. The organism can produce a severe febrile illness, complicated by profound anemia. Untreated, bartonellosis is fatal in 50% of cases. There is no known animal reservoir.

Sand fly fever, also called papatasi fever, is a viral disease seen in the Mediterranean region, central Asia, Sri Lanka, India, and China. *Phlebotomus papatasii* is the main vector for this acute febrile disease, which is characterized by severe frontal headaches, malaise, retro-orbital pain, anorexia, and nausea. Female flies become infected when they feed on viremic individuals. After an incubation period of 7-10 days, the flies become infective and remain so for the rest of their lives.

Leishmaniasis is transmitted by a number of phlebotomine species. Flies initially pick up the parasite while feeding on infected humans or animals. In the fly, the parasite undergoes asexual multiplication, eventually accumulating in the mouthparts, from where it is transmitted to the host when the insect feeds.[6-8]

Control

Phlebotomine sand flies are particularly sensitive to insecticides, and the use of DDT in campaigns against malaria coincidentally controlled these flies and virtually eliminated sand fly-borne diseases in many regions. In areas where malaria has been eliminated or where malaria control programs have been abandoned, the phlebotomine flies have reestablished themselves, and the sand fly-borne diseases have returned.

Sand flies may be controlled with residual or short-lived insecticides applied to breeding sites or houses. Treatment of window screens with insecticides may also be effective. Mosquito repellents can be used to reduce the frequency of sand fly bites.

Simuliidae: Black flies

Members of the family Simuliidae, commonly called Black flies, buffalo gnats, or turkey gnats, are small (1-5 mm long), humpbacked, blood-sucking dipterans that usually breed in fast-flowing streams and rivers. Simuliids are important as vectors of *Onchocerca volvulus*, the causative agent of onchocerciasis. In addition, they present a serious pest problem in many temperate and Arctic areas. Black flies may also serve as vectors of bovine onchocerciasis and protozoan parasites of various species of birds.

Historical information

Black flies first stimulated medical interest in 1910, when it was suggested, incorrectly, that these flies transmitted a malaria-like organism that caused pellagra.[9] Their role in the transmission of onchocerca was demonstrated in 1926.

Life Cycle

Adult female simuliids (Fig. 38.5) lay eggs

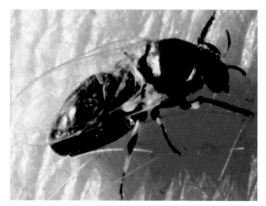

Figure 38.5. Black fly adult feeding on a human host

at or below the surface of moving, well-oxygenated water. Larvae and pupae, equipped with gills for respiration, remain attached to objects below the surface. Larvae are nourished by food filtered from the passing water. They undergo development in five stages. The non-feeding pupae gradually assume adult characteristics while they are enclosed within a cocoon. Adult female simuliids require blood for egg production. They feed primarily during daylight hours. Male simuliids do not feed on blood.

Adult Black flies in temperate areas may emerge synchronously in large numbers. Their bites cause serious damage to humans and animals. Black flies often reach such high population densities that they can kill livestock and wild animals, torment campers and fishermen, and render large areas uninhabitable by humans and animals for long periods of time.

Pathogenesis

The bite of the female simuliid is particularly painful. The insect's mouthparts consist of six blades in the shape of lancets, which tear the skin surface to induce bleeding. The fly feeds from the resulting pool of blood, and the bite wound continues to bleed for some time after the fly has departed. Simuliid bites leave a characteristic point of dried blood at the wound site. The extreme pain of the initial bite is followed by itching and swelling due to reactions to the injected salivary secretions. Blood loss from multiple bites can be considerable. Allergic reactions in previously sensitized individuals are common, and can sometimes reach serious levels, including anaphylaxis. Reports from the Midwestern U.S. in the early part of the 20th century mention human deaths due to swarms of biting black flies.

Control

Control of Black flies is most effectively achieved by the slow dripping of insecticides into rivers or streams. Mass control programs using insecticides applied by fixed-wing aircraft and helicopters have been successful in West African onchocerciasis. Clearing debris from streambeds can also reduce breeding. Repellents containing DEET are recommended for personal protection.

Culicidae: The Mosquitoes

Mosquitoes constitute one of the largest dipteran families and are of major significance as vectors of disease and as biting pests. Their economic, cultural, and evolutionary impact has been devastating. Mosquitoes develop in a wide range of aquatic larval habitats and in all climates from the arctic to the tropics. Adult mosquitoes are generally similar in appearance. They are usually small and have delicate legs, a single pair of wings, long antennae, and elongated mouth parts capable of piercing flesh and sucking blood. Larvae and pupae are aquatic and their development proceeds through complete metamorphosis (Fig. 38.2).

Historical Information

Numerous writers had suggested the association between mosquitoes and various tropical fevers in the past. The association of these fevers with mosquitoes was finally recognized during the nineteenth century. Patrick Manson provided the proof that mosquitoes could transmit diseases in 1878, when he showed that mosquitoes were intermediate hosts of *Wuchereria bancrofti*.

Transmission of malaria by mosquitoes was suggested by Manson as early as 1884, but Ronald Ross and Italian investigators under the direction of Giovanni Grassi were the first to prove that mosquitoes transmitted malaria.[10-12] The incrimination of *Aedes aegypti* in the transmission of yellow fever was suggested by Carlos Finlay in 1880, and proved by Walter Reed and his co-workers in 1900.[13]

Life Cycle

Both major subfamilies of the Culicidae – the Anophelinae and the Culicinae – are involved in transmission of diseases. Members of these subfamilies share a number of basic similarities in their life cycles and development. They lay eggs on or near water or on surfaces that become flooded. Their larvae are always aquatic. The four larval stages are elongate, active "wigglers" that feed by filtering particulate matter from water; they must remain in contact with the surface for respiration. The pupae, known as "tumblers," are comma-shaped and aquatic. They remain at the surface unless disturbed. Adult mosquitoes of most species are good fliers. Males and females feed on nectars and sugars, although females of most species also feed on blood. They require a blood meal for each clutch of eggs, which may contain 100-200 eggs. A female may produce six or more clutches during her lifetime. Eggs require 48-72 hours to develop within the female. They may be deposited almost as soon as they mature. Consequently, a female may take a blood meal every 2-4 days and contact a number of hosts during that period, providing an excellent opportunity for the dissemination of pathogens.

Subfamily Anophelinae

The genus *Anopheles* contains the species responsible for the transmission of human malaria. The anopheline female lays eggs singly, each equipped with floats, usually on the surface of water. Eggs hatch 2-4 days after they are laid. The aquatic larvae attach to the surface and assume a horizontal position. The larval period may last 1-3 weeks, depending on temperature. Anopheline pupae are superficially similar to the pupae of other mosquitoes. The pupal stage lasts 1-3 days. Adult anophelines (Fig. 38.6) are delicate, long-legged mosquitoes. Although some species are capable of extended flight and dispersion from breeding sites, anophelines typically remain close to their food supplies and breeding habitats.

Most anophelines are night feeders, with characteristic peaks of biting activity for each species. Some species are exclusively zoophilic, some are anthropophilic, and others are nonspecific biters. Feeding habits also vary between species. Certain species readily enter houses and feed on sleeping individuals; others feed only outdoors.

In temperate areas, anophelines spend the winter as inseminated adult females. In the tropics, these mosquitoes breed continually,

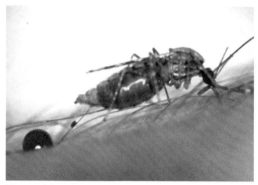

Figure 38.7. *Anopheles stephensi*, a malaria vector found in Asia, particularly India and Pakistan.

although their population levels may fluctuate drastically in relation to rainfall and dry seasons.

Approximately 300 species of *Anopheles* mosquitoes have been described. However, only a small number of species are important as malaria vectors within any geographic area (e.g., *An. gambiae* and *An. funestus* in Sub-Saharan Africa, *An. culicifacies* and *An. stephensi* (Fig. 38.7) on the Indian subcontinent, and *An. quadrimaculatus* and *An. freeborni* (Fig. 38.8) in North America). Populations vary within each species with respect to their competence as vectors and capacity for transmission.

Intense study has led to the division of several well-established species of vectors into morphologically similar but genetically distinct groups or complexes of species. The important vector of malaria in Africa, *An. gambiae*, consists of at least six discrete

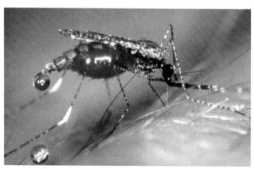

Figure 38.6. *Anopheles dirus*, one of the major malaria vectors in Southeast Asia, performing "plasmapheresis".

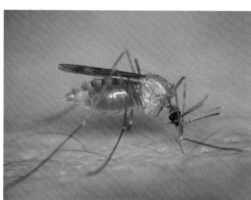

Figure 38.8. *Anopheles freeborni*, a potential malaria vector in California.

but cryptic species, most of which are not major vectors. Similar revision of species has resulted in a clearer definition of the members of the European complex and the Southeast Asian group (Fig. 38.6). It appears that reexamination of most of the anopheline species that occupy large or ecologically diverse geographic areas will lead to the description of closely related but genetically divergent species.

Anophelines also play an important role as vectors of filarial nematodes. *An. gambiae* and *An. funestus* are the main vectors of *Wuchereria bancrofti* in Africa, and *An. hyrcanus* in China and *An. barbirostris* in Southeast Asia are vectors of both *W. bancrofti* and *Brugia malayi*. Although anophelines are not usually involved in the transmission of viruses, *An. gambiae* and *An. funestus* are the vectors of O'nyong-nyong fever.

To learn more about the ecology of anopheline mosquitoes and control programs that take advantage of their biology, see www.medicalecology.org/diseases/malaria/malaria.htm.

Subfamily Culicinae

The subfamily Culicinae consists of more than 1500 species distributed among 20 genera, six of which (*Aedes*, *Ochlerotatus*, *Culex*, *Mansonia*, *Psorophora*, and *Culiseta*) are of major importance to human health. Culicine mosquitoes are primary vectors of a number of viruses and filariae and pose a serious problem as pest insects in many parts of the world.

Several species formerly recognized as members of the genus *Aedes*, the largest of the Culicine genera, have been undergoing a major reorganization. In 2000, the genus was divided into two genera, *Aedes* and *Ochlerotatus*, on the basis of consistent primary characters of the female and male genitalia.[14, 15] These changes have been generally accepted. A more dramatic renaming was suggested where common mosquitoes such as *Aedes aegypti* would be called *Stegomyia aegypti* and *Aedes albopictus* renamed *Stegomyia albopicta*. These changes are being hotly debated.

Mosquitoes of the genera *Aedes* and *Ochlerotatus* remain in the "tribe" Aedini, and are found in all habitats, ranging from the tropics to the Arctic. The typical aedine mosquito (Fig. 38.9) is robust, a strong flier, and usually a vicious biter. Its eggs are laid singly, without floats, on or near the surface of water or in areas likely to be flooded periodically. Unlike the eggs of anopheles or culex mosquitoes, which usually hatch within a few days of deposition, aedine eggs have the capacity for an extended period of dormancy. This dormancy allows the eggs to survive the winter or to delay hatching until conditions are ideal for development. Aedine mosquitoes occupy salt marsh habitats, flood plains, tree holes, irrigated pasturelands, and human-made containers.

Aedine larvae are nourished by food filtered from water. They develop and feed while suspended from the surface of water by a breathing tube. Larvae develop by progressing through four stages over a period of 6-10 days, or longer at lower temperatures. Aedine pupae are typical of those of most mosquitoes; this stage usually lasts less than three days. Adults usually emerge from breeding

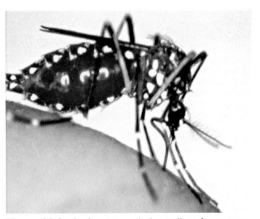

Figure 38.9. *Aedes aegypti*, the yellow fever mosquito, in a typical feeding position.

sites synchronously, followed by mass migrations of females in search of blood.

Aedine species may develop overwhelming populations in salt marshes, tundras, pastures, and floodwater, and they have a severe impact on wildlife, livestock, and humans. If left uncontrolled, the salt-marsh mosquitoes of the East Coast of the United States, *Ochlerotatus. sollicitans* and *Oc. taeniorhynchus*, could deny vast areas of seashore to development and tourism. The floodwater mosquito, *Ae. vexans*, develops after spring rain and flooding; the Arctic species begin hatching with the first melting snows. Populations of Arctic aedes become so great at times that humans and larger mammals do not venture into the tundra area. In some Arctic species, the first egg batch is produced without need of a blood meal, a physiological adaptation termed autogeny.

Aedines, breeding in tree holes in the populated areas of temperate zones (e.g., *Oc. triseriatus*), seldom produce large populations, but can become local pests and important vectors of various viral infections. In tropical regions, populations of aedine mosquitoes are usually much smaller than in the Arctic. *Aedes aegypti* (Fig. 38.9), the yellow fever mosquito, occurs alongside humans throughout the tropics and subtropics. *Ae. aegypti* usually breeds in human-made containers such as discarded auto tires, flower pots, blocked gutters, water jugs, rain barrels, cemetery urns, and tin cans. The mosquito lays eggs above the waterline in these containers, and the eggs remain dormant there, often as long as six months, until the container becomes filled with water. Because this mosquito is closely associated with humans and is almost exclusively anthropophilic, it has most of the characteristics of a good vector. *Ae. aegypti* is the primary vector of yellow fever and dengue in urban environments throughout the world. In the South Pacific, container-breeding members of the *Ae. scutellaris* complex are vectors of certain viruses and *W. bancrofti*. The introduction of *Ae. albopictus* and *Ae. (Ochlerotatus) japonicus* into the United States has added two species with the potential for transmitting dengue. Both of these introduced species are proving to be serious biting pests, particularly in urban and suburban areas of the Eastern and Southeastern U.S. *Ae. albopictus* appears to be out-competing *Ae. aegypti* in many areas, which is not an altogether undesirable effect, since *Ae. aegypti* is much more efficient at transmitting yellow fever and dengue.

The genus *Culex* is the second largest group in the subfamily, best represented by *Cx. pipiens pipiens*, the northern house mosquito found in temperate areas, and *Cx. pipiens quinquefasciatus* (formerly known as *Cx. fatigans*), the southern house mosquito found throughout the sub-tropics and tropics.

Culex mosquitoes deposit their eggs in rafts, which usually contain 50-200 eggs cemented together. The eggs float perpendicular to the water surface and hatch within 2-3 days. The four larval stages develop and feed on nutrients in the water, much like aedine mosquitoes. The siphons of larval culex mosquitoes are usually longer and more slender than those of aedines. The larval period lasts less than two weeks and the pupal stage less than two days. Adults usually feed at night. Many show a preference for avian blood, but most members also feed on humans or other mammals. *Cx. p. quinquefasciatus* is the major vector of *W. bancrofti* throughout the tropics. The species is particularly well-adapted to development in polluted waters, breeding in or near population centers and readily biting humans.

The genus *Mansonia* includes a number of species important as vectors of Brugian filariasis. This genus differs in its development from most other mosquitoes in that its larvae and pupae affix themselves below the surface of water to the stems and roots of aquatic plants and derive oxygen from these plants. Mosquitoes of the genus *Psorophora* can be important biting pests. *Culiseta* includes several species involved in the transmission of arboviruses to humans.

Pathogenesis of the Mosquito Bite

The mouthparts of the adult female mosquito are adapted for piercing flesh and sucking the blood needed by the female for the production of eggs. During the act of feeding, the female repeatedly injects saliva, which produces the reaction that follows the bite.[16]

Although the mechanical damage induced by the feeding mosquito can cause pain and irritation, the immediate and delayed immune reactions are of greater concern. Individuals with no previous exposure to mosquitoes show neither immediate nor delayed reactions. After sensitization, a bite is followed by a small, flat wheal surrounded by a red flare, which appears within a few minutes and lasts about 1 hour, and is mediated by antibodies. The delayed reaction consists of itching, swelling, and reddening of the wound region. It may persist for days. Eventually loss of the delayed reaction and desensitization can develop after repeated exposures. Desensitization to one species does not necessarily extend to other members of the same genus and usually does not include protection against the bites of mosquitoes of other genera. The intense itching, primarily associated with the delayed reaction, encourages scratching and secondary infection of the wound site. Local anesthetics are useful for treating reactions to mosquito bites.[17-19]

Mosquito-Borne Viral Diseases- The New Plagues of the 21st Century

Viral diseases transmitted to and between humans have evolved with humanity from its existence. Yellow fever and its primary vector, *Aedes aegypti,* established itself throughout the tropics with the earliest voyages of exploration and colonization. In the U.S. and Europe, the rapid spread of several previously restricted viral diseases along with the invasion of a least two efficient vector species has occurred over the last 30 years.

Aedes albopictus, the Asian tiger mosquito, is a common species in Japan and Korea. Mosquito eggs, carried in used automobile tires, first invaded Houston, Texas where it was detected in 1985. From there it has spread throughout the continental U.S. and into Hawaii. By 1990, *Ae. albopictus* was established in Italy, by 1999 in France and 2007 in Germany. *Ae. (Ochlerotatus) japonicas,* the Asian rock pool mosquito, is also native to Japan and Korea. This invasive species was first detected in the northeastern U.S. in the late 1990's and has rapidly spread to most states east of the Mississippi River, plus Oregon, Washington and Hawaii and eastern Canada to the shores of Hudson's Bay. It is also established in Germany. Both species have become serious biting pests in urban and suburban backyards in the eastern U.S.

Yellow fever, caused by a flavivirus, has historically been one of the most serious and widespread of the arboviral infections. The virus causes a severe hemorrhagic disease, characterized by high fever, jaundice, and prostration. Case fatality during epidemics may exceed 10%. The yellow fever virus naturally infects monkeys and is maintained in a monkey-to-monkey sylvatic cycle by forest-dwelling mosquitoes. When the sylvatic cycle is disturbed (e.g., by wood cutters), humans can be bitten by one of the monkey-feeding vectors. When these individuals return to their villages and become viremic, the ubiquitous *Ae. aegypti* is able to initiate the urban cycle of transmission from person to person. An effective vaccine for yellow fever is available, and is usually required for travelers to endemic areas.

Dengue, another flavivirus, is an acute, usually non-fatal viral disease characterized by high fever, severe headache, backache, and arthralgia. It is commonly known as "breakbone fever." A hemorrhagic form of dengue is frequently fatal. *Ae. aegypti* is the usual vector of both the typical and the hemorrhagic forms of dengue, although other aedine mosquitoes, particularly *Ae. albopictus* may transmit the organism. In 2015, Brazil recorded over 1.5 million cases of dengue with nearly 500 deaths. There is no verified animal reservoir for dengue; several vaccine candidates, which are effective against all four serotypes of the virus, are being evaluated in clinical and field trials.[20, 21]

In the United States, the mosquito-borne viral encephalitides include St. Louis encephalitis (SLE), eastern equine encephalitis (EEE), and western equine encephalitis (WEE). They are viral diseases of wild birds transmitted by mosquitoes. Under certain conditions, normally ornithophilic mosquito species that had previously fed on viremic birds feed on humans or other mammals. St. Louis encephalitis may be transmitted by members of the *Culex pipiens* complex in urban areas, by *Cx. tarsalis* in rural areas in the western states, and by *Cx. nigripalpus* in Florida. *Cx. tarsalis* is the main vector of WEE in the West, and *Culiseta melanura* is one of the major vectors of EEE in the East.

Japanese encephalitis is transmitted by *Cx. tritaniorhynchus, Ae. togoi* and *Oc. japonicas* in the Orient. In Australia and New Guinea, Murray Valley encephalitis is transmitted by various *Culex* spp.. Rift Valley fever (RVF), an East African disease usually associated with wild animals and livestock, caused a serious epidemic in Egypt in 1977-1978, infecting millions. The viral agent of RVF has been assigned to the sand fly fever group of viruses and is probably transmitted in Egypt by *Cx. pipiens* and by other culex and aedes mosquitoes throughout the rest of Africa.

California group viruses, including LaCrosse virus, rarely cause epidemics. They are transmitted by the tree-hole breeding species *Oc. triseriatus* in the Midwestern United States.

West Nile virus is a member of the flavivirus group responsible for regular epidemics in human populations in Europe and Africa. It can also cause significant epizootics in birds. The 1999 outbreak of human encephalitis in New York associated with the West Nile (WNV) virus was the first isolation of this agent in the New World, and was concurrent with extensive mortality in crows and other corvids. The vector that transmitted WNV to people in the New York City environs was probably *Cu. pipiens.* This is the usual vector for bird-to-bird transmission. WNV has remained endemic in the U.S., and outbreaks in 2003-2004 were the largest on record, infecting an estimated 2 million people and killing countless wild birds. It is hypothesized that dry, hot spells of weather of more than two weeks favor such outbreaks in humans.

West Nile Virus vaccines have been developed for horses and are commercially availalble in the United States. A West Nile Virus vaccine protective for humans is undergoing final clinical evaluation. It has yet to be determined if a human vaccine will ever be mass-produced for general use.

To learn more about the ecology of West Nile virus and the vectors that transmits it, see www.medicalecology.org/diseases/westnile/westnile.htm.

Two serious arboviruses, both of African origin, invaded the Americas in the second decade of the 21st Century. Chikungunya, an alphavirus, had already been seen in Ravenna, Italy in 2007, but appeared in several islands of the Caribbean in 2013. Thereafter, hundreds of cases were imported into the U.S.. Efficient vectors like *Ae. aegypti* and *Ae. albopictus* are present in the U.S. and local transmission is probable. In 2013, Zika virus, another of the flavivirus group was reported in French Polynesia and in 2015 appeared in Mexico and Brazil. This virus is spreading rapidly through the Americas and although symptoms are normally mild, many cases of microcephaly in newborn babies, Guillain-Barre syndrome and acute disseminated encephalomyelitis, (ADEM) have been linked to these infections. Again, the primary vectors are the peridomestic mosquitoes, *Ae. aegypti* and *Ae.albopictus.*

Mosquito Control

The most effective method of mosquito control is reduction at the source (i.e., the elimination or modification of the aquatic sites at which the mosquitoes breed). Control may take the form of draining of impoundments, level control of large bodies of water, the clearing or filling of ditches, or the elimination of human-made containers. Methodology must be tailored to the specific breeding requirements of the species. The general use of chemical insecticides has obvious potential for deleterious side effects. Given the serious nature of many of the mosquito-borne diseases, insecticide use may be required where reduction at the source is inadequate. Larvicides can be applied to breeding sites. Under extreme conditions, pesticides can be directed against adult mosquitoes.

The most common and effective method of malaria control employs insecticides applied to the walls of houses. Anopheline malaria vectors tend to rest on walls after feeding; they then come in contact with the residual insecticide and die. Consequently, insecticides applied to the insides of walls affect only those mosquitoes that have fed on humans and are potentially infected. This scheme does little to reduce mosquito populations and usually has little environmental impact; it does, however, reduce the incidence of malaria by interrupting transmission of the disease. DDT was effectively used in house spraying programs for several decades. In addition to toxicity to resting mosquitoes, this insecticide produced a repellant effect that discouraged mosquitoes from entering treated houses. Bed nets, with or without insecticide impregnation, can provide significant protection from feeding mosquitoes.

The periurban vectors of dengue, chikungunya and Zika virus, *Ae. aegypti, Ae. albopictus* and *Oc. japonicas* are most effectively controlled by removing or destroying their breeding sites. Disposal of used automobile tires and tin cans, clearing gutters of standing water, covering rain barrels, and generally denying water containers to mosquito breeding is an important first step.

Control of *Aedes aegypti*, the primary vector of Zika Virus, has taken a significant leap forward with the demonstration that the release of genetically modified male mosquitos can significantly reduce populations of this species. Field trials of the strategy in Panama, Brazil, and the Cayman Islands have been particularly promising with vector population reductions of over 90%. The U.S. Food and Drug Administration has approved a field trial to be conducted in a suburb of Key West, Florida. In its approval the FDA noted that the program presents "no significant environmental impact". However, a coalition of environmental public interest groups has mounted a major campaign to block the field trials. If successful, the use of genetically modified sterile male mosquitos could provide an environmentally friendly method for controlling this important vector without the use of insecticides.

Recent studies have shown that oral ivermectin given to humans and domestic animals will kill anopheline mosquitoes, notably the major African vector *An gambiae,* and could have a major effect on vector populations and malaria transmission. Systemic ivermectin appears to cause mortality in female *Ae. aegypti* and *Ae.* albopictus, but does not cause mortality in *Culex* mosquitoes.[22]

A number of effective mosquito repellents are available as sprays or lotions. When applied according to direction, they can reduce the annoyance caused by the insects. The most effective repellents usually contain DEET.

Tabanidae: Horse and Deer flies

The Tabanidae are a large family of blood-sucking dipterans with a cosmopolitan distribution. They are robust flies, ranging in size from 7 to 30 mm in length, and are locally referred to as horse flies, deer flies, mango flies, or greenheads. Tabanids are strong fliers, capable of inflicting painful bites, and in some areas of the world are considered serious pests of humans and animals. Flies of the genus *Chrysops* act as vectors of the filarial eye worm *Loa loa* in Africa and may be involved in the mechanical transmission of anthrax, tularemia, and *Trypanosoma evansi*.

Historical Information

Tabanids were implicated in the transmission of anthrax as early as 1874, and of *T. evansi* in 1913. The role of tabanids as intermediate hosts and vectors of *Loa loa* was verified in 1914 by Robert Leiper.[23]

Life Cycle

Tabanids usually lay eggs on vegetation near moist areas. Their larvae develop in water or wet earth and pass through four to nine stages. In some species the larvae remain dormant during the winter. Pupation occurs in dry earth, and the quiescent pupal stage may last 2-3 weeks. Adult females feed on blood and the males on plant juices.

Pathogenesis

Tabanid mouthparts are short and blade-like. During the act of biting, the insect inflicts a deep, painful wound, causing blood to flow. The fly then ingests blood from the freshly formed pool. Individuals can become sensitized to tabanid bites and suffer severe allergic reactions after attack.

Tabanids act as efficient mechanical vectors of several pathogens. They are easily disturbed during feeding. They fly to another host and begin the process anew. Consequently, the fly's mouthparts can readily transfer organisms to the next host after contamination on the first. Bacteria causing anthrax and tularemia, the protozoan *T. evansi*, and the retrovirus agents of bovine leukemia and equine infectious anemia may be transmitted by the tabanid flies, which act as mechanical vectors.

Loa loa is transmitted by African tabanids of the genus *Chrysops*, which include *C. silacea* and *C. dimidiata*. Microfilariae of the worm, ingested by female flies with the blood meal, develop in the flight muscles. When they reach maturity, they migrate to the mouthparts and are deposited on the skin of a new host when the fly feeds again. Infectious larvae burrow into the skin of the host after the fly has abandoned the bite wound.

Control

Tabanids are difficult to control because of their diverse breeding sites. Larvae are sensitive to DDT and other insecticides, but these compounds are seldom used. Sensitive individuals should consider using repellents to avoid bites. Mosquito repellents containing DEET are usually effective.

Muscidae: The Housefly and Its Relatives

The muscoid flies include insects that are important as blood-sucking pests, vectors of diseases, and mechanical vectors of a variety of pathogenic organisms.[24, 25] Some better-known members of this family are the housefly *Musca domestica*, the stable fly *Stomoxys calcitrans*, and the tsetse flies of the genus *Glossina*.

Life Cycle

Musca domestica (Fig. 38.10), the ubiquitous housefly, lays her eggs on any matter that will serve as food for the developing maggots. Animal or human feces, garbage, decaying plant material, and sewage all provide suitable substrates. A single fly lays more than 1,000 eggs during her life span. The development from eggs to adults requires less than 10 days at summer temperatures. As a result of this reproductive potential, summer fly populations can be enormous. These flies can carry viruses, bacteria, protozoa, and the eggs of parasitic worms and are a serious public health problem.[27, 28] The presence of large fly populations is a clear indicator of poor sanitation.

Stable flies

Stomoxys calcitrans is a serious biting pest usually associated with domestic animal husbandry. The fly lays her eggs in moist, decaying vegetable material (e.g., hay, alfalfa, straw, and manure). In suburban communities, moist piles of grass clippings and weeds provide ideal sites for larval development. The egg-to-adult period during the summer lasts about 4 weeks, and a female may lay as many as 400 eggs during her life span.

Although superficially similar in appearance to houseflies, stable flies have a prominent proboscis, which both sexes use effectively for sucking blood. The bite of the stable

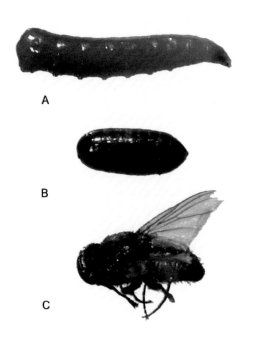

Figure 38.10. *Musca domestica*, the housefly. A. Larva. B. Pupa. C. Adult. The larvae of flies are referred to as maggots.

Most muscoids are fairly large, robust dipterans. They develop from eggs to maggots (larvae), non-motile pupae, and adults by complete metamorphosis. Only the tsetse flies differ, in that their larvae develop singly within the female and are deposited fully developed and ready for pupation.

Historical Information

One of the plagues of Egypt described in the Old Testament consisted of swarms of flies. It appears that humans have been troubled by these insects throughout history. In 1895 David Bruce demonstrated the role of the tsetse fly as the vector of African trypanosomiasis, and the importance of houseflies as disseminators of various pathogens was outlined in 1898 by Veeder.[25, 26]

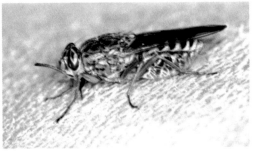

Figure 38.11. *Glossina* spp. tsetse fly feeding on blood. Courtesy of J. Gingrich.

fly is initially painful but usually causes little delayed reaction. Sensitized individuals develop allergic responses to repeated bites. Stomoxys serves as a mechanical vector for anthrax and some trypanosomes of animals.[26]

Tsetse Flies

Tsetse flies of the genus *Glossina* occur in Sub-Saharan Africa, where they are the intermediate hosts and vectors of a number of trypanosomes infecting humans and animals (Fig. 38.11). Tsetse flies differ markedly from muscoid flies, and indeed from most insects, in that they produce only one egg at a time. This single egg is retained within the "uterus" of the female, where it hatches. The larva develops in three stages "in utero" while feeding on "milk" produced by accessory glands of the female. Eventually, a fully mature larva is deposited in a shady location, and it pupates immediately. The pupal stage can last up to 30 days and the resulting adult remains inactive for 1-2 days after emerging before seeking its first blood meal. Both male and female tsetse flies are exclusively hematophagous, and both sexes are capable of transmitting trypanosomes.[29, 30]

A female tsetse produces 10-15 larvae during her life span. Tsetse populations are relatively small and dispersed. *Glossina* hunt by sight and follow animals, humans, or even vehicles for long distances. They feed during the day, usually along paths or riverbanks. *G. palpalis* and *G. tachinoides* are the main vectors of *Trypanosoma brucei gambiense*; *G. morsitans*, *G. swynnertoni*, and *G. pallidipes* are the primary vectors of *T. b. rhodesiense*.

Calliphoridae, Cuterebridae, and Sarcophagidae:

Myiasis-Causing Flies

Not all dipterans inflict damage by the bite of adult flies seeking blood. The larvae

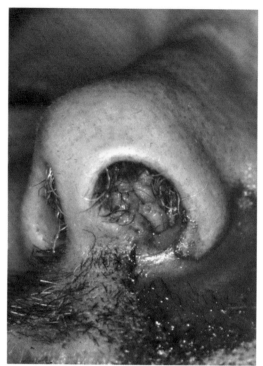

Figure 38.12. *Sarcophaga* larvae *in situ* (Courtesy of Y. Mumcouglu. In Mumcouglu Y, Rufli Th: Dermatologische Entomologie. Perimed Fachbuch, Erlangen, 1982).

of several families are pathogenic during their development within the tissues of the infested host. This infestation with larvae, or maggots, is known as myiasis.[31] Certain species of flies are obligate parasites and require living tissue for development. Other species develop facultatively in either living or dead tissues. A third group can cause accidental myiasis when their eggs, deposited on foodstuffs, are ingested. Cheese-skippers of the family Piophilidae, rat-tailed larvae of the Syrphidae, soldier fly larvae of the Stratiomyidae, and several species of the Muscidae cause gastrointestinal myiasis. Symptoms are proportional to the number of larvae developing and include nausea and vomiting. Diagnosis requires the finding of living or dead maggots in the vomitus, aspirates of gastrointestinal contents, or stool specimens.

Species of flies that normally favor decaying flesh for larval development occasionally deposit eggs or larvae on wounds or ulcers (Fig. 38.12).

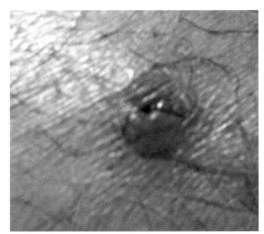

Figure 38.13. Myiasis: note the opening (black spot) in the skin which permits the maggot, burrowing in the tissue below, to breathe.

Maggot therapy is the use of the larvae of certain fly species for selectively debriding non-healing necrotic skin and soft tissue wounds.[32] In 2004, the US Food and Drug Administration began regulating the medicinal use of maggots.[33, 34] In Europe, approximately 30,000 maggot treatments are applied annually.

The flesh flies of the family Sarcophagidae contain several members of the genera *Wohlfahrtia* and *Sarcophaga*, which cause myiasis. Female flies in this family do not lay eggs, but deposit freshly hatched first-stage larvae directly in wounds, ulcers, or even unbroken skin. These feeding larvae may cause considerable tissue damage.

Flies of the family Cuterebridae are obligate parasites, usually of wild and domestic animals. Human myiasis due to infestation with maggots of *Cuterebra*, normally associated with rodents, is not uncommon in the United States. This condition usually presents as individual larvae developing on various parts of the body (Fig. 38.13). *Dermatobia hominis*, the human botfly, parasitizes a number of mammals and is a serious pest of cattle in Central and South America. Flies of this species cause infestation in a unique manner. Female dermatobia flies capture various blood-sucking arthropods (usually mosquitoes or other flies), lay their eggs on

the abdomens of their prey, and release these insects. When the fly or the mosquito carrying the eggs alights on a warm-blooded host, the eggs hatch, immediately liberating larvae onto the skin of the host. These maggots penetrate the skin and develop in the subcutaneous tissue, maintaining contact with the surface through a small opening in the center of an abscess-like swelling (Fig. 38.13). When the larvae complete their development after 6-12 weeks, they emerge, fall to the ground, and pupate. During the phase within the tissues, the maggots can cause intermittent pain and secrete a foul-smelling material from the opening in the skin.

For human infestations, each maggot should be removed surgically. Particular care must be taken not to damage it during the procedure because the patient has usually become sensitized to the antigens of the maggot. The maggots can also be removed by coating their external spiracles with petroleum jelly, which blocks access to oxygen. They are thus forced to crawl to the surface. They may then have to be removed surgically, under local anesthesia, and the wound left open and allowed to heal by secondary intention.

Several species of the family Calliphori-

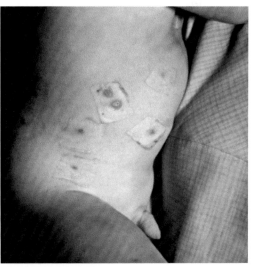

Figure 38.14. Myiasis. Maggots of *Cordylobia anthropophaga* in the flesh of an infant. Note the raised area and opening for the larvae to breath.

dae are obligate parasites, whereas others cause only accidental myiasis. *Cordylobia anthropophaga,* the tumbu fly, is a larval parasite of humans and other animals, especially rats, in Africa. These flies lay eggs on soil contaminated with urine or feces or on similarly soiled bedding or clothing that is set out to dry. The emerging larvae attach themselves to any host with whom they come in contact and penetrate the skin. After penetration, larvae cause individual tender abscess-like swellings from which serous fluid exudes, particularly when pressure is applied to the lesion (Fig. 38.14). Treatment consists in covering the wound with petroleum jelly to force the maggot to the surface in search of oxygen. The maggot can then be gently squeezed out. Surgical excision is necessary for some infestations.

Another African species, the Congo floor maggot, *Auchmeromyia luteola,* feeds preferentially on humans. The fly lays eggs on the floor of huts. The maggots come out of the soil at night to feed on the blood of the inhabitants of the hut who sleep on the floor. The larvae lacerate the victim and suck blood but do not penetrate tissues, returning to the soil after taking their blood meal.

Two species of *Cochliomyia,* the New World screwworm, occasionally cause myiasis in humans in North and South America, although these flies are primarily parasites of animals. Adult females lay their eggs around the edges of wounds, and the larvae invade the wounds and macerate the traumatized tissues. Large numbers of maggots can infest a single wound. Because infestations of the nose can be fatal, the maggots should be removed surgically as soon as they are detected.

Flies of the genus *Chrysomyia,* the Old World screwworm, are important causes of human and animal myiasis throughout Asia and Africa. Chrysomyia larvae penetrate wounds or mucous membranes, primarily affecting areas around the eyes, ears, mouth, and nose.

Green bottle flies (*Lucilia* spp.) and blue bottle flies (*Calliphora* spp.) sometimes infest wounds of humans in Asia, Africa, and the Americas. The larvae of these species prefer dead tissue; in the past, these maggots, reared free of pathogens, were used therapeutically for cleansing septic wounds.[35-37] A number of flies whose larvae are primarily parasites of domestic animals occasionally infest humans. Larvae of the sheep botfly (*Oestrus ovis*) may invade nasal cavities of shepherds and cause severe frontal headaches.[38] Such larvae do not complete their development because humans are aberrant hosts, so the larvae usually exit spontaneously before maturation.

Cattle warbles of the genus *Hypoderma* occasionally infest humans, causing a condition similar to creeping eruption. Larvae penetrate exposed skin and wander aimlessly, causing severe itching, pain, and sleeplessness. Surgical removal of the larvae from the ends of their burrows is recommended.

Larvae of various flies, particularly of the genera *Calliphora, Phaenicia,* and *Cochliomyia,* infest a cadaver in a predictable succession. The science of forensic entomology has developed the use of flies and, to a lesser extent, beetle larvae to determine the manner, time, and place of death; it uses entomologic information to support pathologic findings in

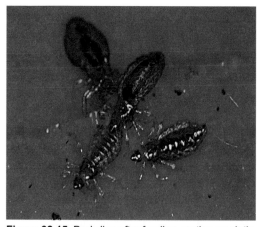

Figure 38.15. Body lice after feeding, resting on cloth.

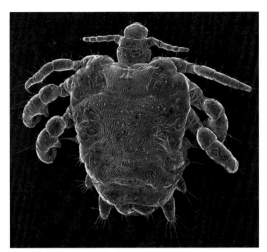

Figure 38.16. Crab louse. Photo David Scharf.

legal proceedings.[24-26, 39-41]

Anoplura: Sucking Lice

Three species of lice infest humans as obligate, blood-feeding ectoparasites. Only one of them, the body louse, is important in human medicine as the vector of the rickettsiae of epidemic typhus and trench fever and the spirochetes of relapsing fever. Louse infestation is known as pediculosis.[42]

The body louse, *Pediculus humanus humanus* (Fig. 38.15), and its close relative, the head louse, *P. humanis capitis*, are wingless, elongate, dorsoventrally flattened insects, 2.5-4.0 mm long. They have three pairs of legs of about equal length. Their mouthparts are adapted for piercing flesh and sucking blood. The crab louse, *Phthirus pubis* (Fig. 38.16), is shorter (0.8-1.2 mm) and, as its common name implies, resembles a crab. Crab lice have somewhat reduced front legs, with the second and third leg pairs stout and strongly clawed. All lice undergo development characterized by incomplete metamorphosis.

Historical Information

The association between humans and lice is an ancient one and probably represents an evolutionary relationship begun by lice and ancestral hominids. Closely related species of lice infest gorillas and monkeys. Humans have certainly been aware of the discomforts of louse infestation from the earliest times, and the condition has been recorded by poets and artists as well as by early writers on science and medicine. The recognition of body lice as disease vectors is more recent. Transmission of typhus and relapsing fever by lice was not demonstrated until the early 1900s.

Lice have been considered variously as unwelcome pests or a sign of unclean habits. They have often been accepted as one of life's unavoidable afflictions. As vectors of diseases, body lice have, on numerous occasions determined the outcome of human history. Zinsser, in 1935, and Busvine, in 1976, chronicled empires and even entire civilizations that were profoundly changed by epidemics of louse-borne typhus.[43, 44]

Life Cycles

The life cycles of the human lice are depicted in Figure 38.17. The crab louse, *P. pubis*, sometimes referred to as *papillion d'amour*, usually inhabits the hairs of the pubic and perianal regions of the body but can also be found on axillary hair or on moustaches, beards, eyebrows, or eyelashes. Adult crab lice are sedentary, often clutching the same hairs for days while feeding for hours at a time. Lice of all stages and both sexes feed solely on blood. They must obtain daily blood meals to survive. The female lays individual eggs or nits (approximately 0.6 mm in length) and attaches them to hairs of the host (Fig. 38.18). They embryonate and hatch over 6-8 days. The louse has three nymphal (pre-adult) stages, lasting 15-17 days, before the final molt to the adult stage. Nymphs are tiny, sexually immature versions of the adults. Adult crab lice live less than one month, and the females usually lay fewer than 50 eggs during their lifetime. The entire life cycle

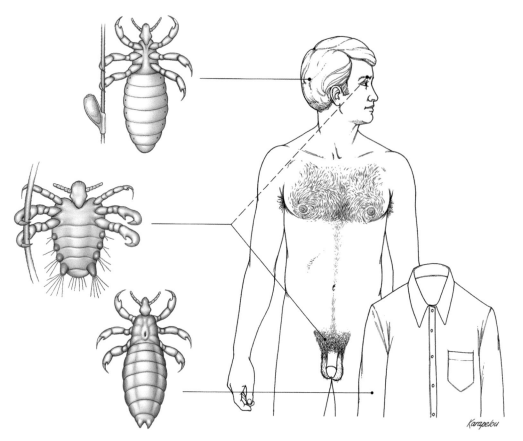

Figure 38.17. Preferred feeding and resting sites of the three species of louse affecting humans. *Pediculus humanus capitis*, the head louse, resides, feeds, and reproduces on the hairs of the head. Eggs are laid individually on hair shafts. *Phthirus pubis*, the crab louse, prefers hair of the pubic regions but is occasionally found on the eyebrows, eyelashes, beard, or moustache. Eggs are attached to the individual hairs. *Pediculus humanus humanus*, the body louse, is usually found on clothing, moving to the body of the human host only to feed. Eggs are laid in masses in the seams of the clothing of the host.

(i.e., egg-to-egg interval) lasts 22-27 days.[32, 45, 46]

Crab lice are most frequently transmitted from one person to another by sexual contact. However, general physical contact or contact with a variety of contaminated objects such as toilet seats, clothing, or bedding can also result in infestation.

The head louse, *P. humanus capitis*, inhabits the hairs of the head, particularly behind the ears and around the occiput. Heavy infestations may force head lice to establish themselves on other hairy parts of the body. Like the crab lice, the head lice are relatively sedentary, feeding for hours at a time while clutching firmly to hair; like the crab lice, they seldom leave the hairy regions voluntarily. The eggs are attached to hair shafts and hatch within approximately one week; the three nymphal stages are completed within less than 14 days. The egg-to-egg cycle lasts about three weeks. A head louse lays 50-150 eggs during her lifetime. Despite the common misperception, head lice are disseminated by physical contact with the hair of an infected person, and tend not to move to inanimate objects. Head lice are not typically spread by sharing of hats, scarves, or by the common storage of garments.[47]

Although head lice have been shown to be capable of transmitting rickettsiae and spirochetes in the laboratory, they are usually not

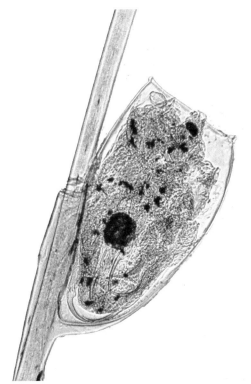

Figure 38.18. Nit of a louse attached to a shaft of hair.

involved in the transmission of these organisms under natural conditions.

The life cycle of the body louse, *P. humanus humanus*, differs significantly from those of the other two in that body lice spend much of their lives on the clothing of infested individuals. Body lice (commonly referred to as "cooties") are usually found on clothing wherever it comes into close contact with the body. Although body lice in all stages of their development must move to the body for regular blood meals, they return to the cloth-

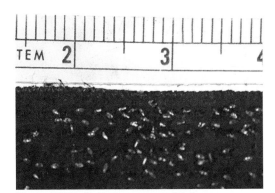

Figure 38.19. Body lice eggs on fabric.

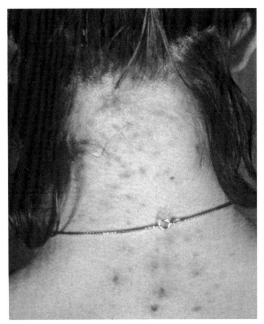

Figure 38.20. Louse bites

ing after feeding. The lice lay eggs along the seams of garments attached to cloth fibers and sometimes attach the eggs to some of the coarser body hairs (Fig. 38.19). Eggs kept near the body hatch within 5-7 days. Nymphs require about 18 days to mature, and the adult lice live for about a month. A body louse lays more than 300 eggs during her lifetime.

Body lice are readily transmitted between individuals by physical contact, exchanges of clothing, or the common storage of infested garments. They are the only vectors of louse-borne relapsing fever, trench fever, and epidemic typhus.

Pathogenesis

Lice inject salivary fluids into the wound during ingestion of blood. These secretions induce varying degrees of sensitization in the human host.

Clinical Disease

The usual characteristic of infestation by all types of lice is intense itching. Constant scratching can lead to secondary bacterial infection of the wound. Crab lice produce characteristic "blue spots", which are often seen around the eyes of individuals with infested lashes. The bites of head lice result in inflammatory papules and impetiginous lesions often associated with lymphadenopathy (Fig. 39.20). Heavy infestations of head lice can cause a condition in which hair, eggs, louse feces, and exudates of bite wounds form a cap-like mass teeming with lice. There may be secondary fungal infection within the mass.[48] Children infested with head lice often appear restless.

Bites by body lice cause pinpoint macules, excoriations, and pigmentation of the skin. "Vagabond's disease" is an extreme condition caused by a combination of persistent heavy infestation and poor personal hygiene. Affected individuals show a generalized bronze pigmentation and hardening of the skin.[49]

Diagnosis

The diagnosis depends on identification of lice or eggs in the hair or in the seams of garments. In the latter, they may be difficult to find. The eggs must be identified by microscopy. For the detection of head lice it is critical to employ the wet combing approach as it has a much higher sensitivity for detecting active infestation.[50]

Treatment

There are several formulations available as dusts, shampoos, lotions, and creams. Some may be obtained as over-the-counter preparations, and others require a prescription. All of the effective products contain low concentrations of insecticides such as benzene hexachloride, pyrethrum, or synthetic pyrethrum analogues.[51]

Head and crab lice can be treated similarly. Infested individuals should remove all clothing, apply the pediculicide, and put on clean clothing after treatment. The procedure should be repeated after 10 days to kill any newly hatched lice, as most treatments do not kill eggs. To prevent re-infestation, the clothing and bedding of infested individuals should be dry-cleaned or washed and dried by exposure to heat. Exposure of infested clothing to temperatures of 70° C for 30 minutes kills lice and eggs. Combs and brushes should also be treated by heat to prevent re-infestation by head lice. Simply washing the head or affected areas with soap does not kill lice or destroy the nits. Currently treatment with permethrin 5% cream applied to the entire body for 8-10 hours is recommended for treatment of body lice. Permethrin 1% is recommended for head lice. Benzene hexachloride (lindane, Kwell), although one of the most effective treatments for head lice, is now reserved for second line therapy due to concerns regarding its toxicity.[52] Oral ivermectin as a systemic insecticide has been suggested as an alternative therapy.[52-57] Insecticides should not be used on crab lice infesting eyebrows or lashes. Petrolatum should be applied thickly and individual lice removed with forceps.

Because body lice inhabit and lay eggs on clothing, regularly changing underwear and garments significantly reduces the infestation. Garments infested by lice should be treated as indicated above. Blankets, bedding, sleeping bags, and other items that might be contaminated should be similarly treated.

Various powdered formulations of pediculicides can be applied directly to clothed individuals. Several of these compounds have been used effectively for mass treatment of large groups of infested individuals to control epidemic typhus. Nit combs, hair combs with teeth spaced closely enough to scrape the louse eggs (nits) from the hair, can be effective if used thoroughly and repeatedly. All nits must be removed to prevent re-infestation.

Epidemiology

The three species of human lice can be considered cosmopolitan in distribution, with infestations recorded throughout tropical, temperate, and Arctic regions. The absence of lice in a population is a result of social or hygienic habits rather than of geographic or climatic factors.

The rates of infestations with crab lice are usually much lower than those for head or body lice. Infestations with head lice can reach epidemic proportions, particularly among schoolchildren.[58, 59]

Infestations with body lice are usually associated with poverty, crowded conditions, social upheavals such as wars, or natural disasters. Because body lice reside and deposit eggs on clothing, conditions that prevent changing and cleaning garments coupled with close contact and crowding foster the spread of these insects.

Louse-Borne Diseases

Body lice are the only vectors involved in infecting humans with *Rickettsia prowazeki*, which causes epidemic typhus, *Rochalimaea quintana*, the rickettsial agent of trench fever; and *Borrelia recurrentis*, the spirochete that causes louse-borne relapsing fever.[60]

The rickettsiae multiply within the louse in the epithelial cells of the midgut, which ultimately rupture, releasing large numbers of these microorganisms. Human infections occur by rubbing infected louse feces into skin abrasions caused by the original louse bites. Scratching often extends these abrasions. Inhalation of fomites containing rickettsiae also causes human infection. Rickettsiae survive dehydration and remain infective for over two months at warm temperatures.

Humans are the usual reservoir for the rickettsiae of epidemic typhus. The organism can remain latent for years, occasionally giving rise to a mild recrudescent form of typhus termed Brill-Zinsser disease. Lice feeding on people with this form of typhus can become infected with the rickettsiae and transmit them to non-immune individuals, giving rise to the primary epidemic form of the disease. Studies have demonstrated a sylvan cycle of *R. prowazeki* in flying squirrels in the United States, but the importance of this rodent reservoir in the spread of typhus is yet to be determined.

Trench fever is a self-limiting disease caused by *Bartonella quintana*. Transmission to humans is similar to that of epidemic typhus. Individuals with trench fever can infect lice from the third day of illness and sometimes for months thereafter. The rickettsiae develop only within the cuticular margin of the louse gut (i.e., not intracellularly) and cause no disease in the insect. Infected feces and crushed lice are the usual sources of infection. The human is the only animal in which this rickettsia causes disease.

Louse-borne relapsing fever is caused by the spirochete *B. recurrentis*. The body louse is the only vector of *B. recurrentis*, although similar spirochetes cause tick-borne relapsing fevers. Lice are infected when feeding on infected individuals during febrile periods. The spirochetes invade the epithelium of the gut and ultimately the blood of the louse. Transmission can occur only when crushed lice are rubbed into a wound or are inhaled. Lice do not pass the spirochete by biting and do not excrete it in feces.

Siphonaptera: The Fleas

The Siphonaptera comprise a small order of insects of generally similar appearance and habits. The adult fleas exist as ectoparasites on warm-blooded animals. The typical adult flea is a brown, laterally compressed, wingless insect with a tough skin, usually less than 3 mm long. Its third pair of legs is adapted for jumping, and it has mouthparts designed for blood-sucking.

Fleas undergo complete metamorphosis in their development, exhibiting markedly different larva, pupa, and adult stages. The larvae are delicate, motile, vermiform creatures; the pupae are encapsulated and quiescent.

Fleas cause diseases in humans as serious biting pests and as vectors of a number of infectious agents, most notably the agent of bubonic plague, *Yersinia pestis*. Fleas usually feed quickly and to repletion at a single site.

Historical Information

Humans have evolved with these "lair" parasites of domestic animals and fellow cave dwellers. Literature is replete with songs, poems, and stories extolling the virtues and vices of fleas and the miseries they cause. The importance of fleas as vectors was not recognized until the final years of the nineteenth century, when they were implicated in the transmission of plague. The historical impact of flea-borne bubonic plague, or Black Death, in the development of civilization, has been well documented.[43, 44]

Life Cycle

The life cycle of a typical flea is shown in Figure 38.3. Fleas are usually parasites of animals inhabiting nests, dens, or caves. The

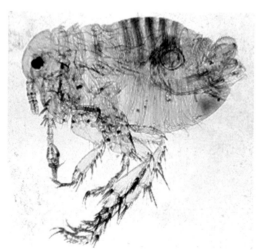

Figure 38.21. *Pulex irritans*

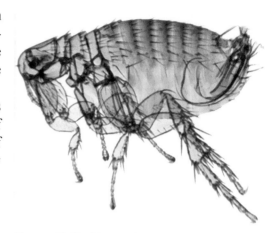

Figure 38.22. *Xenopsylla cheopis*, an important vector of Bubonic Plague.

adult flea is an obligate parasite of its warm-blooded host, feeding only on blood. The flea scatters its eggs in and around the nest of its host. Larval fleas are active, yellowish-white creatures with biting mouthparts. They feed on host feces or on dried blood defected by adult fleas. Under ideal conditions of temperature and humidity, eggs can embryonate and hatch in less than a week; larvae develop to adults in less than two weeks. After the flea has developed through three larval stages, it spins a cocoon and forms a quiescent pupa. The period of pupation, during which the insect gradually develops its adult characteristics, may last from a week to a year depending on the species and the environmental conditions. The pupa, encased in its cocoon, can remain dormant for months. The quiescent adult, encased in the pupal cocoon is stimulated to emerge by detecting vibrations in the local environment, thus giving rise to a hungry adult flea.

Although many species of fleas bite humans if the insects are sufficiently hungry, only a small number are consistent human pests. The combless fleas, so called because they lack prominent spines (ctenidia) on their heads, include several species that regularly feed on humans.

The human flea *Pulex irritans* (Fig. 38.21) is an ectoparasite of humans and animals, particularly swine. *P. irritans* is cosmopolitan in distribution and is the most common flea affecting humans. A closely related species, *P. simulans*, is restricted to the New World. Both species are capable of transmitting plague, but are considered minor vectors of this disease.

The oriental rat flea, *Xenopsylla cheopis* (Fig. 38.22), as the vector of *Y. pestis*, has long been considered one of the great killers of humankind. It is an ectoparasite of rats, feeding on humans only when its customary host is unavailable. Classically, human bubonic plague is a consequence of an epizootic outbreak of plague in the rat population. As rats die in massive numbers, infected fleas leave their dead hosts and seek fresh sources of blood. Under these circumstances, humans are readily attacked and infected.

Xenopsylla acts as an efficient vector because of its association with reservoir rats and its readiness to feed on humans. When a flea takes a blood meal from an infected rat, the plague organism rapidly multiplies within the flea's proventriculus, an organ of the intestinal tract lined with spiny projections. Within three days, the proventriculus is blocked by a gelatinous mass of partially digested blood and bacteria. When the flea feeds again, it is unable to engorge and is forced to regurgitate the blood and bacteria from the proventricu-

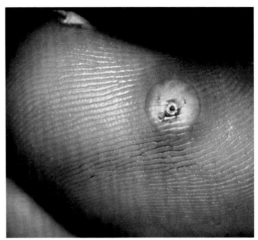

Figure 38.24. *Tunga penetrans* in skin. Courtesy G. Zalar.

lus into the host. Because the flea is unable to feed completely, it moves from host to host, repeatedly attempting to feed without attaining satisfaction, and transmitting the plague organism as it goes. The flea eventually dies of starvation, but not before its role as a vector of plague has been discharged.

The combed fleas also include species that affect humans. The dog and cat fleas, *Ctenocephalides canis* and *C. felis* (Fig. 38.23), are closely related, morphologically similar species, with two sets of prominent combs on the head. Both species feed equally well on dogs and cats, and both bite humans if given the opportunity. Their larvae and pupae are usually found in the places where the animals rest. The fleas can prove particularly annoy-

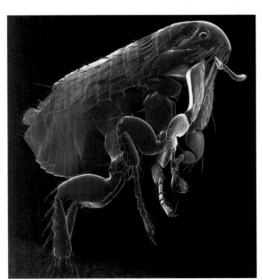

Figure 38.23. *Ctenocephalides felis.* Photo D. Scharf.

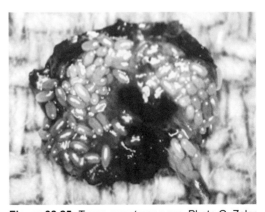

Figure 38.25. *Tunga penetrans* eggs. Photo G. Zalar

ing when the pet leaves the household and the fleas have humans as their only source of blood. Raccoons can also bring dog or cat fleas into homes, often by building their nests in chimneys.

The northern rat flea, *Nosopsyllus fasciatus*, and the squirrel flea, *Diamanus montanus*, are common combed fleas of rodents in North America. They readily bite humans and may be involved in transmission of plague from wild rodents to rats or humans.

Tunga penetrans, known as the chigger flea or chigoe, is a serious pest in the tropical and subtropical regions of the Americas, Africa, and the Indian subcontinent.[61-65] This flea originated in South America and was introduced into Africa during the late nineteenth century. Adult chigoes are less than 1 mm long. Both sexes feed regularly on blood. After insemination, the female flea attaches itself to the skin of the toes, soles of the feet, or the legs, and becomes enveloped by host tissue (Fig. 38.24). Thus protected, the female swells to the size of a pea, produces 150-200 eggs (Fig. 38.25), and dies still embedded in the tissue.[66, 67] The infested tissue can become ulcerated and infected by bacteria, possibly including the clostridia, and cause tetanus or gas gangrene. Auto-amputation of toes is not uncommon. Wearing shoes is usually an effective means of preventing infection with *T. penetrans*. Treatment consists in removing the flea with a sterile instrument and treating the wound locally to prevent infection.

Pathogenesis

The response to repeated flea bites is typical of reactions to most insect bites. Initial exposure produces little or no reaction, but after an individual is sensitized to the salivary antigens of the flea, first delayed reactions and then primary reactions develop.

Clinical Disease

Intense irritation that leads to scratching and secondary bacterial infections is the main manifestation of flea bites. The major health problem caused by fleas is the transmission of infectious agents for which the fleas are vectors.

Diagnosis

The typical fleabite first appears as a single papule. With heavy flea infestations, papules may be grouped along the arms and legs, on the face and neck, or where clothing fits snugly. Precise incrimination of fleas requires capture of one of the offending insects. The species of the flea can be determined with the aid of a dissecting microscope and a key to identifying fleas that affect humans.

Treatment

Pruritus can be treated symptomatically. Secondary bacterial infection is medicated as appropriate.

Control

Fleas can be controlled at the source of the infestation by various commercially available insecticides. Dusts should be applied to the fur and beds of dogs and cats. These dusts are particularly effective against the fleas that dwell in nests, whose larvae feed on particles. Space sprays can be effective against adult fleas. Pets can be treated for flea infestations topically or with systemic compounds that are lethal to the feeding insect. A number of topically applied repellents can protect individuals against fleabites for short periods.

Epidemiology of Flea-Borne Diseases

Fleas serve as primary vectors of *Yersinia*

pestis, the agent of the plague, and *Rickettsia typhi*, which causes murine or endemic typhus. Fleas can serve as intermediate hosts of various cestodes and nematodes that infect mammals, including humans.

Yersinia pestis persists in nature in a so-called sylvan or campestral cycle in which wild rodents are constantly infected by various species of fleas. Foci of naturally infected rodents occur in central Asia, South Africa, South America, and the Russian steppes. In western North America, plague is maintained in a ground squirrel reservoir with the squirrel flea, *Diamanus montanus*, as the vector. A number of other rodent species and flea vectors may also be involved. The United States reports 5-10 autochthonous cases of bubonic plague each year, usually among campers, hunters, and farmers in the western states. As long as plague exists as a disease of field rodents, human cases are rare. When the plague is transferred from wild rodents to peridomestic rats and becomes established in a rat-rat flea cycle, the potential for human infection increases markedly. The epidemiology of murine typhus has been clarified with the demonstration that *R. typhi* can be transmitted transovarially from an infected flea to her progeny.[68]

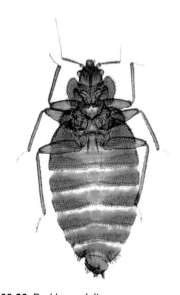

Figure 38.26. Bed bug adult.

Hemiptera: Bugs

Hemiptera include two subclasses, Homopteria and Heteropteria, known as true bugs. This large order contains two families of medical importance. Adults of most heteropterans are winged; the wingless bed bugs, the Cimicidae, are an exception. Bugs have mouthparts modified for piercing and sucking. Their long, slender, segmented beak is usually held along the ventral surface of the body when it is not in use. Most heteropterans are plant feeders, and some are predaceous on other insects; the ones that affect humans, the Reduviidae and Cimicidae are hematophagous. Heteroptera develop by incomplete metamorphosis.

Cimicidae: Bed Bugs

Three closely related species of bed bugs are blood-feeding ectoparasites of humans.[66] The common bed bug (*Cimex lectularius*) and the tropical bed bugs (*C. hemipterus* and *C. boueti*) are morphologically similar; they are oval, flattened, reddish-brown insects with mouth parts well-adapted for piercing flesh and sucking blood. Adult bed bugs (Fig. 38.26) have non-functional reduced wings. They are approximately 5 mm long and 3 mm wide. Their five nymphal stages are smaller, sexually immature copies of the adults.[67]

Bed bugs are cosmopolitan in distribution. *C. lectularius* is widespread throughout temperate and tropical regions. The Indian bed bug, *C. hemipterus*, is restricted to tropical and sub-tropical climates, and *C. boueti* is found in the tropical regions of Africa and South America.

Historical Information

Bed bugs evolved from ectoparasites of cave-dwelling mammals, probably bats, at the time when humans were also cave dwellers. They were first recorded as a problem in the Mediterranean region by early Greek and Roman writers. In northern Europe they were identified much later (e.g., during the eleventh century in England).[32, 44] Bed bugs have been suspected of transmitting a number of human diseases, but no direct evidence of involvement exists. Epidemiologic associations with hepatitis B virus transmission have not been verified experimentally.[69]

Life Cycle

Bed bugs are found in a variety of human habitations, including homes, hotels, dormitories, prisons, barracks, and hospitals. They remain hidden in cracks and crevices in walls, floors, and furniture, usually appearing at night or in dim light to feed on a sleeping host. Humans are the preferred source of blood, but bed bugs feed on a variety of animals if humans are unavailable. They characteristically bite three or four times in succession over a period of a few minutes to engorge themselves.

Adult females lay 2-3 eggs per day for a total of 200-500 during a lifetime. The pearly white eggs are 1 mm long. They are laid individually in crevices, behind loose wallpaper, in cracks in woodwork or furniture, or in mattresses. Hatching depends on temperature but usually occurs after 9-10 days of embryonation. There are five nymphal stages, each requiring a blood meal before molting to the next. The egg-to-egg period, depending on temperature, varies from 7 to 19 weeks, which allows the development of several genera-tions of bugs within a year. Availability of a blood source also influences generation time. Adult bugs feed weekly during the summer, less frequently during the cooler months, and starve during the winter, reappearing to feed again in the spring.

Pathogenesis

Feeding bed bugs inject salivary fluids to sensitize the host. Primary exposure produces little or no reaction. After repeated exposures a severe delayed reaction may develop; continued exposure produces an additional primary reaction. Finally, after a course of regular exposures to bites, the host can become desensitized.

Clinical Disease

Reactions to bites can be mild or severe. Large hemorrhagic bullae form on some sensitized individuals, whereas others develop erythema and local edema, and may experience severe, prolonged pruritus. Scratching can lead to secondary bacterial infections. Heavy bed bug infestations can interfere with sleep.

Diagnosis

The bite wounds are firm, closely spaced papules, appearing as three or four lesions together (Figs. 38.27, 38.28). This grouping

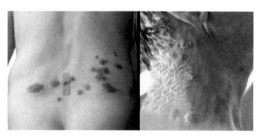

Figures 38.27 and 38.28. Bed bug bites:note hemorrhagic bullae and paired bitemarks.

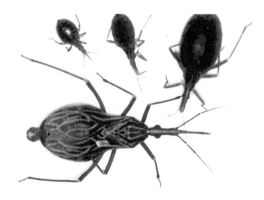

Figure 38.29. Kissing bug family of *Rhodnius prolixus*.

can be used to differentiate predation by bed bugs from the typically single bites of other insects. The final determination that bed bugs are involved depends on finding living or dead bugs or the circumstantial evidence of a characteristically pungent odor associated with the alarm glands of these insects and trails of blood droplets near the hiding places of the bugs.

Treatment

The itching associated with the bites of bed bugs responds to symptomatic therapy.

Control

Control in dwellings is best achieved with chemical insecticides. Residual compounds such as DDT and BHC are effective and long lasting, though generally not recommended. Resistance to these compounds has been reported in a number of areas, particularly in the tropics. Diazinon has been used successfully to treat infested surfaces. Removal of old furniture, mattresses, and loose wallpaper, as well as the patching of wall cracks can deny the bugs resting and breeding places.

Reduviidae: Assassin Bugs

Reduviidae is a large family of predaceous insects collectively referred to as assassin bugs, most members of which are insectivorous. One subfamily, the Triatominae, is found mainly in the New World and is of particular importance because its members are hematophagous and are vectors of Chagas disease.

Bugs of the Triatominae (Fig. 38.29), the so-called kissing bugs, cone-nosed bugs, or vinchucas, are large insects with distinct elongate cone-shaped heads. They possess a long, three-segment proboscis that has been well-developed for piercing skin; all developmental stages feed exclusively on blood. Adults are winged and are good fliers, whereas the nymphal stages are wingless, sexually immature miniatures of the adults, developing through the various stages by incomplete metamorphosis (Fig. 38.1).

Historical Information

The Triatominae received little attention from entomologists before 1909, at which point Carlos Chagas identified them as the vectors of *Trypanosoma cruzi*.[70]

Life Cycle

Three species of Triatominae serve as major vectors of Chagas disease, although several species are important as vectors in restricted areas and a large number of species have been found naturally infected with the parasite. *Panstrongylus megistus, Triatoma infestans*, and *Rhodnius prolixus* are large bugs that feed on humans as well as on wild or domestic animals whenever they are available. These insects abound in the cracks and crevices of the mud and timber houses typical of rural areas in the Latin American tropics. Kissing bugs are usually found in resting places near their source of blood meals. Domestic or peridomestic species that prey on humans are found in cracks and crevices of walls and floors, particularly in sleeping areas.

Adult females require a blood meal before producing a clutch of eggs. They lay eggs singly within the same cracks that harbor the nymphs and adults. The eggs hatch within 10-30 days, and each of the five nymphal stages requires a full blood meal before molting to the next. Kissing bugs are prodigious feeders. First-stage nymphs can ingest 12 times their weight in blood; subsequent stages drink relatively less. Fifth-stage nymphs of *R. prolixus* may ingest more than 300 µl of blood, and adult females may ingest more than 200 µl for each egg batch. The five nymphal stages may last several months before their final molt to the adult stage. Most species have one generation per year.

Pathogenesis

Intense, persistent pain is associated with the bites of some insectivorous assassin bugs, a result of injection of various toxins. The bites of most of the blood-feeding Triatominae are notably painless, enabling these insects to feed undisturbed on sleeping individuals. The habit of feeding around the mouth or eyes of a sleeper accounts for the designation "kissing bug." After sensitization to the salivary fluids of feeding bugs, individuals can develop delayed reactions characterized by itching, swelling, redness, nausea, and, in rare cases, anaphylaxis. This serious responses is a reported risk of xenodiagnosis, usually with *R. prolixus*.[71]

Both nymphs and adult bugs act as vectors of *T. cruzi*. Although bugs may be infected by feeding on human hosts and can transmit the organism from human to human, the usual sources of bug infection are wild and peridomestic animals (e.g., dogs, cats, mice, armadillos, and opossums). *T. cruzi* develops in the hindgut of the bug and does not invade the salivary glands. The bite of the bug does not cause infection. Rather, infectious parasites are passed in the feces of the bug while it feeds. The victim reacts to the irritation of the bite, then rubs the infected feces into the eyes, mouth, or the wound made by the bite. Various triatomine species regularly feed on infected animals, supporting growth of the parasite, but do not defecate until they leave the host. These species usually are not involved in transmission to humans, but may serve to maintain the parasite in an animal reservoir where infected bugs may be eaten by the animal host, which then becomes infected. *T. cruzi* is naturally maintained in wood rats in southern California by such a cycle. Although transmission of *T. cruzi* to humans is rare in

the United States, infected animals are found regularly, and autochthonous cases have been reported.[72-78]

Clinical Disease

Except for the allergic reaction to the bite, the bite itself is innocuous. The well recognized Romaña's sign, a unilateral swelling around the eye, occurs when organisms are introduced into the body through mucous membranes due to a person rubbing them into their eye. This swelling is due to the infecting trypanosomes and not the saliva of the reduviid bug. The importance of these bugs lies in their acting as vectors in Chagas disease.

Diagnosis

The night-feeding kissing bugs are insidious, leaving little initial evidence of their blood meal. Kissing bugs normally feed from one puncture, leaving a single papule. This point distinguishes the lesion from those caused by bed bugs, which also feed at night but whose bites are usually clustered in groups of two or three.

Most of the entomophagous bugs likely to bite humans are large insects; the wheel bug, a common offender with a distinctive cog-like crest on its thorax, is more than 30 mm long. Because they bite during the day, usually when handled, they can be readily identified.

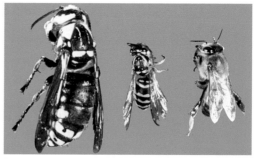

Figure 38.30. Stinging Insects: wasp, yellow jacket, honey bee.

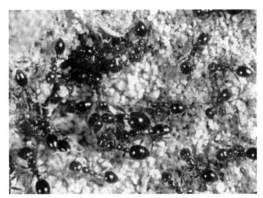
Figure 38.31. Fire ants, *Solenopsis invicta.*

Treatment

Reactions to the bites of kissing bugs require, at most, local symptomatic therapy.

Control

Insecticides applied to houses have been effective for the control of some species of kissing bugs. Environmental control programs work better than even prudent and appropriate application of insecticides. For example, improved housing, in which thatched roofing and adobe walls and flooring are eliminated, helps to greatly reduce breeding sites for the bugs. Indoors, smooth walls with little in the way of pictures, etc. hanging on them also favors the elimination of reduviidae from the local environment. These latter two approaches have been used in many parts of Brazil with a high degree of success. An aggressive vector control program now underway offers the promise of interruption of transmission of Chagas disease throughout most of South America.

Hymenoptera: The Stinging Insects

The stinging insects, including the bees, wasps, hornets (Fig. 38.30), and ants (Fig. 38.31), are members of the Hymenoptera, a large order of highly developed species. Complex social systems, castes, and elaborate hive and nest structures have evolved among the Hymenoptera. The only other insect group to achieve such a level of social development is the termite. In the Hymenoptera, the ovipositor (the apparatus used for egg laying) has been modified to serve as a stinging organ and is used by adult females to capture prey for food or for defense.

The stinging apparati of honeybees, bumblebees, wasps, and hornets are generally similar in structure. They consist of paired acid glands, a single alkaline gland, a poison sac with muscular neck, and the piercing apparatus itself, which includes a pair of stylets and a stylet sheath. The stylets or darts of the honeybee stinger are barbed (Fig. 38.32) and, once inserted by the insect, cannot be withdrawn. Consequently, when a honey bee stings and attempts to fly away, it leaves behind the complete stinging apparatus, virtually disemboweling itself and suffering a mortal wound. The self-contained stinger with its attached poison sac and musculature

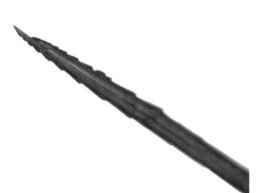
Figure 38.32. Bee stinger – note barbs.

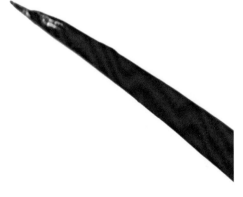
Figure 38.33. Wasp stinger - barbs absent.

continues to pump venom into the wound long after the bee has departed.[79, 80] The stingers of most hymenopterans are not barbed (Fig. 39.33) and are withdrawn after stinging. Wasps, hornets, bumble bees, and ants are capable of multiple stings without losing their stinging apparatus.

It is estimated that in the United States 90-100 people die each year from reactions to stings of the hymenopterans, and even then, there is probably substantial underreporting and some misdiagnosis. Yellow jackets and honeybees are the major causes of such reactions.[81, 82]

Certain behavioral characteristics of bees and yellow jackets result in increased aggressiveness. Honeybees are generally benign unless they are individually molested or provoked to defend their hive. Their venom contains the pheromone isopentyl acetate, which acts as an alarm signal and draws other bees to the site of the original sting, which in turn leads to multiple stings. Dramatic reports of the so-called African killer bees are often exaggerations of reality, although these bees tend to be more aggressive and less predictable than the common bees found in most domestic hives. The range of these "Africanized" honeybees has extended from South America through Central America and Mexico into the southern United States. The ultimate distribution into the United States will be limited by the bees' ability to survive killing temperatures.[82-84]

Yellow jackets are particularly aggressive when their nest areas are approached, at which point they sting without provocation or warning. Their aggressive behavior increases during the late summer and early fall. Gardeners and picnickers are particularly at risk.

Historical Information

The honeybee, *Apis mellifera*, was one of the first insects recorded by humans in writings and art. Bees have long been recognized as sources of honey, and their role as plant pollinators is crucial to agriculture.

Life Cycle

Hymenopterans develop by complete metamorphosis with distinct larva, pupa, and adult stages. Larvae are vermiform and resemble maggots. They are dependent upon adults for food. Pupae, encased in a cocoon, represent an inactive, non-feeding transitional phase. The adults usually have wings and are good fliers. Certain groups with highly developed social systems have evolved non-reproducing worker and soldier castes. Other groups, such as the ants, are wingless as adults except during reproductive periods. Four families of the Hymenoptera contain medically important species, the stings of which can cause severe reactions in humans: Apidae, Vespidae, Formicidae, and Mutillidae.

The bees, or Apidae, include some species that live in complex social organizations such as hives or in less-structured subterranean nests, although most species in this family live as solitary insects. Only the honeybees and bumblebees among the Apidae are of concern to humans because of their ability to sting. The honeybee, *Apis mellifera*, originally an Old World species, is now found worldwide in domestic and wild hives. Bees of this species are raised commercially for their honey and for their role as pollinators of a wide range of plants, including most fruits and legume crops. They construct elaborate hives wherein a single non-foraging queen lays eggs in wax cells. Larvae develop within these cells while being fed by non-reproductive female workers. Adult workers tend the hives and forage for nectar and pollen. The bees tend to sting when their hive or individual insects are disturbed.

Bumblebees of the genus *Bombus* are large, hairy, ungainly, less organized social bees that build simple underground nests.

They sting under the same circumstances as do honey bees.

The Vespidae include the wasps, hornets, and yellow jackets, all of which are capable of inflicting painful stings. Many species in this family build elaborate nests of masticated wood fibers or mud, whereas others construct simple nests underground. The yellow jackets are social hymenopterans with distinctive yellow and black bands on the abdomen, and are often mistaken for bees. They are aggressive insects and a major cause of stings in humans.

Ants belong to the family Formicidae, some members of which can cause damage by biting or stinging. They have a variety of complex social systems, with elaborate behavior patterns, intricate nests, and castes of workers, soldiers, and reproducing insects. Two groups of ants are of concern in the United States.

The harvester ants of the genus Pogonomyrmex readily attack humans and other animals and are capable of inflicting painful stings. They build underground nests, topped by mounds, in warm, dry, sandy areas. When a nest is disturbed, ants come out and swarm over the invader; their stings are repeated and vigorous.

Fire ants of the genus *Solenopsis* are so named because of their sharp, fiery sting. Several native U.S. species are of medical importance, but the imported fire ant, *Solenopsis invicta* (Fig. 38.31), is a particularly dangerous species.[85, 86] It was introduced into the United States around 1930 and since then has spread throughout the southeastern states, where it presents a serious hazard to humans and livestock. These ants build large, hard-crusted mounds, which are well camouflaged and often not seen until they are disturbed. When fire ants attack, they first bite their victim with strong mandibles, and then sting their victim repeatedly. The result is a circle of painful stings around a central bite.

Certain species of tropical ants are notorious for their ability to ravage plants and animals alike as they travel from place to place in colonies or armies numbering millions of individuals.

The so-called velvet ants are not true ants, but wingless wasps of the family Mutillidae. These large, hairy, often brightly colored insects are capable of inflicting a painful sting if they are disturbed. A large black mutillid with scarlet hairs is common in the central United States, where it can cause considerable distress by stinging barefoot bathers. Several other groups of the Hymenoptera have the capacity to sting.

Pathogenesis

During the act of stinging, the aroused insect first inserts the sheath, inflicting a wound, then follows immediately with the inward thrust of the stylets and injection of the venom. The combination of the acid and alkaline venom fluids, designed to kill insect prey, causes extreme pain and inflammation. Venom from 500 stings received within a few minutes can cause death. The inhabitants of a single disturbed beehive can inflict at least that number of stings within a matter of minutes. Sensitization to the venom can result in severe allergic reactions. A number of antigenically active compounds have been identified in venom, phospholipase A being the most important. Others include hyaluronidase, melittin, and apamin.[87, 88]

Clinical Disease

The primary manifestations of the sting are due to mechanical damage and the direct action of the venom. The pain, edema, pruritus, and warmth produced at the site of the sting are transitory. Severe toxic reactions can be caused by as few as 10 stings within a period of a few minutes. Muscle cramps, drowsiness, fever, and headache are characteristic.

Allergic reactions are by far the most serious consequence of the stings of hymenopterans. They may develop in previously sensitized individuals and include three symptom patterns; 1. urticaria associated with pruritus, 2. edematous skin and mucous membranes, and 3. simultaneous bronchospasm and anaphylaxis, followed sometimes by death. In sensitized individuals, even a single sting may bring the most severe reaction. A delayed reaction characterized by urticaria, fever, and arthralgia may occur hours or weeks after a sting.

Although the stinging hymenopterans share a number of common antigens, each possesses one or more unique antigens. Sensitization to stings of one species does not always produce sensitivity to those of other species.

Diagnosis

Individuals with suspected sting sensitivities can undergo skin testing with specific venoms to determine the level of risk. Identification of the species posing the greatest threat to an individual may be critical.[87]

Treatment

Initial treatment for a honeybee sting must include removal of its stinger and the attached venom sac. Removal can be accomplished with a knife blade, a needle, or a fingernail. It is important not to squeeze the site, because such pressure releases more venom from the sac. A non-allergic primary reaction may be treated with ice to lessen edema and pain, and with various local anti-pruritics.

Individuals with known sting sensitivity must be prepared to act quickly to prevent serious reactions. Upon being stung, the individual should remove the stinger immediately.

Emergency kits are available by prescription, and sensitive individuals should be familiar with their use. Such kits contain epinephrine in a syringe, antihistamine tablets, and a tourniquet.

Emergency treatment consists of intramuscular injections of epinephrine and an antihistamine. Obviously, use of these measures presupposes planning; the sensitized person and his or her next of kin must be prepared to carry out the intramuscular injection of epinephrine. In addition, the potential victim should carry an oral antihistamine medication such as diphenhydramine.

Desensitization using whole-body extracts of the insects has been attempted but is ineffective. Purified venoms have been used successfully for desensitization. Successful treatment for severe reactions to fire ant stings has been reported.

Control

Wasp, hornet, and ant nests can be destroyed with a number of commercially available insecticidal compounds, such as carbamates, malathion, and resmithrin. Aerial nests can be destroyed at night, when the insects are quiescent. General avoidance of areas where stinging hymenopterans occur should be a rule for sensitive individuals. There are no effective repellents against these insects.

References

1. Savely, V. R.; Leitao, M. M.; Stricker, R. B., The mystery of Morgellons disease: infection or delusion? *Am J Clin Dermatol* **2006,** *7* (1), 1-5.
2. Koo, J.; Lee, C. S., Delusions of parasitosis. A dermatologist's guide to diagnosis and treatment. *Am J Clin Dermatol* **2001,** *2* (5), 285-90.
3. Peng, Z.; Estelle, F.; Simons, R., Mosquito allergy and mosquito salivary allergens. *Protein Pept Lett* **2007,** *14* (10), 975-81.
4. Ribeiro, J. M. C.; Francischetti, I. M. B., Role of arthropod saliva in blood feeding: Sialome and post-sialome perspectives. *Annu Rev Entomol* **2002,** *48*, 73-88.
5. Theodorides, J., Note historique sur la decouverte de la transmission de la leishmaniose cutanee par les phlebotomes. *Bull Soc Pathol Exot* **1997,** *90*, 177-180.
6. Wenyon, C. M.; J., Some recent advances in our knowledge of leishmaniasis. *School Trop Med* **1912,** *1* 93-98.
7. Lewis, D. J., The biology of Phlebotomidae in relation to leishmaniasis. *Annual review of entomology* **1974,** *19*, 363-84.
8. Valenzuela, J. G.; Garfield, M.; Rowton, E. D.; Pham, V. M., Identification of the most abundant secreted proteins from the salivary glands of the sand fly Lutzomyia longipalpis, vector of Leishmania chagasi. *The Journal of experimental biology* **2004,** *207* (Pt 21), 3717-29.
9. Sambon, L. W.; J., Progress report of investigations of pellagra. *Med* **1910,** *13* 271-287.
10. de Kruif, P., The Microbe Hunters. **1926.**
11. Harrison, G., Mosquitos, Malaria, and Man. **1978.**
12. Shah, S., The Fever: How malaria has ruled mankind for 500,000 years. **2010.**
13. Reed, W.; Carroll, J.; Agremonte, A.; Med, J.; al., e., Etiology of yellow fever, a preliminary note. *Philos* **1900,** *6*, 790-796.
14. Reinert, J. F., New classification for the composite genus Aedes (Diptera: Culicidae: Aedini), elevation of subgenus Ochlerotatus to generic rank, reclassification of the other subgenera, and notes on certain subgenera and species. *Journal of the American Mosquito Control Association* **2000,** *16* (3), 175-88.
15. Reinert, J. F.; Karbach, R. E.; Kithching, I. J.; J., Phylogeny and classification of Aedini (Diptera:Culicidae), based on morphological characters of all life stages. *Zool Soc* **2004,** *142* 289-368.
16. Singh, S.; Mann, B. K., Insect bite reactions. *Indian J Dermatol Venereol Leprol* **2013,** *79* (2), 151-64.
17. Morsy, T. A., Insect bites and what is eating you? *J Egypt Soc Parasitol* **2012,** *42* (2), 291-308.
18. Williams, L. A.; Allen, L. V., Jr., Treatment and prevention of insect bites: mosquitoes. *Int J Pharm Compd* **2012,** *16* (3), 210-8.
19. Steen, C. J.; Carbonaro, P. A.; Schwartz, R. A., Arthropods in dermatology. *J Am Acad Dermatol* **2004,** *50* (6), 819-42, quiz 842-4.
20. Villar, L.; Dayan, G. H.; Arredondo-Garcia, J. L.; Rivera, D. M.; Cunha, R.; Deseda, C.; Reynales, H.; Costa, M. S.; Morales-Ramirez, J. O.; Carrasquilla, G.; Rey, L. C.; Dietze, R.; Luz, K.; Rivas, E.; Miranda Montoya, M. C.; Cortes Supelano, M.; Zambrano, B.; Langevin, E.; Boaz, M.; Tornieporth, N.; Saville, M.; Noriega, F.; Group, C. Y. D. S., Efficacy of a tetravalent dengue vaccine in children in Latin America. *N Engl J Med* **2015,** *372* (2), 113-23.
21. McArthur, M. A.; Sztein, M. B.; Edelman, R., Dengue vaccines: recent developments, ongoing challenges and current candidates. *Expert Rev Vaccines* **2013,** *12* (8), 933-53.
22. Allan, S. A., Susceptibility of adult mosquitoes to insecticides in aqueous sucrose baits. *J Vector Ecol* **2011,** *36* (1), 59-67.
23. Leiper, R. T., Report of the Helminthologist for the Half Year Ending 30 April, . Report of the Advisory Commission on Tropical Diseases Research Fund. **1913,** 1913-1914.
24. Benecke, M., A brief history of forensic entomology. *Forensic Sci Int* **2001,** *120* (1-2), 2-14.
25. Michaud, J. P.; Schoenly, K. G.; Moreau, G., Rewriting Ecological Succession History: Did Carrion Ecologists Get There First? *Q Rev Biol* **2015,** *90* (1), 45-66.

26. Amendt, J.; Richards, C. S.; Campobasso, C. P.; Zehner, R.; Hall, M. J., Forensic entomology: applications and limitations. *Forensic Sci Med Pathol* **2011**, *7* (4), 379-92.
27. Scudder, H. l.; Linda, D. R., Nonbiting flies and disease *Annu Rev Entomol* **1956**, *1*, 323-346.
28. Greenberg, B., Flies and Disease. 1973.
29. Franco, J. R.; Simarro, P. P.; Diarra, A.; Jannin, J. G., Epidemiology of human African trypanosomiasis. *Clin Epidemiol* **2014**, *6*, 257-75.
30. Aksoy, S.; Gibson, W. C.; Lehane, M. J., Interactions between tsetse and trypanosomes with implications for the control of trypanosomiasis. *Adv Parasitol* **2003**, *53*, 1-83.
31. Francesconi, F.; Lupi, O., Myiasis. *Clin Microbiol Rev* **2012**, *25* (1), 79-105.
32. Morley, W. N., Body infestations. *Scottish medical journal* **1977**, *22* (3), 211-6.
33. Steenvoorde, P.; Jacobi, C. E.; Van Doorn, L.; Oskam, J., Maggot debridement therapy of infected ulcers: patient and wound factors influencing outcome - a study on 101 patients with 117 wounds. *Ann R Coll Surg Engl* **2007**, *89* (6), 596-602.
34. Sun, X.; Jiang, K.; Chen, J.; Wu, L.; Lu, H.; Wang, A.; Wang, J., A systematic review of maggot debridement therapy for chronically infected wounds and ulcers. *Int J Infect Dis* **2014**, *25*, 32-7.
35. Mumcuoglu, K. Y.; Davidson, E.; Avidan, A.; Gilead, L., Pain related to maggot debridement therapy. *J Wound Care* **2012**, *21* (8), 400, 402, 404-5.
36. Gilead, L.; Mumcuoglu, K. Y.; Ingber, A., The use of maggot debridement therapy in the treatment of chronic wounds in hospitalised and ambulatory patients. *J Wound Care* **2012**, *21* (2), 78, 80, 82-85.
37. Whitaker, I. S.; Twine, C.; Whitaker, M. J.; Welck, M.; Brown, C. S.; Shandall, A., Larval therapy from antiquity to the present day: mechanisms of action, clinical applications and future potential. *Postgrad Med J* **2007**, *83* (980), 409-13.
38. Gregory, A. R.; Schatz, S.; Laubach, H., Ophthalmomyiasis caused by the sheep bot fly Oestrus ovis in northern Iraq. *Optom Vis Sci* **2004**, *81* (8), 586-90.
39. Lord, W. D.; Burger, J.; J., Collection and preservation of forensically important entomological materials. *Science* **1983**, *28*, 936-944.
40. Greenberg, B., Forensic entomology: case studies. *Bull Entomol Soc Am* **1985**, *31*, 25-28.
41. Greenberg, B.; Kunich, J. C., Entomology and the law. **2002**.
42. Chosidow, O., Scabies and pediculosis. *Lancet (London, England)* **2000**, *355* (9206), 819-26.
43. Zinsser, H., Rats, Lice and History. 1935.
44. Busvine, J. R., Insects, Hygiene, and History. *Athlone Press London* **1976**.
45. Do-Pham, G.; Monsel, G.; Chosidow, O., Lice. *Semin Cutan Med Surg* **2014**, *33* (3), 116-8.
46. Ko, C. J.; Elston, D. M., Pediculosis. *J Am Acad Dermatol* **2004**, *50* (1), 1-12; quiz 13-4.
47. Roberts, R. J., Clinical practice. Head lice. *N Engl J Med* **2002**, *346* (21), 1645-50.
48. Osorio, C.; Fernandes, K.; Guedes, J.; Aguiar, F.; Silva Filho, N.; Lima, R. B.; D'Acri, A.; Martins, C. J.; Lupi, O., Plica polonica secondary to seborrheic dermatitis. *J Eur Acad Dermatol Venereol* **2015**.
49. Nara, A.; Nagai, H.; Yamaguchi, R.; Makino, Y.; Chiba, F.; Yoshida, K. I.; Yajima, D.; Iwase, H., An unusual autopsy case of lethal hypothermia exacerbated by body lice-induced severe anemia. *Int J Legal Med* **2015**.
50. Jahnke, C.; Bauer, E.; Hengge, U. R.; Feldmeier, H., Accuracy of diagnosis of pediculosis capitis: visual inspection vs wet combing. *Arch Dermatol* **2009**, *145* (3), 309-13.
51. Ackerman, A. B., Crabs--the resurgence of Phthirus pubis. *The New England journal of medicine* **1968**, *278* (17), 950-1.
52. Feldmeier, H., Treatment of pediculosis capitis: a critical appraisal of the current literature. *Am J Clin Dermatol* **2014**, *15* (5), 401-12.
53. Burkhart, C. G.; Burkhart, C. N., Oral ivermectin for Phthirus pubis. *J Am Acad Dermatol* **2004**, *51* (6), 1037; author reply 1037-8.
54. Bohl, B.; Evetts, J.; McClain, K.; Rosenauer, A.; Stellitano, E., Clinical Practice Update: Pediculosis Capitis. *Pediatr Nurs* **2015**, *41* (5), 227-34.
55. Walsh, J.; Nicholson, A., Head lice in children--a modern pandemic. *Ir Med J* **2005**, *98* (5), 156-7.
56. Elston, D. M., Treating pediculosis--those nit-picking details. *Pediatr Dermatol* **2007**, *24* (4), 415-

6.

57.   Deeks, L. S.; Naunton, M.; Currie, M. J.; Bowden, F. J., Topical ivermectin 0.5% lotion for treatment of head lice. *Ann Pharmacother* **2013,** *47* (9), 1161-7.

58.   Orion, E.; Matz, H.; Wolf, R., Ectoparasitic sexually transmitted diseases: scabies and pediculosis. *Clinics in dermatology* **2004,** *22* (6), 513-9.

59.   Elgart, M. L., Current treatment for scabies and pediculosis. *Skin Therapy Lett* **2000,** *5*, 1-3.

60.   Raoult, D.; Roux, V., The body louse as a vector of reemerging human diseases. *Clinical infectious diseases : an official publication of the Infectious Diseases Society of America* **1999,** *29* (4), 888-911.

61.   Palicelli, A.; Boldorini, R.; Campisi, P.; Disanto, M. G.; Gatti, L.; Portigliotti, L.; Tosoni, A.; Rivasi, F., Tungiasis in Italy: An imported case of Tunga penetrans and review of the literature. *Pathol Res Pract* **2016.**

62.   Feldmeier, H.; Sentongo, E.; Krantz, I., Tungiasis (sand flea disease): a parasitic disease with particular challenges for public health. *Eur J Clin Microbiol Infect Dis* **2013,** *32* (1), 19-26.

63.   Feldmeier, H.; Keysers, A., Tungiasis - A Janus-faced parasitic skin disease. *Travel Med Infect Dis* **2013,** *11* (6), 357-65.

64.   Grunwald, M. H.; Shai, A.; Mosovich, B.; Avinoach, I., Tungiasis. *The Australasian journal of dermatology* **2000,** *41* (1), 46-7.

65.   Heukelbach, J., Revision on tungiasis: treatment options and prevention. *Expert Rev Anti Infect Ther* **2006,** *4* (1), 151-7.

66.   Huntley, A. C., Cimex lectularius. What is this insect and how does it affect man? *Dermatology online journal* **1999,** *5* (1), 6.

67.   Kolb, A.; Needham, G. R.; Neyman, K. M.; High, W. A., Bedbugs. *Dermatol Ther* **2009,** *22* (4), 347-52.

68.   Farhang-Azad, A.; Traub, R.; Baqar, S., Transovarial transmission of murine typhus rickettsiae in Xenopsylla cheopis fleas. *Science (New York, N.Y.)* **1985,** *227* (4686), 543-5.

69.   Jupp, P. G.; Purcell, R. H.; Phillips, J. M.; Shapiro, M.; Gerin, J. L., Attempts to transmit hepatitis B virus to chimpanzees by arthropods. *South African medical journal = Suid-Afrikaanse tydskrif vir geneeskunde* **1991,** *79* (6), 320-2.

70.   Chagas, C., Nova trypanozomiaze humans: estudos sobre a morfolojiia e o ciclo evalutivo do Schizotripanum cruzi. n genl n sp ajente etiolojico de nova entidade morbida do homen. *Mem Inst Oswaldo Cruz* **1909,** *1* 159-218.

71.   Costa, C. H.; Costa, M. T.; Weber, J. N.; Gilks, G. F.; Castro, C.; Marsden, P. D., Skin reactions to bug bites as a result of xenodiagnosis. *Transactions of the Royal Society of Tropical Medicine and Hygiene* **1981,** *75* (3), 405-8.

72.   Morel, C. M., Chagas' disease, from discovery to control and beyond: history, myths and lessons to take home. *Mem Inst Oswaldo Cruz 94 Suppl* **1999,** *1* 3-16.

73.   Ebrahim, G. J., Eradication of American trypanosomiasis (Chagas' disease): an achievable goal? *Journal of tropical pediatrics* **2004,** *50* (6), 320-1.

74.   Klotz, S. A.; Dorn, P. L.; Mosbacher, M.; Schmidt, J. O., Kissing bugs in the United States: risk for vector-borne disease in humans. *Environ Health Insights* **2014,** *8* (Suppl 2), 49-59.

75.   Bern, C.; Kjos, S.; Yabsley, M. J.; Montgomery, S. P., Trypanosoma cruzi and Chagas' Disease in the United States. *Clin Microbiol Rev* **2011,** *24* (4), 655-81.

76.   Garcia, M. N.; Woc-Colburn, L.; Aguilar, D.; Hotez, P. J.; Murray, K. O., Historical Perspectives on the Epidemiology of Human Chagas Disease in Texas and Recommendations for Enhanced Understanding of Clinical Chagas Disease in the Southern United States. *PLoS Negl Trop Dis* **2015,** *9* (11), e0003981.

77.   Stevens, L.; Dorn, P. L.; Schmidt, J. O.; Klotz, J. H.; Lucero, D.; Klotz, S. A., Kissing bugs. The vectors of Chagas. *Adv Parasitol* **2011,** *75*, 169-92.

78.   Klotz, J. H.; Dorn, P. L.; Logan, J. L.; Stevens, L.; Pinnas, J. L.; Schmidt, J. O.; Klotz, S. A., "Kissing bugs": potential disease vectors and cause of anaphylaxis. *Clin Infect Dis* **2010,** *50* (12), 1629-34.

79.   Tankersley, M. S.; Ledford, D. K., Stinging insect allergy: state of the art 2015. *J Allergy Clin*

Immunol Pract **2015,** *3* (3), 315-22; quiz 323.

80. Touchard, A.; Aili, S. R.; Fox, E. G.; Escoubas, P.; Orivel, J.; Nicholson, G. M.; Dejean, A., The Biochemical Toxin Arsenal from Ant Venoms. *Toxins (Basel)* **2016,** *8* (1).

81. Fitzgerald, K. T.; Flood, A. A., Hymenoptera stings. *Clin Tech Small Anim Pract* **2006,** *21* (4), 194-204.

82. Potiwat, R.; Sitcharungsi, R., Ant allergens and hypersensitivity reactions in response to ant stings. *Asian Pac J Allergy Immunol* **2015,** *33* (4), 267-75.

83. Shaker, M. S.; Hsu, D.; Gruenberg, D. A., An update on venom allergy. *Curr Opin Pediatr* **2013,** *25* (5), 629-34.

84. Winston, M. L., The biology and management of Africanized honey bees *Entomol 547* **1992,** *37 S,* 173-193.

85. Caplan, E. L.; Ford, J. L.; Young, P. F.; Ownby, D. R., Fire ants represent an important risk for anaphylaxis among residents of an endemic region. *The Journal of allergy and clinical immunology* **2003,** *111* (6), 1274-7.

86. Stafford, C. T., Hypersensitivity to fire ant venom. *Annals of allergy, asthma & immunology : official publication of the American College of Allergy, Asthma, & Immunology* **1996,** *77* (2), 87-95; quiz 96.

87. Wong, H. C., Importance of proper identification of stinging insects. *Annals of internal medicine* **2000,** *132* (5), 418.

88. Hoffman, D. R., Insect venom allergy, immunology and immunotherapy. 1984; p 187-223.

39. Arachnids

Introduction

The arachnids comprise a class of arthropods that includes the ticks, mites, scorpions, and spiders. The characteristics of the Arachnida clearly differentiate it from the class Insecta. All arachnids are wingless, have four pairs of legs as adults, and usually show only two distinct body regions: a cephalothorax and an abdomen. Metamorphosis among the arachnids is of the incomplete type. The immature, non-reproductive stages are smaller but morphologically similar to the adults. In many groups, arachnids in the first, or larval, stage may have only three pairs of legs.

The class Arachnida comprises three orders: Acarina, Araneida, and Scorpionida. The order Acarina includes mites and ticks. Ticks are exclusively hematophagous, whereas mites feed on a variety of substances, including insect eggs, cells and blood. The spiders (order Araneida) are mainly insectivorous, feeding on body fluids of captured insects. Some larger tarantulas may feed on small mammals or birds. Scorpions (order Scorpionida) feed on arthropods or small animals that they have immobilized with their stinging apparatus, which is located at the tip of the abdomen.

Most members of these three orders do not affect human health directly. Each order includes some members of medical importance. Ticks and mites injure their victims by their feeding habits and serve as vectors for a number of important diseases (Table 39.1). Spiders inject toxins that can cause severe systemic or tissue reactions, and the toxins injected by the stings of certain species of scorpions can cause severe reactions in affected individuals, rarely death may ensue.

Acarina (Ticks and Mites)

Ticks

The ticks comprise two large families; the Ixodidae (hard ticks) and the Argasidae (soft ticks). Ticks are responsible for damage to livestock, causing considerable weight loss, and for providing opportunities for secondary infection by bacteria or infestation by flies. Many species are capable of transmitting pathogens to domestic animals and humans. The salivary secretions of some species can cause paralysis (tick paralysis) and even death in humans or other mammals.

The consequences of infestations by ticks are enormous in terms of yearly losses in dairy and meat production. In areas of the world where sources of protein are already

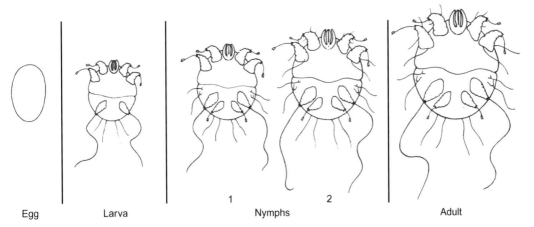

Figure 39.1 Incomplete metamorphosis in the arachnida. Ticks and mites undergo incomplete metamorhosis as typified by the itch mite, *Sarcoptes scabiei*. Larvae have three pair of legs; adults and nymphal stages have four pairs of legs.

scarce, tick infestations have created a crisis situation. Humans are seldom the natural host for any species of tick. Many species will feed on human blood and have the opportunity to become vectors of infections.

Homer recorded the feeding of ticks on humans during the ninth century BCE, as did Aristotle during the fourth century BCE. One of the earliest references to ticks as a possible cause of disease was the suggestion by a 12th-century Persian physician that a fever (probably Crimean-Congo hemorrhagic fever) was transmitted by ticks.[1]

Theobald Smith and Frederick Kilbourne were the first to demonstrate that ticks could transmit disease.[2] They reported that the tick *Boophilus annulatus* carried the bovine protozoan parasite *Babesia bigemina*, a serious pathogen of cattle in the western United States. They further demonstrated that a single infected tick did not pass the parasite from cow to cow; rather, it was transmitted from an infected cow through a female tick to the tick's offspring, transovarially. This mechanism, referred to as vertical transmission, resulted in infection of larval ticks capable of transmitting the parasite at the time of the first feeding. These authors reported their findings in 1893, four years before Ronald Ross completed his studies on the transmission of malaria by mosquitoes. The role of ticks as vectors of spirochetes was shown first with an avian parasite by Émile Marchoux and Alexandre Salimbeni in 1903, and a year later with the spirochete causing human relapsing fever by Ronald Ross and A.D. Milne.[3, 4]

Hard Ticks: Family Ixodidae

Hard ticks (Fig 39.2) (family Ixodidae) are found throughout the world as ectoparasites of a variety of animals. Their name derives from the characteristic tough, leather-like integument that covers most of their body. Their mouthparts are included in a capitulum (Fig. 39.2), but there is no defined head.

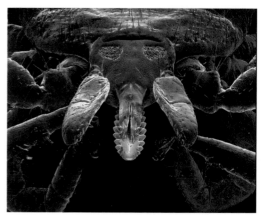

Figure 39.2. Deer tick, *Ixodes scapularis*. Photo D. Scharf

Members of both sexes feed exclusively on blood.

The typical hard tick develops by gradual metamorphosis from the egg through the larva and nymph to the adult. Larvae have three pairs of legs; the nymphs and adults have four pairs. Each stage takes a single blood meal. The larvae and nymphs feed prior to molting and the adult females prior to producing a single batch of eggs. The female tick dies after oviposition.[5]

Hard ticks exhibit one of three life cycles and may be classified as one-, two-, or three-host ticks. A one-host tick spends its life on a single animal. It attaches to the skin of its host as a larva, feeds, and then molts to the nymph stage. After feeding again, it molts a second time, developing into the adult. The adults mate, after which the female engorges with blood, falls to the ground, and lays her

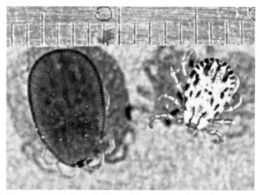

Figure 39.3. Soft (left) and hard ticks (right)

Table 39.1. Arthropods of medical importance.

Order and representative species	Common name	Geographic distribution	Effects on humans
Acarina (ticks and mites)			
Argasidae: various genera and species	Soft ticks	Worldwide	Skin reactions to bite, tick paralysis, vectors of relapsing fever
Ixodidae: various genera and species	Hard ticks	Worldwide	Skin reactions to bite; tick paralysis; vectors of rickettsia, viruses, bacteria, and protozoa
Dermanyssidae *Allodermanyssus sanguineus*	House mouse mite	Worldwide	Vector of *Rickettsia akari*, the cause of rickettsial pox
Various genera and	Mites	Worldwide	Occasional dermatitis from bite species
Demodicidae *Demodex folliculorum*	Follicle mite	Worldwide	Found in sebaceous glands and hair follicles, occasional skin reactions
Trombiculidae *Trombicula* spp.	Chigger, red bug	Worldwide	Intense itching at site of attachment
Trombicula akamushi		Southeast Asia, India, Pacific Islands	Vector of *Rickettsia tsutsugamushi*, the cause of scrub typhus
Sarcoptiae *Sarcoptes scabiei*	Human itch mite	Worldwide	Burrows in skin causing severe itching
Araneidae (spiders)			
Latrodectus mactans	Black widow spider	Americas	Bite usually painless; delayed systemic reaction
Latrodectus spp.	Widow spider	Worldwide	
Loxoceles reclusa	Brown recluse spider	North America	Initial blister at wound site followed by sometimes-extensive necrosis and slow healing
Loxoceles laeta		South American	
Scorpionida (scorpions)			
Various genera and species	Scorpion	Tropics and subtropics	Initially painful sting often followed by systemic reactions

eggs. Larvae begin to hatch within 30 days, and await a new host to begin the cycle again. Two-host ticks usually spend their larva and nymph stages on one host, drop to the ground, molt, and await a second host of another species for completion of the adult phase of the cycle. Each of the three stages of a three-host tick develops on a separate host. The immature stages are usually found on small rodents. The adults feed and mate on larger animals.

Hard ticks display remarkable longevity, with adults of many species surviving up to two years without a blood meal. One-host ticks have the shortest egg-to-egg life cycles, sometimes lasting less than a year. Three-host ticks require 2-3 years to complete their life cycles.

Hard ticks feed slowly, requiring 7-9 days to become completely engorged. After attaching to a suitable host, the tick searches for a feeding site often well concealed by hair. Once in place, it inserts its mouthparts armed with re-curved teeth, secretes a cement-like substance, and begins to feed. After engorging it easily detaches and moves away. In general, the act of feeding is painless to the host, who is often unaware of the tick.[5, 6]

There are 11 genera within the Ixodidae, some of which include species of ticks that feed on humans, and so are of medical importance. *Amblyomma americanum* and *A. cajennense* prey on a variety of animals, feed avidly on humans, and are serious pests in the southern and southwestern states of the United States and in Mexico. They are capable of transmitting the rickettsiae that cause Rocky Mountain spotted fever (*Rickettsia rickettsii*).

Dermacentor variabilis (Fig. 39.4), the American dog tick, is the major vector of Rocky Mountain spotted fever in the eastern and central United States. It is involved in the transmission of tularemia and can cause tick paralysis in humans and dogs. *D. variabilis*

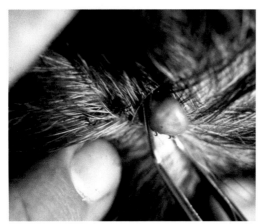

Figure 39.4. Blood-engorged adult female American dog tick, *Dermacentor variabilis*. Courtesy W. Burgdorfer.

is a three-host tick. The larvae and nymphs feed on small rodents, and the adults feed and mate on larger mammals. The dog is the most common host for adults of this species, but humans are readily targeted as well.

Dermacentor andersoni (Fig. 39.5), the Rocky Mountain wood tick, is a common species in the western and northern United States. It transmits Rocky Mountain spotted fever and Colorado tick fever (Colorado tick fever virus), and it causes tick paralysis in humans. This three-host tick feeds on a variety of small mammals as a larva or nymph. As an adult, it feeds on large wild or domes-

tic animals and humans. Both nymphs and adults are capable of over-wintering, and the life cycle of this species is usually greater than two years. *D. albipictus* and *D. occidentalis*, found in the western United States, are capable of transmitting Rocky Mountain spotted fever and Colorado tick fever, but they attack humans only infrequently.[5-11]

Ixodes scapularis (Fig. 39.6) is a three-host tick common throughout the eastern United States. It readily attacks humans and can inflict painful bites. In New England, it had been suggested that a distinct species, *I. dammini*, was responsible for the transmission of human babesiosis and later for being the vector of Lyme disease.[7, 8] Subsequent studies determined that a single species, *I. scapularis*, was involved throughout the area.[9] *I. pacificus* is a common pest of deer and cattle in California. It readily bites humans as well, and has been implicated in the transmission of the Lyme spirochete (*Borrelia burgdorferi*).[10] *I. holocyclus* is an important cause of tick paralysis in Australia.

Rhipicephalus sanguineus, the brown dog tick, is a cosmopolitan ectoparasite of dogs. Although this species does not readily bite humans, it can be a serious nuisance around

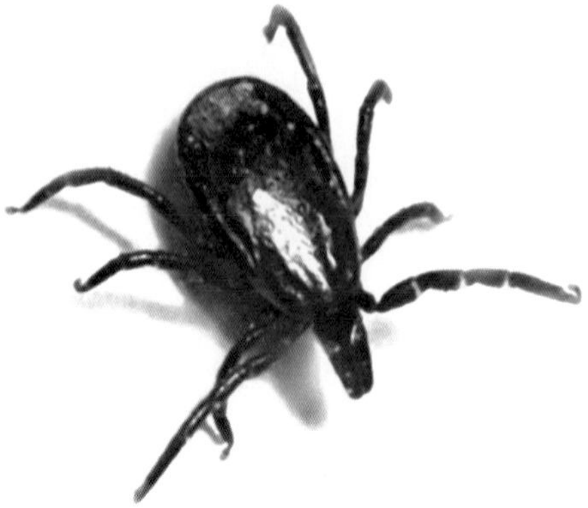

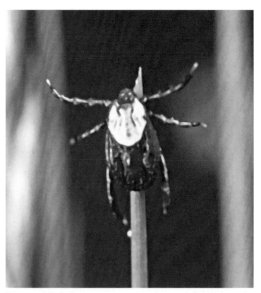

Figure 39.5. Ixodes scapularis. The adult feeds on deer. Nymphs transmit spirochetes and babesia to humans.

Figure 39.6. *Dermacentor andersoni.* Adult female on vegetation, awaiting a host. Courtesy W. Burgdorfer.

homes. Female ticks recently engorged on the blood of domestic dogs drop off and deposit eggs in houses or kennels. The newly hatched larvae tend to crawl up vertical surfaces, literally covering walls or furniture. *R. sanguineus* is considered the major vector of the rickettsia that causes boutonneuse fever (*Rickettsia conorii*).

Hyalomma and *Boophilus* are genera of ticks whose members are ectoparasites of animals and play important roles in transmitting pathogens in animal populations. Occasionally, these ticks act as vectors of human diseases.

Soft Ticks: Family Argasidae

Ticks of the family Argasidae are soft-bodied arthropods covered by a wrinkled, often granulated tegument (Fig. 39.3). They do not have a distinct head region, and their mouthparts are located on the ventral surface, not visible from above. Soft ticks are found throughout the world, usually as ectoparasites of birds, although some species normally feed on bats and other small mammals. Several species attack humans if given the opportunity.

Soft ticks differ from the hard ticks in their feeding behavior, habitat, and life cycles. Soft ticks normally inhabit the nesting site of their hosts, moving onto the host to feed and returning to the nest when satisfied. They are completely engorged within a matter of minutes or a few hours at most, usually feeding at night while the host is asleep.

The typical life cycle of a soft tick consists of a single six-legged larval stage, two or more eight-legged nymph stages, and the eight-legged adult stage. Some species require several blood meals before each molt, and adult females feed repeatedly, producing a small batch of eggs after each meal.

Three genera of soft ticks affect humans as pests or as vectors of pathogens. The fowl tick *Argas persicus* is an important cosmopol-

itan ectoparasite that preys on poultry. It bites humans as well, particularly if the normal fowl hosts are unavailable. Ticks of the genus *Otobius* occasionally infest human ears.

Ticks of the genus *Ornithodorus* are important pests and vectors of the spirochetes, causing tick-borne relapsing fevers. *O. moubata* attacks a number of wild and domestic animals, but humans are its major host. This tick inhabits huts, feeding at night on the sleeping inhabitants. It is found throughout southern and central Africa reaching as far north as Ethiopia, and it is the major vector of African relapsing fever caused by various *Borrelia* spp. Epidemiologic evidence suggests that *O. moubata*, the tampan tick, may be involved in the transmission of Hepatitis B virus in Africa, but direct experimental evidence is lacking.[11]

Several species of *Ornithodorus* are vectors of relapsing fevers in both the New World and the Old World. Most of these species, however, are ectoparasites of rodents and other mammals, feeding on humans only occasionally.

Pathogenesis and Treatment of Tick Bites

Most ticks attach themselves firmly to the skin of the host before beginning the blood meal. The mouthparts and injected salivary secretions provoke inflammation of the surrounding tissue, characterized by local hyperemia, edema, hemorrhage, and thickening of the stratum corneum.[12] Although the initial bite and insertion of the mouthparts may be painless, irritation often develops later, followed by necrosis and secondary infection at the wound site.

It is important to remove ticks from the skin of the host as soon as they are detected, as early removal often prevents firm attachment and makes transmission of the pathogens less likely. It also limits the infusion of toxins that cause tick paralysis, as these toxins are released slowly.

Numerous methods have been suggested for the removal of firmly attached ticks. Traditionally, ticks have been treated with chloroform, ether, benzene, turpentine, or petrolatum, each of which, it has been suggested, irritates the tick, causing it to withdraw. The U.S. Public Health Service recommends mechanical removal without chemical aids. Many genera of ticks, especially *Dermacentor*, may be removed by gently but firmly, pulling the tick away from its attachment. Ixodes and amblyomma, which have longer mouthparts that do not detach easily, may require the use of instruments for removal. These ticks should be pulled gently away from the host so the skin surrounding the mouthparts forms a tent. A sterile needle or scalpel can then be inserted under the mouthparts and used to tease them away from the tissue. In all cases, care should be taken to avoid leaving any tissue from the tick, as it will induce intense inflammation. The tick should not be crushed or damaged, thereby preventing the release of pathogenic organisms onto the wound site. Subsequent thorough cleaning of the wound is recommended.[13]

Tick Paralysis

More than 40 species in 10 genera of both hard and soft ticks secrete salivary toxins that cause paralysis in humans and a number of other animals. It is not a universal property of any one species, though, suggesting that salivary secretions are characteristic of individual ticks.[14-18]

The affected patient becomes irritable, is restless, and experiences numbness and tingling in the extremities, face, lips, and throat. Soon, the patient develops symmetric, flaccid paralysis that is ascending in nature and can lead to bulbar palsy. Sensory loss is rare. There is no fever. Death results from respiratory paralysis. The laboratory findings (complete blood count, urinalysis, and cerebrospinal fluid examination) are normal. Differen-

tial diagnosis includes poliomyelitis, Guillain-Barre syndrome, transverse myelitis, and spinal cord tumors. The diagnosis depends on the patient's clinical history and finding the tick. Treatment consists in removing the feeding tick. Recovery follows rapidly. The usual causes of human tick paralysis are *D. andersoni* and *D. variabilis* in the United States and *I. holocyclus* in Australia. A number of species of *Dermacentor*, *Ixodes*, *Amblyomma*, *Rhipicephalus*, *Argas*, and *Ornithodorus* often cause paralysis in animals, but only occasionally affect humans. A vaccine for tick paralysis is under development.[19-23]

Tick-Borne Diseases in Humans

Ticks transmit a broad array of viruses, rickettsiae, bacteria, and protozoa, which may cause disease in their human hosts.

Viral Diseases

Colorado tick fever is the most common tick-borne viral disease in humans in the United States. A benign disease transmitted by the bite of *D. andersoni*, it is maintained in nature as an enzootic infection of rodents spread by the same vector. Transovarial (vertical) transmission of the virus (Colorado tick fever virus) has not been demonstrated. Colorado tick fever is characterized by sudden onset of chills, headache, severe myalgia, and fever.[24]

In the Old World, hard ticks are vectors of a number of viral diseases grouped as hemorrhagic fevers or tick-borne encephalitides. Among them are Russian spring-summer encephalitis, Kyasanur Forest disease, Crimean-Congo hemorrhagic fever, and Omsk hemorrhagic fever.

Rickettsial Diseases

Rocky Mountain spotted fever is an acute, sometimes fatal, febrile, exanthematous disease caused by *Rickettsia rickettsii*. It most frequently affects children and is characterized by fever, headache, musculoskeletal pain, and a generalized rash that appears first on the wrists and ankles and often becomes hemorrhagic.

Although initially described from the Rocky Mountain region of the United States and distributed throughout much of North and South America, the infection is of particular importance in the "tick belt" states of Maryland, Virginia, North Carolina, South Carolina, and Georgia. In these states, the incidence of the disease has been rising steadily over the last 10 years (see www.cdc.gov/ncidod/dvrd/rmsf.htm). The main vector in the eastern United States is *D. variabilis*, the American dog tick; in the western states it is *D. andersoni*. Other tick species that are considered minor vectors have the capacity to transmit the organism to humans, but may be primarily important as vectors that infect reservoir hosts.

In areas where Rocky Mountain spotted fever is prevalent, regular inspection for ticks should be undertaken. Children especially should be examined twice daily. The tick must be attached to the host for several hours before it transmits the pathogen; therefore its expeditious removal can prevent infection. No vaccine against Rocky Mountain spotted fever is currently available, but infections can easily be treated with doxycycline. Untreated cases have a mortality rate of 2-5%.[13, 24, 25]

Old World tick-borne typhus has different regional names: boutonneuse fever, Kenya typhus, and South African tick bite fever. It is a relatively mild disease, presenting with chills, fever, and generalized body rash. *Rhipicephalus sanguineus*, the brown dog tick, is the main vector of boutonneuse fever in the Mediterranean region; other hard ticks are involved elsewhere.

Q fever is a self-limited infection. The disease consists of fever, headache, constitutional symptoms, and often pneumonitis. Caused by the rickettsia *Coxiella burnetii*, it is usually contracted by inhalation. Ticks are involved in maintaining the infection in the animal reservoir host and can transmit the organism to humans.

Anaplasmosis is a tick-borne rickettsiosis, first described in Japan in 1954, that resembles other tick-borne diseases such as "spotless" Rocky Mountain spotted fever. This generally mild infection may be mistaken for pyelonephritis, hepatitis-C or D, gastroenteritis, or unexplained febrile illnesses with leukopenia or thrombocytopenia. Treatment is similar to that for other rickettsial diseases.[26, 27] Co-infection with more than one tick-borne pathogen in a single individual has been reported.[28]

Bacterial Diseases

Tularemia is a bacterial disease caused by *Franciscella tularensis* and characterized by a focal ulcer at the site of entry of the organism, enlargement of regional lymph nodes, fever, prostration, myalgia, and headache. *Dermacentor andersoni* and *D. variabilis* are the ticks most frequently involved in the transmission of this infection from small mammals, particularly rabbits, to humans. A number of tick species maintain the infection in the reservoir population.

The relapsing fevers form a group of diseases with a similar clinical pattern; they are caused by spirochetes of the genus *Borrelia*, all of which are transmitted by arthropod vectors. Lice transmit epidemic louse-borne relapsing fever, and soft ticks transmit endemic tick-borne relapsing fever.[29] The human relapsing fevers are described as acute infections with toxemia and febrile periods that subside and recur over a period of weeks. Ticks of the genus *Ornithodoros* transmit tick-borne relapsing fevers. In the Western Hemisphere, *O. hermsi*, *O. turicata*, and *O. rudis* are the most important vectors. A close association between humans, vector ticks, and rodents infected with spirochetes, usually in a rural setting, is the typical condition necessary for human infections. In Africa, *O.*

moubata, which feeds primarily on humans and lives in human dwellings, maintains transmission of relapsing fever from human to human.

Lyme arthritis and erythema chronicum migrans, or Lyme disease, as these conditions are known collectively, is caused by the spirochete *Borrelia burgdorferi,* which is transmitted by a number of ixodid ticks. *I. scapularis* (Fig. 39.7) is the primary vector in the eastern United States, while *I. pacificus* is the main vector on the West Coast, and *I. ricinus* is primarily responsible for transmission in Europe.[30-34]

The spirochete is commonly found in rodents, especially white-footed mice. In its immature stages, the tick vector feeds on this rodent reservoir host, and on deer in its adult stage. The range of the tick is limited by the range of the deer populations (see www.medicalecology.org/diseases/lyme/lyme_disease.htm).

Human infection with this spirochete usually results from a bite of the nymphal tick, though adult ticks are also capable of transmitting it. Before the tick has fed, the spirochete is found in its gut. After the tick has attached to a host and has begun feeding, the spirochetes disseminate throughout the hemocele, invade the salivary glands, and infect the host. This process takes about a day, so prompt removal of the tick reduces the chance of infection.

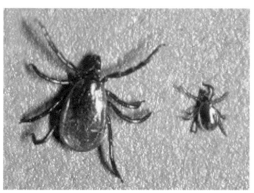

Figure 39.7. Adult female and nymph of *Ixodes scapularis*. Courtesy of A. Spielman and P. Rossignol.

Protozoal Diseases

Babesiosis, a protozoal disease, is seen in a variety of animals but rarely appears in humans. The focus of human cases on Nantucket and other islands Island off Cape Cod, Massachusetts has spread to the mainland.[14]

Prevention and Control of Tick-Transmitted Infections

The best measure of tick control is avoidance of areas where ticks are known to exist. Wide-scale chemical control of tick populations is impractical, although various compounds have been used. Tick control on dogs can be achieved with systemic compounds, topically applied chemicals, or available tick collars. Dusts have proved useful for preventing the introduction of brown or American dog ticks into homes. Permethrin, sprayed on clothing, appears to be most effective and may last at least a week or more.[35] Diethyltoluamide (DEET) has been shown to be generally ineffective as a tick repellent. Careful examination for ticks is still necessary after traveling through   infested areas. Because deer are the primary hosts of the tick vector, control of the over-abundant deer populations can be efficacious. Total elimination of a deer population on an isolated island eliminated the tick vector and stopped transmission of the Lyme spirochaete. Significant reduction of deer populations at other sites had a major effect on density of tick populations and the frequency of transmission.[36, 37] In one study, feeding ivermectin-medicated food had a significant effect on a population of vector ticks.[38]

Mites

Within the Order Acarina, the term "mite" is applied to members of several large families of minute arthropods, most free-living but many existing as ecto- or endoparasites of vertebrates and invertebrates. Mites affect humans by causing dermatitis. They serve as vectors of a number of diseases and as a source of allergens that can lead to serious hypersensitivity reactions.

Mites, as described by Aristotle, were well-known to ancient civilizations. Their function as ectoparasites was not recognized until about the year 1000 CE, when scabies was first recorded. Although scabies continued to be described in the early medical literature, and physicians and naturalists repeatedly noted the association of a mite with this skin condition, the causal relation was largely ignored by the medical profession. The unequivocal demonstration that a mite was indeed the cause of scabies took place in 1834 when a Corsican medical student recovered mites from affected individuals.[39]

Human Itch Mite: *Sarcoptes scabiei*

Scabies is a human skin disease caused by the mite *Sarcoptes scabiei* (Figs. 39.1, 39.8). It is usually associated with crowded living conditions, and its outbreaks often accompany wars, famine, and human migrations. Currently, scabies has reached pandemic proportions.[39]

The condition first presents as nocturnal itching, usually on the webbing and sides of the fingers, later spreading to the wrists, elbows, and the rest of the body. The buttocks, breasts of females, and genitalia of men are occasionally affected. Lesions appear as short, sinuous, slightly raised, cutaneous burrows.

Infections begin when fertile female mites (Fig. 39.9) are transferred from infected individuals by direct contact. The female mite finds a suitable site, burrows into the skin, and tunnels through the upper layers of the epidermis, depositing fertile eggs. Six-legged larvae hatch from these eggs, leave the tunnel, and wander about the skin before re-invading it and starting new burrows. Once in place, the larvae eat, molt, and transform into eight-legged nymphs. Larvae destined to become

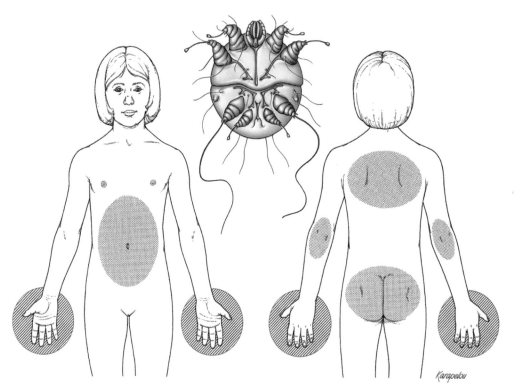

Figure 39.8. The itch mite, *Sarcoptes scabiei*. The stippled areas represent regions of the body where the rash is found. The mites themselves are found predominantly between the fingers and on the wrists (hatched areas).

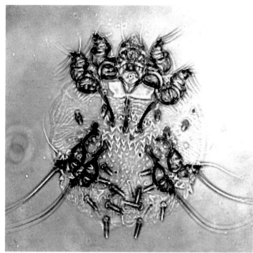

Figure 39.9. Adult female itch mite, *Sarcoptes scabiei*.

females molt again into a second nymph stage. Those destined to become males molt directly to the adult form. After fertilization, young adult females begin construction of a new tunnel. The egg-to-egg life cycle may be as short as two weeks. A typical infection usually involves only 10-15 adult female mites.[40-43]

With primary infections, itching and skin eruption are usually delayed for several

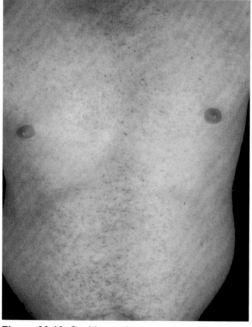

Figure 39.10. Scabies rash.

weeks. As sensitization develops, the typical scabies rash appears on various parts of the body that do not necessarily correspond to the location of active adult female mites, but represent a generalized response to the allergens (Fig. 39.10).

The face and scalp may be affected in infants and children, whereas adults seldom have lesions in these areas. A rare condition known as Norwegian, or crusted, scabies may result from hyper-infection with thousands to millions of mites (Fig. 39.11). The consequence is a crusted dermatosis of the hands and feet and often much of the body. This condition is characteristic of infected individuals who cannot take care of themselves and is often reported in custodial institutions such as mental hospitals.[44, 45] It is highly contagious because of the large number of loosely attached, easily transferred mites present in the exfoliating skin. Crusted scabies has also been reported in individuals treated with immunosuppressive drugs (Fig. 39.12). Secondary infections of lesions, particularly as a result of scratching, are common; and post-streptococcal glomerulonephritis has been reported.[46]

A diagnosis of scabies can be confirmed by picking up adult female mites at the ends of their burrows or by scraping the affected skin lightly covered with mineral oil. The scrapings are then examined under a microscope for immature or adult mites or for eggs.

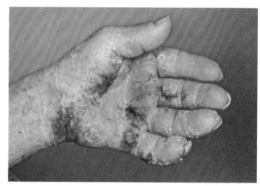

Figure 39.11. Patient with Norwegian scabies showing numerous lesions. Millions of mites may be present. Courtesy of Y. Mumcouglu.

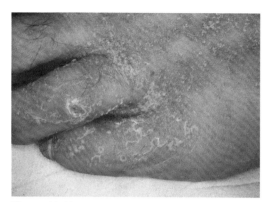

Figure 39.12. Large numbers of scabies mites and lesions on an immunosupressed patient.

Skin biopsy reveals mites in tissue sections. The presence of infection in several members of a family is reasonable circumstantial evidence for a diagnosis of scabies in those not yet examined.

Lindane, the γ-isomer of benzene hexachloride, and permethrin are the most effective treatments available for treatment of scabies, but lindane may have significant neurotoxicity. Lindane is available as a lotion or cream, which is applied once to the affected areas. Permethrin 5% cream is applied and left on for 8 to 14 hours. Benzyl benzoate in a 25% emulsion is an alternative drug, but must be applied to the whole body. Treatment of all members of a family may be necessary to prevent reinfection. Systemic treatment with ivermectin has proven particularly efficacious, but should still be used with care.[47, 48]

Animal Scabies

The itch and mange mites of various domestic animals (horses, pigs, dogs, cats, camels) can infest humans. These mites are often morphologically indistinguishable from the human parasites and are fully capable of penetrating human skin. The infection is usually self-limited because these mites do not form tunnels and cannot complete their life cycles. Humans may react with severe papular urticaria to these transitory infestations.

Chigger Mites

The chiggers, or redbugs, (Fig. 39.13) of the family Trombiculidae comprise an important group of annoying human ectoparasites. In some geographic areas, they act as vectors of the organism, causing scrub typhus (*Orientalis tsutsugamushi*).

In the United States, the chigger mites include three species of *Trombicula*. Among the chiggers, only the six-legged larvae feed on humans and other mammals, whereas the nymphs and adults usually feed on arthropods or arthropod eggs. Chigger larvae are usually picked up in brush frequented by rodents or other small mammals, which serve as normal hosts of the larvae. These mites tend to attach to skin where clothing is tight or restricted. The ankles, waistline, armpits, and perineal skin are common areas of infestation. Chiggers insert their capitula but do not burrow into the skin. The host reacts to the mouthparts and the injected saliva by forming a tube-like "stylosome" partially engulfing the feeding mites. The chigger does not feed on blood, rather, it ingests a mixture of partially digested cells and fluids formed within the

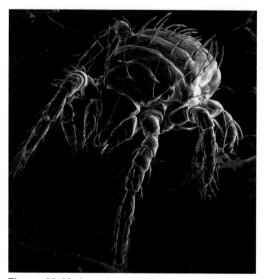

Figure 39.13. Larval stage of the common chigger *Trombicula alfreddugesi*. It is the larva, with three pairs of legs, that feeds on vertebrates. Photo by D. Scharf.

stylosome. After feeding for several days, the engorged chigger withdraws and drops to the ground.[49, 50]

The intense itching and discomfort associated with chigger "bites" often begins after the chiggers have withdrawn and departed. Irritation may be so severe as to cause fever and loss of sleep. Local anesthetics may be useful for relieving itching, and antibiotics may be needed to treat secondary bacterial skin infections.[51]

In areas where chiggers are common, repellents containing DEET applied to skin and clothing can be effective. Scrubbing exposed or infested areas of the body with soap and water removes even well-attached chiggers.

Scrub typhus (*Orientalis tsutsugamushi*) is a chigger-borne gram-negative coccobacillus zoonotic disease found in Southeast Asia, certain islands in the Indian and Pacific Oceans, and Australia that is antigenically distinct from rickettsiae. The causative agent is *Orientalis tsutsugamushi*, and the usual vectors are larvae of the chigger *Trombicula akamushi* and *T. deliensis*. Rodents are the normal reservoir hosts for this pathogen.[52]

Follicle Mites

The ubiquitous follicle mite *Demodex folliculorum* are normal inhabitants of our sebaceous glands and hair follicles, particularly around the nose and eyelids. Follicle mites are minute (<0.4 mm long), atypically vermiform arthropods that seldom cause discomfort.[53-55] In rare cases, the skin of the scalp becomes heavily infected. Follicle mites have been implicated as the cause of some forms of rosacea and blepheritis. Treatment consists of a topical application of ivermectin cream.[56] Closely related species of *Demodex*, which cause mange in dogs and other mammals, may cause a transitory burning reaction in individuals handling heavily infested animals.

Mites and Dermatitis

A number of species of mites, either parasitic for animals or free living, occasionally infest humans and cause dermatitis. Mites associated with straw, flour, grain, dried fruits, vanilla, copra, and cheese can produce serious but transitory skin irritation in persons contracting large numbers of these acarines. Bird and rodent mites may also cause serious annoyance when they attempt to feed on humans, but they do so only occasionally. Bird mites may be particularly bothersome if their normal avian hosts depart and they are forced to forage for food.

The tropical rat mite, *Ornithonyssus bacoti,* is a parasite of rodents that can attack humans and cause dermatitis.[41, 57] The house mite *Allodermanyssus sanguineus* is a common ectoparasite of mice, but readily feeds on humans. These mites have been shown to transmit rickettsial pox (*Rickettsia akari*), a mild exanthematous disease related to Rocky Mountain spotted fever found in the eastern United States and Russia.[52]

Allergies Caused by Mites

Certain mites of the genus *Dermatophagoides* have been incriminated as sources of antigens associated with allergies to house dust.[43] House dust mite allergens are a common cause of asthma attacks in sensitized individuals, particularly children. Desensitization has been successful.[58-63]

Araneida (Spiders)

The spiders constitute a large, distinctive order of arachnids whose bodies are divided into two regions: cephalothorax and abdomen. Four pairs of walking legs, pedipalps, and chelicerae with poison fangs all arise from the cephalothorax. All spiders produce venom in anterior venom glands that is capable of immobilizing prey. Although most species are unable to pierce human skin, several groups of spiders do occasionally bite humans. The consequences of these bites may include transitory pain, necrotic lesions, systemic reactions, or even death.[64]

Tarantulas

The name tarantula is loosely applied to a number of large, hairy spiders, some of which belong to the family Theraphosidae. These spiders are common in tropical and subtropical regions. Although they are much feared, few tarantulas bite humans. Those that do may inflict a painful wound, but the symptoms are not long lasting, and no fatalities have been reported. Tarantulas are kept as house pets by many individuals and are regularly bred in captivity.

Black Widow Spiders

Spiders of the genus *Latrodectus* are found throughout the world, primarily in warm climates. At least six species that bite humans have been reported. They inflict painful and rarely fatal wounds (mostly in children).[65-67]

Latrodectus mactans, the black widow, hourglass, or shoe-button spider, (Fig. 39.14) is widespread throughout the United States and southern Canada. Related species are found throughout the temperate and tropical regions of all continents. The adult female black widow spider is usually black with a characteristic crimson hourglass marking on the underside of its globose abdomen. The coloration (various shades of black, gray, or brown) and the shape of the hourglass may vary. The typical mature female is about 40 mm long with its legs extended. Black widow spiders are normally reclusive in behavior, but females bite if disturbed and are particularly aggressive when they are gravid or defending their egg cases. These spiders frequent wood and brush piles, old wooden buildings, cellars, hollow logs, and vacant rodent burrows. The pit privy is a preferred site for webs, and a significant number of human spider bites have taken place in these locations.

Bites of the black widow spider may be initially painless, sometimes appearing only as two small red puncture marks at the site. Subsequently, pain at the site increases, spreads, reaching a maximum within 1-3 hours, and later subsides. Generalized muscle pain, abdominal rigidity, tightness in the chest, difficulty with breathing and speaking, nausea, and sweating may occur within an hour of the bite. Most symptoms pass after 2-3 days without treatment. In severe cases, paralysis and coma may precede cardiac or respiratory failure. The toxin has been identified as a low-molecular-weight protein. Its mode of action involves the inhibition of fusion of neurotransmitter vesicles with membranes leading to depolarization of synapses.[68-71] Treatment usually consists of measures designed to relieve pain and reduce muscle spasms. Anti-venom is available in locales where bites are common.[72, 73] Control of black widow spiders with the use of insecticides such as malathion, particularly in privies, is effective.

Nectrotic Arachnidism

Five species of the genus *Loxoceles* in the New World attack when they are disturbed. Their bites may produce severe tissue reactions. *Loxoceles reclusa* (Fig. 39.15) is found

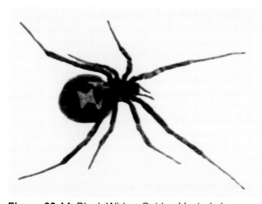

Figure 39.14. Black Widow Spider. Ventral view.

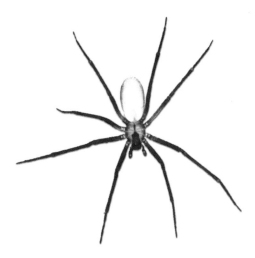

Figure 39.15. *Loxoceles reclusa*, the brown recluse spider. Dorsal view. Note "fiddle" pattern.

in the southern and central United States; *L. unicolor* and *L. arizonica* are found in the western states; and *L. laeta* and *L. intermedia* are seen in South America. These spiders are of medium size, are yellow to brown in color, and have a body length of 10-15 mm.[74]

Loxoceles reclusa, the brown recluse spider of the United States, is a non-aggressive arachnid found outdoors in woodpiles and debris in warm climates, and in basements or storage areas in cooler regions. Humans are typically bitten only when they disturb them (e,g., when entering a sleeping bag, or putting on shoes or clothing).[51]

The South American brown spiders, *L. laeta* and *L. intermedia*, are common domestic species found in closets, corners of rooms, or behind pictures. Humans are often bitten while sleeping or dressing, but only when the spider is threatened or disturbed. *L. laeta* has been introduced into the United States on at least one occasion.[75]

The bite of loxoceles tends to be initially painless. Several hours later, itching, swelling, and tenderness may develop in the area of the bite. The wound site may turn violaceous and then black and dry. In other cases, a blister may form over the bite. Necrosis may begin within 3-4 days, and tissue destruc-

tion may be extensive (Fig. 39.16). Healing may take eight weeks or longer. Some of the more serious lesions require surgery and skin grafts. The venom of loxoceles appears to work by inactivating hemolytic components of complement.[76-82] An antiserum for treatment of loxoceles bites is being evaluated in Brazil. Loxoceles spiders may be controlled in dwellings with insecticide compounds containing γ-benzene hexachloride or malathion.

Chiracanthium mildei is the most common spider found in houses in the eastern United States; usually in bathrooms, kitchens, and bedrooms. It attacks when disturbed, and its bite can cause a mild necrotizing skin lesion.[83-90] Spiders of the genera *Phoneutria* in Brazil and Chile are capable of inflicting severe bites, sometimes with fatal results.

The spider fauna of Australia is particularly robust and contains many dangerous species, but only the male Atrax spider is capable of inflicting a lethal bite in humans. The venom is neurotoxic and causes nausea, vomiting, abdominal pain, diarrhea, profuse sweating, salivation, and lacrimation. There may also be severe hypertension and cardiac arrest.

Scorpionida (Scorpions)

The scorpions belong to the order Scorpionida of the class Arachnida, with all members generally similar in appearance (Fig.

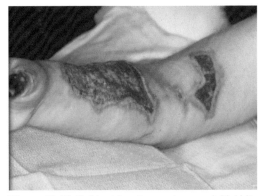

Figure 39.16. Spider bite - *Loxoceles* spp. initial bite on the tip of the thumb.

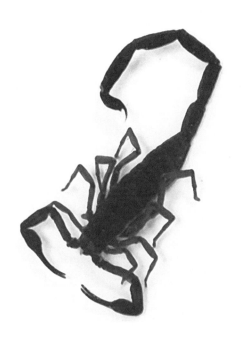

Figure 39.17. Scorpion.

39.17). The typical scorpion is an elongate arthropod with stout, crab-like claws (pedipalps), four pairs of walking legs, and a distinctly-segmented abdomen ending in a hooked stinger.[91]

Scorpions are reclusive, nocturnal animals in behavior that feed primarily on other arthropods and sometimes on small rodents. While feeding, the scorpion holds its prey with its pedipalps and repeatedly stings its victim with over-the-back thrusts of its stinger. When the scorpion is disturbed, it uses the stinger for defense, which is the manner in which humans are stung. Most species of scorpions are unable either to penetrate human skin or inject sufficient toxin to cause damage. The few species that do sting humans are capable of inflicting a painful wound, precipitating a severe reaction and sometimes causing death. These species present a significant hazard to public health in many tropical and sub-tropical regions.[92]

Scorpions produce two types of venom: hemolytic and neurotoxic. The first induces local reactions characterized by a burning sensation, swelling, and necrosis at the wound site. The second produces intense pain at the site of the sting and causes chills, cold perspiration, thirst, excessive salivation, and vomiting. Other systemic symptoms may include generalized numbness, difficulty with speech and swallowing, paralysis, convulsions, tachycardia, and myocarditis. Death may result from respiratory paralysis, often within two hours of the sting.

Children under five years of age are particularly susceptible to the adverse effects of scorpion stings, and case fatality rates of 5% in Mexico, 25% in Trinidad, and 60% in the Sudan have been reported. Multiple stings, stings around the head, and stings of debilitated individuals are also particularly serious. Scorpion stings are not uncommon in the western U.S..[93]

Since the venom is injected into the subcutaneous tissues, initial treatment of scorpion stings should be designed to delay absorption of the toxin into the lymphatic vessels. The affected limb should be immobilized and the sting area cleaned with soap and water. Ice should be applied to the wound site and the patient kept calm. Specific scorpion antisera are available in areas where stings are common.[94-97]

Programs to reduce scorpion populations with wide-scale or focal application of persistent chemical pesticides have met with limited success. Elimination of rubbish piles around dwellings can reduce favored hiding and breeding places of scorpions.

References

1. Bowman, A. S.; Nuttall, P. A., Ticks: Biology, Disease and Control. Cambridge University Press. **2009**.
2. Sonenshine, D. E., Biology of Ticks Volume 2. **2013**.
3. Smith, T.; Kilobourne, F. L., Investigations into the Nature, Causation, and Prevention of Texas or Southern Cattle Fever. **1893**.
4. Marchoux, E.; Salimbeni, A., La spirillose des poules. *Ann Inst Pasteur Paris* **1903**, *17*, 569-580.
5. Ross, P. H.; Milne, A. D., "Tick Fever.". *British medical journal* **1904**, *2* (2291), 1453-4.
6. Bratton, R. L.; Corey, R., Tick-borne disease. *Am Fam Physician* **2005**, *71* (12), 2323-30.
7. de la Fuente, J.; Estrada-Pena, A.; Venzal, J. M.; Kocan, K. M.; Sonenshine, D. E., Overview: Ticks as vectors of pathogens that cause disease in humans and animals. *Front Biosci* **2008**, *13*, 6938-46.
8. Meagher, K. E.; Decker, C. F., Other tick-borne illnesses: tularemia, Colorado tick fever, tick paralysis. *Dis Mon* **2012**, *58* (6), 370-6.
9. Pujalte, G. G.; Chua, J. V., Tick-borne infections in the United States. *Prim Care* **2013**, *40* (3), 619-35.
10. Buckingham, S. C., Tick-borne diseases of the USA: Ten things clinicians should know. *J Infect* **2015**, *71 Suppl 1*, S88-96.
11. Anderson, J. F., The natural history of ticks. *Med Clin North Am* **2002**, *86* (2), 205-18.
12. Spielman, A.; Clifford, C. M.; Piesman, J.; Corwin, M. D., Human babesiosis on Nantucket Island, USA: description of the vector, Ixodes (Ixodes) dammini, n. sp. (Acarina: Ixodidae). *Journal of medical entomology* **1979**, *15* (3), 218-34.
13. Colyar, M., Tick removal techniques. *Adv Nurse Pract* **2006**, *14* (5), 26-7.
14. Spielman, A.; Wilson, M. L.; Levine, J. F.; Piesman, J., Ecology of Ixodes dammini-borne human babesiosis and Lyme disease. *Annual review of entomology* **1985**, *30*, 439-60.
15. Oliver, J. H., Jr.; Owsley, M. R.; Hutcheson, H. J.; James, A. M.; Chen, C.; Irby, W. S.; Dotson, E. M.; McLain, D. K., Conspecificity of the ticks Ixodes scapularis and I. dammini (Acari: Ixodidae). *J Med Entomol* **1993**, *30* (1), 54-63.
16. Burgdorfer, W.; Lane, R. S.; Barbour, A. G.; Gresbrink, R. A.; Anderson, J. R., The western black-legged tick, Ixodes pacificus: a vector of Borrelia burgdorferi. *The American journal of tropical medicine and hygiene* **1985**, *34* (5), 925-30.
17. Jupp, P. G.; Purcell, R. H.; Phillips, J. M.; Shapiro, M.; Gerin, J. L., Attempts to transmit hepatitis B virus to chimpanzees by arthropods. *South African medical journal = Suid-Afrikaanse tydskrif vir geneeskunde* **1991**, *79* (6), 320-2.
18. Sen, S. K., The mechanism of feeding in ticks. *Parasitology* **1935**, *27*, 355-368.
19. Greenstein, P., Tick paralysis. *Med Clin North Am* **2002**, *86* (2), 441-6.
20. Pecina, C. A., Tick paralysis. *Semin Neurol* **2012**, *32* (5), 531-2.
21. Vedanarayanan, V. V.; Evans, O. B.; Subramony, S. H., Tick paralysis in children: electrophysiology and possibility of misdiagnosis. *Neurology* **2002**, *59* (7), 1088-90.
22. Diaz, J. H., A Comparative Meta-Analysis of Tick Paralysis in the United States and Australia. *Clin Toxicol (Phila)* **2015**, *53* (9), 874-83.
23. Felz, M. W.; Smith, C. D.; Swift, T. R., A six-year-old girl with tick paralysis. *N Engl J Med* **2000**, *342* (2), 90-4.
24. Burgdorfer, W., Tick-borne diseases in the United States: Rocky Mountain spotted fever and Colorado tick fever. A review. *Acta tropica* **1977**, *34* (2), 103-26.
25. Burgdorfer, W.; J., A review of Rocky Mountain spotted fever (tick-borne typhus), its agent, and its tick vectors in the United States. *Entomol* **1979**, *12*, 269-278.
26. McDade, J. F.; Olson, J. G.; Ehrlichiosis, Q.; Gorbach, S. L.; Bartlett, J. G.; Blacklow, N. R., Erhlichiosis, Q fever, typhus, rickettsialpox, and other rickettsioses. 1998; p 1599-1611.
27. Ijdo, J. W.; Meek, J. I.; Cartter, M. L.; Magnerelli, L.; J., The emergence of another tick-borne infection in the 12-town area around Lyme, Connecticut: Human Granulocytic Ehrlichiosis. *Dis 181* **2000**, *4*.

28. Diuk-Wasser, M. A.; Vannier, E.; Krause, P. J., Coinfection by Ixodes Tick-Borne Pathogens: Ecological, Epidemiological, and Clinical Consequences. *Trends Parasitol* **2016**, *32* (1), 30-42.

29. Burgdorfer, W.; Johnson, R. C.; Orlando, F. L., The epidemiology of relapsing fevers. 1976; p 191-200.

30. Burgdorfer, W.; Barbour, A. G.; Hayes, S. F.; Benach, J. L.; Grunwaldt, E.; Davis, J. P., Lyme disease-a tick-borne spirochetosis? *Science (New York, N.Y.)* **1982**, *216* (4552), 1317-9.

31. Burgdorfer, W.; Barbour, A. G.; Hayes, S. F.; Péter, O.; Aeschlimann, A., Erythema chronicum migrans--a tickborne spirochetosis. *Acta tropica* **1983**, *40* (1), 79-83.

32. Basler, E. M.; Coleman, J. L.; al, e., Natural distribution of Ixodes dammini spirochete *Science* **1983**, *220* 321-322.

33. Lane, R. S.; Piesman, J.; Burgdorfer, W., Lyme borreliosis: relation of its causative agent to its vectors and hosts in North America and Europe. *Annual review of entomology* **1991**, *36*, 587-609.

34. Steere, A. C.; Grodzicki, R. L.; Kornblatt, A. N.; Craft, J. E.; Barbour, A. G.; Burgdorfer, W.; Schmid, G. P.; Johnson, E.; Malawista, S. E., The spirochetal etiology of Lyme disease. *The New England journal of medicine* **1983**, *308* (13), 733-40.

35. Pages, F.; Dautel, H.; Duvallet, G.; Kahl, O.; de Gentile, L.; Boulanger, N., Tick repellents for human use: prevention of tick bites and tick-borne diseases. *Vector Borne Zoonotic Dis* **2014**, *14* (2), 85-93.

36. Kilpatrick, H. J.; LaBonte, A. M.; Stafford, K. C., The relationship between deer density, tick abundance, and human cases of Lyme disease in a residential community. *J Med Entomol* **2014**, *51* (4), 777-84.

37. Rand, P. W.; Lubelczyk, C.; Holman, M. S.; Lacombe, E. H.; Smith, R. P., Jr., Abundance of Ixodes scapularis (Acari: Ixodidae) after the complete removal of deer from an isolated offshore island, endemic for Lyme Disease. *J Med Entomol* **2004**, *41* (4), 779-84.

38. Pound, J. M.; Miller, J. A.; George, J. E.; Oehler, D. D.; Harmel, D. E., Systemic treatment of white-tailed deer with ivermectin-medicated bait to control free-living populations of lone star ticks (Acari:Ixodidae). *J Med Entomol* **1996**, *33* (3), 385-94.

39. Busvine, J. R., Insects, Hygiene, and History. *Athlone Press London* **1976**.

40. Mellanby, K., Transmission of Scabies. *Br Med J* **1941**, *2* (4211), 405-6.

41. Rosamilia, L. L., Scabies. *Semin Cutan Med Surg* **2014**, *33* (3), 106-9.

42. Walton, S. F.; Holt, D. C.; Currie, B. J.; Kemp, D. J., Scabies: new future for a neglected disease. *Advances in parasitology* **2004**, *57*, 309-76.

43. Romani, L.; Steer, A. C.; Whitfeld, M. J.; Kaldor, J. M., Prevalence of scabies and impetigo worldwide: a systematic review. *Lancet Infect Dis* **2015**, *15* (8), 960-7.

44. Hatter, A. D.; Soler, D. C.; Curtis, C.; Cooper, K. D.; McCormick, T. S., Case report of individual with cutaneous immunodeficiency and novel 1p36 duplication. *Appl Clin Genet* **2016**, *9*, 1-4.

45. Karthikeyan, K., Crusted scabies. *Indian J Dermatol Venereol Leprol* **2009**, *75* (4), 340-7.

46. Guldbakke, K. K.; Khachemoune, A., Crusted scabies: a clinical review. *J Drugs Dermatol* **2006**, *5* (3), 221-7.

47. Goldust, M.; Rezaee, E.; Hemayat, S., Treatment of scabies: Comparison of permethrin 5% versus ivermectin. *J Dermatol* **2012**, *39* (6), 545-7.

48. Romani, L.; Whitfeld, M. J.; Koroivueta, J.; Kama, M.; Wand, H.; Tikoduadua, L.; Tuicakau, M.; Koroi, A.; Andrews, R.; Kaldor, J. M.; Steer, A. C., Mass Drug Administration for Scabies Control in a Population with Endemic Disease. *N Engl J Med* **2015**, *373* (24), 2305-13.

49. Sasa, M., Biology of chiggers. *Annu Rev Entomol* **1961**, *6* 221-244.

50. Audy, J. R., Red Mites and Typhus. *Athlone Press London* **1968**.

51. Schulert, G. S.; Gigante, J., Summer penile syndrome: an acute hypersensitivity reaction. *J Emerg Med* **2014**, *46* (1), e21-2.

52. Fuller, H. S.; J., Studies of rickettsial pox: Life cycle of the mite vector Allodermanyssus sanguineus. *I Am* **1954**, *59*, 236-239.

53. Elston, C. A.; Elston, D. M., Demodex mites. *Clin Dermatol* **2014**, *32* (6), 739-43.

54. Chen, W.; Plewig, G., Human demodicosis: revisit and a proposed classification. *Br J Dermatol* **2014**, *170* (6), 1219-25.

55.   Cheng, A. M.; Sheha, H.; Tseng, S. C., Recent advances on ocular Demodex infestation. *Curr Opin Ophthalmol* **2015**, *26* (4), 295-300.

56.   Ali, S. T.; Alinia, H.; Feldman, S. R., The treatment of rosacea with topical ivermectin. *Drugs Today (Barc)* **2015**, *51* (4), 243-50.

57.   Cafiero, M. A.; Raele, D. A.; Mancini, G.; Galante, D., Dermatitis by Tropical Rat Mite, Ornithonyssus bacoti (Mesostigmata, Macronyssidae) in Italian city-dwellers: a diagnostic challenge. *J Eur Acad Dermatol Venereol* **2015**.

58.   Arlien, L. G.; Morgan, M. S., Biology, ecology, and prevelance of dust mites. *Immunol Allergy Clin North Am* **2003**, *23*, 443-468.

59.   Milian, E.; Diaz, A. M.; Sci, J.; R., P., Allergy to house dust mites and asthma. **2004**, *23* 47-57.

60.   Bessot, J. C.; Pauli, G., Mite allergens: an overview. *Eur Ann Allergy Clin Immunol* **2011**, *43* (5), 141-56.

61.   Huss, K.; Adkinson, N. F., Jr.; Eggleston, P. A.; Dawson, C.; Van Natta, M. L.; Hamilton, R. G., House dust mite and cockroach exposure are strong risk factors for positive allergy skin test responses in the Childhood Asthma Management Program. *J Allergy Clin Immunol* **2001**, *107* (1), 48-54.

62.   Raulf, M.; Bergmann, K. C.; Kull, S.; Sander, I.; Hilger, C.; Bruning, T.; Jappe, U.; Musken, H.; Sperl, A.; Vrtala, S.; Zahradnik, E.; Klimek, L., Mites and other indoor allergens - from exposure to sensitization and treatment. *Allergo J Int* **2015**, *24* (3), 68-80.

63.   Ken, K. M.; Shockman, S. C.; Sirichotiratana, M.; Lent, M. P.; Wilson, M. L., Dermatoses associated with mites other than Sarcoptes. *Semin Cutan Med Surg* **2014**, *33* (3), 110-5.

64.   Juckett, G., Arthropod bites. *Am Fam Physician* **2013**, *88* (12), 841-7.

65.   Vetter, R. S.; Isbister, G. K., Medical aspects of spider bites. *Annu Rev Entomol* **2008**, *53*, 409-29.

66.   Isbister, G. K.; Fan, H. W., Spider bite. *Lancet* **2011**, *378* (9808), 2039-47.

67.   Kang, J. K.; Bhate, C.; Schwartz, R. A., Spiders in dermatology. *Semin Cutan Med Surg* **2014**, *33* (3), 123-7.

68.   Nicholson, G. M.; Graudins, A., Spiders of medical importance in the Asia-Pacific: atracotoxin, latrotoxin and related spider neurotoxins. *Clin Exp Pharmacol Physiol* **2002**, *29* (9), 785-94.

69.   Maretic, Z.; North, I.; Bucherl, W.; Buckley, E. E., Venomous Animals and Their Venoms. 1971; p 299-309.

70.   Russell, F. E., Venom Poisoning. *Rational drug therapy* **1971**, *5* (8), 1-7.

71.   Sudhof, T. C., alpha-Latrotoxin and its receptors: neurexins and CIRL/latrophilins. . *Annu Rev Neurosci* **2001**, *24*, 933-62.

72.   Monte, A. A., Black widow spider (Latrodectus mactans) antivenom in clinical practice. *Curr Pharm Biotechnol* **2012**, *13* (10), 1935-9.

73.   Monte, A. A.; Bucher-Bartelson, B.; Heard, K. J., A US perspective of symptomatic Latrodectus spp. envenomation and treatment: a National Poison Data System review. *Ann Pharmacother* **2011**, *45* (12), 1491-8.

74.   Furbee, R. B.; Kao, L. W.; Ibrahim, D., Brown recluse spider envenomation. *Clin Lab Med* **2006**, *26* (1), 211-26, ix-x.

75.   Levi, H. W.; Spielman, A.; J., Biology and control of the South American brown spider Loxosceles laeta (Nicolet) in a North American focus. *Am Med Hyg* **1964**, *13*, 132-136.

76.   Rhoads, J., Epidemiology of the brown recluse spider bite. *J Am Acad Nurse Pract* **2007**, *19* (2), 79-85.

77.   Wendell, R. P., Brown recluse spiders: a review to help guide physicians in nonendemic areas. *South Med J* **2003**, *96* (5), 486-90.

78.   Vetter, R. S.; Barger, D. K., An infestation of 2,055 brown recluse spiders (Araneae: Sicariidae) and no envenomations in a Kansas home: implications for bite diagnoses in nonendemic areas. *J Med Entomol* **2002**, *39* (6), 948-51.

79.   Vetter, R., Identifying and misidentifying the brown recluse spider. *Dermatology online journal* **1999**, *5* (2), 7.

80.   Swanson, D. L.; Vetter, R. S., Bites of brown recluse spiders and suspected necrotic arachnidism. *The New England journal of medicine* **2005**, *352* (7), 700-7.

81. Williams, S. T.; Khare, V. K.; Johnston, G. A.; Blackall, D. P., Severe intravascular hemolysis associated with brown recluse spider envenomation. A report of two cases and review of the literature. *American journal of clinical pathology* **1995,** *104* (4), 463-7.

82. Zeglin, D., Brown recluse spider bites. *Am J Nurs* **2005,** *105* (2), 64-8.

83. Spielman, A.; Levi, H. W., Probable envenomation by Chiracanthium mildei; a spider found in houses. *The American journal of tropical medicine and hygiene* **1970,** *19* (4), 729-32.

84. Nimorakiotakis, B.; Winkel, K. D., The funnel web and common spider bites. *Aust Fam Physician* **2004,** *33* (4), 244-51.

85. Isbister, G. K.; Graudins, A.; White, J.; Warrell, D., Antivenom treatment in arachnidism. *J Toxicol Clin Toxicol* **2003,** *41* (3), 291-300.

86. Isbister, G. K.; Gray, M. R.; Balit, C. R.; Raven, R. J.; Stokes, B. J.; Porges, K.; Tankel, A. S.; Turner, E.; White, J.; Fisher, M. M., Funnel-web spider bite: a systematic review of recorded clinical cases. *Med J Aust* **2005,** *182* (8), 407-11.

87. Isbister, G. K.; Gray, M. R., Bites by Australian mygalomorph spiders (Araneae, Mygalomorphae), including funnel-web spiders (Atracinae) and mouse spiders (Actinopodidae: Missulena spp). *Toxicon* **2004,** *43* (2), 133-40.

88. Graudins, A.; Padula, M.; Broady, K.; Nicholson, G. M., Red-back spider (Latrodectus hasselti) antivenom prevents the toxicity of widow spider venoms. *Ann Emerg Med* **2001,** *37* (2), 154-60.

89. White, J., Envenoming and antivenom use in Australia. *Toxicon : official journal of the International Society on Toxinology* **1998,** *36* (11), 1483-92.

90. Currie, B. J., Clinical toxicology: a tropical Australian perspective. *Therapeutic drug monitoring* **2000,** *22* (1), 73-8.

91. Keegan, H. L., Scorpions of medical importance. 1980.

92. Del Brutto, O. H., Neurological effects of venomous bites and stings: snakes, spiders, and scorpions. *Handb Clin Neurol* **2013,** *114,* 349-68.

93. LoVecchio, F.; McBride, C., Scorpion envenomations in young children in central Arizona. *J Toxicol Clin Toxicol* **2003,** *41* (7), 937-40.

94. Tuuri, R. E.; Reynolds, S., Scorpion envenomation and antivenom therapy. *Pediatr Emerg Care* **2011,** *27* (7), 667-72; quiz 673-5.

95. Bawaskar, H. S.; Bawaskar, P. H., Scorpion sting: update. *J Assoc Physicians India* **2012,** *60,* 46-55.

96. Bosnak, M.; Levent Yilmaz, H.; Ece, A.; Yildizdas, D.; Yolbas, I.; Kocamaz, H.; Kaplan, M.; Bosnak, V., Severe scorpion envenomation in children: Management in pediatric intensive care unit. *Hum Exp Toxicol* **2009,** *28* (11), 721-8.

97. Chippaux, J. P., Emerging options for the management of scorpion stings. *Drug Des Devel Ther* **2012,** *6,* 165-73.

40. Arthropods of Minor Importance

Butterflies and Moths: Order Lepidoptera

Several species of larvae or caterpillars of the order Lepidoptera are covered with hollow, sharply pointed hairs containing a toxin that may cause severe dermatitis. Contact occurs when an individual handles the caterpillars or inhales the "hairs," which are blown about after the larva molts. In the northeastern United States, the gypsy moth, *Lymantria dispar*, has been responsible for defoliation of enormous areas of forest. The "population explosion" of the caterpillars of this species has led to periodic outbreaks of pruritic dermatitis, primarily among school children.[1] Similar outbreaks of dermatitis have been reported from the southeastern and south central states, attributed to the caterpillars of the puss moth *Megalopyge opercalis*. In a Mexican outbreak, severe dermatitis was initially attributed to scabies, but eventually associated with contact with adult moths of the species *Hylesia alinda*. Populations of this normally rare species rapidly expanded after its natural predators were killed by a hurricane sweeping the island.[2]

Individuals working with lepidopterans may become sensitized to the scales of adult moths or butterflies. Repeated exposure may produce severe bronchospasm and even asthma. There is an increasing awareness of the ubiquity and potential serious consequences of exposure to a wide range of these larvae.[3-5]

Beetles: Order Coleoptera

Within the order Coleoptera, which comprises a large group of insects, only a few families contain members of medical importance. Certain scavenger beetles of the families Dermestidae, Silphidae, and Staphylinidae feed on feces and carrion and mechanically transmit pathogenic organism. Adult beetles of the family Meloidae, the blister beetles, produce a vesicant (cantharidin) that may cause blistering or a severe burning sensation on contact with the skin or mucous membranes. Inadvertent ingestion of beetle larvae, a condition termed canthariasis, may produce transient gastrointestinal discomfort.

Many beetles, particularly those that feed on feces, act as intermediate hosts for helminthic parasites of humans and other animals. Members of the family Scarabaeidae are intermediate hosts of the spiny-headed worm *Macracanthorhynchus hirudinaceus*, a parasite of pigs, which rarely infects humans. The tapeworms *Hymenolepis nana* and *H. diminuta* develop in grain beetles of the family Tenebrionidae.

Cockroaches: Order Orthoptera

Orthoptera is a large, diverse order of primitive, successful insects (over 4,000 species, worldwide) that includes the grasshoppers and crickets, as well as cockroaches. The cockroaches are included in a single family, the Blattidae, with several members closely associated with human habitations. All members of this group have chewing mouthparts.

The female cockroach encloses her eggs in a bean-shaped case called an ootheca. Some species retain the ootheca internally until the eggs hatch, others carry it externally for several weeks, and still others drop the ootheca soon after it is formed. After hatching, the young, wingless, feeding nymphs begin to undergo staged development. Some species progress through as many as 13 nymph stages, each being wingless and somewhat larger than its predecessor, until the final molt produces the winged adult. With its series of wingless nymph stages, the cockroach is a classic example of an insect developing by incomplete metamorphosis.

Most cockroach species do not invade homes, confining themselves to outdoor habitats, although in the United States eleven species of cockroaches do invade human habitats. The most common is the German cockroach or croton bug, *Blatella germanica*, a small (<16 mm), light brown species. The American cockroach or palmetto bug, *Periplaneta americana*, is in fact an African species now found worldwide. It is a large (30-40 mm) reddish-brown insect with long wings. It is found in and around homes, farms, restaurants, stores, and warehouses. Other species that may infest homes are the Oriental cockroach *Blatta orientalis*, the Australian cockroach *P. australasiae*, and the brown-banded cockroach, *Supella longipalpa*.

Most of these species are cosmopolitan, having been distributed by ship traffic starting with the earliest voyages. In general, domestic species are omnivorous. They feed on a wide variety of nutrients, paper, book bindings, and human and animal feces. They serve as mechanical vectors of pathogens, carrying infectious agents from feces to food.[6]

The presence of cockroaches is usually associated with a breakdown of general sanitation. Exposed foods or poor packaging and storage, open garbage, darkness and moisture are all conducive to the development of large cockroach populations. Initial infestations may be introduced with foodstuffs or migration from adjoining dwellings. In apartment buildings, the insecticide treatment of one apartment may cause the migration of cockroaches to adjoining, untreated apartments.

Although cockroaches are resistant to a number of insecticides in some areas, compounds for control are commercially available. Coupled with improved housekeeping, treatment with these agents can be sufficient, although heavy infestations require repeated treatments by professional exterminators.

Cockroaches, because of their close association with sewage and garbage, may serve as paratenic hosts for various pathogens.[6]

Long-term exposure to cockroaches or to their shed exoskeletons can induce asthma-like symptoms.[7, 8]

Centipedes: Class Chilopoda

The centipedes of the class Chilopoda are worm-like, segmented creatures with a distinct head and paired appendages on each of 15-100 or more segments. They have a pair of poisonous claws, or maxillipeds, on the first segment after the head, which are used for capturing prey. Most centipedes are predaceous insectivores, and humans are sometimes bitten accidentally. Centipede bites may be locally painful, causing transient swelling at the site of the bite. No long-term complications are usually associated with these bites.[9]

Crustacea

The crustacea include many species that serve as intermediate hosts of parasites of humans and other animals. These organisms are discussed in the other, relevant chapters.

Tongue Worms: Class Pentastomida

The pentastomids, or tongue worms, of the class Pentastomida are a small group of parasites of uncertain origin and affinity. Because their larvae superficially resemble the larvae of mites, they have been included among the Arthropoda, but they probably evolved early from annelid or arthropod ancestral stocks. They were first noted in the nasal cavities of dogs and horses during the eighteenth century and were later described in human autopsy material as insect larvae.

The adult tongue worms are blood sucking, endoparasitic, legless vermiform inhabitants of the respiratory system of reptiles, birds, and mammals. Eggs fertilized within the host emerge through the respiratory tract. After being eaten by an intermediate host, they hatch in the gut, yielding a migratory larva that pierces the stomach wall and encysts in host tissue. When the intermediate host is eaten by the definitive host, the larvae mature.[10]

In humans, encysted larvae have been found in the lungs, liver, intestine, spleen, and other internal organs.[11, 12] There may be rare cases of symptomatic human disease from infection with tongue worms, but most cases are usually identified at autopsy without prior attributable symptoms.[11-15]

References

1.   Allen, V. T.; Miller, O. F., 3rd; Tyler, W. B., Gypsy moth caterpillar dermatitis--revisited. *J Am Acad Dermatol* **1991,** *24* (6 Pt 1), 979-81.

2.   Fernandez, G.; Morales, E.; Beutelspacher, C.; Villanueva, A.; Ruiz, C.; Stetler, H. C., Epidemic dermatitis due to contact with a moth in Cozumel, Mexico. *The American journal of tropical medicine and hygiene* **1992,** *46* (5), 560-3.

3.   Diaz, J. H., The evolving global epidemiology, syndromic classification, management, and prevention of caterpillar envenoming. *The American journal of tropical medicine and hygiene* **2005,** *72* (3), 347-57.

4.   Hossler, E. W., Caterpillars and moths. *Dermatol Ther* **2009,** *22* (4), 353-66.

5.   Hossler, E. W., Caterpillars and moths: Part II. Dermatologic manifestations of encounters with Lepidoptera. *J Am Acad Dermatol* **2010,** *62* (1), 13-28; quiz 29-30.

6.   Graczyk, T. K.; Knight, R.; Tamang, L., Mechanical transmission of human protozoan parasites by insects. *Clin Microbiol Rev* **2005,** *18* (1), 128-32.

7.   Gao, P., Sensitization to cockroach allergen: immune regulation and genetic determinants. *Clin Dev Immunol* **2012,** *2012,* 563760.

8.   Pomes, A.; Arruda, L. K., Investigating cockroach allergens: aiming to improve diagnosis and treatment of cockroach allergic patients. *Methods* **2014,** *66* (1), 75-85.

9.   Sanaei-Zadeh, H., Centipede bite. *Eur Rev Med Pharmacol Sci* **2014,** *18* (7), 1106-7.

10.   Drabick, J. J., Pentastomiasis. *Rev Infect Dis* **1987,** *9,* 1087-1094.

11.   Tappe, D.; Buttner, D. W., Diagnosis of human visceral pentastomiasis. *PLoS Negl Trop Dis* **2009,** *3* (2), e320.

12.   Tappe, D.; Dijkmans, A. C.; Brienen, E. A.; Dijkmans, B. A.; Ruhe, I. M.; Netten, M. C.; van Lieshout, L., Imported Armillifer pentastomiasis: report of a symptomatic infection in The Netherlands and mini-review. *Travel Med Infect Dis* **2014,** *12* (2), 129-33.

13.   Latif, B.; Omar, E.; Heo, C. C.; Othman, N.; Tappe, D., Human pentastomiasis caused by Armillifer moniliformis in Malaysian Borneo. *Am J Trop Med Hyg* **2011,** *85* (5), 878-81.

14.   Sulyok, M.; Rozsa, L.; Bodo, I.; Tappe, D.; Hardi, R., Ocular pentastomiasis in the Democratic Republic of the Congo. *PLoS Negl Trop Dis* **2014,** *8* (7), e3041.

15.   Tappe, D.; Sulyok, M.; Rozsa, L.; Muntau, B.; Haeupler, A.; Bodo, I.; Hardi, R., Molecular Diagnosis of Abdominal Armillifer grandis Pentastomiasis in the Democratic Republic of Congo. *J Clin Microbiol* **2015,** *53* (7), 2362-4.

Appendix A: Procedures for Collecting Clinical Specimens for Diagnosing Protozoan and Helminthic Parasites

There is no substitute for a well-trained laboratory diagnostic technician, even with the advent of sensitive and specific serological and molecular diagnostic methods, such as ELISA, PCR, and NAAT. But even the best-trained personnel cannot make up for an improper sample delivered to the laboratory in the expectation of securing the diagnosis. Stool, blood, urine and tissue samples must be treated as the most important link between the patient and the correct diagnosis of their parasitic illness. The following advice outlines standard procedure for insuring that the diagnostic laboratory receives the right amount and type of patient specimen.

Stool Specimens

Proper collection and delivery of stool specimens is a critical aspect of any diagnostic procedure relying on stool examination. The clinician can control the quality of this aspect, and in doing so, will insure both the reliability and accuracy of any test they recommend, regardless of whether that test is carried out in-house or at a regional diagnostic facility.

1. Fresh, unpreserved feces should be obtained and transported to the laboratory immediately. Fresh specimens are preferred for examinations for trophozoites, and are required when tests for *Strongyloides stercoralis* larvae are to be performed.
2. Unpreserved feces should be examined within one hour after passage, especially if the stool is loose or watery, and might contain trophozoites of pathogenic amoebae. Examination of formed stool may be delayed for a short time, but must

be completed on the day on which the specimen is received in the laboratory. If prompt examination or proper fixation cannot be carried out, formed specimens may be refrigerated for 1-2 days.
3. If specimens are delayed in reaching the laboratory, or if they cannot be examined promptly (such as those received at night, on weekends, or when no parasitologist is available), portions should be preserved in fixatives such as 8% aqueous formalin or formol-saline, or with polyvinyl alcohol (PVA). Formalin preserves cysts, eggs and larvae for wet-mount examination or for concentration tests. PVA-fixative preserves trophozoites, cysts, and eggs for permanent staining. A ratio of one part feces to three parts of fixative is recommended. The specimen may be placed in fixatives in the laboratory, or the patient may be provided with fixatives and instructions for collection and preservation of their own specimens.

Stool Examination

Stool specimens may be successfully examined by any one of the three methods listed below. The advantages and limitations of each technique must be recognized.

1. Saline mounts are of value primarily for demonstrating the characteristic motility of amoebae and flagellates. In addition, seeing red cells inside a trophozoite of an amoeba is indicative of infection with *Entamoeba histolytica*. These organisms may be found in fresh stools, or occasionally in bloody mucus adhering to the surface of formed stools. Material should be obtained from several parts of the specimen. An iodine stain (a drop of 1% iodine in 2% potassium iodide) mixed with a stool suspension in saline solution facilitates identification of

protozoan cysts, but it kills and distorts trophozoites.

2. Concentration techniques, useful for detecting small numbers of cysts and helminth eggs, may be used on unpreserved stool specimens, those preserved in aqueous formalin or formol-saline, or on PVA-fixed material.

3. Stained, thin smears of feces should be made if possible on all specimens obtained fresh or fixed in PVA. If properly prepared, they comprise the single most productive stool examination for protozoa. Smears may be stained with Wheatly-Gomori's Trichrome solution or with iron-hematoxylin (see Appendix B for colors of each). Any outstanding examples of positive specimens should be retained in a permanent file and used for future reference.

Number of Specimens Examined and Appropriate Intervals

1. To detect amoebae, a minimum of three specimens should be examined; if these samples (obtained preferably at intervals of 2-3 days) are negative and amoebic infection remains a diagnostic consideration, additional specimens should be examined.

2. With suspected giardiasis, nucleic amplification testing and antigen capture ELISA are the currently recommended tests. When employing light microscopy, three specimens should initially be examined. If they are negative, additional specimens should be obtained at weekly intervals for three weeks.

3. A single concentrate from one day's worth of stool is frequently sufficient to detect intestinal helminthic infections of clinical importance. With very light infections due to *Schistosoma* spp., few or no eggs may be found in the feces or urine. *Strongyloides stercoralis* may also require concentrating the specimen for diagnosis, but this method is not always reliable; various fecal culture methods may also be used.

4. Examination after treatment, under most circumstances, should be delayed until one month after completion of therapy (three months after treatment for schistosomiasis or tapeworms).

Examination of Blood

1. Smears for malaria should consist of both thick and thin films. It is important that all involved laboratory personnel be aware of the technique for making thick films as they are useless if improperly made. Smears should be stained with Giemsa solution and a minimum of 100 contiguous microscopic fields examined before a specimen is reported as "negative." If the first specimen is negative, additional thick and thin films should be taken every six hours for the first 24 hours after admission.

2. When examining for filarial infection, the possibility of diurnal or nocturnal periodicity of microfilariae in the peripheral blood must be taken into account, and specimens should be taken every six hours for the first 24 hours after admission, as with malaria. Thick smears or blood concentration methods are most likely to demonstrate infection. Smears should be done in conjunction with the Knott Test (see Appendix B).

Serologic Methods

A variety of immunodiagnostic methods may serve as useful adjuncts to the clinical diagnosis of parasitic infections. In some cases, serologic methods may be the only laboratory recourse for making a diagnosis. Certain serologic tests provide a high degree of diagnostic accuracy; however, mixed infections, cross reacting antigens by related and unrelated parasites, and other diseases or physiologic conditions may interfere with the diagnostic accuracy of a given test.

Western blot analysis and ELISA will undoubtedly continue to offer the clinician sensitive, reliable methods for diagnosing parasitic infections. Positive tests revealing the presence of specific antibodies are indirect evidence of infection, no matter how good the method. Tests employing antibody capture techniques, in which monoclonal antibodies are used to select for a single class of immunoglobulin increases the likelihood of a true positive result.

Most serum specimens may be shipped frozen or preserved with thimerosal to a final concentration of 1:10,000 to a state public health laboratory for forwarding to the Centers for Disease Control and Prevention in Atlanta, Georgia. The vial, containing at least 2 ml of serum, should indicate the preservative used.

Nucleic Acid Amplification Tests (NAAT) and Polymerase chain reaction (PCR)

The advent of amplifying parasite DNA in stool, blood, and tissue samples has widened the range of parasite detection methods. Reliable NAAT tests have been developed for malaria, most species that cause leishmaniasis, toxoplasmosis, giardiasis, amoebiasis (*Entamoeba histolytica* and *E. dispar*), trypanosomiasis, and many others, as well. These tests have already become the primary diagnostic tests in many clinical centers.

Appendix B: Laboratory Diagnostic Methods

In recent years, a battery of cutting-edge diagnostic modalities have emerged, making the identification of many infectious diseases straightforward, without requiring any more skill than being able to read the instructions and to execute them. Microscopy training is not needed in these instances. Each of the preceding chapters attests to this fact, with a robust sampling of modern serological and molecular diagnostic strategies.

The vast majority of parasitology laboratories in hospitals and outpatient health clinics throughout the world continue to rely on more traditional approaches for the diagnosis of eukaryotic parasites. In these instances, microscopy remains the gold standard for pathogen identification. This chapter serves as a standard reference for these time-honored laboratory procedures.

Part I deals with unpreserved specimens and Part II with preserved specimens. There is no single method that efficiently renders all stages of all parasites available for microscopic identification; several tests must often be performed to obtain optimal results.

Unpreserved Stool Specimens

Ideally, stool specimens should be less than one hour old when first examined, although this may not always be possible. Stools that are up to 24 hours old may still be useful for recovering protozoan cysts, larvae and eggs of helminthes, but trophozoites rarely survive that long. A confounding factor when examining specimens left at room temperature for more than 24 hours is that some parasites can grow and develop. Refrigeration helps prevent this problem. Stools should not be frozen, as that would alter the morphology of the organisms examined.

Because of day-to-day variability in the quantity of various stages of parasite shed by an infected individual, parasites may not be present in a single specimen, particularly when the infection is light. A total of three specimens collected on consecutive days are suggested when attempting to detect most enteric infections by visual microscopy. Some parasites (e.g., the schistosomes and *Giardia lamblia*) often require more specimens for detection or the use of more sensitive diagnostic modalities.

Barium or mineral oil interferes with identification of parasites. Patients should not be subjected to radiographic studies involving barium or given laxatives containing mineral oil until the stool specimens have been obtained.

Direct Examination

Gross examination:
1. Observe and record the appearance of the entire specimen, noting the color, consistency, and odor.
2. Examine the specimen for the presence of living parasites.
3. Perform a microscopic examination.
4. Examine a direct smear of the material.

The direct examination is effective for diagnosing living parasites (e.g., *Entamoeba histolytica, Giardia lamblia, Strongyloides stercoralis*), and should be performed on loose, diarrheic, or purged stool. When motile amoebae are found on a direct smear, a stained preparation should also be examined for the definitive diagnosis. If the amoeba contains erythrocytes within the cytoplasm, it is indicative of infection caused by *E. histolytica*.

If the specimen appears negative, as may occur with light infections, the sample should be concentrated.

1. Dip a wooden applicator stick into the

specimen to coat the tip of it with stool.

2. Smear the stool onto a clear glass microscope slide on which a drop of normal saline solution has been placed and overlay with a coverslip. Smears must be thin enough to facilitate microscopic examination.

Staining the Direct smear

The Wheatly-Gomori trichrome (WGT) reagent stains the protozoan nuclei red to dark blue, the cytoplasm a lighter blue, and the background material green. Trophozoites and cysts tend to shrink away from the background material and are therefore relatively easy to locate.

The WGT reagent consists of 6.0 g chromotrope 2R, 0.5 g aniline blue CI42755, and 0.25 g dodecatungstophosphoric acid AR in 3 ml glacial acetic acid. WGT stain is applied to a thin smear of stool on a coverslip, and the coverslip is immersed sequentially in the solutions enumerated below for the prescribed lengths of time.

Solution	Time
Schaudinn's fixative	5 minutes at
50+°C, or 1 hour at room temperature	
Ethanol-iodine 70%	1 minute
Ethanol 70%	1 minute
Ethanol 70%	1 minute
Trichrome stain	2-8 minutes
Ethanol 90%	10-20 secs
(acidified)	

To remove excess stain, briefly dip the coverslip in destaining solution once or twice. Rinse in 90% ethanol to stop the process. Thin smears destain quickly; thicker ones may require three or four dips to obtain optimal differentiation. The process is as follows.

Solution	Time
Ethanol 95% or 100%	Two rinses
Ethanol 100%	1 minute
Xylol	1 minute

Mount the coverslip in an appropriate mounting medium and examine under a microscope.

Concentration Methods

Sedimentation by Centrifugation: Formaldehyde-Ethyl Acetate Method.

Sedimentation by concentration and exposure to formaldehyde-ethyl acetate concentrates cysts and eggs of parasites, but debris and ether-soluble materials localize in the formaldehyde-ether interface or the ether layer in the top of the tube. This process destroys trophozoites, as they disintegrate in ethyl acetate.

1. Mix stool 1:10 with H_2O.
2. Strain through a single layer of gauze into a 15-ml centrifuge tube.
3. Centrifuge the strained stool (1 minute at 2000 rpm) and discard the supernatant.
4. Wash the sediment once with H_2O.
5. Repeat steps 3 and 4.
6. Discard the supernatant and save the sediment.
7. Add 10 ml of 7.5% formaldehyde to the sediment.
8. Let stand 10-30 minutes.
9. Add approximately 3 ml of ethyl acetate, plug the tubes with stoppers, and agitate the mixture vigorously.
10. Remove the stoppers and centrifuge the tubes at 1500 rpm for 1 minute.
11. Gently loosen the debris from the tube wall with an applicator stick, being careful not to disturb the pellet.
12. Discard the supernatant.
13. Examine the sediment microscopically.
14. Add a drop of 70% ethanol-iodine solution (Lugol's solution) and examine

again if internal structures of cysts are not recognized on first examination.

Sedimentation by Gravity:

The water sedimentation test is used primarily for the concentration and recovery of *Schistosoma mansoni* and *Schistosoma japonicum* eggs, and it is effective for determining their viability. An entire day's worth of stool should be examined in a single test because schistosome eggs are shed sporadically.

1. Emulsify the entire stool sample in H_2O.
2. Strain the specimen through a single layer of gauze into conical sedimentation flasks.
3. Allow the sediment to settle (approximately 20 minutes) and discard the supernatant.
4. Resuspend the sediment in water.
5. Repeat steps 3 and 4 until the supernatant is clear.
6. Discard final supernatant and save the sediment.
7. Examine the entire sediment microscopically.

The entire water sedimentation procedure should be done within two hours of starting, since prolonged exposure of schistosome eggs to water stimulates them to hatch. If hatching occurs, the empty shells remain in the sediment and the ciliated miracidia can be seen moving about rapidly.

Baerman Sedimentation Method.

This method is extremely useful for concentrating and recovering larvae of *Strongyloides stercoralis*. The test requires a funnel with a piece of rubber tubing attached to it. An adjustable clamp is applied across the tubing, and the entire apparatus is suspended from a ring stand in a 37°C incubator. Larvae concentrate in the

sediment that accumulates in the base of the rubber tube connected to the funnel, and the fluid containing them is expressed into a test tube for microscopic identification

1. Emulsify the entire stool sample in H2O.
2. Strain the specimen through a single layer of gauze into conical sedimentation flasks.
3. Allow the sediment to settle (approximately 20 minutes) and discard the supernatant.
4. Resuspend the sediment in water.
5. Repeat steps 3 and 4 until the supernatant is clear.
6. Discard final supernatant and save the sediment.
7. Examine the entire sediment microscopically.

Floatation by Centrifugation:

Floatation methods concentrate various stages of parasites by taking advantage of their specific gravity. The unwanted debris sediments to the bottom of the tube during centrifugation, but the diagnostic forms float to the surface. Cysts and most eggs can be recovered in large quantities by this method, but trophozoites, operculated eggs, and schistosome eggs are either destroyed, or sediment to the bottom of the tube.

Zinc Sulfate Floatation Method
1. Mix 1 part stool in 15 ml H_2O in a 15-ml centrifuge tube.
2. Centrifuge for 1 minute at 2500 rpm; decant the supernatant.
3. Add zinc sulfate solution (specific gravity1.18) until the tube is half full and resuspend the sediment with a wooden applicator stick.
4. Fill the tube to the top with more zinc sulfate solution.
5. Centrifuge the suspension for 1 minute at 2500rpm. Do not apply the brake to the centrifuge or jar the tube, as

either maneuver causes any eggs or cysts accumulated at the liquid-surface interface to sink.

6. Using a bacteriologic loop, remove two aliquots from the surface and place them on a clean glass slide.

7. Examine microscopically. A small drop of Lugol's iodine solution can be added to provide contrast.

Sugar (Sheather's) Floatation Method.

The recovery of *Cryptosporidium parvum* oocysts is facilitated by this method.

1. Filter stool through three pieces of cheesecloth.

2. Place 2 ml of stool filtrate in a conical tube.

3. Fill the tube to the top with sucrose solution.

4. Place a coverslip on top of the tube.

5. Centrifuge at 1000 rpm for 5 minutes. If the stool sample is watery, no centrifugation is necessary. Let the coverslip rest on the top of sucrose solution for 20 minutes.

6. Examine the coverslip microscopically at 400 X. The focal plane is important, because the oocysts are located on the inner surface of the coverslip, rather than on the slide itself. The oocysts appear slightly pink in color without the addition of any stain. They are ovoid to spherical in shape, range in size from 5 to 6 um in diameter and are usually not sporulated.

Blood

Fresh, heparinized, or citrated blood samples are best for examination. Delays reduce the chances of finding the parasites.

Place a drop of blood on a slide, overlay with a coverslip, and examine microscopically for living microfilariae or trypanosomes. Both groups of parasites are motile and can be seen swimming among the formed blood elements. Motility is significantly decreased if the blood sample is refrigerated. If an organism is seen, the smears should be prepared and stained, preferably with Giemsa solution.

Urine

Gross Examination

Observe and record the degree of turbidity and the color of the specimen.

Microscopic Examination

1. Take a drop of urine with a Pasteur pipette, preferably from the bottom of the container, and transfer it to a glass slide.

2. Examine microscopically.

If *Trichomonas vaginalis* is suspected, the specimen must be fresh (<1 hour old), as the trophozoites quickly lose their characteristic morphology and motility.

Sedimentation by Centrifugation

1. Divide the entire urine specimen into 15-ml conical glass centrifuge tubes.

2. Sediment at 1000 rpm for 5 minutes.

3. Discard the supernatant.

4. Re-suspend the pellets with a Pasteur pipette and examine microscopically.

Sputum

Gross Examination

Observe and record the appearance of the specimen.

Microscopic Examination

1. Transfer a small amount of sputum with a wooden applicator stick to a clean glass slide.

2. Add a drop of normal saline solution.

3. Examine microscopically.

Sedimentation by Centrifugation

1. Mix sputum with equal parts of 3% NaOH.
2. Let stand 5 minutes.
3. Sediment at 1000 rpm for 5 minutes and examine microscopically.

Tissues

Place a small piece of tissue between two clean glass slides using forceps, press to flatten, then examine under a microscope.

To examine skin scrapings:

1. Place the scrapings on a clean glass slide.
2. Add a drop of normal saline solution and overlay with a coverslip.
3. Let stand 30 minutes.
4. Press the coverslip gently to break up the skin pieces and then examine microscopically.

Whole tapeworms must be carefully examined for the presence of a scolex. It is located at the narrowest end of the strobila. If only proglottids are available for observation, they must first be preserved in 10% formaldehyde. Then, the central uterus is injected with India ink using a 25-gauge needle. It is then placed between two glass slides, compressed, and examined with the aid of a dissection microscope. With taenia segments, the lateral branches on one side of the main uterine stem are counted (see *Taenia saginata* and *T. solium*).

Arthropods are best identified preserved. The specimen should be placed in 70% ethanol and transferred to a Petri dish for examination when no longer motile.

Aspirated Fluids

Sedimentation by Centrifugation

1. Centrifuge clear fluid aspirates at 1000 rpm for 5 minutes in a conical centrifuge tube.
2. Decant supernatant.
3. Examine the pellet microscopically.
4. Stain by the Wheatly-Gomori trichrome procedure.

Miscellaneous Tests

Tape test for *Enterobius vermicularis* (Pinworm)

Clear tape preparations of various types, available commercially, are routinely used in the diagnosis of pinworm infection. The tape is placed with the sticky side down on the perineum, and eggs or adult worms adhere to it. The tape is then examined microscopically. Adult pinworms are also occasionally found on the surface of formed stool samples. Occasionally, eggs of *Taenia* spp. are seen on sticky tape tests.

Preserved Specimens

Whenever a delay of 24 hours or longer is anticipated, the specimen should be preserved. The preservative to be employed depends on the type of test selected.

Stool: Direct Smear

Merthiolate-iodine-formaldehyde Method (MIF). a solution of merthiolate, iodine, and formaldehyde (MIF) preserves and stains trophozoites and cysts. The organisms develop an orange color, but this stain does not last. Therefore, a permanent stain should also be done on the same stool sample. MIF is not acceptable for other staining procedures, such as the Wheatly-Gomori trichrome stain.

1. Emulsify 1 g of stool sample in 10 ml of MIF solution.
2. Place a drop of stool-MIF-emulsion on a clean glass slide and examine microscopically.

Stools preserved in MIF can be concentrated by sedimentation using the formaldehyde-ethyl acetate method.

Wheatly-Gomori Trichrome Stain for PVA-Preserved Stool

Stool specimens preserved in polyvinyl alcohol (PVA) can be stained by the Wheatly-Gomori trichrome method, which is the same as that for unpreserved stools, except that Schaudinn's fixative is not necessary and the staining time differs.

Solution	Time
Ethanol-iodine 70%	1 0 - 2 0 minutes
Ethanol 70%	3-5 minutes
Ethanol 70%	3-5 minutes
Trichrome stain	8-10 minutes
Ethanol 90% (acidified)	1-10 seconds

Dip the coverslip in the destaining solution once or twice. Rinse in 95% alcohol to stop the process. Thin smears destain quickly; thicker smears require three to five dips.

Solution	Time
Ethanol 95%	Rinse
Ethanol 95%	5 minutes
Xylol	10 minutes

Mount the stained coverslip and examine microscopically.

Blood

Microscopic Examination

A thick smear consists of several drops of blood on a slide, dried in air, and hemolyzed by immersion in a hypotonic solution. This process concentrates the parasites. A thin smear is prepared by making a film of blood analogous to that used for a differential count of the white cells. Giemsa staining is recommended for both preparations.

1. Immerse the slide in 100% ethanol or methanol for 2-3 minutes.
2. Make a solution consisting of 1 drop of concentrated Giemsa stain per 1 ml of distilled water (pH 7.4) and fill a Copeland jar with 50 ml of the mixture.
3. Stain for 10-30 minutes.
4. Wash in distilled H2O.
5. Air dry the slide.
6. Examine microscopically under oil immersion. View 100 contiguous fields of a thin smear.

Concentration by Sedimentation: Knott Test

The Knott technique concentrates and preserves filarial microfilariae, which can be stained by Giemsa solution and identified morphologically.

1. Mix I ml of heparinized blood with 9 ml of 2% formaldehyde.
2. Centrifuge at 2,000 rpm for 10 minutes.
3. Decant the supernatant.
4. Examine the sediment microscopically.

If microfilariae are present, they are stained as follows.

1. Spread the sediment on a clean glass slide.
2. Dry overnight.
3. Stain with Giemsa solution (1 ml of concentrated Giemsa stain in 50 ml of distilled water at pH 7.4).
4. Destain 10-15 minutes in H2O.
5. Air dry.
6. Examine microscopically.

Solutions

Schaudinn's Fixative

- H_gCl_2, saturated aqueous solution: 666 ml (add 80 g H_gCl_2 to 1 liter de-ionized H_2O; stir 3-4 hours and then filter)
- Ethyl alcohol 95%: 333 ml
- Ethanol-iodine solution 70%. Add enough crystalline iodine to 70% ethanol to turn the solution deep amber-brown; filter before using.

Wheatly-Gomori Trichrome Stain

Chromotrope 2R   0.6 g
Light green SF   0.3 g
Phosphotungstic acid   0.7 g
Mix with 1 ml of glacial acetic acid and stir gently for 20 minutes. Add 100 ml of distilled H2O, then store in dark brown bottle.

Buffered Formaldehyde

Formaldehyde solution 37-40% 100ml
Sodium phosphate (monobasic, 4.0 g anhydrous)
Sodium phosphate (dibasic, 6.5 g anhydrous)
H_2O 900 ml
Adjust the pH of the solution to 7.0

Zinc Sulfate

Zinc sulfate   333 g
Water (50°-55°C)   1000 ml
Adjust the specific gravity to 1.18 by adding either more H_2O or more zinc sulfate crystals.

Sugar Solution (Sheather's Method)

Sucrose   500 g
Water   320 ml
Phenol   6.5 g

Merthiolate-Iodine-Formaldehyde Solution

Tincture of Merthiolate No. 99 (Lilly)
     1:1000 100 ml
Formaldehyde solution 37-40%
     25 ml
Glycerol
     5 ml
H_2O
     250 ml
Store solution in a dark bottle.

Lugol's Iodine Solution

Iodine   5 g
Potassium iodide   10 g
H_2O 100 ml

Polyvinyl alcohol

Polyvinyl alcohol is available
     commercially.

Schaudinn's fixative   935 ml
Glycerol   15 ml
Glacial acetic acid   50 ml
Polyvinyl alcohol (powder) 50 g
H_2O 1000 ml

Appendix C: Diagnostic Color Atlas of Protozoa and Helminths

This atlas is intended as a pictorial reference for the diagnostic laboratory. It is important to be reminded that the laboratory obtains the most relevant information regarding a given parasitic infection. The physician must act according to the findings of the laboratory. Pattern recognition is the key to becoming a competent parasitology diagnostic technician. Space only permits a single example to be shown of each relevant stage of the major parasites infecting the human host. Our atlas can only serve as a guide for a much broader range of variation in both size and shape for any given diagnostic stage. When an object is encountered under the microscope, the parasitic stage usually looks as it is depicted here. Occasionally, even the most experienced laboratory technician may be unsure of or express some doubt about the identity of some objects. A few commonly encountered artifacts are shown for comparison. Suggested readings to more comprehensive atlases are listed,

in case more visual examples are desired for comparison with the object in question. Internet resources for each parasite stage have become an invaluable resource for helping with identification. There is no shortcut to becoming familiar with each parasite. Only by co-observing patient samples with an accomplished technician can the skills necessary for advancement to the front lines of the diagnostic laboratory be developed.

It is very helpful to have a camera (preferably a digital image capturing device) attached to the diagnostic microscope. Images can then be stored on a computer and recalled on-demand. This allows for the accumulation of a permanent record of interesting objects encountered under the microscope throughout the year. Such images are extremely helpful during training sessions for beginning parasitology technicians. Digital images can be sent via email, permitting instant consultation with any expert group, such as the Centers for Disease Control and Prevention, in Atlanta, Georgia.

The majority of the protozoa depicted

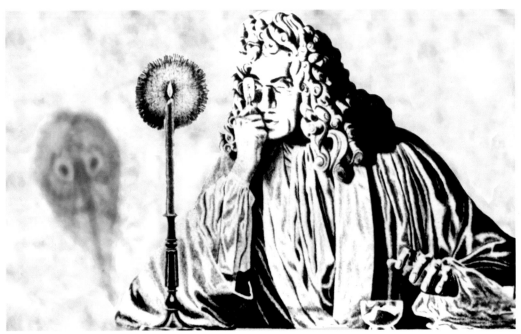

Anton van Leeuwenhoek, microscopist extraordinaire. Discoverer of the trophozoite of *Giardia lamblia*.

here have been stained with either iron-hematoxylin (blue-gray stain) or Wheatly and Gomori's trichrome stain (green and red stain). Helminth eggs are as they appear in unstained, concentrated stool samples. Their yellow-brown tints attest to the fact that they have encountered bile pigments. Microfilariae have all been stained with Giemsa (blue and red stain), as have the malaria parasites. The tissue section of the Nurse cell-parasite complex of *Trichinella spiralis* is stained with hematoxylin and eosin.

Protozoa

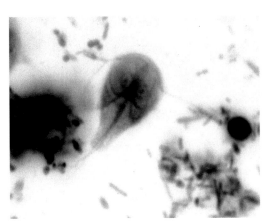

Figure C.1. *Giardia lamblia* trophozoite
15 µm

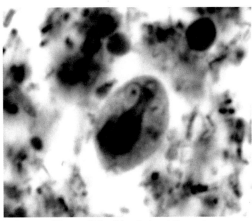

Figure C.2. *Giardia lamblia* cyst
15 µm

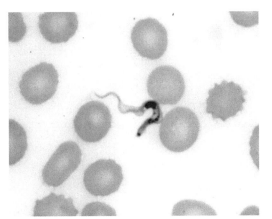

Figure C.3. *Trypanosoma brucei rhodesiense*
25 µm x 3 µm

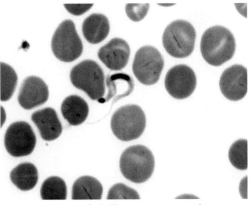

Figure C.4. *Trypanosoma cruzi*
20 µm x 3 µm

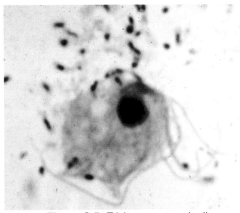

Figure C.5. *Trichomonas vaginalis*
20 µm x 10 µm

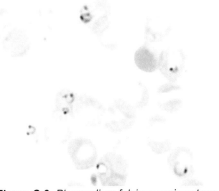

Figure C.6. *Plasmodium falciparum* ring stage

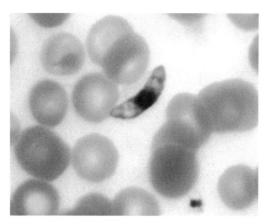

Figure C.7. *Plasmodium falciparum* macrogametocyte

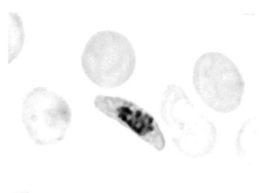

Figure C.8. *Plasmodium falciparum* microgametocyte

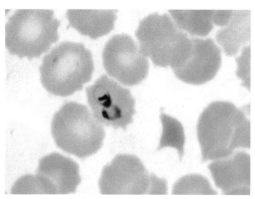

Figure C.9. *Plasmodium vivax* ring stage

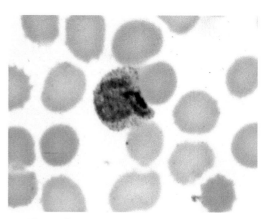

Figure C.10. *Plasmodium vivax* trophozoite

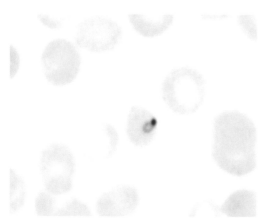

Figure C.11. *Plasmodium malariae* ring stage

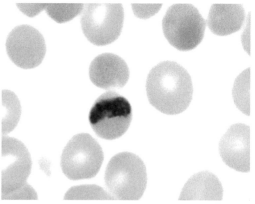

Figure C.12. *Plasmodium malariae* trophozoite

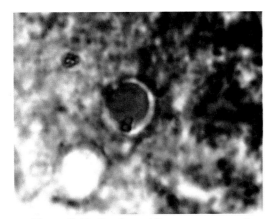

Figure C.13. *Cryptosporidium parvum* oocyst
(acid-fast stain) 5 μm

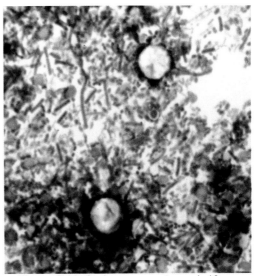

Figure C.14. *Cyclospora cayetanensis* 10 μm

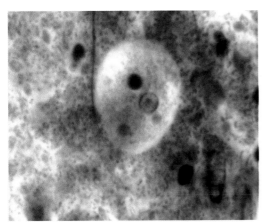

Figure C.15. *Entamoeba histolytica trophozoite*
(note red cell in cytoplasm)

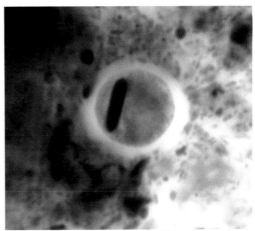

Figure C.16a. *Entamoeba histolytica* cyst
Note smooth-ended chromatoidal bar
15 μm

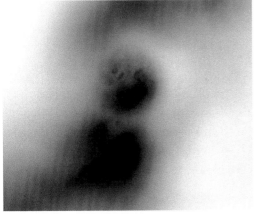

Figure C.16b. *Entamoeba histolytica* cyst
(Through-focus #1):
Note two nuclei
15 μm

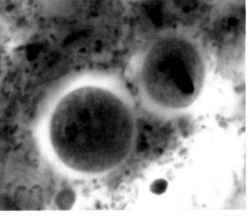

Figure C.16c. *Entamoeba histolytica* cyst
(Through-focus #2):
Note smooth-ended chromatoidal bar

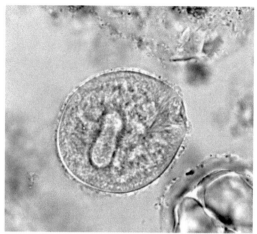

Figure C.17. *Balantidium coli* trophozoite
150 μm x 65 μm (unstained)

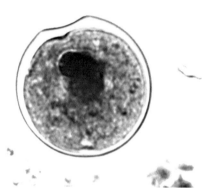

Figure C.18. *Balantidium coli* cyst
65 μm

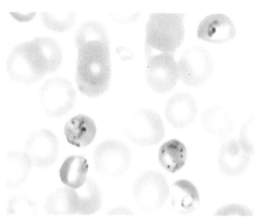

Figure C.19. *Babesia* spp. Bloodsmear

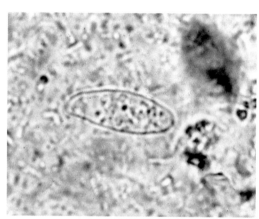

Figure C.20. *Cytoisospora belli* unsporulated
oocyst
25 μm x 15 μm

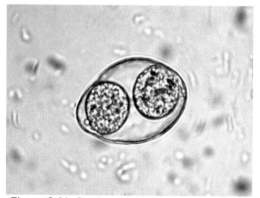

Figure C.21. *Cytoisospora belli* sporulated oocyst
25 μm x 15 μm

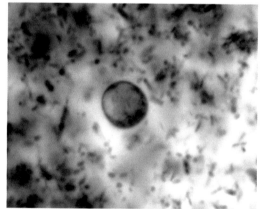

Figure C.22. *Blastocystis hominis*
6 μm

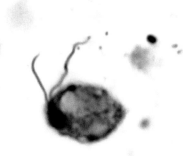

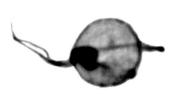

Figure C.23. *Trichomonas hominis*
10 µm x 8 µm

Figure C.24. *Trichomonas tenax*
7 µm x 3 µm

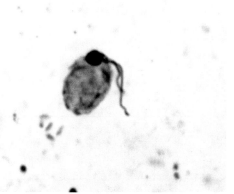

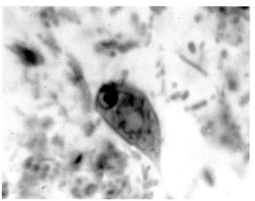

Figure C.25. *Retortamonas hominis*
6 µm x 2 µm

Figure C.26. *Chilomastix mesnili* trophozoite
15 µm x 12 µm

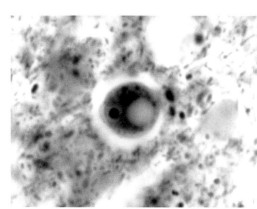

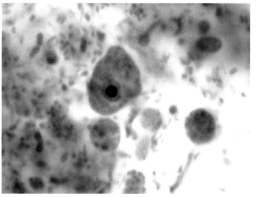

Figure C.27. *Chilomastix mesnili* cyst
8 µm x 5 µm

Figure C.28. *Endolimax nana* trophozoite
10 µm x 4 µm

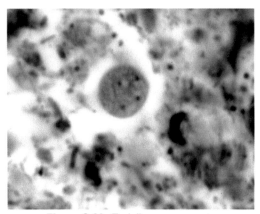

Figure C.29. *Endolimax nana* cysts
Note four nuclei
8 μm x 6 μm

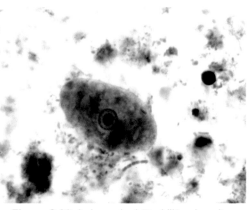

Figure C.30. *Iodamoeba bütschlii* trophozoite
18 μm

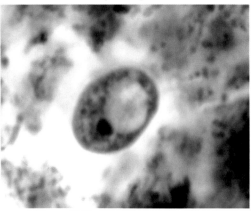

Figure C.31. *Iodamoeba bütschlii* cyst
12 μm x 8 μm

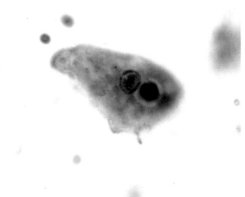

Figure C.32. *Entamoeba gingivalis* trophozoite
30 μm

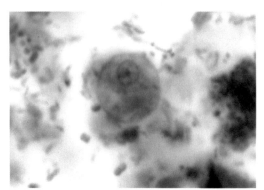

Figure C.33. *Entamoeba hartmanni* trophozoite
10 μm

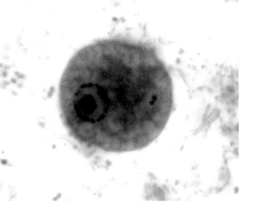

Figure C.34. *Entamoeba coli* trophozoite
35 μm

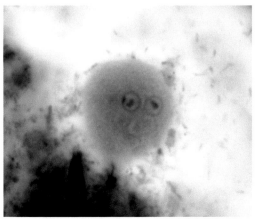

Figure C.35a. *Entamoeba coli* cyst
(Through-focus #1): Two nuclei can be seen
30 µm

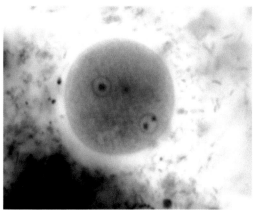

Figure C.35b. *Entamoeba coli* cyst
(Through-focus #2): Two nucleus can be seen

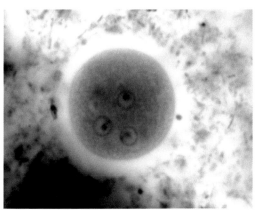

Figure C.35c. *Entamoeba coli* cyst
(Through-focus #3): Three nucleus can be seen

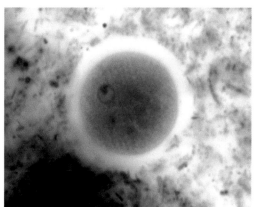

Figure C.35d. *Entamoeba coli* cyst
(Through-focus #4): One nuclei can be seen
A total of eight nuclei are present in the cyst

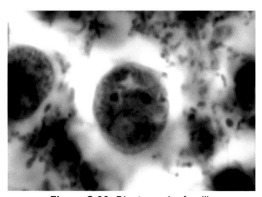

Figure C.36. *Dientamoeba fragilis*
10 µm

Nematodes

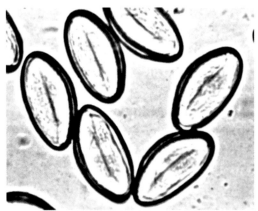

Figure C.37. *Enterobius vermicularis*
55 µm x 25 µm

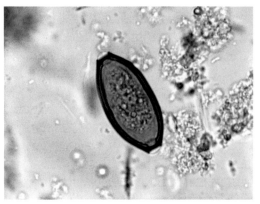

Figure C.38. *Trichuris trichiura*
50 µm x 20 µm

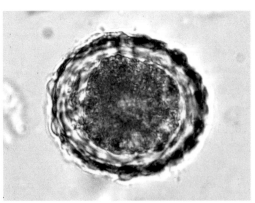

Figure C.39. *Ascaris lumbricoides*
(fertilized)
60 µm x 35 µm

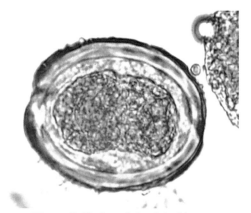

Figure C.40. *Ascaris lumbricoides*
(fertilized, decorticated)
50 µm x 30 µm

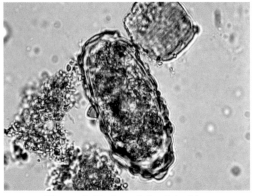

Figure C.41. *Ascaris lumbricoides*
(unfertilized)
Size variable; 70 µm x 30 µm

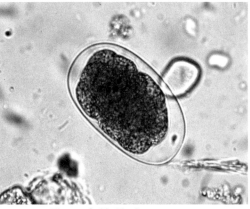

Figure C.42. Hookworm ovum
70 µm x 40 µm

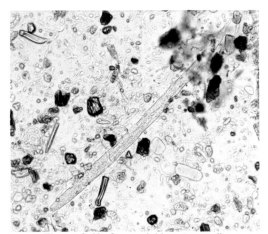

Figure C.43. *Strongyloides stercoralis*
(rhabditiform larvae)
500 µm x 15 µm

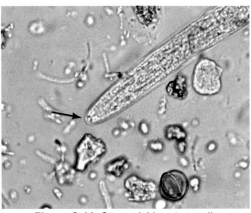

Figure C.44. *Strongyloides stercoralis*
(rhabditiform larvae)
Note short buccal cavity (arrow)

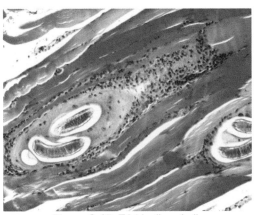

Figure C.45. *Trichinella spiralis*
Larva in muscle

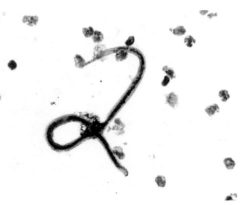

Figure C.46. *Wuchereria bancrofti* microfilaria
260 µm x 9 µm

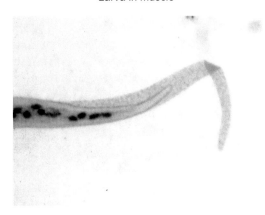

Figure C.47. *Wuchereria bancrofti* microfilaria
Note sheath and nuclei, which do not extend to end
of tail

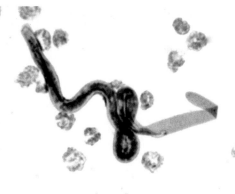

Figure C.48. *Brugia malayi* microfilaria
200 µm x 6 µm

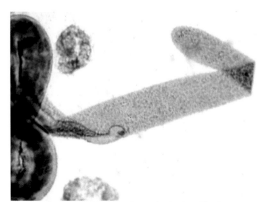

Figure C.49. *Brugia malayi* microfilaria
Note nucleus at tip of tail and sheath

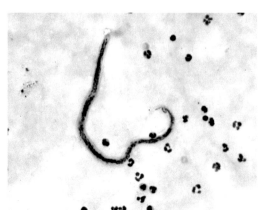

Figure C.50. *Loa loa* microfilaria
Note sheath
35 mm x 40 µm

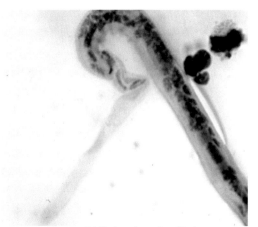

Figure C.51. *Loa loa* microfilaria
Note sheath and nuclei, which extend to end of tail

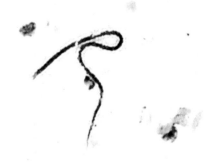

Figure C.52. *Mansonella ozzardi*
190 µm x 4 µm

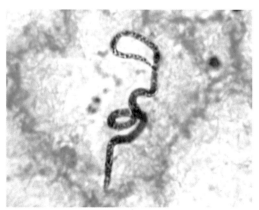

Figure C.53. *Mansonella perstans*
200 µm x 4 µm

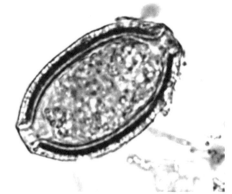

Figure C.54. *Capillaria philippinensis*
40 µm x 20 µm

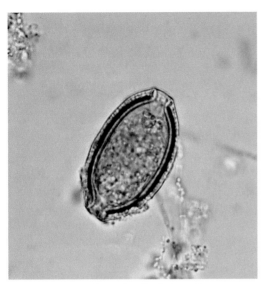

Figure C.55. *Capillaria hepatica*
60 μm x 30 μm

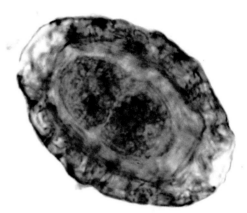

Figure C.56. *Dioctophyma renale*
70 μm x 45 μm

Cestodes

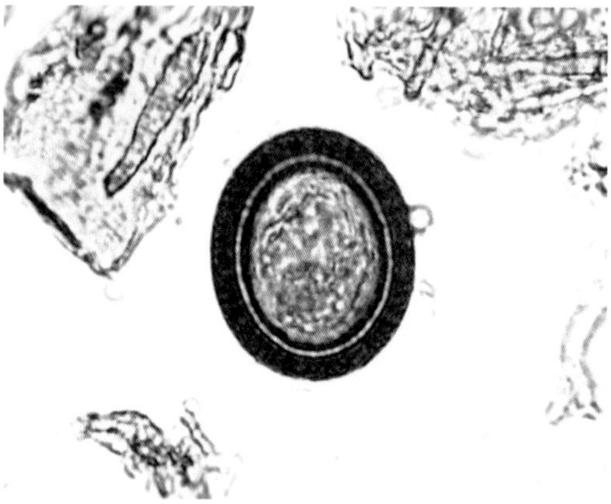

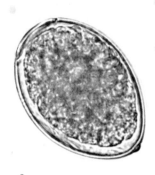

Figure C.57. *Taenia* spp. ovum
40 µm x 30 µm

Figure C.58. *Diphyllobothrium latum*
65 µm x 45 µm

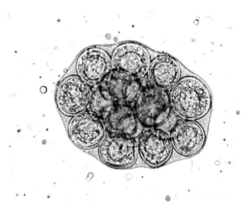

Figure C.59. *Dipylidum caninum* egg cluster
Each egg measures 35 µm

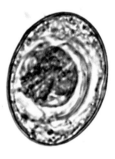

Figure C.60. *Hymenolepis nana*
45 µm x 30 µm

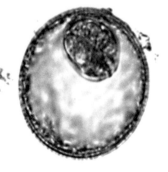

Figure C.61. *Hymenolepis diminuta*
75 µm x 70 µm

Trematodes

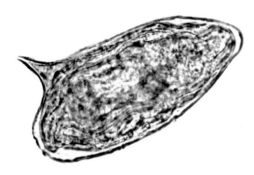

Figure C.62. *Schistosoma mansoni*
160 µm x 60 µm

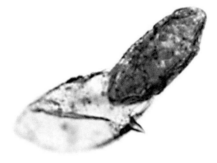

Figure C.63. *Schistosoma mansoni*
Hatching egg

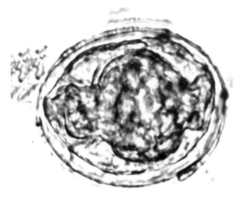

Figure C.64. *Schistosoma japonicum*
85 µm x 60 µm

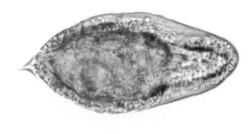

Figure C.65. *Schistosoma haematobium*
170 µm x 60 µm

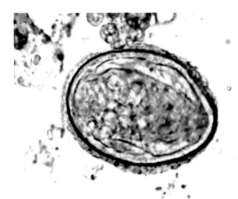

Figure C.66. *Schistosoma mekongi*
60 µm x 45 µm

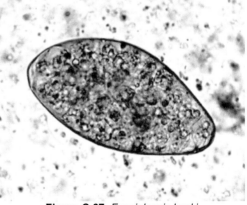

Figure C.67. *Fasciolopsis buski*
135 µm x 80 µm

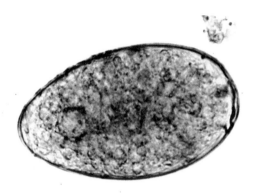

Figure C.68. *Fasciola hepatica*
140 μm x 75 μm

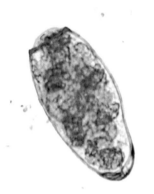

Figure C.69. *Paragonimus westermani*
110 μm x 60 μm

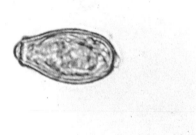

Figure C.70. *Clonorchis sinensis*
30 μm x 16 μm

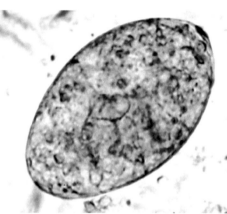

Figure C.71. *Echinostoma ilocanum*
130 μm x 60 μm

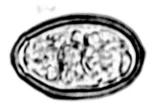

Figure C.72. *Heterophyes heterophyes*
20 μm x 15 μm

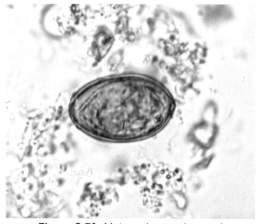

Figure C.73. *Metagonimus yokogawai*
30 μm x 15 μm

Miscellaneous

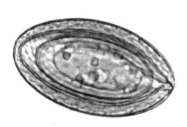

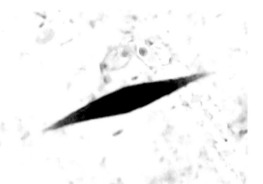

Figure C.74. *Macrocanthorynchus hirudinaceus*
60 μm x 20 μm

Figure C.75. Charcot-Leyden crystal
10 μm x 2 μm

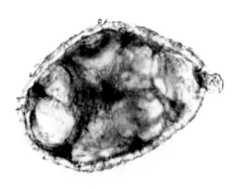

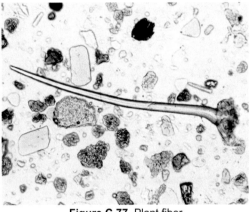

Figure C.76. Digested vegetable matter
(Artifact)

Figure C.77. Plant fiber
(Artifact)

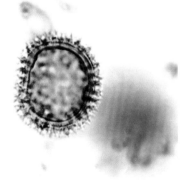

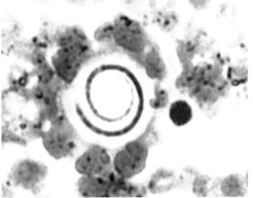

Figure C.78. Pollen grain
(Artifact)

Figure C.79. *Helicosporum* spp. (fungus)
(Artifact)

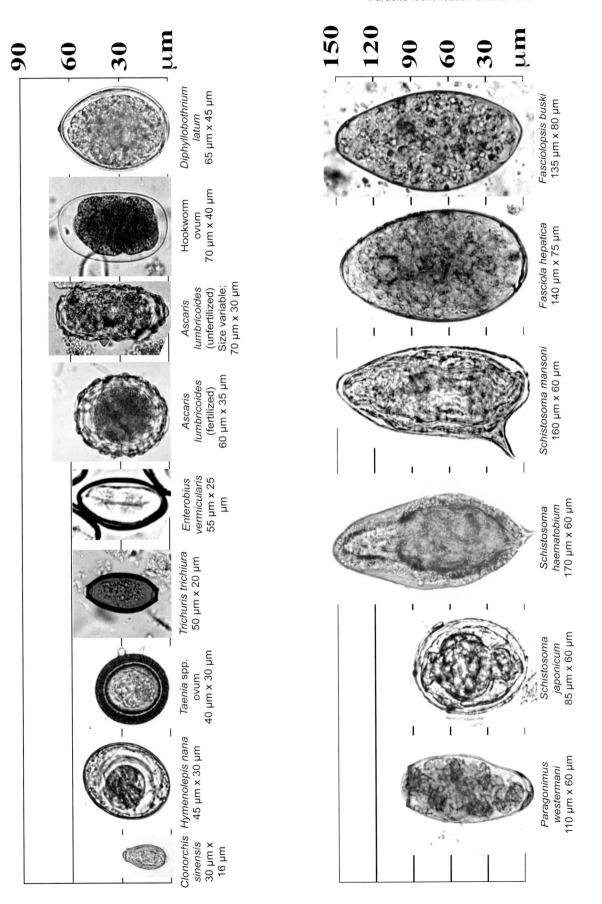

90
60
30
μm

Diphyllobothrium latum
65 μm × 45 μm

Hookworm ovum
70 μm × 40 μm

Ascaris lumbricoides (unfertilized)
Size variable;
70 μm × 30 μm

Ascaris lumbricoides (fertilized)
60 μm × 35 μm

Enterobius vermicularis
55 μm × 25 μm

Trichuris trichiura
50 μm × 20 μm

Taenia spp. ovum
40 μm × 30 μm

Hymenolepis nana
45 μm × 30 μm

Clonorchis sinensis
30 μm × 16 μm

150
120
90
60
30
μm

Fasciolopsis buski
135 μm × 80 μm

Fasciola hepatica
140 μm × 75 μm

Schistosoma mansoni
160 μm × 60 μm

Schistosoma haematobium
170 μm × 60 μm

Schistosoma japonicum
85 μm × 60 μm

Paragonimus westermani
110 μm × 60 μm

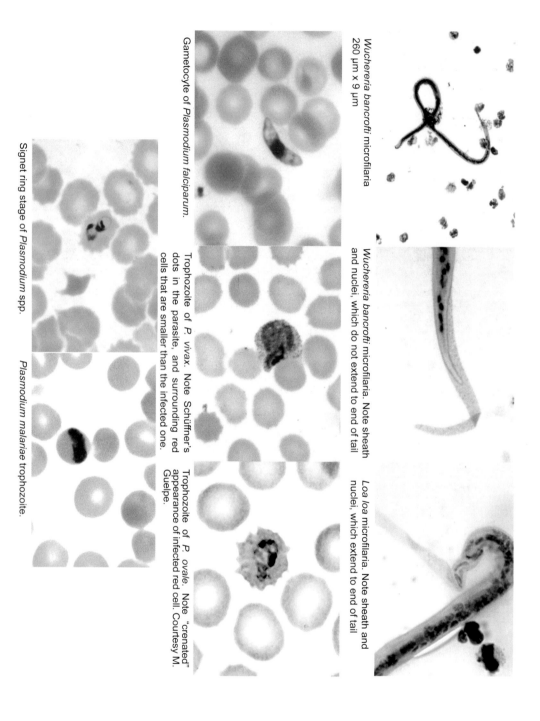

Wuchereria bancrofti microfilaria
260 μm x 9 μm

Wuchereria bancrofti microfilaria. Note sheath and nuclei, which do not extend to end of tail

Loa loa microfilaria. Note sheath and nuclei, which extend to end of tail

Gametocyte of Plasmodium falciparum.

Trophozoite of P. vivax. Note Schüffner's dots in the parasite, and surrounding red cells that are smaller than the infected one.

Trophozoite of P. ovale. Note "crenated" appearance of infected red cell. Courtesy M. Guelpe.

Signet ring stage of Plasmodium spp.

Plasmodium malariae trophozoite.

Giardia lamblia

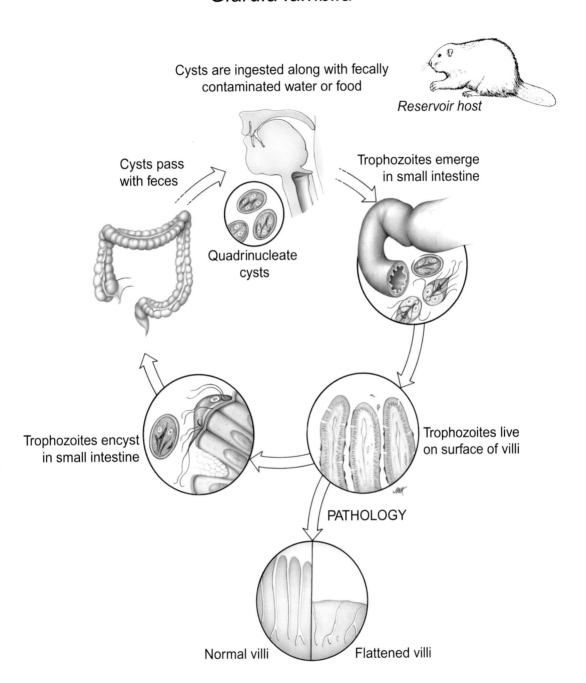

Cysts are ingested along with fecally
contaminated water or food

Reservoir host

Cysts pass
with feces

Trophozoites emerge
in small intestine

Quadrinucleate
cysts

Trophozoites encyst
in small intestine

Trophozoites live
on surface of villi

PATHOLOGY

Normal villi   Flattened villi

Leishmania tropica

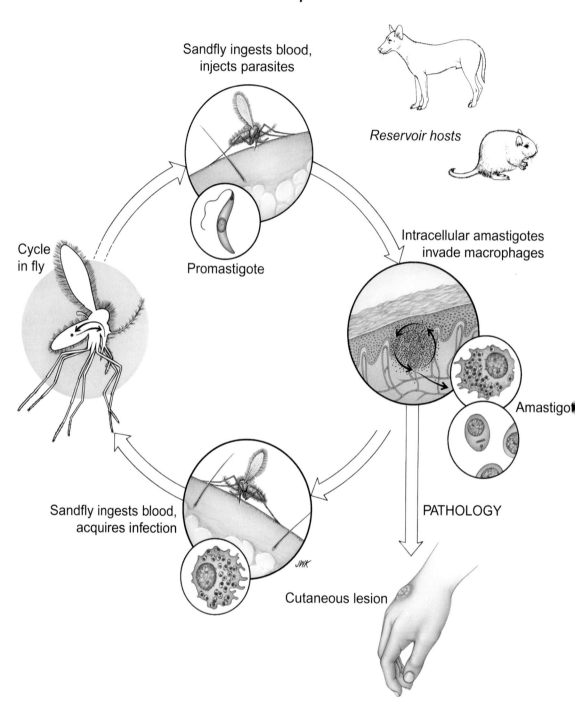

Sandfly ingests blood, injects parasites

Reservoir hosts

Promastigote

Cycle in fly

Intracellular amastigotes invade macrophages

Amastigo[te]

Sandfly ingests blood, acquires infection

PATHOLOGY

Cutaneous lesion

Parasitic Diseases 6th Ed. Parasites Without Borders www.parasiteswithoutborders.com

Leishmania braziliensis

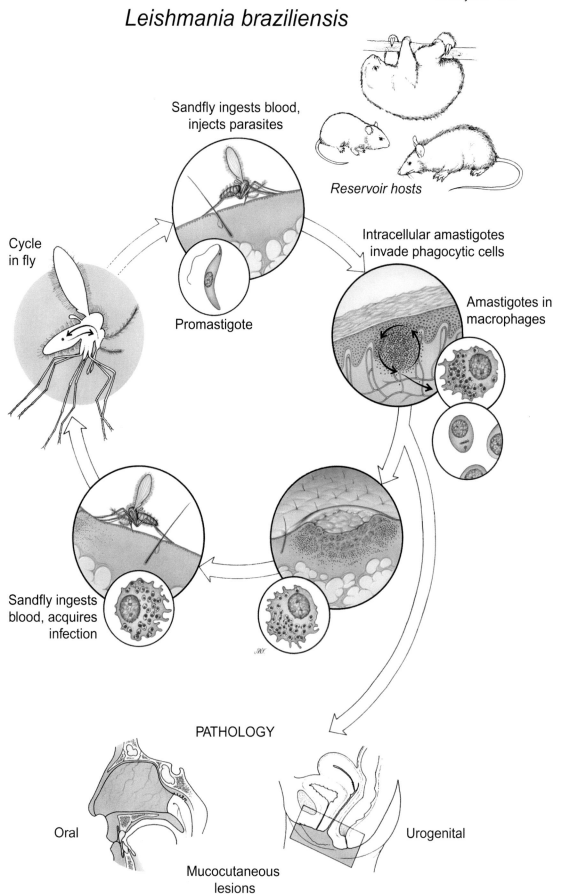

Sandfly ingests blood, injects parasites

Reservoir hosts

Cycle in fly

Promastigote

Intracellular amastigotes invade phagocytic cells

Amastigotes in macrophages

Sandfly ingests blood, acquires infection

PATHOLOGY

Oral

Urogenital

Mucocutaneous lesions

Leishmania donovani

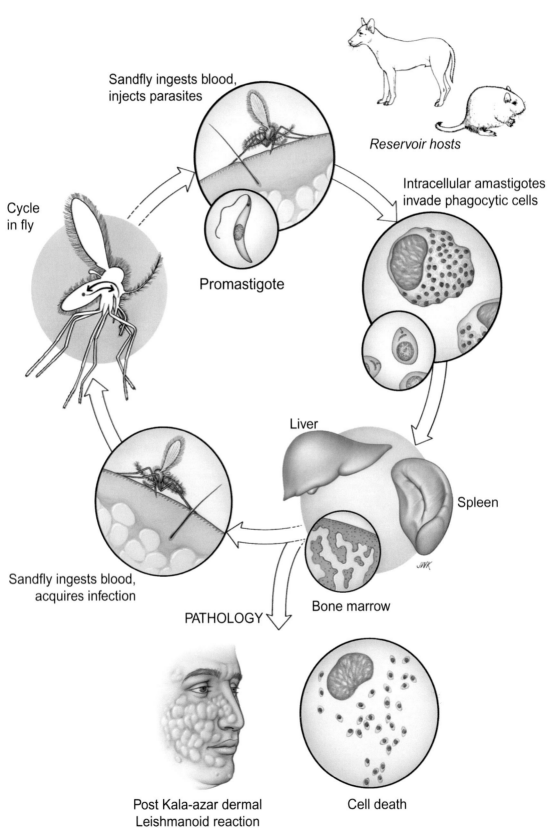

Sandfly ingests blood, injects parasites

Reservoir hosts

Cycle in fly

Promastigote

Intracellular amastigotes invade phagocytic cells

Liver

Spleen

Bone marrow

Sandfly ingests blood, acquires infection

PATHOLOGY

Post Kala-azar dermal Leishmanoid reaction

Cell death

Trypanosoma brucei gambiense and *T. b. rhodesiense*

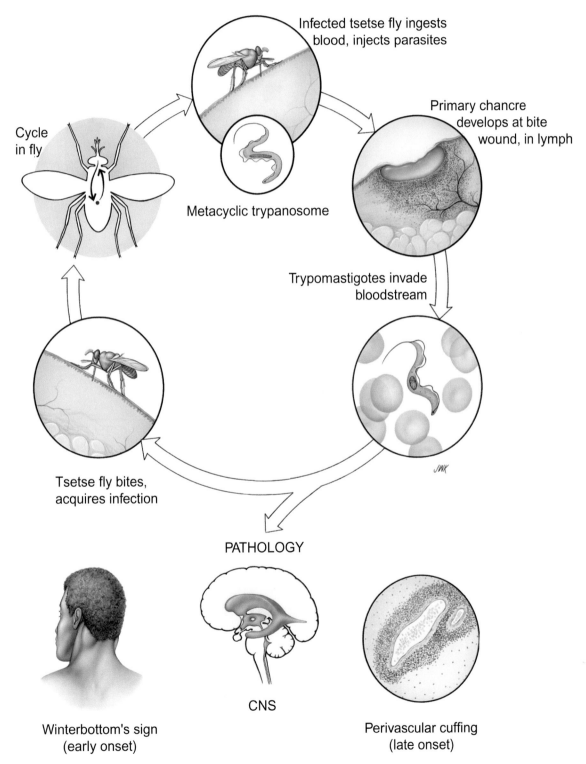

Infected tsetse fly ingests blood, injects parasites

Metacyclic trypanosome

Cycle in fly

Primary chancre develops at bite wound, in lymph

Trypomastigotes invade bloodstream

Tsetse fly bites, acquires infection

PATHOLOGY

Winterbottom's sign (early onset)

CNS

Perivascular cuffing (late onset)

Trypanosoma cruzi

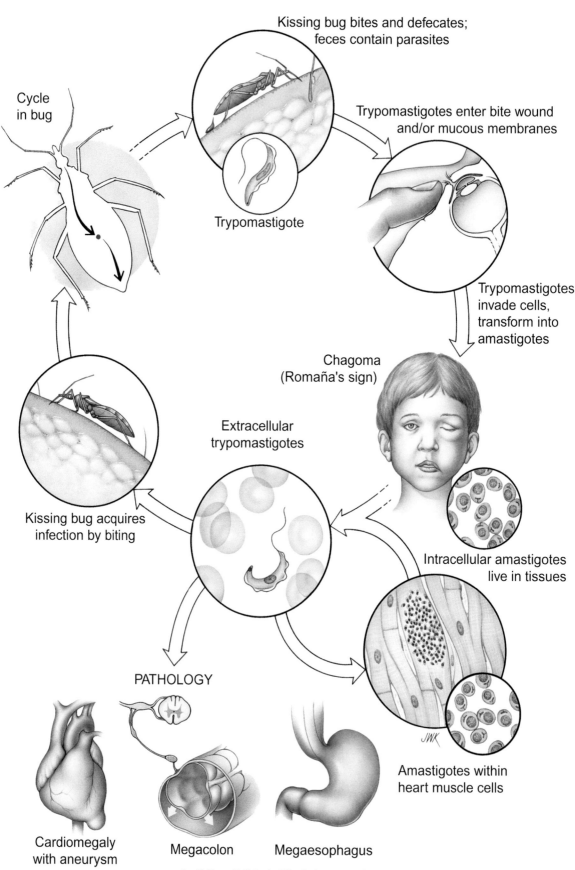

Kissing bug bites and defecates; feces contain parasites

Cycle in bug

Trypomastigote

Trypomastigotes enter bite wound and/or mucous membranes

Trypomastigotes invade cells, transform into amastigotes

Chagoma (Romaña's sign)

Extracellular trypomastigotes

Kissing bug acquires infection by biting

Intracellular amastigotes live in tissues

Amastigotes within heart muscle cells

PATHOLOGY

Cardiomegaly with aneurysm

Megacolon

Megaesophagus

JWK

Parasitic Diseases 6th Ed. Parasites Without Borders wwww.parasiteswithoutborders.com

Trichomonas vaginalis

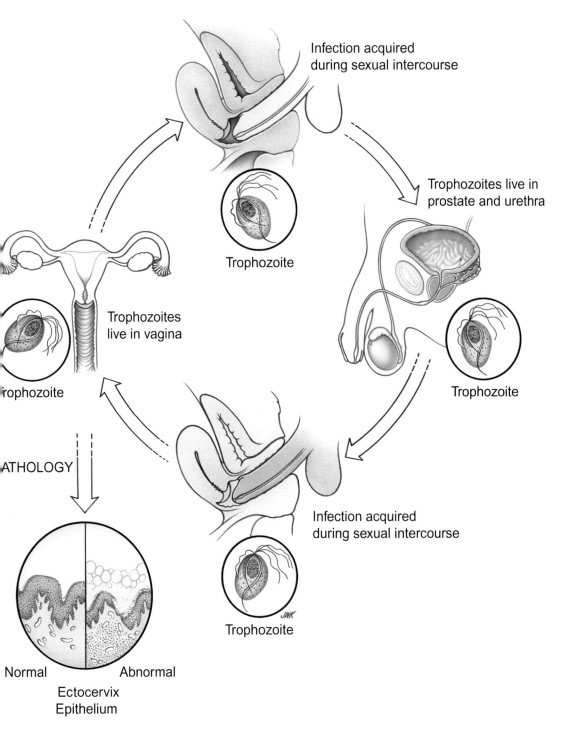

Infection acquired
during sexual intercourse

Trophozoites live in
prostate and urethra

Trophozoite

Trophozoite

Trophozoites
live in vagina

Trophozoite

PATHOLOGY

Infection acquired
during sexual intercourse

Trophozoite

Normal   Abnormal

Ectocervix
Epithelium

Mosquito Cycle (Sporogony)

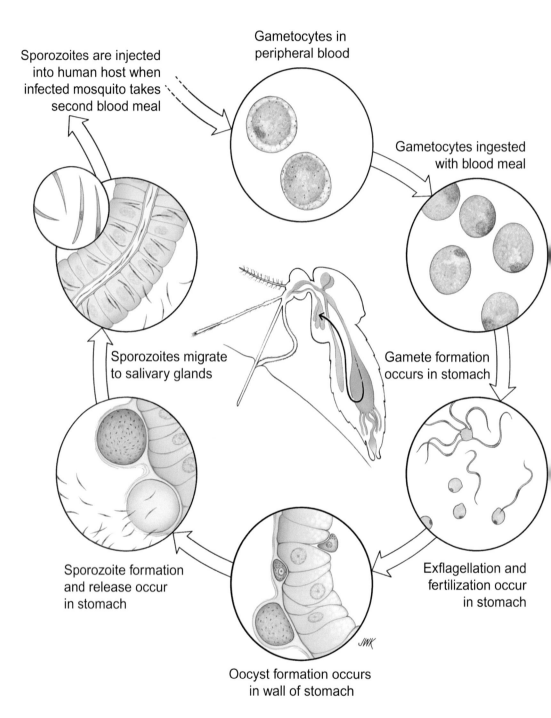

Sporozoites are injected into human host when infected mosquito takes second blood meal

Gametocytes in peripheral blood

Gametocytes ingested with blood meal

Gamete formation occurs in stomach

Sporozoites migrate to salivary glands

Exflagellation and fertilization occur in stomach

Sporozoite formation and release occur in stomach

Oocyst formation occurs in wall of stomach

Parasitic Diseases 6th Ed. Parasites Without Borders www.parasiteswithoutborders.com

Plasmodium falciparum

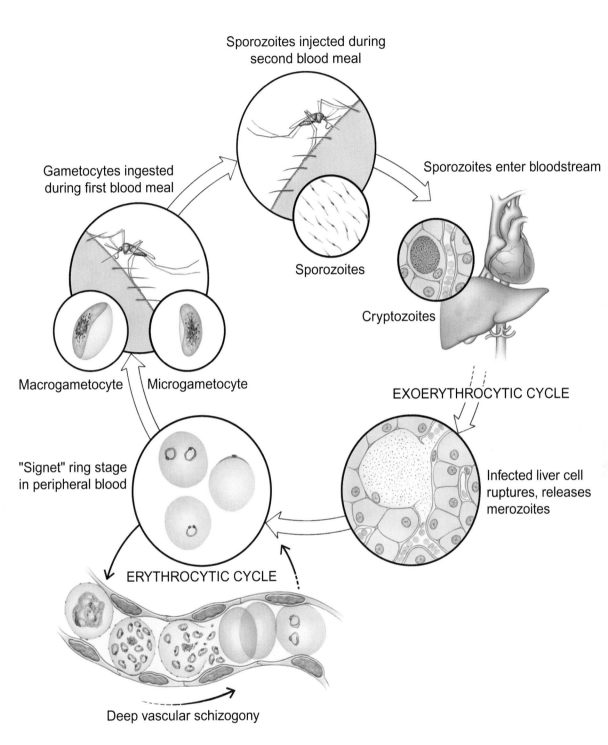

Sporozoites injected during
second blood meal

Gametocytes ingested
during first blood meal

Sporozoites enter bloodstream

Sporozoites

Cryptozoites

Macrogametocyte   Microgametocyte

EXOERYTHROCYTIC CYCLE

"Signet" ring stage
in peripheral blood

Infected liver cell
ruptures, releases
merozoites

ERYTHROCYTIC CYCLE

Deep vascular schizogony

Parasitic Diseases 6th Ed. Parasites Without Borders www.parasiteswithoutborders.com

Plasmodium vivax

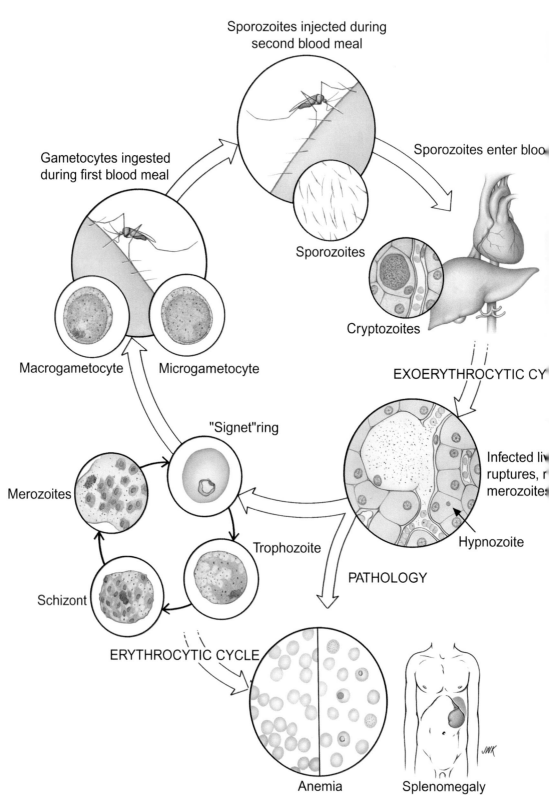

Sporozoites injected during second blood meal

Gametocytes ingested during first blood meal

Sporozoites enter bloo

Sporozoites

Cryptozoites

Macrogametocyte

Microgametocyte

EXOERYTHROCYTIC CY

"Signet"ring

Merozoites

Infected li ruptures, r merozoite

Trophozoite

Hypnozoite

Schizont

PATHOLOGY

ERYTHROCYTIC CYCLE

Anemia

Splenomegaly

Cryptosporidium parvum

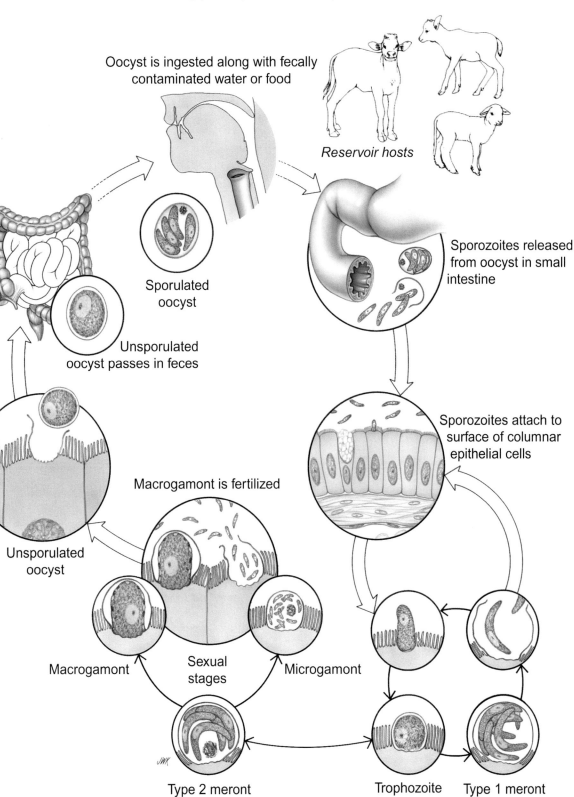

Oocyst is ingested along with fecally contaminated water or food

Reservoir hosts

Sporulated oocyst

Unsporulated oocyst passes in feces

Sporozoites released from oocyst in small intestine

Sporozoites attach to surface of columnar epithelial cells

Macrogamont is fertilized

Unsporulated oocyst

Macrogamont

Sexual stages

Microgamont

Type 2 meront

Trophozoite

Type 1 meront

Toxoplasma gondii

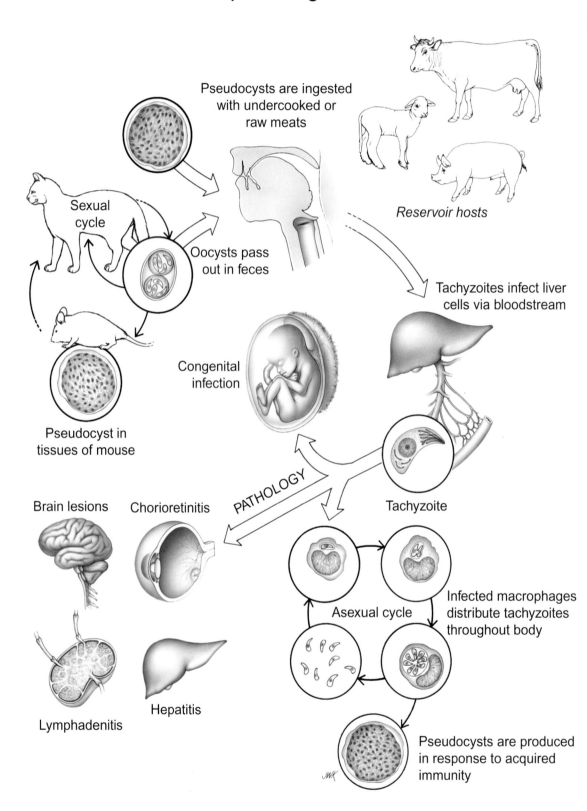

Pseudocysts are ingested with undercooked or raw meats

Reservoir hosts

Sexual cycle

Oocysts pass out in feces

Tachyzoites infect liver cells via bloodstream

Pseudocyst in tissues of mouse

Congenital infection

PATHOLOGY

Brain lesions

Chorioretinitis

Tachyzoite

Lymphadenitis

Hepatitis

Asexual cycle

Infected macrophages distribute tachyzoites throughout body

Pseudocysts are produced in response to acquired immunity

Entamoeba histolytica

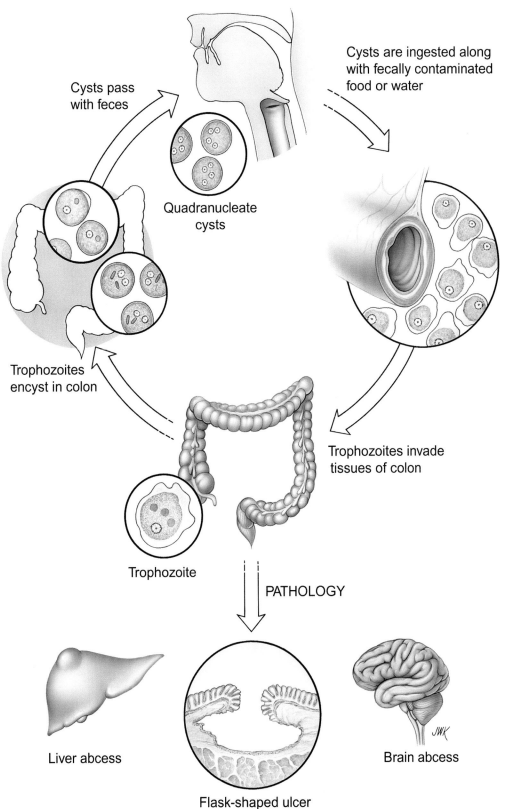

Cysts pass with feces

Quadranucleate cysts

Cysts are ingested along with fecally contaminated food or water

Trophozoites encyst in colon

Trophozoites invade tissues of colon

Trophozoite

PATHOLOGY

Liver abcess

Flask-shaped ulcer

Brain abcess

Balantidium coli

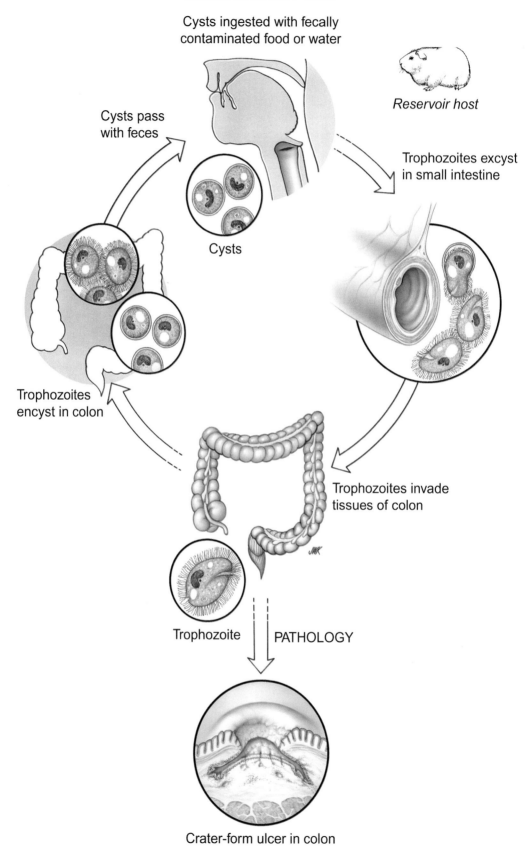

Cysts ingested with fecally
contaminated food or water

Reservoir host

Cysts pass
with feces

Cysts

Trophozoites excyst
in small intestine

Trophozoites
encyst in colon

Trophozoites invade
tissues of colon

Trophozoite

PATHOLOGY

Crater-form ulcer in colon

Enterobius vermicularis

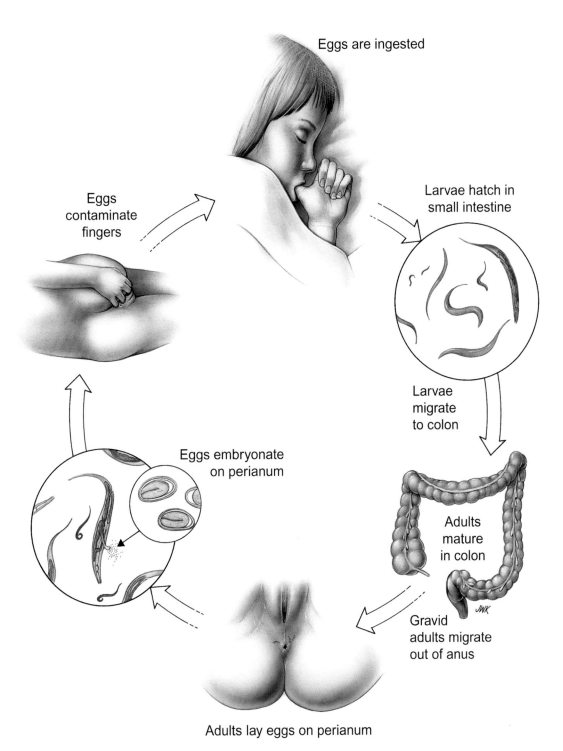

Eggs are ingested

Eggs contaminate fingers

Larvae hatch in small intestine

Larvae migrate to colon

Eggs embryonate on perianum

Adults mature in colon

Gravid adults migrate out of anus

Adults lay eggs on perianum

Trichuris trichiura

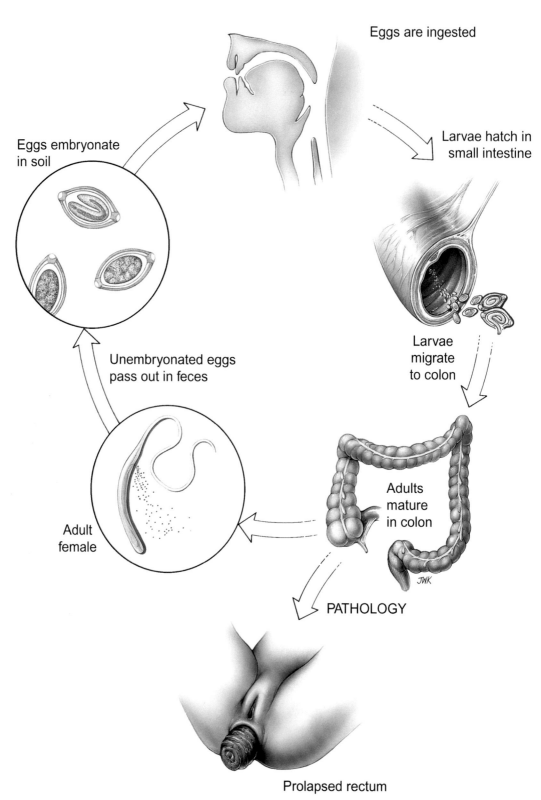

Eggs are ingested

Eggs embryonate in soil

Larvae hatch in small intestine

Larvae migrate to colon

Unembryonated eggs pass out in feces

Adults mature in colon

Adult female

JWK

PATHOLOGY

Prolapsed rectum

Ascaris lumbricoides

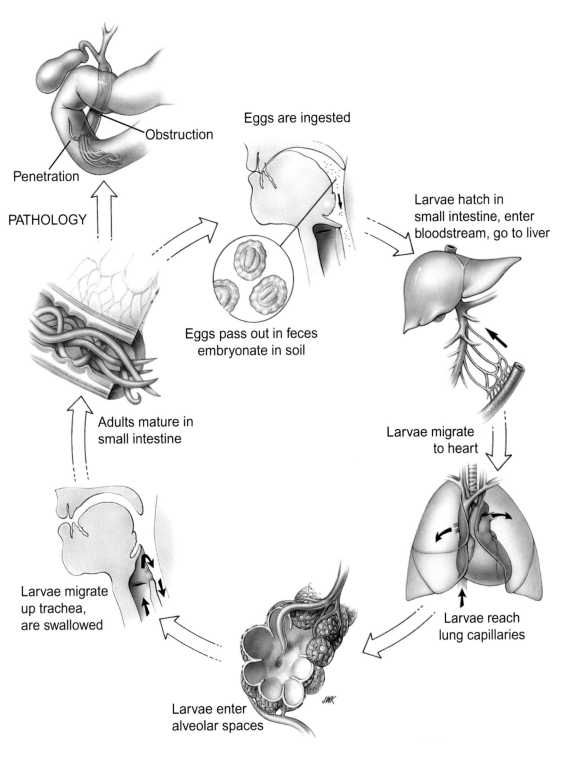

Obstruction

Penetration

PATHOLOGY

Eggs are ingested

Eggs pass out in feces
embryonate in soil

Larvae hatch in
small intestine, enter
bloodstream, go to liver

Larvae migrate
to heart

Larvae reach
lung capillaries

Larvae enter
alveolar spaces

Larvae migrate
up trachea,
are swallowed

Adults mature in
small intestine

Necator americanus

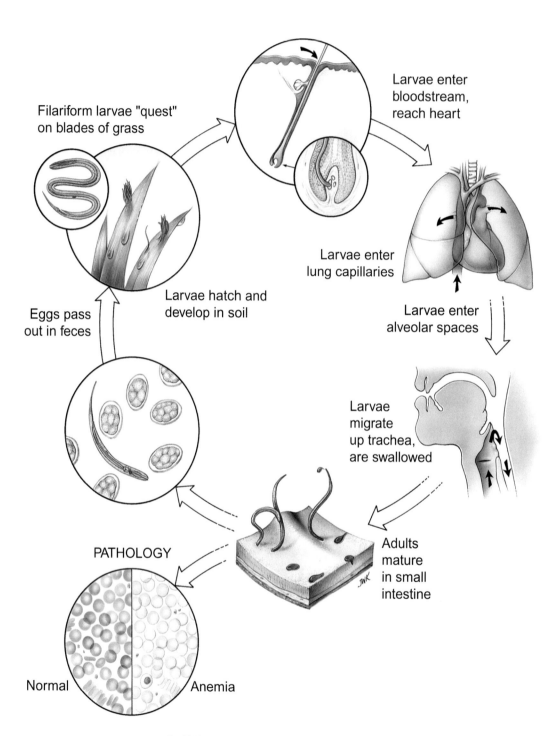

Filariform larvae "quest" on blades of grass

Larvae enter bloodstream, reach heart

Larvae enter lung capillaries

Larvae enter alveolar spaces

Eggs pass out in feces

Larvae hatch and develop in soil

Larvae migrate up trachea, are swallowed

Adults mature in small intestine

PATHOLOGY

Normal

Anemia

Strongyloides stercoralis

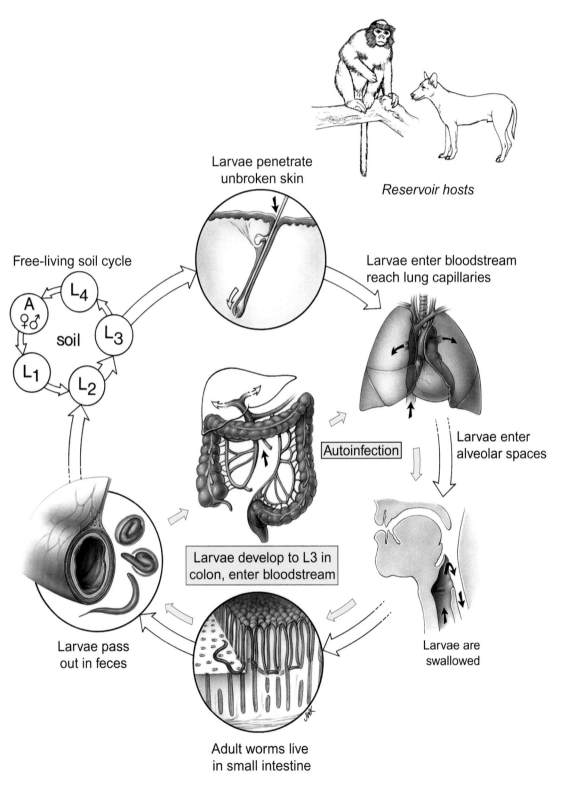

Reservoir hosts

Larvae penetrate
unbroken skin

Larvae enter bloodstream
reach lung capillaries

Free-living soil cycle

soil

Autoinfection

Larvae enter
alveolar spaces

Larvae develop to L3 in
colon, enter bloodstream

Larvae pass
out in feces

Larvae are
swallowed

Adult worms live
in small intestine

Trichinella spiralis

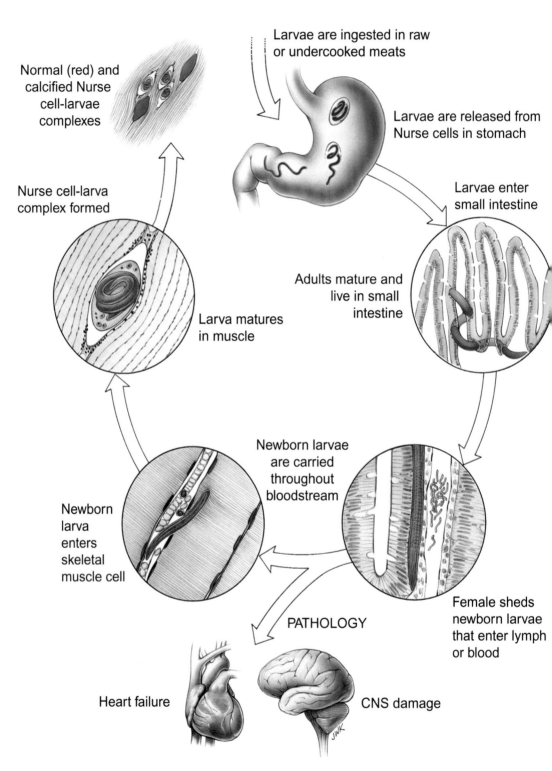

Larvae are ingested in raw or undercooked meats

Normal (red) and calcified Nurse cell-larvae complexes

Larvae are released from Nurse cells in stomach

Nurse cell-larva complex formed

Larvae enter small intestine

Larva matures in muscle

Adults mature and live in small intestine

Newborn larvae are carried throughout bloodstream

Newborn larva enters skeletal muscle cell

Female sheds newborn larvae that enter lymph or blood

PATHOLOGY

Heart failure

CNS damage

Wuchereria bancrofti

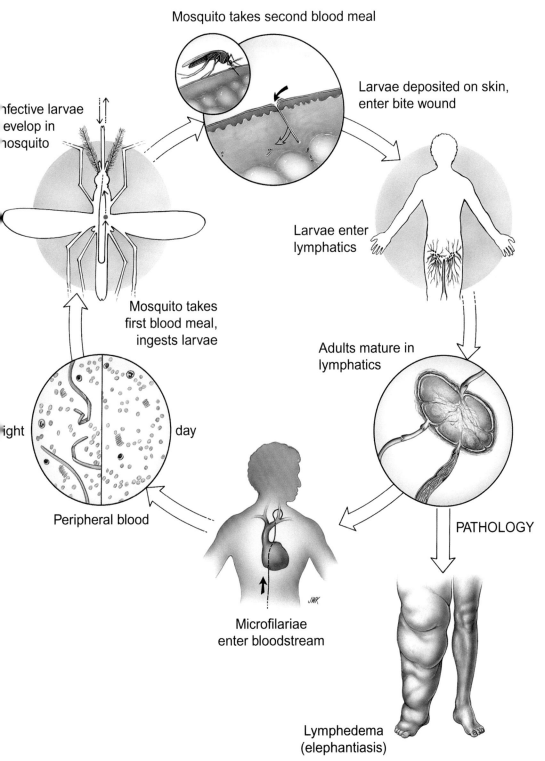

Mosquito takes second blood meal

Larvae deposited on skin, enter bite wound

Infective larvae develop in mosquito

Larvae enter lymphatics

Mosquito takes first blood meal, ingests larvae

Adults mature in lymphatics

night

day

Peripheral blood

PATHOLOGY

Microfilariae enter bloodstream

Lymphedema (elephantiasis)

Parasitic Diseases 6th Ed. Parasites Without Borders www.parasiteswithoutborders.com

Onchocerca volvulus

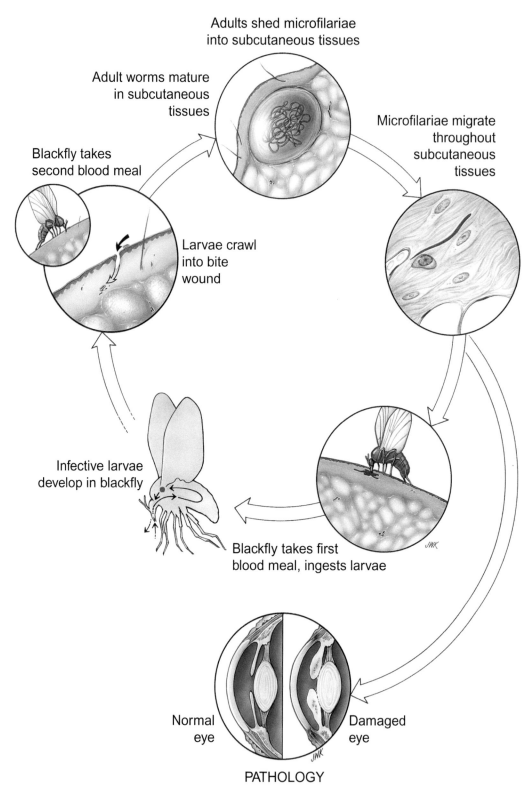

Adults shed microfilariae into subcutaneous tissues

Adult worms mature in subcutaneous tissues

Microfilariae migrate throughout subcutaneous tissues

Blackfly takes second blood meal

Larvae crawl into bite wound

Infective larvae develop in blackfly

Blackfly takes first blood meal, ingests larvae

Normal eye

Damaged eye

PATHOLOGY

Loa loa

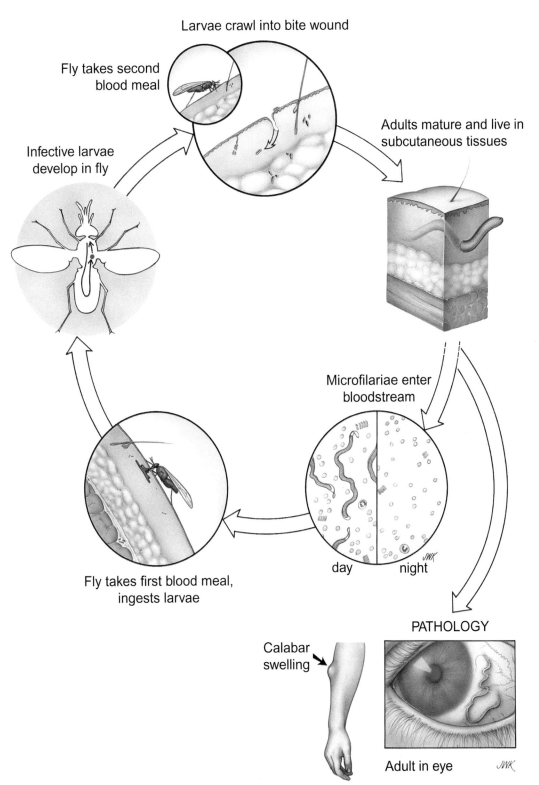

Larvae crawl into bite wound

Fly takes second blood meal

Infective larvae develop in fly

Adults mature and live in subcutaneous tissues

Microfilariae enter bloodstream

day   night

Fly takes first blood meal, ingests larvae

PATHOLOGY

Calabar swelling

Adult in eye

Dracunculus medinensis

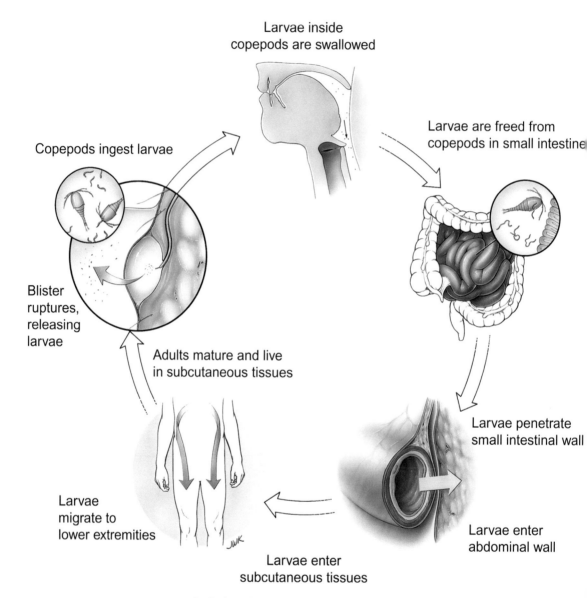

Larvae inside copepods are swallowed

Larvae are freed from copepods in small intestine

Copepods ingest larvae

Blister ruptures, releasing larvae

Adults mature and live in subcutaneous tissues

Larvae migrate to lower extremities

Larvae penetrate small intestinal wall

Larvae enter abdominal wall

Larvae enter subcutaneous tissues

Parasitic Diseases 6th Ed. Parasites Without Borders wwww.parasiteswithoutborders.com

Toxocara canis and Toxocara cati

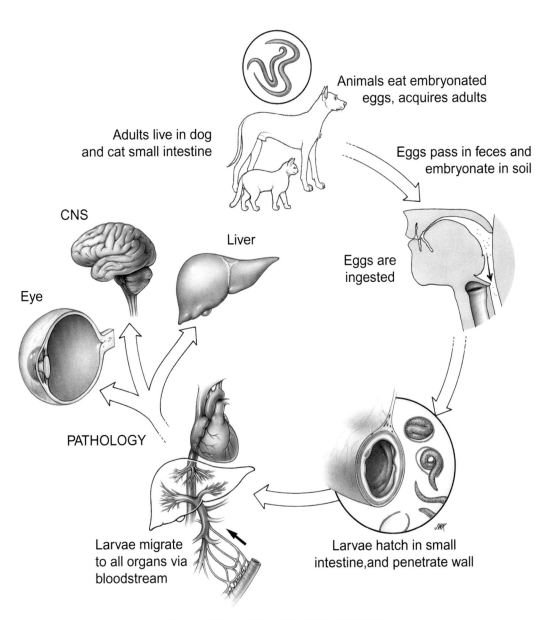

Animals eat embryonated eggs, acquires adults

Adults live in dog and cat small intestine

Eggs pass in feces and embryonate in soil

CNS

Liver

Eggs are ingested

Eye

PATHOLOGY

Larvae migrate to all organs via bloodstream

Larvae hatch in small intestine, and penetrate wall

Taenia saginata

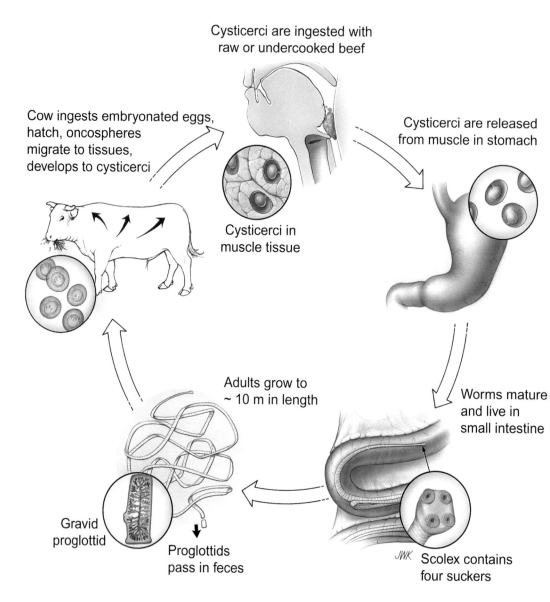

Cysticerci are ingested with raw or undercooked beef

Cow ingests embryonated eggs, hatch, oncospheres migrate to tissues, develops to cysticerci

Cysticerci are released from muscle in stomach

Cysticerci in muscle tissue

Worms mature and live in small intestine

Adults grow to ~ 10 m in length

Gravid proglottid

Proglottids pass in feces

Scolex contains four suckers

Parasitic Diseases 6th Ed. Parasites Without Borders www.parasiteswithoutborders.com

Cysticercosis
(Taenia solium)

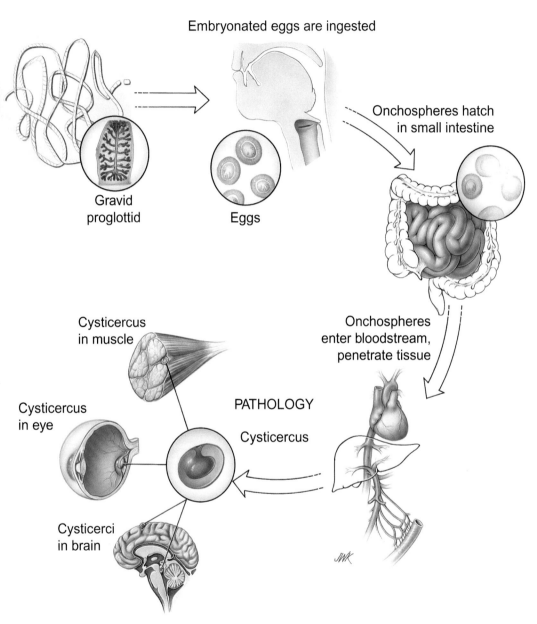

Embryonated eggs are ingested

Onchospheres hatch
in small intestine

Gravid
proglottid

Eggs

Onchospheres
enter bloodstream,
penetrate tissue

Cysticercus
in muscle

Cysticercus
in eye

PATHOLOGY

Cysticercus

Cysticerci
in brain

Cysticercosis
(Taenia solium)

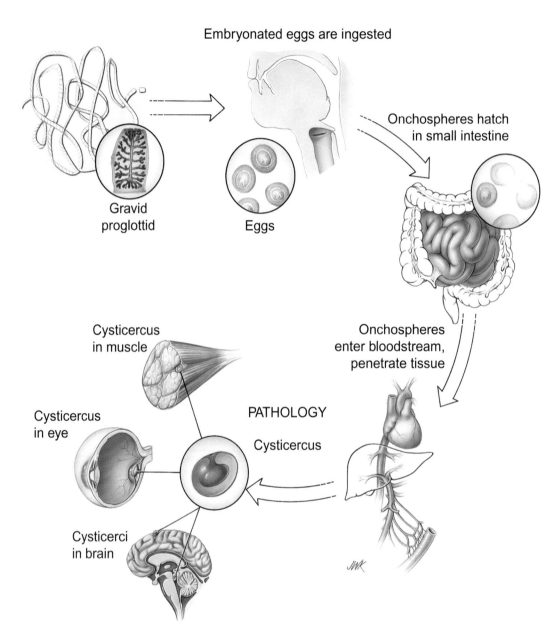

Embryonated eggs are ingested

Gravid proglottid

Eggs

Onchospheres hatch in small intestine

Onchospheres enter bloodstream, penetrate tissue

Cysticercus in muscle

Cysticercus in eye

PATHOLOGY

Cysticercus

Cysticerci in brain

Diphyllobothrium latum

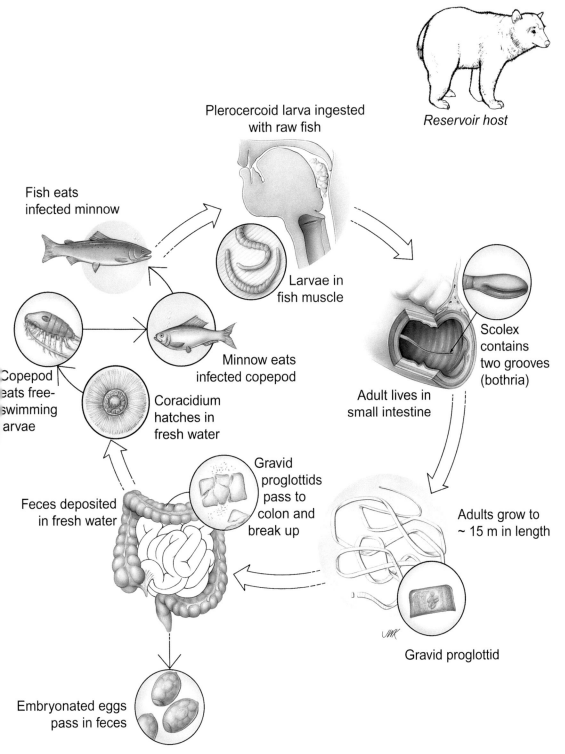

Reservoir host

Plerocercoid larva ingested
with raw fish

Fish eats
infected minnow

Larvae in
fish muscle

Scolex
contains
two grooves
(bothria)

Minnow eats
infected copepod

Adult lives in
small intestine

Copepod
eats free-
swimming
larvae

Coracidium
hatches in
fresh water

Gravid
proglottids
pass to
colon and
break up

Adults grow to
~ 15 m in length

Feces deposited
in fresh water

Gravid proglottid

Embryonated eggs
pass in feces

Echinococcus granulosus

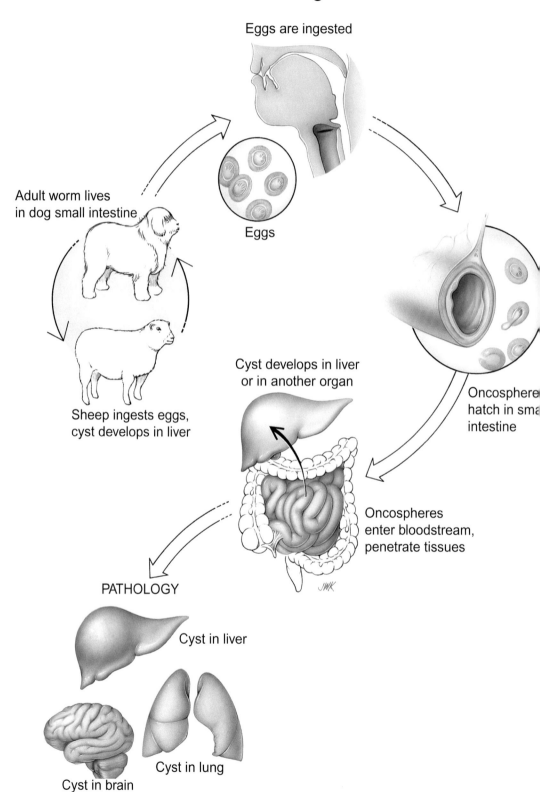

Eggs are ingested

Eggs

Adult worm lives
in dog small intestine

Sheep ingests eggs,
cyst develops in liver

Oncosphere
hatch in sma
intestine

Cyst develops in liver
or in another organ

Oncospheres
enter bloodstream,
penetrate tissues

PATHOLOGY

Cyst in liver

Cyst in lung

Cyst in brain

JWK

Schistosoma mansoni

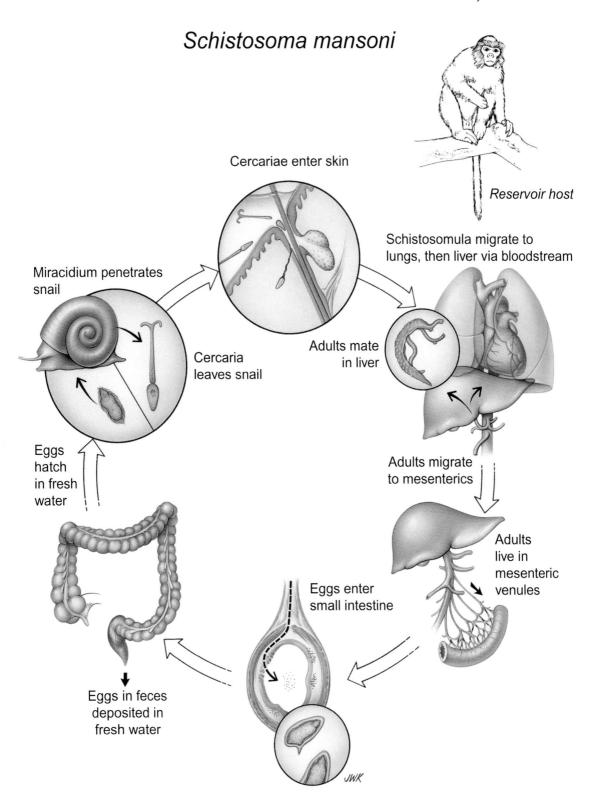

Cercariae enter skin

Reservoir host

Miracidium penetrates snail

Cercaria leaves snail

Schistosomula migrate to lungs, then liver via bloodstream

Adults mate in liver

Eggs hatch in fresh water

Adults migrate to mesenterics

Adults live in mesenteric venules

Eggs enter small intestine

Eggs in feces deposited in fresh water

JWK

Schistosoma japonicum

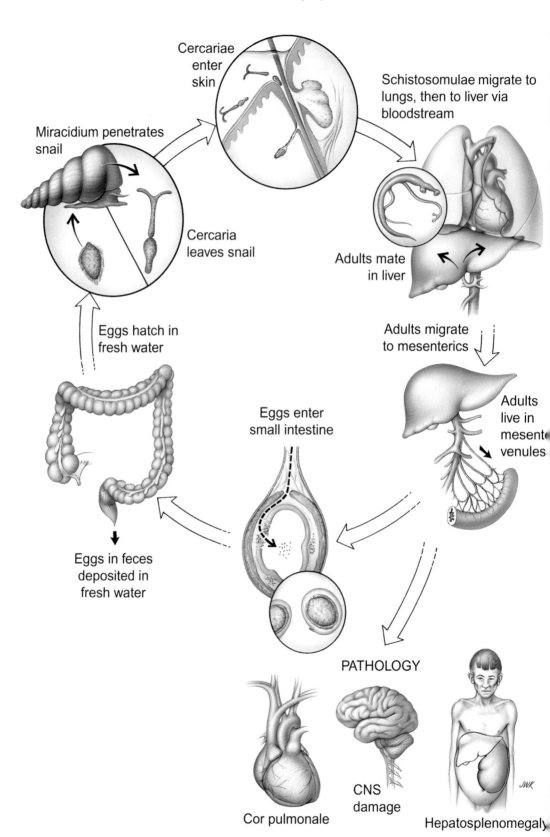

Cercariae enter skin

Schistosomulae migrate to lungs, then to liver via bloodstream

Miracidium penetrates snail

Cercaria leaves snail

Adults mate in liver

Adults migrate to mesenterics

Eggs hatch in fresh water

Eggs enter small intestine

Adults live in mesenteric venules

Eggs in feces deposited in fresh water

PATHOLOGY

Cor pulmonale

CNS damage

Hepatosplenomegaly

Schistosoma haematobium

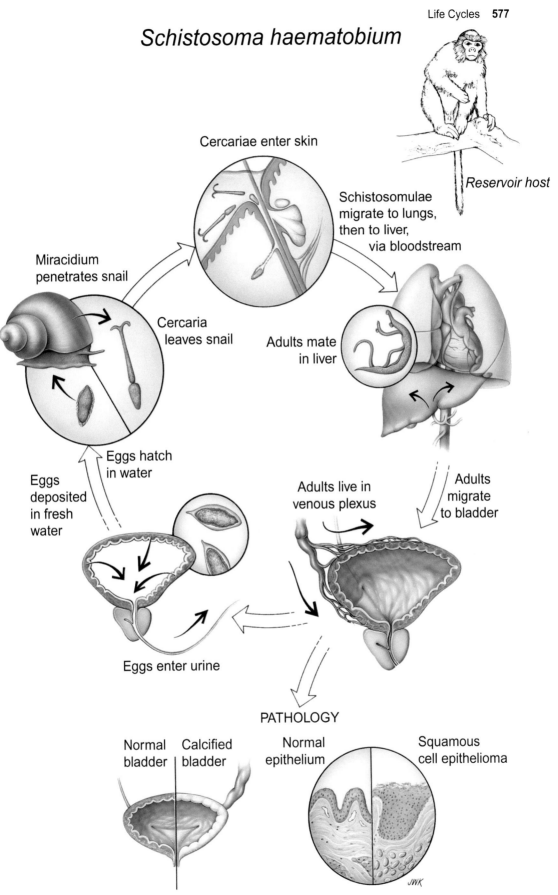

Reservoir host

Cercariae enter skin

Schistosomulae migrate to lungs, then to liver, via bloodstream

Miracidium penetrates snail

Cercaria leaves snail

Adults mate in liver

Eggs hatch in water

Eggs deposited in fresh water

Adults live in venous plexus

Adults migrate to bladder

Eggs enter urine

PATHOLOGY

Normal bladder | Calcified bladder

Normal epithelium

Squamous cell epithelioma

JWK

Clonorchis sinensis

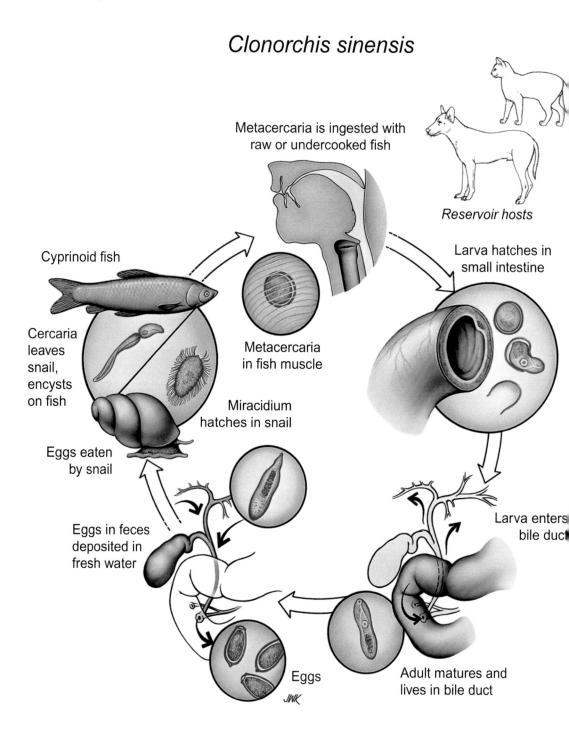

Metacercaria is ingested with raw or undercooked fish

Reservoir hosts

Cyprinoid fish

Larva hatches in small intestine

Cercaria leaves snail, encysts on fish

Metacercaria in fish muscle

Miracidium hatches in snail

Eggs eaten by snail

Larva enters bile duct

Eggs in feces deposited in fresh water

Eggs

Adult matures and lives in bile duct

JWK

Parasitic Diseases 6th Ed. Parasites Without Borders www.parasiteswithoutborders.com

Fasciola hepatica

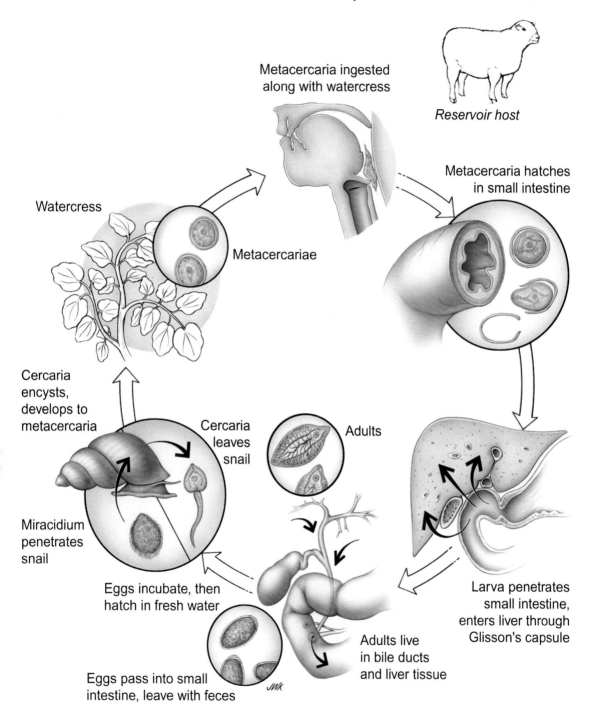

Metacercaria ingested along with watercress

Reservoir host

Watercress

Metacercariae

Metacercaria hatches in small intestine

Cercaria encysts, develops to metacercaria

Cercaria leaves snail

Adults

Miracidium penetrates snail

Larva penetrates small intestine, enters liver through Glisson's capsule

Eggs incubate, then hatch in fresh water

Adults live in bile ducts and liver tissue

Eggs pass into small intestine, leave with feces

JWK

Paragonimus westermani

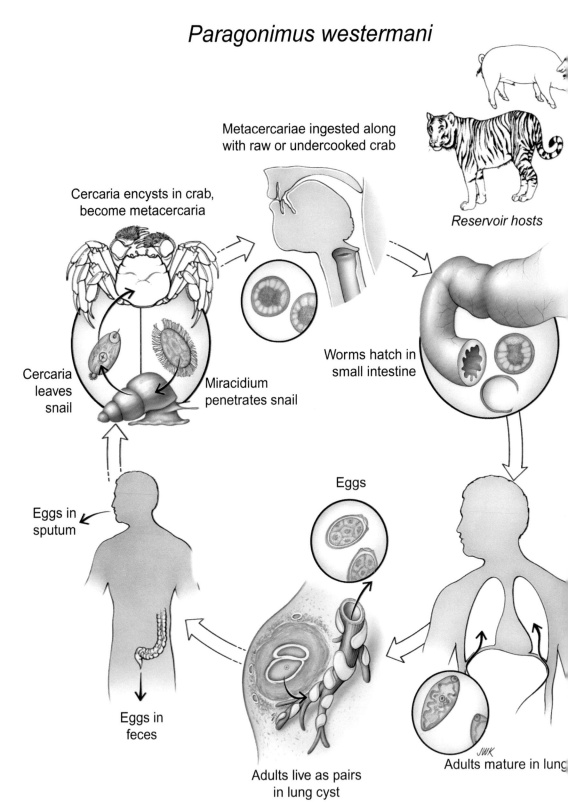

Metacercariae ingested along
with raw or undercooked crab

Reservoir hosts

Cercaria encysts in crab,
become metacercaria

Worms hatch in
small intestine

Cercaria
leaves
snail

Miracidium
penetrates snail

Eggs

Eggs in
sputum

Adults mature in lung

Eggs in
feces

Adults live as pairs
in lung cyst

Index

Y

Z